T0206352

REPRODUCTIVE ECOLOGY AND HUMAN EVOLUTION

REPRODUCTIVE ECOLOGY AND HUMAN EVOLUTION

PETER T. ELLISON
EDITOR

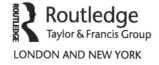

Routledge
Taylor & Francis Group

LONDON AND NEW YORK

First published 2011 by Transaction Publishers

Published 2017 by Routledge
2 Park Square, Milton Park, Abingdon, Oxon OX14 4RN
711 Third Avenue, New York, NY 10017, USA

Routledge is an imprint of the Taylor & Francis Group, an informa business

Library of Congress Catalog Number: 2001022083

Library of Congress Cataloging-in-Publication Data

Reproductive ecology and human evolution / Peter T. Ellison [editor].
    p. cm. - (Evolutionary foundations of human behavior)
  ISBN 0-202-30657-7 (cloth : alk. paper)
  ISBN 0-202-30658-5 (pbk.: alk. paper)
    1. Reproduction.   2. Human evolution.   3. Human ecology.
  I. Ellison, Peter Thorpe. II. Series.

QP251 .R444485 2001
612.6—dc21

                                   2001022083

ISBN 13: 978-0-202-30658-2 (pbk)
ISBN 13: 978-0-202-30657-5 (hbk)

To Irven DeVore,
teacher, mentor, friend, and inspiration
to a generation of biological anthropologists.

Contents

Contributors

Helen L. Ball, Department of Anthropology, University of Durham, U.K.

Gillian R. Bentley, Department of Anthropology, University College, London, U.K.

Fred B. Bercovitch, Center for the Reproduction of Endangered Species, Zoological Society of San Diego, Calif.

Jesper L. Boldsen, Danish Demographic Research Center, Center for Health and Social Policy, Odense University, Denmark

Richard G. Bribiescas, Department of Anthropology, Yale University, New Haven, Conn.

Diane K. Brockman, Department of Biological Anthropology and Anatomy, Duke University, Durham, N.C.

Benjamin C. Campbell, Department of Anthropology, Boston University, Boston, Mass.

Kenneth L. Campbell, Department of Biology, University of Massachusetts at Boston, Mass.

Peter T. Ellison, Department of Anthropology, Harvard University, Cambridge, Mass.

Kim Hill, Department of Anthropology, University of New Mexico, Albuquerque, N.Mex.

Darryl J. Holman, Department of Anthropology, University of Washington, Seattle, Wash.

A. Magdalena Hurtado, Department of Anthropology, University of New Mexico, Albuquerque, N.Mex.

Grazyna Jasienska, Institute of Public Health, Jagiellonian University, Krakow, Poland

Hillard Kaplan, Department of Anthropology, University of New Mexico, Albuquerque, N.Mex.

Cheryl Knott, Department of Anthropology, Harvard University, Cambridge, Mass.

Jane Lancaster, Department of Anthropology, University of New Mexico, Albuquerque, N.Mex.

Lynnette Leidy Sievert, Department of Anthropology, University of Massachusetts at Amherst, Mass.

Susan F. Lipson, Department of Anthropology, Harvard University, Cambridge, Mass.

William D. Lukas, Department of Anthropology, Boston University, Boston, Mass.

Martin N. Muller, Department of Anthropology, Harvard University, Cambridge, Mass.

Richard R. Paine, Department of Anthropology, University of Utah, Salt Lake City, Utah

Catherine Panter-Brick, Department of Anthropology, University of Durham, U.K.

Ivy L. Pike, Department of Anthropology, Ohio State University, Columbus, Ohio

Ned J. Place, Department of Zoology, University of Washington, Seattle, Wash.

Karen B. Strier, Department of Anthropology, University of Wisconsin at Madison, Madison, Wis.

Claudia R. Valeggia, Department of Anthropology, Harvard University, Cambridge, Mass.

Virginia J. Vitzthum, Department of Anthropology, State University of New York at Binghamton, Binghamton, N.Y.

Samuel K. Wasser, Department of Zoology, University of Washington, Seattle, Wash.

Patricia L. Whitten, Departments of Anthropology and Biology, Emory University, Atlanta, Ga.

James W. Wood, Department of Anthropology and the Population Research Institute, Pennsylvania State University, University Park, Pa.

Richard W. Wrangham, Department of Anthropology, Harvard University, Cambridge, Mass.

INTRODUCTION
Ecology, Reproduction, and Human Evolution

PETER T. ELLISON

THE ECOLOGY OF HUMAN REPRODUCTION

At the center of Darwin's theory of evolution by natural selection is the concept of adaptation. Evolution is the name we give to the process of biological change through time. Natural selection is a mechanism that can drive such change. But it is not the only such mechanism. Random events from the molecular to the planetary level can also be mechanisms of biological change. Natural selection, however, remains the only scientific theory of adaptation, the demonstrable "fit" between an organism and the challenges of its specific environment. In Darwinian terms, evolution is the process, natural selection is the mechanism, and adaptation is the result. But organisms do not display adaptations in the abstract; they display adaptations *to* specific conditions. The study of Darwinian evolution thus necessarily involves the study of ecology, the relationship of organism to environment. It is in that relationship that the power of natural selection becomes discernible and a manifest object of inquiry.

Because biological evolution is cumulative, however, organisms in the present must be viewed as products of the selective forces of past environments. The study of adaptation thus often involves inferences about formative ecological relationships that may no longer exist, or not in the same form. Making such inferences depends on carefully weighing a broad range of evidence drawn from studies of contemporary ecological variation, comparative studies of related taxa, and paleontological and genetic evidence of evolutionary history. The result of this inquiry sheds light not only on the functional aspects of an organism's contemporary biology but also on its evolutionary history and the selective forces that have shaped it through time.

1

The study of human reproductive ecology represents an important new development in human evolutionary biology. Its focus is on the physiology of human reproduction and evidence of adaptation, and hence the action of natural selection, in that domain. But at the same time the study of human reproductive ecology provides an important perspective on the historical process of human evolution, a lens through which we may view the forces that have shaped us as a species. In the end, all actions of natural selection can be reduced to variation in the reproductive success of individuals. Even survival only has selective value insofar as it leads to some individual's greater genetic representation in future generations, a representation that must ultimately be gained through reproduction. Although variation in reproductive physiology is not the only pathway through which variation in reproductive success occurs, it is a very important one, and one in which we might logically expect to see expressed the ecological influences that are the stuff of adaptation.

Yet despite its logical importance, the study of human reproductive ecology has flourished only recently. Serious attention to reproductive physiology by those interested in human evolution probably began with the pioneering work of Melvin Konner and Carol Worthman (1980) in arguing for the importance of breastfeeding patterns in regulating the interbirth intervals of the !Kung San. Roger Short (1987) was able to use this evidence in providing a comparative evolutionary framework within which to understand human reproductive biology, a framework that brought the mechanisms of reproductive physiology together with the ultimate explanations of life history theory. From the very beginning, however, human reproductive ecology has provided an active arena of contesting hypotheses. Nancy Howell (1979) in her landmark volume, *The Demography of the Dobe !Kung*, argued for an alternative explanation of !Kung interbirth intervals based on different physiological mechanisms linking female fecundity to female nutritional status. The debate over the relative importance of nursing patterns versus nutritional status as potential regulators of natural human fertility has continued ever since, stimulating a wide range of important and influential empirical work. But the domain of inquiry encompassed by human reproductive ecology has also expanded, and as it has expanded it has created a broad interface with adjacent disciplines in both the social and biological sciences, such as demography, endocrinology, medicine and public health, growth and developmental biology, exercise and sports science, primatology and conservation biology, gerontology and embryology, and life history theory. One result of this expansion and interdisciplinary encounter has been an invigorating infusion of ideas and perspectives creating exactly the sort of intellectual synergy that interdisciplinary efforts so often promise but fail to deliver. Among the recent important volumes that serve as testimonies to both the continuity and the advancement of this field are James Wood's *Dynamics of Human Reproduction: Biology, Biometry, Demography* (1994a), stressing the interface between reproductive physiology and demography, and Kim Hill and Magdalena Hurtado's *Ache Life History* (1996), stressing the relationship of ecology to formal life history theory. In addition, a number of conferences and symposia resulting in published volumes have bridged traditional disciplinary boundaries in focusing attention on human reproduction and its ecological context (Campbell and Wood 1994; Dunbar 1995; Rosetta and Mascie-Taylor 1996). In a separate volume, *On Fertile Ground* (Ellison 2001), I have provided a synthesis of my own thinking.

An additional important element in the expansion of the field of human reproductive ecology has been the development of new techniques for the study of reproductive physiology under field conditions. The pioneering work of Konner and Worthman (1980) involved the collection of serum samples in the field, samples that could be collected only occasionally from willing subjects, that had to be spun with hand centrifuges in the field and transported in liquid nitrogen back to laboratory facilities in the United States. In recent years the development of less invasive, less cumbersome field techniques based on collection of saliva, urine, and blood spots (Campbell 1994; Ellison 1988; Worthman and Stallings 1997) has dramatically increased the range and scope of empirical studies. It is now possible to monitor variation in key aspects of the reproductive physiology of individuals and populations longitudinally with minimal disruption to normal routines of daily life. Comparable methods are now being adopted and modified by primatologists, supporting a new level of sophistication in the study of reproductive ecology among wild primates (Brockman et al. 1995; Knott 1996; Strier and Ziegler 1994; Strier et al. 1999; Wasser 1996).

In many ways the central concept of reproductive ecology is *reproductive effort*, the allocation of resources to reproduction rather than to other competing biological functions such as growth or maintenance. In evolutionary studies, reproductive effort is a variable the value of which is strategically determined depending on specific constitutional and ecological circumstances. This fact alone distinguishes the evolutionary perspective from the medical perspective in which reproduction is presumed to have only one optimum level of function. Reproductive ecology is the study of reproductive effort from an evolutionary perspective with the operating assumption that the allocation of reproductive effort has been shaped by natural selection. Reproductive effort can be adjusted both behaviorally and physiologically; thus reproductive ecology properly involves the study of both behavior and physiology.

The present volume focuses on the physiology of reproductive effort, the ways in which the reproductive systems of humans and nonhuman primates display evidence of adaptive responses to constitutional and

environmental conditions. Paradoxically, the study of physiological variation in human reproductive effort has lagged behind the study of behavioral variation since the beginning of modern evolutionary biology. There
are numerous reasons for this bias. Darwin himself, when addressing the
question of human evolution, stressed the importance of sexual selection
in which behavioral mechanisms predominate (Darwin 1871). Social scientists adopted the standard medical view of an invariant reproductive
physiology, except for the effects of pathology, a view embraced by
Malthus (1798), whose influence Darwin explicitly acknowledged. In the
twentieth century, evidence of the role of behavioral changes in the modern demographic transition to low birth rates reinforced the view that variation in human reproductive effort is primarily modulated through
behavioral channels. The first important challenge to this view, presented
by the French demographer Louis Henry, who demonstrated the existence
of significant variation in human fertility that was not the result of conscious behavior, seemed to be turned aside by early work on natural birth
spacing which emphasized breastfeeding behavior. More recently, the renaissance of Darwinian theory in behavioral biology has stimulated a proliferation of new research on the behavioral regulation of human
reproductive effort that has stressed ecological approaches and life history
theory (Betzig, Borgerhoff Mulder, and Turke 1988).

Research into the physiological regulation of human reproductive effort
until recently suffered from relative neglect stemming both from the aversion of social scientists to biological explanations and from the preoccupa-
tion of evolutionary biologists with behavioral biology. But the debate over
natural birth spacing brought physiology back into the explanatory fore-
ground. The recognition of the importance of lactation in regulating female
fecundity did not arise from the work of social scientists and demographers. Indeed, such influential mid-twentieth century contributions as
Frank Lorimer's *Culture and Fertility* (1954) and Kingsley Davis and Judith
Blake's "Social structure and fertility: an analytical framework" (1956)
include no mention of lactation as a regulator of human fertility. Rather, the
theory of nursing frequency as a modulator of postpartum female fecundity was derived from new data on the hormonal control lactation that was
collected in the 1970s and 1980s (Delvoye et al. 1977; Howie and McNeilly
1982; Konner and Worthman 1980; Tyson 1977). At the same time Rose
Frisch and her colleagues advanced a theory of female menstrual function
that stressed a connection between female energetic status and female
fecundity (Frisch 1978; Frisch and McArthur 1974; Frisch and Revelle 1970,
1971). Although Frisch's specific formulation was severely criticized on
empirical grounds (see Ellison 2001), her approach also stimulated new
research into the determinants of female ovarian function (Ellison 1990).
While the role of female energetics and that of lactation are sometimes set

in opposition to each other in discussions of human reproductive effort (Bongaarts 1980; Wood 1994a, 1994b), that opposition is forced and basically false (Ellison 2001), since the evolutionary logic behind both theories stresses the avoidance of excessive reproductive effort in the form of energetic investment. This logic has in fact led to a productive dialectic between evolutionary life history theory and the new approach to human reproductive physiology that is identified by the term *reproductive ecology* (Ellison et al. 1993; Hill and Hurtado 1996; Short 1987).

ORGANIZATION OF THE VOLUME

Reproductive Ecology and Human Evolution represents an offering of contemporary research and thinking in this vigorously developing field. The volume has been composed to give readers a useful cross-section of current issues and controversies. While it aims at broad representation, it still samples only a portion of the research activity that is current and the researchers engaged in it. Within this sample, however, are contained many of the important themes and voices that are pushing the field forward. The contributors include some of the original pioneers of the field as well as many of the newer researchers who are setting the contemporary research agenda. Also included are contributions from the field of primate reproductive ecology to emphasize the broad, comparative context in which human and primate evolutionary studies must be situated. The focus of the volume is on reproductive physiology, rather than reproductive behavior, demography, or life history theory, but these other aspects of reproductive ecology are inextricably bound up with the content of many of the contributions in the volume. Finally, in assembling the volume emphasis was placed on investigators engaged in empirical field research. Despite this empirical focus, contributors were encouraged to be theoretically bold and to consider the larger implications of their research for our understanding of human evolution.

The organization of the volume groups contributions with reference to certain general contexts of inquiry and explanation. This sorting is heuristic only to a point, however, since many of the contributions crosscut this classification scheme. The first section, "Physiological Context," includes contributions that highlight central physiological mechanisms important to human reproductive physiology which are also foci of investigation in reproductive ecology. Darryl Holman and James Wood review the evidence for variation in rates of pregnancy loss between individuals and populations and the mechanisms responsible for it. Their chapter includes presentation of the results of a large field study of pregnancy loss in Bangladesh, the first substantial study of this aspect of human reproduction in a nonwestern context. Ivy Pike reviews the physiology of human pregnancy from an evolutionary perspective, drawing attention to the potential for ecological variation in this crucial component of female reproductive investment. In addition to reviewing other studies, she draws upon her own research with the Turkana of northern Kenya. Grazyna Jasienska provides an important theoretical approach to the impact of energy expenditure on female ovarian function based upon both her own research with Polish farm women and the growing literature on exercise and reproductive function. Claudia Valeggia and I offer a contemporary perspective on the still open question of the mechanisms and nature of lactational amenorrhea, including discussion of a new field study among the Toba of northern Argentina. Finally, Richard Bribiescas presents a new approach to male reproductive ecology stressing the role of the male reproductive axis in modulating male somatic investment. His contribution surveys both the clinical and field-based literature as well as presenting results of his own research among the Ache of Paraguay.

The second section, "Ecological Context," includes contributions that highlight particular aspects of the interaction between the environment and human reproductive physiology. Samuel Wasser and Ned Place review the evidence for the impact of the social environment on the reproductive system. Drawing on a broad research literature ranging from primate studies to clinical infertility research, Wasser and Place argue that the human reproductive system demonstrates sensitivity to cues regarding the likelihood and quality of social support important to reproductive success. Benjamin Campbell, William Lukas, and Kenneth Campbell review the relationship between male reproduction and immune system function, a relationship that links human reproduction to environmental disease burden. Their review makes use of both clinical and field studies and includes new research results from Zimbabwe. Virginia Vitzthum considers the impact of chronic energy shortage on female reproductive physiology, arguing that female fecundity shows different responses to acute and chronic energetic stresses. Her carefully constructed theoretical argument is supported on a wealth of empirical evidence including her own recent research in Bolivia. Finally, Gillian Bentley, Richard Paine, and Jesper Boldsen present a critical review of the evidence for and against shifts in reproductive ecology associated with the adoption of agriculture. Their review integrates comparative research on contemporary societies characterized by different subsistence strategies with paleodemographic evidence from archaeological studies.

The third section, "Developmental Context," stresses the interrelationship of reproductive ecology with developmental processes and different human life stages, as well as with life history theory more generally. Susan Lipson presents an argument regarding developmental effects on female reproductive function that leads her to different conclusions from those of Vitzthum. Also included in her contribution is a review of contemporary research on mechanisms that link energy metabolism to ovarian function. Helen Ball and Catherine Panter-Brick present an evolutionary perspective on maternal investment and child survival in the postnatal period. Their review includes work from the domains of social anthropology and contemporary child-centered approaches to the biology of infancy and childhood. Lynnette Leidy Sievert focuses her contribution on issues of aging and reproductive senescence. The relationship of declining fecundity to increasing age, the proximate and ultimate causes of female menopause, and variation in reproductive senescence between individuals and populations are all covered in this review that synthesizes the medical and anthropological literature, including Leidy Sievert's own recent work in Mexico. Finally, Hillard Kaplan, Kim Hill, Magdalena Hurtado, and Jane Lancaster present a broad and encompassing approach to human life history evolution that stresses the enhanced capacity of humans to embody experience through increased cognitive capacity, ultimately tied to selection for increased brain size and central nervous system complexity. Although not focused narrowly on questions of reproduction, their synthesis provides a context in which to view selective forces acting on human reproductive maturation, the distribution of somatic investment between different tissues, and reproductive constraints on human brain development.

The last section, "Comparative Context," includes contributions on the reproductive ecology of nonhuman primates. The contributors to this section include many of the leading pioneers in the development and application of new field techniques for the study of primate reproductive ecology. Patricia Whitten and Diane Brockman review the reproductive ecology of prosimians, drawing on their own research with sifakas and other Malagasy lemurs. Karen Strier reviews the reproductive ecology of New World monkeys, providing broad taxonomic coverage but highlighting distinctive features of strepsirrhine reproductive biology. Her own pioneering work on the reproductive ecology of muriquis in Brazil is included in her review. Fred Bercovitch provides a review of Old World monkey reproductive ecology that focuses on key areas of theoretical importance and current research, including sexual dimorphism in maturation, sexual advertisement, and maternal investment. Martin Muller and Richard Wrangham review the reproductive ecology of male hominoids, stressing current field research on the relationship of male reproductive physiology to both reproductive and social behavior. Included in their review are results of their own recent research on testosterone and the behavior of male chimpanzees in Uganda. Finally, Cheryl Knott reviews the reproductive ecology of female hominoids, focusing in particular on the linkages between female energetics and female reproduction. Her own pioneering research with orangutans in Borneo is combined with a thorough review of the literature to provide a framework that links the reproductive ecology of humans to that of our closest taxonomic relatives.

REPRODUCTIVE ECOLOGY AND HUMAN EVOLUTION

As befits any area of active research, the conclusions and perspectives of the various contributors do not always coincide and, in some cases, provide competing alternatives. The tension between guiding hypotheses, empirical results, and provisional syntheses is the mainspring from which energetic research emerges. The ecological, cultural, temporal, and taxonomic diversity of the studies that are presented and the range of empirical and analytical tools that they bring to bear provide for an incredibly rich intellectual ferment, stimulating creative ideas and new approaches. The central purpose of this volume is to provide readers with a sense of the breadth and excitement of the field of human reproductive ecology as well as an introduction to its important practitioners, its innovative techniques, its questions and controversies, and its future directions.

While the study of human and primate reproductive ecology is still young and vigorously growing, it already casts new light on the traditional questions of human evolution. One can ask, for example, what aspects of reproductive physiology and associated aspects of life history have most likely changed during the course of human evolution. Using chimpanzee reproductive characteristics as a reference point, the list might include the following:

1. increased neurological altriciality at birth despite a relatively large full-term brain size, and an associated pattern of extended postnatal brain growth
2. remodeling of the female pelvis to accommodate both bipedal locomotion and the passage of a large fetal cranium at birth
3. increased difficulty in parturition, leading to the frequent intercession of conspecifics and the general enhancement of the role of social support during labor and delivery
4. enhanced infant and child survivorship, perhaps reflecting increased investment on the part of parents and other relatives, including increased paternal investment
5. a longer period of reproductive immaturity
6. a more exaggerated adolescent growth spurt in advance of reproductive maturation

7. shorter birth intervals, both absolutely and relative to the imma-
    ture period, with the result of a common pattern of overlapping
    dependent offspring
8. increased fat deposition in both sexes, but particularly in females,
    starting at reproductive maturity and coupled to ovarian function
9. decreased muscle mass in both sexes, but still with sexual dimor-
    phism in muscle mass favoring males, starting at reproductive
    maturity and coupled to testicular function
10. increased longevity without a concomitant increase in reproduc-
    tive span (certainly in females, probably in males as well) leading
    to a common extended period of postreproductive life

Understanding human evolution involves understanding the emergence
of this new pattern of reproduction and life history. Unfortunately, physiology leaves even fewer clues in the fossil and archaeological record than
behavior, so that we must rely heavily on the study of contemporary patterns of reproductive ecology to extrapolate the past. It may well be that
many of the changes listed above will ultimately be traceable to a few key
changes in ecology. A shift to a more open habitat with a more scattered and
less predictable resource base may have selected for bipedality and increased fat storage. A later shift to a more dependable food supply of higher
caloric density, perhaps associated with fire and cooking, could have
selected for increased reproductive effort and shorter birth intervals while,
in conjunction with a physiology of efficient energy storage and mobilization, supporting increased fetal and postnatal brain growth. Increased fetal
brain size in a bipedal hominid may have resulted in more difficult labor
and delivery, selecting for increased social support at parturition. Selective
pressure for a sufficiently large female pelvis may have led to a longer
period of prereproductive growth even while increased parental investment led to shorter birth intervals. Increased social support and more reliable resources, together with increasingly complex social life, might simultaneously have led to lower mortality and an increasing postreproductive
survivorship. Postreproductive life would have generated tremendous
selective presssure for continued, indirect reproductive effort through support for younger reproductive relatives. It is possible that all of these
changes reflect linkages between hominid ecology and hominid reproductive physiology (Ellison 2001). Testing the hypotheses that underlie such
hypotheses and linking the results with the rest of the evidence pertaining
to human evolutionary history are both the challenge and the promise of
human reproductive ecology.

Ultimately the study of human and primate reproductive ecology has
the potential to illuminate our understanding of human evolution and our

place in nature. But in addition to this broad intellectual contribution are many applied consequences as well. The future conservation of endangered primate species, especially the other great apes, depends crucially on our fuller understanding of their reproductive ecology and the linkages between habitat and population persistence (Jones 2000). A fuller understanding of human reproductive ecology also promises to contribute to a better understanding of reproductive cancers (Ellison 1999; Jasienska et al. 2000), age-related infertility (Ellison 1996), and senescence itself (Hawkes et al. 1998; O'Rourke et al. 1996). Evolutionary studies and the study of adaptation provide deeply satisfying insights into the history of life and humanity. But they also provide, through a clearer appreciation for the road we have traveled, a new appreciation for the road ahead.

REFERENCES CITED

Betzig L, Borgerhoff Mulder M, Turke P (Eds) (1988) *Human Reproductive Behavior: A Darwinian Perspective* (New York, Cambridge University Press).

Bongaarts J (1980) Does malnutrition affect fecundity? A summary of evidence. *Science* 208:564–569.

Brockman DK, Whitten PL, Russell E, Richard AF, Izard MK (1995) Application of fecal steroid techniques to the reproductive endocrinology of female Verreaux's sifaka, *Propithecus verreauxi. American Journal of Primatology* 36:313–325.

Campbell KL (1994) Blood, urine, saliva and dip-sticks: experiences in Africa, New Guinea, and Boston. *Annals of the New York Academy of Sciences* 709:312–330.

Campbell KL, Wood JW (Eds) (1994) *Human Reproductive Ecology: Interactions of Environment, Fertility, and Behavior* (New York, New York Academy of Sciences).

Darwin C (1871) *The Descent of Man and Selection in Relation to Sex* (London, Murray).

Davis K, Blake J (1956) Social structure and fertility: an analytic framework. *Economic Development and Cultural Change* 4:211–235.

Delvoye P, Demaegd M, Delogne-Desnoeck J, Robyn C (1977) The influence of the frequency of nursing and of previous lactation experience on serum prolactin in lactating mothers. *Journal of Biosocial Science* 9:447–451.

Dunbar RIM (Ed) (1995) *Human Reproductive Decisions: Biological and Social Perspectives* (New York, St. Martin's Press).

Ellison PT (1988) Human salivary steroids: methodological considerations and applications in physical anthropology. *Yearbook of Physical Anthropology* 31:115–132.

Ellison PT (1990) Human ovarian function and reproductive ecology: new hypotheses. *American Anthropologist* 92:933–952.

Ellison PT (1996) Age and developmental effects on adult ovarian function. In L Rosetta, CGN Mascie-Taylor (Eds) *Variability in Human Fertility: A Biological Anthropological Approach* (Cambridge, Cambridge University Press), 69–90.

Ellison PT (1999) Reproductive ecology and reproductive cancers. In C Panter-Brick, C Worthman (Eds) *Hormones and Human Health* (Cambridge, Cambridge University Press), 184–209.

Ellison PT (2001) *On Fertile Ground* (Cambridge, Massachusetts, Harvard University Press).

Ellison PT, Panter-Brick C, Lipson SF, O'Rourke MT (1993) The ecological context of human ovarian function. *Human Reproduction* 8:2248–2258.

Frisch RE (1978) Population, food intake, and fertility. *Science* 199:22–30.

Frisch RE, Revelle R (1970) Height and weight at menarche and a hypothesis of critical body weights and adolescent events. *Science* 169:397–399.

Frisch RE, Revelle R (1971) Height and weight at menarche and a hypothesis of menarche. *Archives of Disease in Childhood* 46:695–701.

Frisch RE, McArthur JW (1974) Menstrual cycles: fatness as a determinant of minimum weight for height necessary for their maintenance or onset. *Science* 185:949–951.

Hawkes K, O'Connell JF, Blurton-Jones NG, Alvarez H, Charnov EL (1998) Grandmothering, menopause, and the evolution of human life histories. *Proceedings of the National Academy of Sciences* 95:1336–1339.

Hill K, Hurtado AM (1996) *Ache Life History* (New York, Aldine de Gruyter).

Howell N (1979) *Demography of the Dobe !Kung* (New York, Academic Press).

Howie PW, McNeilly AS (1982) Effect of breast feeding patterns on human birth intervals. *Journal of Reproduction and Fertility* 65:545–557.

Jasienska G, Thune I, Ellison PT (2000) Energetic factors, ovarian steroids, and the risk of breast cancer. *European Journal of Cancer Prevention* 9:231–239.

Jones J (2000) *Cycling in the Slow Lane: Applications of Evolutionary Demography to Biological Anthropology* (PhD dissertation, Harvard University).

Knott CD (1996) Field collection and preservation of urine in orangutans and chimpanzees. *Tropical Biodiversity* 4:95–102.

Konner M, Worthman C (1980) Nursing frequency, gonadal function, and birth spacing among !Kung hunter-gatherers. *Science* 207:788–791.

Lorimer F (Ed) (1954) *Culture and Human Fertility* (Paris, UNESCO).

Malthus T (1798) *An Essay on the Principle of Population as It Affects the Future Improvement of Society with Remarks on the Speculations of Mr. Godwin, M. Condorcet, and Other Writers.* (London, Murray).

O'Rourke MT, Lipson SF, Ellison PT (1996) Ovarian function in the latter half of the reproductive lifespan. *American Journal of Human Biology* 8:751–760.

Rosetta L, Mascie-Taylor CGN (Eds) (1996) *Variability in Human Fertility: A Biological Anthropological Approach* (Cambridge, Cambridge University Press).

Short RV (1987) The biological basis for the contraceptive effects of breast feeding. *International Journal of Gynaecology and Obstetrics* 25(Suppl):207–217.

Strier KB, Ziegler TE (1994) Insights into ovarian function in wild muriqui monkeys *(Brachyteles arachnoides). American Journal of Primatology* 32:31–40.

Strier KB, Ziegler TE, Wittwer D (1999) Seasonal and social correlates of fecal testosterone and cortisol levels in wild male muriquis *(Brachyteles arachnoides). Hormones and Behavior* 35:125–134.

Tyson JE (1977) Neuroendocrine control of lactational infertility. *Journal of Biosocial Science* 4(Suppl):23–40.

Wasser SK (1996) Reproductive control in wild baboons measured by fecal steroids. *Biology of Reproduction* 55:393–399.

Wood JW (1994a) *Dynamics of Human Reproduction: Biology, Biometry, Demography* (New York, Aldine de Gruyter).

Wood JW (1994b) Maternal nutrition and reproduction: why demographers and physiologists disagree about a fundamental relationship. *Annals of the New York Academy of Sciences* 709:101–116.

Worthman CM, Stallings JF (1997) Hormone measures in finger-prick blood spot samples: new field methods for reproductive endocrinology. *American Journal of Physical Anthropology* 104:1–21.

Part I

PHYSIOLOGICAL CONTEXT

1

Pregnancy Loss and Fecundability in Women

DARRYL J. HOLMAN and JAMES W. WOOD

Compared to other mammals, reproduction in women is characterized by low lifetime fertility, a slow pace of reproduction, and a large investment in each offspring. The reproductive span begins relatively late in life; births tend to be spaced at increasingly longer intervals until they stop altogether. Many women then live well beyond ages at which reproduction is possible, something that is rarely seen in other mammals. Making sense out of this pattern of reproduction has been a goal of anthropologists, demographers, physiologists, and evolutionary biologists.

In this chapter, we examine one aspect of this pattern: the way that births are spaced across the female reproductive life span. The timing of births is a complex outcome of many physiological, cultural, and behavioral factors, but our focus will be on two of the components that play an important role in shaping female fecundity and birth spacing. These components are pregnancy loss, which is defined as the loss of any product of conception prior to birth, and fecundability, defined as the monthly or cycle-wise probability of conception. We pay particular attention to some of the methodological difficulties that are encountered in trying to measure fecundability and pregnancy loss, and how these difficulties have limited or distorted our understanding of age-related changes in female fecundity. We propose new methods to overcome the difficulties and apply the methods to data collected in rural Bangladesh.

The physiological changes associated with menarche and menopause explain much of the lower levels of natural fertility at the extremes of the reproductive span. Between these two points substantial changes in fertility can be observed as an increase in the average length of birth intervals. A universal finding from studies among natural fertility populations is that female fecundity initially increases to a peak in the early twenties and then declines with a woman's age.[1] These age-related changes in birth spacing can be fruitfully explored by dividing the reproductive life course into a series of smaller components (Figure 1.1). At the top level, the reproductive life course is a series of events, including menarche, menopause, and a number of birth intervals. The time from marriage to first birth defines the first birth interval, and each subsequent birth defines the start of a new birth interval. Each birth interval can be subdivided into four meaningful events separated by three waiting times (Figure 1.1, row 2). A live birth is followed by a waiting time until the return of fecundity. This is followed by a *fecund waiting time* to the next conception, which is some number of months or menstrual cycles until a conception occurs. Finally, a conception is followed by a period of gestation which, in the absence of pregnancy loss, terminates in a live birth.

The role that pregnancy loss plays in shaping birth intervals can be understood from the third row of Figure 1.1. At the time a pregnancy is lost, some period of gestation leading up to that point has been added to the current birth interval. The distribution of these partial gestations is

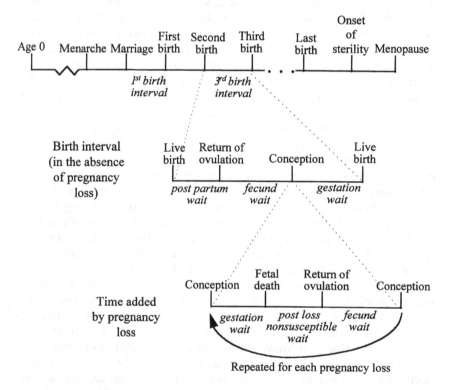

Figure 1.1.   A schematic of events that occur in the female reproductive life course. The vertical lines represent *events*, and events are separated by *waiting times* (after Bongaarts and Potter 1983).

determined by the gestational age-specific risk (or hazard) of pregnancy loss.

After a pregnancy is lost, three new waiting times are added to the birth interval. The first is a *post loss nonsusceptible wait*, which is a period of time in which a woman is not susceptible to conception. A pregnancy lost immediately after conception will add little to this waiting time. Wilcox and colleagues (1988) report the lengths of menstrual cycles following 43 subclinical pregnancy losses that were detected, on average, by day 11. Menstrual cycles were lengthened by an average of two days, which represents the *combined* effects of the length of gestation that preceded the loss and any delays added through the follicular phase of the following cycle. One third of the subjects who experienced an early pregnancy loss conceived in the next cycle (compared with 25% for the study on the whole), so it appears that these early losses do not lead to a high probability of anovulation in the following cycles. Studies of resumption of menses in women who never breast-feed provide information about the other extreme. About six weeks lapse from a live birth to first ovulation in non-breastfeeding women (Gray et al. 1987; Jones 1989). Aside from these two extremes, little is known about the distribution of times from pregnancy loss until the return of fecundity.

The second time added by a pregnancy loss is a new fecund waiting time until the next conception. There has been little investigation of this waiting time, but it is reasonable to suppose that it is similar to the initial waiting time to conception in the second panel. Finally, a new period of gestation follows the fecund waiting time.

Within one birth interval, a woman may become pregnant and lose the pregnancy any number of times. The total number of pregnancies lost within a single birth interval will depend on the probability of loss for each conception. If this probability is high, multiple pregnancy losses can occur within one birth interval, each time adding three new waiting times and resulting in a substantially lengthened birth interval. On the other hand, if the probability of pregnancy loss is very low, then the additional waiting times are rarely added even once per birth interval. Wood (1994:261) gives a mathematical treatment of the relationship between pregnancy loss, the waiting times added by pregnancy loss, and the distribution of birth interval lengths.

Throughout the rest of this chapter, we examine in more detail three of the components that make up birth intervals. First we examine fecundability, which determines the fecund waiting time to the next conception. Then we examine the distribution of gestational ages at which pregnancies are lost and the overall probability of pregnancy loss. As will be clear from the discussion that follows, all three components must be treated together for a complete understanding of any one component.

FECUNDABILITY

Fecundability is defined as the monthly or cycle-wise probability of conception for a couple that is sexually active, not contracepting, and capable
of getting pregnant (Gini 1924). This probability directly determines the
waiting time to next conception. In the simplest case, if fecundability is
homogenous among and within women, then it is simply the inverse of
the mean waiting time to conception (Sheps and Menken 1973).

A number of different methods have been devised for estimating
fecundability. It has been estimated from the fraction of couples conceiving in a month (Gini 1924; Henry 1972; Potter 1961; Sheps 1965; Tietze et
al. 1950), waiting times to a recognized conception (Henry 1972; Jain 1969;
Majumdar and Sheps 1970; Potter and Parker 1964; Sheps 1964; Sheps and
Menken 1973; Strassmann and Warner 1998), and waiting times from marriage to the first birth (Bongaarts 1975; Gini 1924; Wood et al. 1994). At the
most detailed level, fecundability is found as a function of daily probabilities of conception given coitus for each day near ovulation (e.g., Barrett
and Marshall 1969; Weinberg et al. 1994).

A fundamental difficulty with all measures of fecundability is that early
pregnancies cannot be detected by any current noninvasive technology.
Thus any pregnancies that terminate before being detected lead to under-
estimation of fecundability. Demographers have defined fecundability in
a number of ways in order to take into account this difficulty. *Total fecundability* is defined as the true monthly or cycle-wise probability of conception, *apparent fecundability* is the monthly or cycle-wise probability of
conception using a particular technology to detect a pregnancy, and *effective fecundability* is the monthly or cycle-wise probability of conception that
results in a live birth.

Total fecundability cannot be measured by existing technology; yet, it is
conceptually the most important measure because it completely disentan-
gles fecundability from the effects of pregnancy loss (which is a measure
of mortality). We will revisit issues of how total fecundability and pregnancy loss are confounded as well as age-specific total fecundability after
we examine pregnancy loss in more detail. Both apparent and effective
fecundability are measures that confound total fecundability and pregnancy loss. Effective fecundability discounts pregnancy loss altogether.
Apparent fecundability is more difficult to interpret, since we must consider the technology being used for detecting pregnancies and how early
pregnancies are detected by the method.

The effect of age on apparent fecundability is fundamental for an
understanding of birth spacing. The observed pattern of age-specific
apparent fecundability based on earlier data shows a rapid increase from
zero in the teens to a peak in the early twenties. Thereafter fecundability

declines steadily with age until reaching zero in the mid-forties (Wood 1994). It is important to keep in mind that the age-specific decline in apparent fecundability may be biased by an age-related increase in early (i.e., undetectable) pregnancy loss. The extent of this bias can only be known by measuring total fecundability.

PREGNANCY LOSS

In trying to evaluate the effect of pregnancy loss on the human life course, we run into the same difficulty that we had for fecundability. Since some pregnancies may terminate before they can be detected, empirical studies underenumerate the true number of pregnancies and therefore the number of pregnancies that are lost. Again, the extent of this underenumeration depends on the characteristics (particularly the sensitivity) of the methods used to diagnose pregnancy. For this reason, it will prove useful to use the modifiers *total* and *apparent* with pregnancy loss in the same sense they were used for fecundability. Total pregnancy loss refers to all pregnancy loss from conception through term, and apparent pregnancy loss refers to losses that occur after a pregnancy is diagnosed.

As with fecundability, comparisons among studies of pregnancy loss are problematic. Even so, it is helpful to examine the results of broadly similar studies, and to see the effects that the study methods have on apparent pregnancy loss.

Community Surveys

The earliest large-scale population-based studies of pregnancy loss were community surveys that relied on subjects' self-reports of pregnancy. The apparent probability of pregnancy loss found in these studies are in the range of 12% to 15% per conception. Details and summaries of some of these studies can be found elsewhere (Boklage 1990; Kline et al. 1989; Leridon 1977; Wood 1994). Determining pregnancy by self-reports is not a very sensitive assay method, so that all of these community-based studies grossly underestimated the probability of total pregnancy loss. Still, when properly analyzed, these studies provide a useful picture for the risk of pregnancy loss at later gestational ages.

hCG-based Studies

A number of biochemical changes that take place early in pregnancy can be used to diagnose pregnancy (reviewed in Grudzinskas and Nysenbaum 1985). To date, the only method that has been refined, validated, and used extensively for studies of pregnancy loss involves assays for the hormone human chorionic gonadotropin (hCG) in maternal blood or urine. These hCG-based methods show a high sensitivity and are capable of detecting pregnancies before the end of the second week after fertilization. Even so, the most sensitive assays of this type cannot detect pregnancies until about seven days after conception (Lenton 1988) and fail to detect half of all true pregnancies up to about 10–14 days after ovulation (Holman et al. 1998).[2]

Another important characteristic of a pregnancy assay is its specificity, defined as the probability that the assay will correctly diagnose a non-pregnant woman as not pregnant.[3] Extremely sensitive pregnancy assays tend to have lower specificity because they pick up low levels of background hCG that occur naturally in non-pregnant women (Alfthan et al. 1987; Armstrong et al. 1984; Stenman et al. 1987). Some hCG-based assays have low specificity for another reason: they cross-react with molecules that are similar to hCG, particularly luteinizing hormone (LH). High specificity is extremely important for studies of pregnancy loss, as many assays will be carried out for every early pregnancy loss detected, so that even a small false-positive rate will bias upward the probability of pregnancy loss (Weinberg et al. 1992).

The first large-scale study of apparent pregnancy loss using hCG-based pregnancy assays was that of Miller and colleagues (1980), who measured urinary hCG concentrations in first morning urines taken every other day over the luteal phase of 197 women (mean age 27.5 years) who were discontinuing nonhormonal contraception. The hCG assay they used showed "very little" cross-reaction to LH. Unfortunately, additional details on specificity were not provided, and they did not use a pool of non-pregnant women to test the specificity of the assay under the conditions of study. The limit of detection of the assay was 10 IU/L hCG, and their criterion for pregnancy was a concentration above 20 IU/L hCG in two successive samples or a single sample over 50 IU/L hCG. The probability of pregnancy loss was 0.427 for all pregnancies they could detect, and 0.139 for pregnancies that were detectable by standard clinical methods. These surprisingly high rates of pregnancy loss must be interpreted with some caution because of the lack of controls and the possibility of false positive diagnoses of pregnancies.

Edmonds and colleagues (1982) studied pregnancy loss using the same assay as was used by Miller et al. (1980). However, they paid careful attention to issues of specificity. Subjects collected first morning urines every other day beginning with cycle day 21. A series of 18 women who had undergone a tubal ligation served as controls; their samples were assayed to determine the maximum concentration of hCG that could be detected in non-pregnant women. From this, they arrived at an extremely conservative cutoff of 56 IU/L hCG, which provided a specificity of 99.99%. They also demonstrated that cross-reaction to physiological levels of LH was negligible. Eighty-two women (mean age 27 years) discontinuing nonhormonal contraception contributed 198 ovulatory cycles. Despite the very conservative cutoff for a pregnancy diagnosis, a remarkable 62% of pregnancies were lost and the probability of clinically recognized pregnancies ending in loss was 0.12.

Edmonds and colleagues' findings (1982) are perplexing because about one third of the early pregnancy losses were diagnosed on day 6 or 7 after (estimated) ovulation, and half of the early losses were diagnosed before day 9. But the relatively low sensitivity of their assay and the extremely conservative hCG cutoff they used should have made such early detection of pregnancy unlikely. Lenton (1988) showed that only 5% of spontaneous conception cycles produce hCG in concentrations exceeding 5 IU/L by day 8 and 16% by day 9; likewise, studies by O'Connor et al. (1994) and Wilcox et al. (1985, 1988) suggest that hCG concentrations rarely exceed 50 IU/L before about the first missed menses. Wilcox et al. (1985) further examined this issue by comparing two highly sensitive and specific assays, including the SB6 antibody–based assay used by Edmonds et al. (1982). Several possible difficulties were found for the SB6 assay, including some cross-reaction with LH. One subject showed a consistent nonspecific immunoreactivity by the SB6 assay that was not found with the other assay. In this way, estimates of pregnancy loss in the Edmonds et al. (1982) study may have been biased by one or more difficulties with their assay.

Wilcox et al. (1988) studied pregnancy loss in 221 women (mean age was 29 years; 707 cycles) discontinuing contraception. A control group of 31 women who had undergone tubal ligation provided samples to develop a pregnancy criterion of 0.035 ng/ml (≈0.45 IU/L) hCG for three days. The hCG assay used a polyclonal antibody (R525) that was highly sensitive and specific (Wilcox et al. 1985). This study measured a probability of apparent pregnancy loss of 0.32, and the probability of pregnancy loss in clinically recognized pregnancies of 0.22.

Hakim et al. (1995) studied infertility and early pregnancy loss in 148 women (mean age about 32 years; 679 menstrual cycles) who worked in a semiconductor manufacturing plant. About 60% of the subjects reported no past or present fertility problems. They used a highly sensitive and specific monoclonal antibody–based hCG assay. The overall probability of pregnancy loss for women without fertility problems was 0.38, and the probability of pregnancy loss following a clinically recognized pregnancy was 0.21.

The hCG-based studies all provide broadly consistent estimates for the probability of *clinically* recognized pregnancy loss even though the more sensitive assay methods yielded loss rates from 0.32 to over 0.60. The large range reflects, in part, methodological differences in assays characteristics, criteria for pregnancy diagnosis, and the sampling methods used.

Anatomical Studies

Hertig et al. (1956, 1959) studied early pregnancy loss by direct micro-scopic examinations of conceptuses. In this remarkable study, conducted from 1938 to 1954, uteri and oviducts were surgically removed from 211 women of proven fertility. Prior to surgery, the women attempted to get pregnant. One hundred and seven cases were deemed optimal for finding an early conceptus, based on ovarian signs of a recent ovulation and removal of the uterus between ovulation and the next menses. The oviducts and uteri were carefully flushed and 34 conceptuses of known gestational age were found, of which 10 appeared to be morphologically abnormal. Four of eight conceptuses recovered prior to implantation were abnormal. Of the remaining 26 conceptuses, six were abnormal. James (1970) reviewed the results of Hertig et al. (1959) and another small anatomical study, and the results of the community-based study of French and Bierman (1962). By estimating the proportion of fertilized ova that were missed in the Hertig study, he estimated a probability of total preg-nancy loss of 0.49.

Age-Specific Pregnancy Loss

Biomedical and demographic research suggests that the risk of preg-nancy loss varies considerably among women within a population. An important source of this variation appears to be maternal age. The pattern that has emerged from a number of studies suggests the risk of pregnancy loss changes with age according to a U-shaped distribution. The risk of pregnancy loss declines in the years immediately following menarche, is lowest around age 20, and then increases regularly with age thereafter.

Wood and Weinstein (1988) compiled results from nine studies examin-ing the effects of age on risk of pregnancy loss. The distribution from each study was rescaled to a common rate of 150 pregnancy losses for 1,000 con-ceptions to account for differences among studies in methods of preg-nancy determination. Apparent pregnancy loss showed a steady rise with age, increasing from a probability of 0.15 at age 20 to a peak of 0.40 toward the end of the reproductive span. From the hCG-based studies discussed above, we can conclude that the true overall rate of pregnancy loss is likely to be substantially higher at each maternal age; it is the overall shape of the curve that is of interest.

Several authors have suggested that the increased risk of pregnancy loss by maternal age or gravidity is, to some extent, a statistical artifact (Casterline 1989; Leridon 1977; Resseguie 1974; Santow and Bracher 1989; Wilcox and Gladen 1982). A bias toward higher risk of loss at older ages results from examining risk of pregnancy loss in non–natural fertility pop-ulations. If there is heterogeneity in risk of pregnancy loss among women in the population, then the group of women still attempting to reproduce at older ages may increasingly be made up of those at higher risk of pregnancy loss. In other words, in studies of pregnancy loss in contracepting populations, older subjects are those women who have not yet met their family size goals, perhaps because they are at higher risk of pregnancy loss. This selectivity hypothesis has received some empirical support (e.g., Santow and Bracher 1989); but, as Wood (1994) points out, the same elevation in risk of loss is found in studies among natural fertility populations such as the Amish (Resseguie 1974) and rural Indian women (Potter et al. 1965).[4]

Bishop's Theory of Pregnancy Loss

Beginning in the early 1960s, the first cytogenetic studies of spontaneous abortions were undertaken. These studies uncovered the role of lethal trisomies (Edwards et al. 1960; Patau et al. 1960) and triploidies (Delhanty et al. 1961; Penrose and Delhanty 1961) in pregnancy loss. These case studies were soon followed by larger cytogenetic studies of aborted material (Carr 1963; Clendenin and Benirschke 1963; Thiede 1969).

Marcus Bishop (1964) summarized the cytogenetic studies of human abortuses and his own work on the cytogenetics of bull sperm, and put together a theory of pregnancy loss. Bishop proposed that *(a)* the majority of pregnancy losses resulted from chromosomal abnormalities, *(b)* chromosomal abnormalities would increase with the age of parents,[5] and *(c)* many unobserved losses would occur during the earliest parts of the pregnancy. Since Bishop's theory was first formulated, a number of lines of research have substantiated the basic elements. In particular, numerous cytogenetic studies of spontaneous abortions (reviewed in Boué et al. 1985; Jacobs 1991; Thiede 1969; Warburton 1987) confirmed the prediction that chromosomal abnormalities are the single most common cause of human pregnancy death in conceptuses that survive long enough for the pregnancy to be recognized.

Risk of pregnancy loss may vary among women for reasons other than the increase in chromosomal errors associated with maternal age. These factors include environmental chemicals (Brent and Beckman 1994; Pernoll 1986), endocrine factors (Coulam and Stern 1994; Maxson 1986), implantation factors (Hunt and Roby 1994; McIntyre and Faulk 1986), uterine and other maternal defects (Crenshaw 1986; Patton 1994; Rock and Murphy 1986), maternal infection (Benirschke and Robb 1987; Byrn and Gibson 1986; Sever 1980), and immunological causes (Branch 1987; del Junco 1986; Silver and Branch 1994). Although these nonchromosomal causes may be important in a medical context, they share the common characteristics that each cause is individually rare.

Probability of Pregnancy Loss across Gestation

Ideally, we want to know the risk of pregnancy loss at each gestational age. The gestational-age-specific risk of pregnancy loss defines both the ages when pregnancies are lost as well as the overall probability of pregnancy loss. Kline et al. (1989) summarized the data from Hertig et al. (1959), Wilcox et al. (1988), and French and Bierman (1962) to arrive at an aggregate distribution for the risk of pregnancy loss across gestation that shows the risk being highest immediately after fertilization and declining at all later gestational ages. Wood (1989, 1994) and Boklage (1990) took another approach to this question. They independently developed a parametric model of pregnancy loss, which captures much of the underlying theory of Bishop's model. Under the Wood-Boklage model pregnancies fall into one of two risk groups—a chromosomally abnormal group for which risk of pregnancy loss is high, and a chromosomally normal group for which risk of pregnancy loss is low. The hazard for each risk group is considered constant across gestation, corresponding to a negative exponential distribution of deaths in each subgroup. A third parameter of the model is the initial fraction of conceptuses in the high-risk group.

Results from previous studies were analyzed by Wood (1989, 1994) and Boklage (1990). The parametric and etiologic nature of the model gave them the means to extrapolate the risk of pregnancy loss back to conception and thus to estimate the probability of total pregnancy loss. Wood reanalyzed the French and Bierman community survey data and found the proportion of conceptuses in the abnormal group was 0.29; the abnormal subgroup had a hazard of loss of 0.169 and the normal group had a hazard of 0.001. Mathematically, these estimates imply a probability of total pregnancy loss of 0.30, of which 8% constitute those that die before clinical detection. In the high-risk group, 99.8% of the conceptuses perished before birth, and 3.4% of the low-risk group died before birth.

Boklage (1990) used results from five hCG-based studies of natural conceptions, adjusted for each study to a common probability of 0.287 at clinical detection, and then estimated the parameters of the model. The estimated fraction of abnormal conceptuses was 73%. The hazard for the abnormal subgroup group was 0.155, and the hazard for the normal subgroup was 0.00042. The estimates give a probability of total pregnancy loss of 0.733. The chromosomally abnormal subgroup constituted almost all of the pregnancy losses; only about 1.1% of the normal conceptuses were expected to be lost.

Wood's and Boklage's estimates primarily differ in the initial proportion of abnormal conceptuses. The subgroup hazards are remarkably similar, despite the very different regimes of pregnancy detection. Wood's original estimates are almost certain to have underestimated the fraction of abnormal conceptuses because the French and Bierman (1962) data used in the analysis were based on self-reports of pregnancy loss, implying that pregnancies had to survive to fairly late gestational ages to be ascertained.

MEASURING TOTAL FECUNDABILITY AND TOTAL PREGNANCY LOSS

As should be clear from the preceding discussion, most previous work has treated pregnancy loss alone or fecundability alone. The result is that *apparent* fecundability and pregnancy loss have been estimated rather than *total* fecundability and pregnancy loss. In this section, we develop an approach for estimating both quantities together. First we examine in detail the way in which pregnancy loss and fecundability are confounded. Then we extend the Wood-Boklage model and use it as the basis of a new model to estimate total fecundability and total fetal loss.

Suppose we were to conduct a study using a pregnancy assay with perfect sensitivity. Some number of women would be followed prospectively and a test for pregnancy made within each menstrual cycle. The results of this study might look like Figure 1.2 (top panel), in which some number of menstrual cycles are observed along the *y*-axis. Cycles that result in a pregnancy are followed to term along the *x*-axis. The horizontal line indicates the number of cycles in which fertilization occurred, and the dashed curve represents the numbers of ongoing pregnancies that survive to each gestational age. After all pregnancies have terminated in this study, each menstrual cycle can be classified as a non-conception cycle, a cycle that ended in the loss of the pregnancy, or a cycle that resulted in a live birth. We could then directly compute total fecundability as described in the figure caption.

Since we cannot detect pregnancies at fertilization, a more realistic portrayal for this fictitious study is shown in the lower panel of Figure 1.2. The vertical line labeled "detection" represents the imperfect sensitivity of the pregnancy assay. The assay cannot detect any pregnancy before this point, and it detects all pregnancies that survive beyond this point. Now each menstrual cycle must be classified in one of three ways: cycles in which a pregnancy was not detected, cycles in which a detected pregnancy is lost, and cycles that end in a live birth. The incomplete sensitivity means that we do not know the proper denominator to compute total fecundability and we do not know the proper numerator or denominator to compute the probability of total pregnancy loss.

Figure 1.2 illustrates why direct measurement of total fecundability and pregnancy loss is impossible when the earliest pregnancies cannot be detected, but it also suggests a way to get around the difficulty. Suppose we had a parametric model for the gestational-age-specific risk of pregnancy loss. We could use the observations of pregnancy loss taken from the point of detection forward to estimate the entire distribution of pregnancy loss.

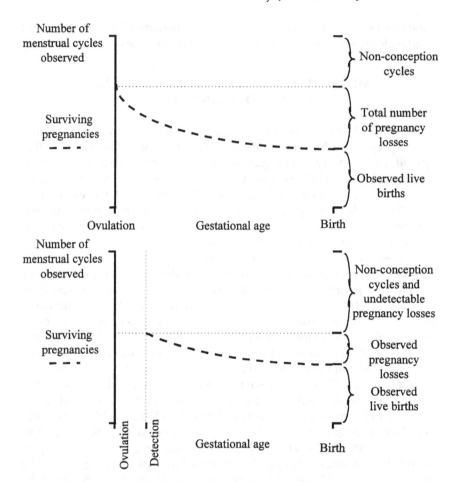

Figure 1.2.   The way in which total pregnancy loss and total fecundability are confounded by incomplete sensitivity of pregnancy assays. The y axis represents
some number of menstrual cycles under study, and the x axis is time from ovulation to birth. The upper panel shows classification of each cycle as if exact information were known. Fecundability is computed as (pregnancy losses + births) /
(number of menstrual cycles), and the probability of pregnancy loss is computed
as (pregnancy losses) / (pregnancy losses + births). The bottom panel shows what
happens when pregnancy detection cannot occur until sometime after fertilization. The mean gestational age at which the assay can detect a pregnancy is
labeled "detection." Now, the earliest pregnancy losses and the nonconception
cycles cannot be differentiated. The proper numerator for fecundability is not
known, and the proper numerator and denominator for estimating the total probability of pregnancy loss are not known (Holman 1996).

The resulting distribution could be used to compute total pregnancy loss, which, in turn, provides a basis for estimating total fecundability. This procedure involves projecting the distribution of pregnancy loss back to the start of the pregnancy, so the model for risk of pregnancy loss needs to be an accurate reflection of the most important biological mechanisms involved in pregnancy loss.

The Wood-Boklage model is suitable for this purpose. The model captures the most important components of pregnancy loss as envisioned by Bishop (1964). It is parameterized by defining h_h as the hazard for the abnormal (high-risk) subgroup and h_l as the hazard for the normal (low-risk) subgroup. Both parameters are constant across gestation. The fraction of abnormal conceptuses surviving to gestational age t is $\exp(-h_h t)$. Likewise, the fraction of normal conceptuses surviving to t is $\exp(-h_l t)$. At fertilization, a certain fraction of conceptuses is chromosomally abnormal; the fraction is denoted p_h. This percentage declines over the course of gestation because abnormal conceptuses are lost at a greater rate.[6]

The Wood-Boklage model was used as the basis for a new model to estimate both age-specific total pregnancy loss and age-specific total fecundability. The data required to estimate parameters of the model are a series of menstrual cycles along with results of pregnancy assays within each cycle. The mathematical details of the model are given elsewhere (Holman 1996), and only an overview is given here. The model incorporates the effects of both assay sensitivity and assay specificity, incorporates interval-censored and right-censored observations, and statistically estimates a nonsusceptible fraction of women (i.e., those who are not at risk of getting pregnant). Controlling for the nonsusceptible fraction means that a fecundability of 1 will be estimated for at least one age.

The observations we used to test the model are twice weekly urine samples assayed for the presence of hCG one or more times within each ovarian cycle (Holman et al. 1998). The start of each "cycle" was taken as the estimated day of ovulation. Each cycle ended when one of three events occurred: the next menses (which includes both non-conception cycles as well undetected pregnancy losses), a pregnancy terminated, or a live birth occurred. From observations of this type, maximum likelihood estimates were found for total fecundability (ρ_0), total pregnancy loss (p_h, h_h, and h_l), the gestational-age-specific sensitivity of the pregnancy assay, and maternal age effects on fecundability and pregnancy loss. Assay specificity (0.94) was a constant in the model.

The underlying logic of the method is seen in Figure 1.3. Events are occurring probabilistically from one pregnancy assay to the next within a single cycle according to the branches and branch weights of this tree. All we can observe are the positive or negative assay results shown at the branch tips. At ovulation (time t_0), a fraction of women will be pregnant with probability ρ_0 (which is the estimate of total fecundability). For women who are not pregnant (probability $1 - \rho_0$), the left branch of the tree is traversed. A pregnancy assay given at the first observation after ovulation (time t_1) will give a true negative diagnosis with specificity q, and a false positive diagnosis with probability $(1 - q)$. For the women who are pregnant, fraction $1 - P_1$ will experience a pregnancy loss in the interval $[t_0, t_1]$; P_k arises directly from the Wood-Boklage model as $P_k = S(t_k)/S(t_{k-1})$ and incorporates parameters p, h_h, and h_l and covariate parameters. Again specificity q probabilistically changes the outcome of the pregnancy assays. For women who do not experience pregnancy losses (with probability P_1), some fraction of their pregnancies will be detected with probability equal to sensitivity D_1. Likewise, fraction $1 - D_1$ pregnancies will not be detected; specificity q probabilistically can then change the result.

The tree yields four routes to a positive assay result, and three routes to a negative result for the first pregnancy assay at time t_1. For all women who have positive results, we can now compute ρ_1, the probability that they are truly pregnant at time t_1, as the sum of the two "pregnant" branches that yield positive results divided by the sum of all four "positive" branches, which is $\rho_1 = \rho_0 P_1[1 - q(1 - D_1)]/[1 - q(1 - \rho_0 D_1 P_1)]$. The probability that these women are not pregnant given a positive assay is $1 - \rho_1$. For women who have negative assay results, the probability that they are pregnant (but the assay could not detect it) is $\rho_1 = \rho_0 P_1(1 - D_1)/(1 - \rho_0 D_1 P_1)$.

The left and right branch of the tree are weighted by probability ρ_1 between the first pregnancy assay and the second pregnancy assay. The tree is probabilistically traversed again and the assay result is used to compute ρ_2 given ρ_1. The tree is traversed this way for all intervals between pregnancy assays, always computing the value of ρ_k from ρ_{k-1}.

We have given the preceding description as though values for p_h, h_h, h_l, ρ_0, D, and covariate parameters are known, whereas the goal is to estimate these parameters from observations. Because the model was specified as a series of probabilistic events, maximum likelihood methods can be used to find the parameters. Details of the model, estimation methods, statistical validations, and results are given elsewhere (Holman 1996).

TOTAL PREGNANCY LOSS AND TOTAL FECUNDABILITY IN BANGLADESHI WOMEN

We collected data from a near-natural fertility population in rural Bangladesh in order to estimate parameters of the fecundability and fetal loss model (Holman 1996). The field study was conducted from February through December 1993 in Matlab thana, a rural subdistrict of Bangladesh

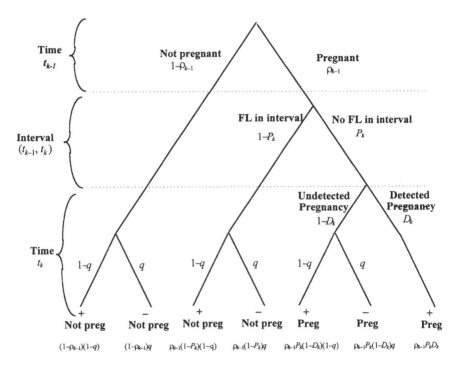

Figure 1.3. Probability tree showing the relationship among pregnancy assay results, characteristics of the assays, and probability of pregnancy loss across the interval (t_{k-1}, t_k); ρ_k is the probability of pregnancy at time k; P_k is the probability of no pregnancy loss occurring in the interval; D_k is the sensitivity of the assay at gestational age t_k; q is the specificity of the assay. At the terminal branches, $+$ and $-$ indicate whether the result of the pregnancy test is positive or negative; *Preg* and *Not preg* refer to whether the individual is pregnant or not. The probability of arriving at each of the seven outcomes is given along the bottom (Holman 1996).

about 50 km southeast of Dhaka. For the first month of the study, female field-workers conducted one-time interviews of almost all married women ages 18 to 48 who permanently resided with their husbands in 28 villages ($N = 3,290$). The 17 villages with the lowest contraceptive prevalence were selected for the nine-month prospective portion of the study. The sample included married women of all reproductive statuses, including those who were pregnant or breastfeeding at the start of the study. In this way, we did not select for subfecundity by eliminating those of proven fecundity (i.e., breastfeeding or pregnant women). Women using any form of contraception were excluded from the pool of potential participants. At any time during the prospective portion of the study, 320 subjects were enrolled. As subjects dropped out of the study or became ineligible (e.g., because of divorce), replacements were randomly selected from the pool of eligible subjects. Subjects were interviewed twice weekly about menses, pregnancy, breastfeeding, and contraception, and at the same time a urine specimen was collected. By the end of the field study, over 19,000 paired interview and urine specimens were collected from 494 subjects who participated in the study for one to nine months. Urine samples taken during the last one-third of all menstrual cycles were assayed for hCG to detect early pregnancies (Holman et al. 1998 provide details on the sensitivity and specificity of the pregnancy assay). The final set of observations consisted of 4,400 pregnancy assays in 1,561 menstrual cycles. A total of 329 pregnancies were followed: 81 pregnancies were ongoing at the end of the study (right-censored), 151 pregnancies went to term, 84 pregnancies were biochemically detected and ended in an early pregnancy loss, 10 pregnancies were lost after the subjects were aware of the pregnancy, and 3 pregnancies ended by induced abortion.

Maternal age effects were modeled on the risk of pregnancy loss in three ways: as affecting the initial fraction of abnormal conceptuses, as changing the risk of loss for abnormal conceptuses, and as changing the risk of loss for normal conceptuses. Maternal age did not significantly affect the risk of pregnancy loss for either the normal or abnormal subgroups. The only significant effect of age, as assessed by likelihood ratio tests, was to increase the probability that a conceptus was abnormal. This result is consistent with the predictions of Bishop (1964), and it supports his idea that the primary mechanism acting over the reproductive life course is an age-related increase in the proportion of chromosomally abnormal conceptuses.

The hazard of pregnancy loss over the course of early pregnancy is shown in Figure 1.4. The top panel shows the fit independent of maternal age for the parametric model and a life table model. The fits are similar, except at the earliest gestational ages when the pregnancy assays were unable to detect all pregnancies reliably. The parametric model makes use of the observed ranges of data and fits the entire distribution. Most of the abnormal pregnancies have terminated by day 100 so the hazard approaches that of the normal subgroup. The lower panel shows the gestational-age-specific risk expected at four different maternal ages, and at the mean age in this study.

The effect of maternal age on fecundability and pregnancy loss is shown in Figure 1.5. Total fecundability was constant over most of the reproductive life span. Age showed little effect from 20 to 36 years of age. At about 40 years of age, fecundability declined rapidly until approaching zero near age 46. The probability of pregnancy loss increases by maternal age: 20-year-old women are expected to lose about 55% of their pregnancies, the percentage increases to 84% at age 30 and 96% at age 40. These results are

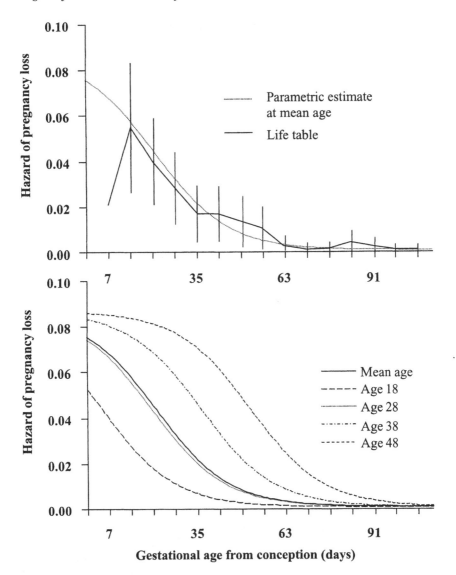

Figure 1.4. Hazard of pregnancy loss in early pregnancy. The top panel shows the fit to the parametric model at the mean age compared to life table estimates (± one standard error). The bottom panel shows the parametric distribution at five different ages (Holman 1996).

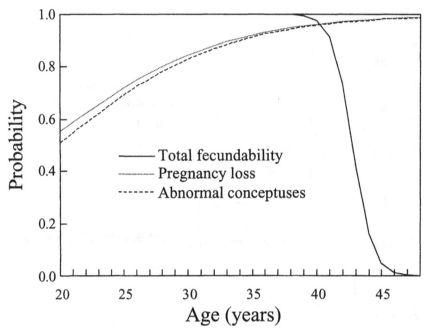

Figure 1.5. Estimates of maternal age-specific total fecundability and pregnancy
loss in Bangladeshi women (Holman 1996).

similar to those of Boklage (1990), who estimated a probability of 0.73 over
all ages.

DISCUSSION

The results of this study provide a rather unexpected picture of fecundability and pregnancy loss. The age-related decline in female apparent
fecundability has traditionally been interpreted as a true decline in
fecundability resulting from declining coital frequency by age or marital
duration (James 1981), a deteriorating uterine environment (Gosden 1985;
Gostwamy et al. 1988; Naeye 1983), declining ovarian function, or an
increase in the age-specific prevalence of sterility (Wilson et al. 1988). The
results presented here suggest that most of the age-related decline in
apparent fecundability results from an age-related increase in pregnancy
loss, not from the decline in total fecundability per se. These other factors
appear to be less important until after about age 40, when total fecundability declines sharply.

These findings provide a number of significant insights into the human
pattern of reproduction. One clear implication is for our view of repro-

ductive aging and the end of the reproductive life span. Reproductive aging appears to be a gradual process dominated primarily by pregnancy loss, followed by a rapid decline in fecundability only after age 40. By the age at which menopause is reached, fecundity is already nearly zero. In other words, menopause plays almost no role in reproductive aging and the cessation of reproduction. Because of pregnancy loss, reproductive cessation effectively occurs some time before menopause, explaining the lag of about five years between the average age of women at their last birth and the onset of menopause in natural fertility populations (Wood 1994). Hence, menopause is unlikely to affect reproductive success directly. From an evolutionary perspective, this means that menopause itself has no direct effect on fitness and therefore requires no special pleading to explain its regular occurrence in humans.[7] For a further discussion of these issues see Leidy Sievert (chapter 12, this volume).

This argument, of course, merely shifts the evolutionary question from "why menopause?" to "why the rapid age-related increase in the risk of pregnancy loss?" At present we have no firm suggestions to make. Bishop (1964) suggested that, because pregnancy loss is selective with respect to chromosomal aberrations, it serves an important "editing" function in the production of viable offspring. This idea may have some merit, but it ignores the fact that high rates of pregnancy loss add substantial time to the total length of the interbirth interval and therefore reduce overall reproductive success (Wood 1994). It has never been shown that the editing role of pregnancy loss is enough to offset this fitness cost.

Instead of considering reproductive cessation per se as adaptive, we ask the question, why does the human life span extend so far beyond the age at which female fecundity approaches zero? Or, asked another way, why does female fecundity decline so early in life? This question is complex, and we can only speculate briefly here. Our first response is that this may be a purely demographic question. Small decreases in age-specific mortality, particularly infant mortality, can dramatically increase the fraction of individuals who survive beyond age 40. It is not implausible that human cultural practices, which have likely decreased age-specific rates of mortality and the variance in mortality, are largely responsible for this pattern.

A second, and closely related, possibility is that there may be severe physiological constraints to the further evolution of the mechanism needed to extend the viability of oocytes. Alternatively, there is too little genetic variability in these systems upon which natural selection can act. As the human life span lengthened, whether through biological evolution or cultural practice, the evolution of fecundity has lagged behind. This idea leads to some predictions. First, it suggests that the heritability of age-specific rates of pregnancy loss resulting from chromosomal abnormalities should be very low, as any substantial genetic variability would be acted on by selection. A direct test of this idea would be difficult and invasive, but the indirect methods developed in this paper could be adapted for examining correlations among relatives. The second prediction is that these same constraints will be found in other long-lived primates, so that other species will show a similar pattern of high and increasing rates of chromosomal abnormalities at later reproductive ages.

We gratefully acknowledge support from the National Institute on Aging (RO1AG15141), the National Institute of Child Health and Human Development (F32HD07994), the National Science Foundation (DBS9218734), and the Population Council. Research in Bangladesh was supported by the Hill Foundation; the American Institute of Bangladesh Studies; the Centre for Development Research, Bangladesh; the International Centre for Diarrhoeal Disease Research, Bangladesh; and a Dissertation Research Grant on International Demographic Issues made on behalf of the Andrew W. Mellon Foundation to the Population Research Institute. We thank Robert Jones, Kenneth Campbell, Kathleen O'Connor, Matthew Steele, and Michael Strong for comments and assistance.

NOTES

1.   Natural fertility populations are those in which effective methods of contraception are not used to limit reproduction. See Wood 1994 for a technical definition and discussion of the concept of natural fertility. Natural fertility populations provide an ideal experimental system in which to examine the physiological and behavioral components of human birth spacing (Henry 1961). For this reason, discussions of the reproductive life course and components of birth spacing in this paper are restricted to conditions of natural fertility.

2.   The sensitivity of a pregnancy assay refers to the gestational-age-specific probability (from fertilization on) that the hCG assay will detect a true pregnancy. This definition of sensitivity is appropriate for qualitative assays, such as those used to diagnose a pregnancy. A different definition of sensitivity is used for quantitative assays, such as those that quantify the concentrations of hCG. An hCG assay can be used as a pregnancy assay by defining one or more criteria that must be met before the result is considered a positive indication of pregnancy.

3.   One minus the specificity is the probability of a false positive pregnancy diagnosis. Typically, the specificity of a particular assay is determined by quantifying the number of false pregnancies diagnosed in a series of women who have had tubal ligations.

4.   The apparent increase in risk of fetal loss at the youngest ages may result from a bias toward earlier initiation of sexual relations in women who experience menarche at younger ages (Wood 1994).

5.   Discussions of age-related changes in the risk of pregnancy loss tend to focus on maternal age rather than paternal age. Several analyses support the claim that it is primarily maternal age, not paternal age, that is most important for pregnancy loss (Antonarakis et al. 1991; Hassold et al. 1980; Hatch 1983). Even so, parental ages tend to be highly correlated, so that statistical models will have difficulty teasing apart maternal and paternal age effects.

6.   The overall fraction of surviving conceptuses at gestational age t is $S(t) = p_h \exp(-h_h t) + (1 - p_h)\exp(-h_l t)$. The proportion of abnormal conceptuses at gestational age t is $p(t) = p_h \exp(-h_h t)/S(t)$. The hazard for the combined subgroups at gestational age t is $h(t) = p(t)h_h + [1 - p(t)]h_l$. We model covariates, such as maternal

age, as affecting h_h and h_l using a proportional hazard specification. For the p_h parameter, a logistic specification is used to model the effect of covariates.

7. This idea is supported by the otherwise puzzling findings on heritability (h^2) in age at menopause: Liqun et al. (1990) estimated an h^2 of 0.70 for age at menopause from 216 mother- daughter pairs, Peccei (1999) estimated an h^2 of 0.37 (95% CI 0.10 to 0.62) in 117 mother-daughter pairs, Snieder et al. (1998) estimated an h^2 of 0.63 (95% CI 0.53 to 0.71) from a study of 260 twin pairs, and Do et al. (2000) estimated an h^2 of 0.51 from 426 twin pairs. Taken together, these studies suggest high heritability for age at menopause, and high heritability is usually considered evidence that a trait is not closely related to fitness (Hartl and Clark 1997).

REFERENCES

Alfthan H, Haglund C, Dabek J, Stenman U-H (1987) Concentrations of human choriogonadotropin, its β-subunit, and the core fragment of the β-subunit in serum and urine of men and nonpregnant women. *Clinical Chemistry* 38:1981–1987.

Antonarakis SE and the Down Syndrome Collaborative Group (1991) Parental origin of the extra chromosome in Trisomy 21 as indicated by analysis of DNA polymorphisms. *New England Journal of Medicine* 324:872–876.

Armstrong EG, Ehrlich PH, Birken S, Schlatterer JP, Siris E, Hembree WC, Canfield RE (1984) Use of a highly sensitive and specific immunoradiometric assay for detection of human chorionic gonadotropin in urine of normal, nonpregnant, and pregnant individuals. *Journal of Clinical Endocrinology and Metabolism* 59:867–874.

Barrett JC, Marshall J (1969) The risk of conception on different days of the menstrual cycle. *Population Studies* 23:455–461.

Benirschke K, Robb JA (1987) Infectious causes of fetal death. *Clinical Obstetrics and Gynecology* 30:284–294.

Bishop MWH (1964) Paternal contribution to embryonic death. *Journal of Reproduction and Fertility* 7:383–396.

Boklage CE (1990) Survival probability of human conceptions from fertilization to term. *International Journal of Fertility* 35:75–94.

Bongaarts J (1975) A method for the estimation of fecundability. *Demography* 12:645–660.

Bongaarts J, Potter RG (1983) *Fertility, Biology and Behavior: An Analysis of the Proximate Determinants* (New York, Academic Press).

Boué A, Boué J, Gropp A (1985) Cytogenetics of pregnancy wastage. *Advances in Human Genetics* 14:1–57.

Branch DW (1987) Immunologic disease and fetal death. *Clinical Obstetrics and Gynecology* 30:295–311.

Brent RL, Beckman DA (1994) The contribution of environmental teratogens to embryonic and fetal loss. *Clinical Obstetrics and Gynecology* 37:646–670.

Byrn FW, Gibson M (1986) Infectious causes of recurrent pregnancy loss. *Clinical Obstetrics and Gynecology* 29:925–940.

Carr DH (1963) Chromosome studies in abortuses and stillborn infants. *Lancet* 2:603.

Casterline JB (1989) Maternal age, gravidity, and pregnancy spacing effects on spontaneous pregnancy mortality. *Social Biology* 36:186–212.

Clendenin TM, Benirschke K (1963) Chromosome studies in spontaneous abortions. *Laboratory Investigations* 12:1281–1292.

Coulam CB, Stern JJ (1994) Endocrine factors associated with recurrent spontaneous abortion. *Clinical Obstetrics and Gynecology* 37:730–744.
Crenshaw C Jr (1986) Preterm premature rupture of the membranes. *Clinical
Obstetrics and Gynecology* 29:735–738.
del Junco DJ (1986) Association of autoimmune conditions with recurrent
intrauterine death. *Clinical Obstetrics and Gynecology* 29:959–975.
Delhanty JDA, Ellis JR, Rowley PT (1961) Triploid cells in a human embryo. *Lancet*
1:1286.
Do K-A, Broom BM, Kuhnert P, Duffy DL, Todorov AA, Treloar SA, Martin NG
(2000) Genetic analysis of the age at menopause by using estimating equations
and Bayesian random effects models. *Statistical Medicine* 19:1217–1235.
Edmonds DK, Lindsay KS, Miller JF, Williamson E, Woods PJ (1982) Early embryonic mortality in women. *Fertility and Sterility* 38:447–453.
Edwards JH, Harnden DG, Cameron AH, Cross VM, Wolff OH (1960) A new tri-
somic syndrome. *Lancet* 1:787.
French FE, Bierman JE (1962) Probabilities of pregnancy mortality. *Public Health
Reports* 77:835–847.
Gini C (1924) Premières recherches sur la fécondabilité de la femme. *Proceedings of
the International Mathematics Congress* 2:889–892.
Gosden RG (1985) Maternal age: a major factor affecting the prospects and outcome of pregnancy. *Annals of the New York Academy of Sciences* 442:45–57.
Gostwamy RK, Williams G, Steptoe PC (1988) Decreased uterine perfusion: a cause
of infertility. *Human Reproduction* 3:955–959.
Gray RH, Campbell OM, Zacur HA, Labbok MH, MacRae SL (1987) Postpartum
return of ovarian activity in nonbreastfeeding women monitored by urinary
assays. *Journal of Clinical Endocrinology and Metabolism* 64:645–650.
Grudzinskas JG, Nysenbaum AM (1985) Failure of human pregnancy after implan-
tation. *Annals of the New York Academy of Sciences* 442:38–44.
Hakim RB, Gray RH, Zacur H (1995) Infertility and early pregnancy loss. *American
Journal of Obstetrics and Gynecology* 172:1510–1517.
Hartl DL, Clark AG (1997) *Principles of Population Genetics,* third edition (Sunder-
land MA, Sinauer Associates).
Hassold T, Chen N, Funkhouser J, Jooss T, Manuel B, Matsuura J, Matsuyama A,
Wilson C, Yamane JA, Jacobs PA (1980) A cytogenetic study of 1000 sponta-
neous abortions. *Annals of Human Genetics* 44:151–178.
Hatch MC (1983) *Paternal Risk Factors for Spontaneous Abortion* (PhD dissertation,
Columbia University, New York).
Henry L (1961) Some data on natural fertility. *Social Biology* 8:81–91.
Henry L (1972) *On the Measurement of Human Fertility: Selected Writings, Louis
Henry,* MC Sheps, E Lapierre-Adamcyk (Eds) (Amsterdam, Elsevier).
Hertig AT, Rock J, Adams EC (1956) A description of 34 human ova within the first
17 days of development. *American Journal of Anatomy* 98:435–493.
Hertig AT, Rock J, Adams EC, Menkin MC (1959) Thirty-four fertilized human ova,
good, bad, and indifferent, recovered from 210 women of known fertility: a
study of biologic wastage in early human pregnancy. *Pediatrics* 23:202–211.
Holman DJ (1996) *Total Fecundability and Pregnancy Loss in Rural Bangladesh* (PhD
dissertation, Pennsylvania State University).
Holman DJ, Rasheed FN, Stroud CM, Brindle E, O'Connor KA and Campbell KL
(1998) A commercial pregnancy test modified for field studies of pregnancy
loss. *Clinica Chimica Acta* 271:25–44.
Hunt JS, Roby KF (1994) Implantation factors. *Clinical Obstetrics and Gynecology*
37:635–645.

Jacobs PA (1991) The chromosome complement of human gametes. *Oxford Reviews of Reproductive Biology* 11:47–72.

Jain AK (1969) Fecundability and its relation to age in a sample of Taiwanese women. *Population Studies* 23:69–85.

James WH (1970) The incidence of spontaneous abortion. *Population Studies* 24:241–245.

James WH (1981) Distributions of coital rates and of fecundability. *Social Biology* 28:334–341.

Jones RE (1989) Breast-feeding and post-partum amenorrhoea in Indonesia. *Journal of Biosocial Science* 21:83–100.

Kline J, Stein Z, Susser M (1989) *Conception to Birth: Epidemiology of Prenatal Development* (Oxford, Oxford University Press).

Lenton EA (1988) Pituitary and ovarian hormones in implantation and early pregnancy. In M Chapman, G Grudzinskas, T Chard (Eds) *Implantation Biological and Clinical Aspects* (London, Springer-Verlag), 17–29.

Leridon H (1977) *Human Fertility: The Basic Components* (Chicago, University of Chicago Press).

Liqun W, Roufu D, Zili W (1990) Studies of the change and heretability [sic] of menopausal age. *Acta Anthropologica Sinica* 9:45–54.

Majumdar H, Sheps MC (1970) Estimators of a type 1 geometric distribution from observations on conception times. *Demography* 7:349–360.

Maxson WS (1986) Hormonal causes of recurrent abortion. *Clinical Obstetrics and Gynecology* 29:941–952.

McIntyre JA, Faulk WP (1986) Trophoblast antigens in normal and abnormal human pregnancy. *Clinical Obstetrics and Gynecology* 29:976–998.

Miller JF, Williamson E, Glue J, Gordon YB, Grudzinskas JG, Sykes A (1980) Pregnancy loss after implantation. *Lancet* 2:554–556.

Naeye RL (1983) Maternal age, obstetric complications, and the outcome of pregnancy. *Obstetrics and Gynecology* 61:210–216

O'Connor JF, Birken S, Lustbader JW, Krichevsky A, Chen Y, Canfield RE (1994) Recent advances in the chemistry and immunochemistry of human chorionic gonadotropin: impact on clinical measurements. *Endocrine Reviews* 15:650–683.

Patau K, Smith DW, Therman E, Inhorn L, Wagner HP (1960) Multiple congenital anomaly caused by an extra autosome. *Lancet* 1:790.

Patton PE (1994) Anatomic uterine defects. *Clinical Obstetrics and Gynecology* 37:705–721.

Peccei JS (1999) First estimates of heritability in the age of menopause. *Current Anthropology* 40:553–558.

Penrose LS, Delhanty JDA (1961) Triploid cells cultures from a macerated foetus. *Lancet* 1:1261.

Pernoll ML (1986) Abortion induced by chemicals encountered in the environment. *Clinical Obstetrics and Gynecology* 29:953–958.

Potter RG (1961) Length of the fertile period. *Milbank Memorial Fund Quarterly* 39:132–162.

Potter RG, Parker MP (1964) Predicting the time required to conceive. *Population Studies* 18:99–116.

Potter RG, Wyon JB, New M, Gordon JE (1965) Pregnancy wastage in eleven Punjab villages. *Human Biology* 37:262–273.

Resseguie LJ (1974) Pregnancy wastage and age of mother among the Amish. *Human Biology* 46:633–639.

Rock JA, Murphy AA (1986) Anatomic abnormalities. *Clinical Obstetrics and Gynecology* 29:886–911.

Santow G, Bracher M (1989) Do gravidity and age affect pregnancy outcome? *Social Biology* 36:9–22.

Sever JL (1980) Infectious causes of human reproductive loss. In IH Porter, EB Hood (Eds) *Human Embryonic and Fetal Death* (New York, Academic Press), 169–176.

Sheps MC (1964) On the time required for conception. *Population Studies* 18:85–97.

Sheps MC (1965) An analysis of reproductive patterns in an American isolate. *Population Studies* 19:65–80.

Sheps MC, Menken JA (1973) *Mathematical Models of Conception and Birth* (Chicago, University of Chicago Press).

Silver RM, Branch DW (1994) Recurrent miscarriage: autoimmune considerations. *Clinical Obstetrics and Gynecology* 37:745–760.

Snieder H, MacGregor AJ, Spector TD (1998) Genes control the cessation of a woman's reproductive life: a twin study of hysterectomy and age at menopause. *Journal of Clinical Endocrinology and Metabolism* 83:1875–1880.

Stenman U-H, Alfthan H, Ranta T, Vartiainen E, Jalkanen J, Seppälä M (1987) Serum levels of human chorionic gonadotropin in nonpregnant women and men are modulated by gonadotropin-releasing hormone and sex steroids. *Journal of Clinical Endocrinology and Metabolism* 64:730–736.

Strassmann BI, Warner JH (1998) Predictors of fecundability and conception waits among the Dogon of Mali. *American Journal of Physical Anthropology* 105: 167–184.

Thiede HA (1969) Cytogenetics and abortion. *Medical Clinics of North America* 53:773–794.

Tietze C, Guttmacher AF, Rubin S (1950) Time required for conception in 1727 planned pregnancies. *Fertility and Sterility* 1:338–346.

Warburton D (1987) Chromosomal causes of fetal death. *Clinical Obstetrics and Gynecology* 30:268–277.

Weinberg CR, Gladen BC, Wilcox AJ (1994) Models relating the timing of intercourse to the probability of conception and the sex of the baby. *Biometrics* 50:358–367.

Weinberg CR, Hertz-Picciotto I, Baird DD, Wilcox AJ (1992) Efficiency and bias in studies of early loss. *Epidemiology* 3:17–22.

Wilcox AJ, Gladen B (1982) Spontaneous abortion: the role of heterogeneous risk and selective fertility. *Early Human Development* 7:165–178.

Wilcox AJ, Weinberg CR, O'Connor JF, Baird DD, Schlatterer JP, Canfield RE, Armstrong EG, Nisula BC (1988) Incidence of early loss of pregnancy. *New England Journal of Medicine* 319:189–194.

Wilcox AJ, Weinberg CR, Wehmann RE, Armstrong EG, Canfield RE, Nisula BC (1985) Measuring early pregnancy losses: laboratory and field methods. *Fertility and Sterility* 44:366–374.

Wilson C, Oppen J, Pardoe M (1988) What is natural fertility? The modeling of a concept. *Population Index* 54:4–20.

Wood JW (1989) Fecundity and natural fertility in humans. *Oxford Reviews of Reproductive Biology* 11:61–109.

Wood JW (1994) *Dynamics of Human Reproduction: Biology, Biometry, Demography* (Hawthorne NY, Aldine de Gruyter).

Wood JW, Weinstein M (1988) A model of age-specific fecundability. *Population Studies* 42:85–113.

Wood JW, Holman DJ, Yasin A, Peterson RJ, Weinstein M, Chang M-c (1994) A multistate model of fecundability and sterility. *Demography* 31:403–426.

2

The Evolutionary and Ecological Context of Human Pregnancy

IVY L. PIKE

Pregnancy is arguably the most important factor in defining an individual's reproductive success. From a demographic standpoint, pregnancy represents a crude dichotomy: the production of a live birth or intrauterine death with no live birth. But as a complicated physiological process, pregnancy is never as simple as the successful or unsuccessful production of a live birth. Indeed, pregnancy and the perinatal period may represent one of the defining moments for natural selection. Adequate fetal growth influences short-term outcomes such as postnatal growth, development, and survival. Over the long term, intrauterine growth predicts risk for adult onset chronic diseases (Barker et al. 1993), can impact adult reproductive function in females (Kline et al. 1989), and plays a crucial role in overall survival rates (Kramer 1987). In turn, adequately meeting the metabolic demands of gestation and the spacing of pregnancies have short- and longer-term consequences on the mother's health and fitness.

Gestation is a complex physiological process, but commonly it is the larger social and physical environment that constrains or enhances a woman's ability to meet the metabolic demands of pregnancy successfully. Thus, there are three complementary sections of this chapter. First, the evolution and physiology of pregnancy are examined. Second, gestation is discussed as one event in a woman's reproductive span. Third, ecological variables such as seasonality and subsistence practices are discussed as determinants of pregnancy outcome. The common thread that connects these three sections is the assertion that gestation is a defining moment for natural selection and overall reproductive success.

EVOLUTION AND THE PHYSIOLOGY OF PREGNANCY

Maternal Trade-off and Reproductive Potential

In general, the mammalian reproductive strategy includes substantial female investment in reproduction. For primates, body size is generally a good predictor of female life histories, including overall reproductive rates, gestational duration, and interbirth intervals (Ross 1991). Prolonged fetal nourishment is characteristic of primate investment in gestation and is commonly attributed to increased encephalization (Fleagle 1999; Martin 1990). This prolonged fetal nourishment translates into an average gestational duration of 228–264 days for great apes and 267 days for larger-brained humans (Napier and Napier 1967). Gestation is followed by a period of extended infant dependency and prolonged development. For example, free-ranging orangutans suckle for an average of 6 years (Galdikas and Wood 1990). Therefore, the primate reproductive strategy generally includes considerable female investment in gestation and lactation and is linked to primate evolutionary adaptations that include mechanisms for nourishing large-brained offspring that develop slowly.

Pregnancy induces critical and energetically expensive maternal adjustments. Physiological adjustments and requirements combined with the nourishment and development of the products of conception place important demands on the maternal system. These demands are even more difficult to meet in environments where food shortages are common and disease burdens variable. From an evolutionary standpoint, seasonal variability in exploitable resources have been important characteristics of our evolutionary past (Foley 1993). Consequently, total reproductive success should balance the expense of maternal investment and current maternal condition by weighing these considerations against the potential reproductive value of each conception (Peacock 1991).

Conception may be deferred if the overall costs to the maternal system are too high (Peacock 1991). There is ample evidence to suggest that fecundity changes in response to maternal condition (Ellison 1990; Ellison et al. 1993). For example, ovarian function responds to changes in maternal energy balance (Ellison 1990), physical exercise (Ellison and Lager 1986; Panter-Brick et al. 1993), health (McFalls and McFalls 1984), and psychosocial stress (Jeong et al. 1999). In turn, such changes are strongly associated with alterations in environmental circumstances. Marginally nourished women do conceive and often deliver viable offspring, but both may experience a host of negative consequences (Martorell 1995). Thus, an important trade-off occurs if women conceive and maintain a pregnancy when marginally nourished or in poor health.

Maternal investment in individual pregnancies is also unwise if, regardless of maternal condition, the viability or quality of a zygote is low (Haig 1993, 1999). Many researchers have suggested a screening mechanism which allows maternal recognition of offspring quality (Anderson 1990; Erickson 1978). Direct evidence for this mechanism is limited, although human chorionic gonadotropin (hCG) (Haig 1993) and alpha fetoprotein (AFP) (Cuckle 1995) have been proposed. Indirect evidence of a screening mechanism is derived from several related lines of inquiry (Forbes 1997). First, incidence of early (< 4 weeks) fetal deaths is relatively high (Roberts and Lowe 1975; Wilcox et al. 1988). Higher incidences of fetal deaths early in pregnancy not only suggest a screening mechanism but also have the advantage of demanding fewer maternal resources (Wood 1994). Second, the majority of these losses are chromosomally abnormal, with a high frequency of autosomal trisomies (Guerneri et al. 1987; Kline et al. 1989). Third, with increasing age, the risk for delivering a chromosomally abnormal offspring increases (Bray 1998; Drugan et al. 1999). Some researchers suggest this increase in delivering chromosomally abnormal offspring represents a "relaxing" of the maternal screen as opportunity for reproduction decreases (Haig 1993; Kline et al. 1989; Peacock 1991).

Maintaining a pregnancy is a balancing act among maternal resources, future reproductive potential, and the viability of the zygote. As part of the primate strategy of prolonged fetal nourishment, maternal investment in gestation is expensive. Changes in maternal condition alter reproductive function, thereby potentially avoiding a pregnancy when the impact on maternal resources could compromise future reproductive events or her survival. Additional mechanisms may exist that monitor zygote quality and viability, thereby enhancing reproductive outcomes. Over the course of a woman's reproductive span the threshold for tracking maternal condition and offspring screening mechanisms may change owing to the decreased opportunity for reproduction.

Genetic Conflicts in Pregnancy

In an article that reconceptualizes the maternal-fetal relationship, Haig (1993) extends Trivers's (1974) ideas regarding parent-offspring conflict to human pregnancy. Drawing on the idea of self-promoting elements (i.e., selfish, ultra-selfish genes) (Hurst et al. 1996), Haig (1993) argues that human pregnancy represents a fundamental genetic conflict. Given the cost of human pregnancy, maternal and fetal demands may directly oppose one another, particularly in unpredictable environmental settings. Thus, conflicts during pregnancy may exist between maternal genes and fetal genes, particularly those fetal genes that are paternally derived. A conflict may also occur within the fetal genome between maternally and paternally derived genes; this conflict is referred to as genomic imprinting (Haig 1993). Evolutionary processes may select paternally derived fetal genes that enhance fetal growth and survival while maternal genes may be selected based on longer-term maternal reproductive success and survival. In short, Haig (1993) argues that maternal and fetal genes may engage in a process of "evolutionary escalation" whereby fetal actions trigger maternal countermeasures, with cooperation occurring in some instances (coevolution) and conflict (antagonistic coevolution) occurring in other instances.

Conflict theories of genomic imprinting have met with considerable enthusiasm and critical appraisal (Hurst and McVean 1997; Spencer et al. 1999). While there are many other theories of the evolution of genomic imprinting (Hurst 1997; Hurst and McVean 1997), conflict theory provides a framework for examining the differential impact of paternally and maternally derived fetal genes on the capture of maternal resources. One test of this hypothesis includes an examination of the relationship between uniparental disomies (defined as receiving both copies of a chromosome, or part thereof, from one parent) and embryonic growth (Haig and Graham 1991). Uniparental disomies are, by definition, imprinted genes, and they would be predicted to limit fetal growth if derived from the mother but enhance fetal growth if paternally derived. Haig and Graham (1991) suggest a review of the literature supports this hypothesis. However, Hurst and McVean (1997) arrive at a slightly different conclusion. For example, a review of maternally derived disomies for 13 chromosomes found inconclusive support: not all maternally derived disomies restrict fetal growth. For paternally derived disomies, the results are similarly equivocal. Barlow (1995) has suggested, however, that in general more of the imprinted genes are related to embryonic and fetal growth than would be expected by chance alone. Hurst and McVean (1997) argue that the conflict and genomic imprinting model may not be correct as initially formulated, but owing to the complex nature of embryonic and fetal growth and development there is a need for more refined tests to examine such intriguing evolutionary relationships. Future research in this area promises to provide greater insight into the evolution of human pregnancy.

Gestational Duration and Survival

Given the impact of pregnancy on maternal resources, subtle shifts in the timing of delivery could be beneficial, particularly when maternal condition is marginal. While such a shift has important consequences, it could theoretically enhance the chances for maternal survival, fetal survival, or both. Peacock (1991) suggests that a facultative adjustment in length of gestation may be a maternal strategy for coping with marginal resources during pregnancy. A nutritionally stressed mother may benefit from avoiding the last few weeks of pregnancy when fetal fat accumulation is most dramatic. The functional consequences of delivering one to two weeks early may be a trade-off that increases the newborn's chances of short- and long-term morbidity and even mortality but reduces the physiological impact on a marginally nourished mother. Peacock argues that shifting from pregnancy to lactation allows a marginally nourished woman to draw on energy reserves rather than continue the active nutrient transfer associated with pregnancy. From a maternal-fetal conflict perspective, decreases in the length of gestation would be advantageous to the mother and longer gestational duration would benefit the fetus (Haig 1993, 1999). Both Haig and Peacock frame the timing of delivery in similar, complementary ways; each suggest that at a certain point, following extrauterine viability, there may be advantages to the mother, the fetus, or both by modifying gestational duration. Interestingly, very recent clinical research suggests both researchers conceptualized the problem appropriately. Whether of shorter or longer duration, the regulation of the timing of delivery begins early in gestation and is controlled by what has been termed "the placental clock" (McLean et al. 1995). This new research merits further elaboration.

Preterm labor is a heterogenous condition and is linked to multiple potential causal mechanisms (Romero et al. 1994). Parturition, whether preterm, term, or post-term, occurs as a result of a common terminal pathway triggered by anatomical, biochemical, and endocrinological events (Challis and Olson 1988). However, in preterm labor, the early activation of the terminal pathway is typically due to pathological events (Romero et al. 1994). These events include premature rupture of membranes (Hediger et al. 1995) intrauterine infection (Romero and Mazor 1988), systemic maternal infection (Benedetti et al. 1976), and even food withdrawal (Berkowitz and Papiernik 1993). Understanding the events that trigger the initiation of the common terminal pathway leads to a better understanding of the mechanisms that regulate the timing of deliveries, which until recently have been poorly understood (Hediger et al. 1995).

Endocrine factors associated with parturition become established early in gestation and are regulated by maternal and feto-placental feedback mechanisms. Important hypothalamus-pituitary-adrenal axis messengers include corticotropin releasing hormone (C-RH), adrenocorticotropic hormone (ACTH), and glucocorticoids, especially cortisol. C-RH is a multi-functional stress response protein that is produced in the maternal hypothalamus, fetal hypothalamus, and the placenta (Clifton and Challis 1997; McLean and Smith 1999). Corticotropin releasing hormone stimulates the release of ACTH from the pituitary (Fuchs 1983). In turn, ACTH activates the release of cortisol, with cortisol acting in a negative feedback loop with C-RH in the mother (Fuchs 1983). In the feto-placental unit, these mechanisms work in a slightly different manner. Placental C-RH is stimulated by cortisol, unlike in the hypothalamus where it is inhibitory. Moreover, placental C-RH can directly target the fetal pituitary, fetal adrenals, and the myometrium (McLean and Smith 1999). When placental C-RH targets the fetal pituitary, ACTH is released. In turn, ACTH secretion stimulates the release of fetal adrenal cortisol, which stimulates fetal organ development, particularly the lungs (McLean and Smith 1999). Fetal ACTH also triggers the release of dehydroepiandrosterone sulphate (DHEA-S) (Fuchs 1983). The release of DHEA-S is important because it is a major substrate for placental estrogen synthesis (McLean and Smith 1999). Placental estrogen, released in the blood, initiates important myometrial changes in preparation for parturition (Challis and Olson 1988).

Research pinpoints C-RH as a critical factor in the regulation of maturation. Infusing fetal sheep with C-RH throughout pregnancy prematurely activates organ development and induces preterm spontaneous delivery (McLean and Smith 1999). Experiments with spadefoot toads reveal similar results (Denver 1997). Spadefoot toads reside in desert environments and spawn in ephemeral puddles. If the sun appears and the puddle begins to dry up, C-RH levels increase and act as mediators that accelerate development. Controlled laboratory studies that progressively reduced the levels of water in a tank found elevated C-RH levels and accelerated growth and development (Denver 1997). Denver (1997) argues that environmental stress triggers a cascade of phenotypic plasticity that comes at a cost to fitness but certainly enhances survival. Based on these toad experiments and their research on C-RH, McLean et al. (1995) argue that placental C-RH plays an important role in regulating maturation and may even be a primitive trait (McLean et al. 1995).

In addition to regulating the tempo of maturation, C-RH, synthesized in the placenta, regulates the timing of delivery (McLean et al. 1995). From approximately 16–18 weeks gestation, maternal plasma levels of C-RH begin to increase exponentially across the remainder of gestation (McLean et al. 1995). In a sample of 485 women, preterm delivery was associated with elevated levels of corticotropin releasing hormone (C-RH); post-term delivery was associated with lower than average C-RH levels (McLean et al. 1995). At least one subsequent study found strikingly similar results (Wadhwa et al. 1998). There is evidence to suggest that increased levels of C-RH output from the placenta, as is found in women who delivered preterm, is a response to fetal stress, particularly hypoxia and undernutrition (McLean and Smith 1999). Moreover, McLean et al. (1995) identified these different C-RH levels as early as 16–20 weeks gestation, or as soon as placental C-RH is detectable in maternal blood. Therefore, they argue that the timing of parturition is linked to events that occur early in pregnancy and that parturition is the culmination of a longitudinal process of the feto-placental unit. This longitudinal process is activated at a predetermined stage of gestation, thereby suggesting the presence of a placental clock that shifts to the left in response to an inadequate intrauterine environment or fetal stress.

Higher C-RH levels explain 40% of the spontaneous preterm deliveries in McLean et al.'s (1995) economically homogenous sample, thereby reinforcing the multiple etiologies of preterm delivery. To date, such research has not been conducted in populations that experience chronic physiological stressors such as undernutrition and infectious disease. Thus, we have no knowledge of how placental C-RH levels vary within and between populations. Such research would require careful controlling for maternal dietary intake, preconception weight, gestational weight gain, and disease with C-RH levels throughout gestation. Moreover, precise mechanisms that trigger the elevated C-RH levels in the second trimester have not been fully elucidated. While fetal stress, including hypoxia and undernutrition, or subtle differences in the genetic make-up of C-RH–producing cells of the placenta have been proposed to explain the variation in C-RH levels (McLean and Smith 1999), continued research on fetal condition, C-RH levels, and genetic differences is required. For example, at least one study suggests that maternal psychosocial stress impairs fetal growth and increases the risk for preterm labor (Wadhwa et al. 1993). Linking the results of maternal psychosocial stress with changes in the feto-placental unit and thus C-RH levels is intriguing and the next logical step. Identifying the array of potential mechanisms that elevate C-RH, thereby shifting fetal development and the placental clock to a faster pace when confronted with a less than desirable intrauterine environment, has considerable evolutionary and public health implications.

LIFESPAN PERSPECTIVES ON FEMALE REPRODUCTIVE SUCCESS

A lifespan perspective on reproduction requires that individual reproductive events, such as pregnancy, be seen as one part of an unfolding process. Moreover, sexual maturation is not the starting point; reproduction begins with a female's experience in utero and even extends to her mother's experience in utero (Kline et al. 1989). In fact, a lifespan perspective suggests that reproduction, as one component of an individual's lifespan, is shaped by biological, environmental, and cultural influences that begin at an individual's conception but extend to previous and subsequent generations. Thus, a lifespan perspective requires us to ask different questions about reproductive function by examining development, growth, maturation, and senescence across an individual's life as well as across generations (Leidy 1996).

Phenotypic plasticity is an important adaptive response to life in unpredictable or diverse environments. However, a trade-off that occurs earlier in an individual's life can have immediate and longer-term consequences that may enhance immediate survival but lower fitness. There are abundant examples of such compromises in human reproduction. Preterm delivery is a good example; fetal stress leads to preterm delivery with a resulting increase in the risk for morbidity and mortality in the short term (Kramer 1987). Longer-term consequences of being delivered preterm include an increased risk for experiencing preeclampsia during a first pregnancy (Innes et al. 1999), which in turn is associated with poorer fetal outcomes and increased risk for chronic diseases later in a woman's life (Institute of Medicine 1990). Similarly, experiencing growth restriction in utero strongly predicts infant mortality (Kramer 1987). However, among the survivors myriad consequences may ensue. These potential consequences include compromised immune function, altered patterns of growth, permanently altered metabolism, and increased risk for delivering a growth-restricted newborn in the next generation (Barker et al. 1993; Ferro-Luzzi et al. 1998; Stein et al. 1995). Early developmental concessions affect longer-term fitness, health, and survival.

Just as reproductive function reflects a woman's previous developmental experiences (Ellison 1996), reproductive events interact with her age and reproductive history. A woman's first reproductive cycle (defined as pregnancy and lactation) is determined by many factors, including age at menarche, duration of adolescent subfecundity, and cultural influences that regulate entry into a sexual union and timing of births. Being younger (<18) or older (≥35) at first pregnancy is linked to poorer pregnancy outcome (Kline et al. 1989; Kramer 1987). Researchers argue that younger women, particularly adolescents, must compete with the fetus for growth and development (Scholl et al. 1994). However, not all studies found strong links between maternal and fetal competition for growth except among the youngest gravida, particularly those less than two years postmenarche (Kline et al. 1989). Conversely, older women are more likely to deliver chromosomally abnormal babies, experience longer waits to conception, and are at higher risk for fetal deaths (Kline et al. 1989; Wood 1994).

Maternal physiology also appears to change from the first pregnancy to subsequent pregnancies. Primiparous women give birth to smaller babies, on average, than multiparous women do (Kline et al. 1989). One suggested explanation for this epidemiological pattern is that the placentation process is less complete in primigravids and improves with subsequent pregnancies (Haig 1993). First and second pregnancies are at higher risk for severe placental parasitemia in areas with endemic malaria, and subsequent pregnancies are less affected (Meuris et al. 1993). Conversely, Rh incompatibility between mother and fetus increases damage to the fetus in successive pregnancies owing to a progressively sensitized maternal immune system (Kline et al. 1989). Therefore, physiology interacts with maternal age and previous reproductive experiences differentially to influence gestational outcomes.

In addition to examining age, parity, and gravidity as independent predictors of reproductive success, it is also important to examine the interacting relationship of age and repeated reproductive cycles across the reproductive years. Repeated cycles of reproduction have nutritional consequences (Merchant et al. 1990). The consequences are particularly marked among marginally nourished populations who often continue to breast-feed during the next pregnancy (Gray 1996; Merchant et al. 1990; Siega-Riz and Adair 1993). Such fertility-related changes in maternal energy reserves have been termed *maternal depletion* (Jelliffe and Maddocks 1964). The magnitude of the effect is linked to a woman's general nutritional status prior to and during the reproductive cycle, birth spacing, and the interaction between nutritional condition and birth spacing (Winkvist et al. 1992). Even subtle intrapopulation differences in wealth (Tracer 1991), dietary intake (Little et al. 1992), breastfeeding practices (Merchant et al. 1990; Tracer 1991), and fecundity (Pike 1999) can result in variation in the presence of fertility-related decreases in energy reserves. Future studies that examine differences in maternal condition, regardless of age or parity, must closely control for heterogeneity in women's ability to buffer nutritional stress (e.g., reduced activity, wealth differences). To date, few studies have endeavored to control nutritional stress resulting from closely spaced births and repeated reproductive cycles versus insufficient dietary intake during reproductive events (Winkvist et al. 1992). Studies that assess finer-grained mechanisms of differential maternal investment, such as increased nutrient transfer or modified metabolism, may provide clearer answers for this debate.

ECOLOGICAL DETERMINANTS

A single pregnancy is just one component of the larger reproductive span, and the success of an individual pregnancy is strongly linked to the physical and social environment in which a woman lives. A woman's social position and autonomy changes through her life span, thereby influencing her ability to meet her needs and the needs of her children (Das Gupta 1995). In natural fertility populations, women may spend the majority of their reproductive years in repeated cycles of pregnancy and lactation. Reproductive demands are energetically expensive and often coexist with the energetic demands of seasonally variable subsistence production. Subsistence populations often experience a host of stressors, including seasonal fluctuations in nutritional status and infectious disease burdens (Ulijaszek and Strickland 1993). Maternal nutritional status, physical activity levels, and infectious disease independently affect pregnancy outcome (Barnes et al. 1991; McFalls and McFalls 1984; Prentice et al. 1996).

Clearly, such interacting stressors influence reproductive outcomes and women's health; thus, understanding the heterogeneity in the array of coping strategies available to women has important implications for both women and their children.

Environmental Factors

Characteristics of the physical environment act as both proximal and distal determinants of pregnancy outcome. One proximal environmental stressor is hypoxia. Hypoxic stress is strongly associated with fetal growth restriction (Moore et al. 1998). The physiological mechanisms that are responsible for this relationship may vary from one high-altitude population to the next, but overall, hypoxia does place additional metabolic demands on the pregnant woman (Moore et al. 1998). Heat stress may also directly affect early pregnancy, although this relationship is poorly understood (Bronson 1995). Seasonality, as a cluster of environmental factors, may represent the single most important environmental determinant of pregnancy outcome. Seasonality directly affects diet, activity, and disease, and in turn, these variables have a profound impact on reproduction. Seasonal differences in diet, activity, and disease influence the timing of conceptions and births (Bailey et al. 1992; Huss-Ashmore 1988; Leslie and Fry 1989; Panter-Brick 1996), gestational weight gain (Roberts et al. 1982), and the adequacy of fetal growth (Ceesay et al. 1997).

Disease

Seasonal variation in infectious disease represents an important stressor for the mother and fetus. In temperate climates, immune function, mediated by the pineal hormone melatonin, elevates in response to the onset of winter (Nelson and Drazen 1999). Seasonality and immune function in the tropics remain poorly studied and require careful controlling for the synergism between endemic disease and marginal nutritional levels (Shell-Duncan 1995; Tomkins 1993). In general, maternal infections during gestation have been associated with an array of short-term negative consequences, including preterm delivery (Berkowitz and Papiernik 1993) and fetal deaths (McFalls and McFalls 1984). Longer-term consequences, such as an increased likelihood of developing type I diabetes (insulin dependent diabetes mellitus) (Samuelsson et al. 1999) and perhaps dyslexia (Livingston et al. 1993), have also been linked to maternal infections in utero.

One particularly important seasonal disease stressor is malaria, particularly *Plasmodium falciparum*. Acquired immunity is common in endemic areas, but pregnant women, particularly during first and second pregnancies, encounter more-frequent and higher-density infections than non-pregnant women (Bouvier et al. 1997; Steketee et al. 1996). A malaria infection in pregnancy alters maternal immune function and is associated with fetal growth restriction (Bouvier et al. 1997; Meuris et al. 1993; Steketee et al. 1996). Previous research suggested that malaria infections were linked to increased risk for preterm delivery and fetal deaths (McFalls and McFalls 1984). However, Steketee and colleagues (1996) suggest that the limited data on fetal deaths indicate no association and the studies examining preterm delivery are plagued by imprecise gestational age assessment. Despite recent advances, there is still much to learn about maternal and fetal physiological responses to gestational malaria.

Nutrition and Dietary Intake

Pregnancy represents a period of heightened nutritional requirements. A woman's prepregnancy nutritional status, including macronutrient status, micronutrient status, and energy stores, dictates the actual nutritional requirements needed to meet the demands of maternal tissue expansion and the products of conception (Institute of Medicine 1990). For marginally nourished women, dietary stress associated with perturbations in food quantity and quality compromises fetal growth and development and increases the risk for delivering preterm (Kramer 1987). For example, a longitudinal study in The Gambia clearly connected seasonal increases in agricultural workloads and decreased maternal dietary intake with reduced birth weights (Lawrence and Whitehead 1988). Additional studies in Taiwan found similar seasonal reductions in maternal nutrition and corresponding reductions in birth weight (Adair and Pollitt 1983, 1985). Maternal dietary stress yields fetal responses (i.e., growth restriction and preterm delivery) that are strongly linked to short- and long-term survival (Kramer 1987).

Seasonal fluctuations in food availability result in important modifications in the micronutrient content of the diet. For example, studies in The Gambia and Guatemala found seasonal variation in intakes of vitamin A, vitamin C, folate, and iron (Bates et al. 1994; Tejero et al. 1994). Research indicates that dietary composition is of equal importance to quantity of intake (Susser 1991). Indeed, maternal micronutrient status, especially during the periconceptional period, plays an important role in determining maternal and fetal outcomes (McArdle and Ashworth 1999; Scholl et al. 1997). For example, inadequate folic acid reserves during the first two months of pregnancy, when palate development occurs, are associated with an increased risk for orofacial clefts (Berry et al. 1999; Czeizel et al. 1999). Vitamin A is not only important for night vision but also appears to be an integral component of the immune system (McArdle and Ashworth 1999). One study suggests that adequate vitamin A status reduces the risk for maternal mortality (West et al. 1999; cf. Ronsmans et al. 1999; Sachdev 1999). Depressed maternal vitamin A status during pregnancy increases the progression of disease in her HIV-1 infected infant and risk of death during the first 18 months of life (Rich et al. 2000). The precise mechanisms through which micronutrients influence fetal growth, development, and maternal outcome are being illuminated. Given the importance of micronutrient status on maternal and fetal outcomes, increasing our understanding of seasonal differences in micronutrient intake deserves a high priority for future research.

Recent studies provide important new clues on the longer-term consequences of compromised maternal nutrition on fetal growth. Epidemiological studies link inadequate fetal growth to adult onset chronic diseases such as cardiovascular disease and non-insulin dependent diabetes mellitus (Barker 1997). Barker and colleagues' findings connect patterns of low birth weight (<2500 grams) in impoverished areas of the U.K. to higher resting heart rate and slightly higher plasma cortisol concentrations (Phillips and Barker 1997). In turn, heart rate and cortisol concentrations were related to systolic blood pressure, plasma triglyceride levels, and insulin resistance (Phillips et al. 1998). Neuroendocrine research suggests that maternal stress, including undernutrition, increases fetal exposure to excess glucocorticoids (Dodic et al. 1999). These results indicate that at critical periods of development, particularly early in the first trimester, exposure to glucocorticoids alters growth and results in fetal metabolic imprinting that permanently modifies sympathetic nerve activity (Phillips et al. 1998). In animal studies, metabolic imprinting occurs irrespective of the mechanism by which fetal growth is restricted, including maternal anemia, reduced caloric intake, and reduced protein intake (Dodic et al. 1999). Programming might operate on several different systems, including the renin-angiotensin system, central nervous system, and pancreatic β cells (Dodic et al. 1999). Important questions for future research include quantifying the range of maternal stress that precipitates altered fetal programming, identifying the critical periods of exposure, and identifying the mechanisms that induce the metabolic changes (Dodic et al. 1999). In addition, few studies have assessed these relationships in developing countries where the prevalence of maternal physiological stress and low birth weight is high. In keeping with the placental clock research, these findings suggest that fetal responses to maternal stress include compromises that may enhance survival but have consequences across all stages of the life cycle.

Nutritional deficiency may be the most important determinant of immune function worldwide, yet the degree to which this interaction impairs pregnancy outcome is poorly understood (Gennaro and Fehder 1996). In addition, interactions among psychosocial stress, nutrition, and immune function remain poorly understood. The degree to which micronutrient status modifies the stress response and immune function requires further elucidation. Examining the synergistic relationship among these variables and the impact on reproductive outcomes remains an important challenge, particularly for populations in developing countries that experience seasonal stress.

Physical Activity Levels

In subsistence-level societies, seasonal fluctuations in work demands are potentially important stressors for pregnant women. Maternal activity levels modify nutritional requirements during pregnancy (Institute of Medicine 1990) and can independently influence pregnancy outcome (Barnes et al. 1991; Hatch et al. 1998). Physiological mechanisms that directly link maternal activity to pregnancy outcome are poorly understood (Hatch et al. 1998). Many women in subsistence-level societies are unable to reduce their workloads. Gambian women reduced household activities during the final stages of pregnancy, but not agricultural work (Roberts et al. 1982). Pregnant women in Nepal did not significantly reduce activity levels during the monsoon season (Panter-Brick 1993). Alternatively, activity reduction can serve as an important energy-sparing mechanism during pregnancy. Among pregnant Colombian women, Dufour et al. (1999) found that women reduce energetically expensive activities in favor of energy-conserving activities. Reducing workloads may improve pregnancy outcome, but such measures may diminish household economic well being (Baksh et al. 1994). Subtle modifications in workloads may be important strategies for ameliorating work stress during pregnancy but are notoriously difficult to quantify and observe (Ulijaszek 1995). Considering the inter- and intrapopulation variations that exist in women's ability to modify work patterns, further research on the positive and negative consequences for pregnancy outcome and household economy are necessary.

Coping and Psychosocial Stress

Pregnancy induces important biological and emotional responses in women. Many studies document the role of psychosocial stress, coping, and social support during parturition, but very few have examined this relationship in pregnancy. Yet there is evidence that women from diverse populations worry about how they will care for their children and maintain their households throughout their pregnancies (Senturia 1997). Clinical research from western populations suggest a strong link between maternal stress and preterm delivery, with growing evidence for fetal growth restriction (Paarlberg et al. 1999; Sandman et al. 1997; Wadhwa et al. 1993). Direct pathways between maternal psychosocial stress and pregnancy outcomes include increases in stress-dependent hormones and stimulation of psycho-immunologic factors (Paarlberg et al. 1999). Wadhwa et al. (1998) found that maternal psychosocial factors were associated with elevated plasma levels of ACTH, beta E, and cortisol, with psychosocial factors explaining 36%, 22%, and 13% of the variance, respectively. Psychosocial factors also affect immune function (Dantzer and Kelley 1989). Pregnant women with higher anxiety levels experience lower levels of immunoglobulin A (IgA), irrespective of nutrition or exercise (Gennaro and Fehder 1996). Decreased immune function coupled with pregnancy-induced immunosuppression may increase the risk for contracting an infectious disease, potentially resulting in impaired utero-placental function (Paarlberg et al. 1999).

Despite recent advances in our understanding of psychosocial stress and pregnancy outcome, data examining this relationship in developing countries are exceedingly rare. The obstacles for collecting such information among populations that experience variable levels of nutrition, physical activity, and disease demand careful control of confounding factors. Moreover, assessing psychosocial stress and major life event stress has relied on highly structured survey instruments that may be inappropriate in nonwestern populations. Flinn's (1999) work in Jamaica suggests that close, longitudinal monitoring of individuals within their social and ecological context yields the most reliable results, yet such studies demand a considerable financial and time commitment. Examining psychosocial stress in nonwestern populations remains an exciting but difficult challenge for the future.

CONCLUSIONS/FUTURE DIRECTIONS FOR RESEARCH

Many opportunities and challenges confront future studies in the evolution and ecological context of pregnancy. Improved molecular techniques have refined our understanding of embryology and neurological development. Genetic evidence for natural selection in populations exposed to chronic stressors, such as hypoxia, is also accumulating. In addition, biomedical research continues to offer clues about the evolutionary mechanisms that shape fetal and maternal responses to stress. However, the challenge remains to examine the range of variation present in diverse populations. Technological advancements will not solve all of the problems facing future research projects. For example, despite methodological advances in assessing physical work output, intensive monitoring of an individual's daily, monthly, and seasonal patterns of activity greatly improves data quality and helps establish the magnitude of work stress or buffering. The same obstacles hold true for psychosocial stress data and dietary intake information. Closer scrutiny of variation in behavioral buffering of environmental, physiological, and psychosocial stress in pregnancy remains a high priority for future research.

Reproductive success requires a careful balance among current and future offspring, and the ability to balance these needs varies within and between populations. Improvements in our understanding of mechanisms that allow for variation in maternal investment in individual pregnancies will help situate reproductive success within the larger context of the lifespan. Shifts in maternal investment in reproduction with changing reproductive potential align with predictions of life history theory. However, carefully controlled studies are required to tease apart physiological changes in maternal investment in poorly nourished populations. Genetic factors, intergenerational well-being, growth and development trajectories from conception to the onset of reproduction, and variation in women's physical and emotional ability to meet the needs of current and future offspring interact to influence lifetime reproductive success.

REFERENCES

Adair LS, Pollitt E (1983) Seasonal variation in pre- and postpartum maternal body measurements and infant birth weights. *American Journal of Physical Anthropology* 62:325–331.

Adair LS, Pollitt E (1985) Outcome of maternal nutritional supplementation: a comprehensive review of the Bacon Chow Study. *American Journal of Clinical Nutrition* 41:948–978.

Anderson D (1990) On the evolution of human brood size. *Evolution* 44:438–440.

Bailey RC, Jenike MR, Ellison PT., Bentley GR, Harrigan AM, Peacock NR (1992) The ecology of birth seasonality among agriculturalists in Central Africa. *Journal of Biosocial Science* 24:393–412.

Baksh M, Neumann CG, Paolisso M, Trostle RM, Jansen AA (1994) The influence of reproductive status on rural Kenyan women's time use. *Social Science and Medicine* 39:345–354.

Barker D (1997) Fetal nutrition and cardiovascular disease in later life. *British Medical Bulletin* 53:96–108.

Barker D, Gluckman P, Godfrey K, Harding J, Owens J, Robinson J (1993) Fetal nutrition and cardiovascular disease in adult life. *Lancet* 341:938–1001.

Barlow D (1995) Gametic imprinting in mammals. *Science* 270:1610–1613.

Barnes DL, Adair LS, Popkin BM (1991) Women's physical activity and pregnancy outcome: a longitudinal analysis from the Philippines. *International Journal of Epidemiology* 20:162–172.

Bates CJ, Prentice AM, Paul AA (1994) Seasonal variations in vitamins A, C, riboflavin and folate intakes and status of pregnant and lactating women in a rural Gambian community: some possible implications. *European Journal of Clinical Nutrition* 48:660–668.

Benedetti T, Valle R, Ledger W (1976) Antepartum pneumonia in pregnancy. *American Journal of Obstetrics and Gynecology* 144:143.

Berkowitz G, Papiernik E (1993) Epidemiology of preterm birth. *Epidemiological Review* 15:414–443.

Berry RF, Li Z, Erickson JD, Li S, Moore CA, Wang H, Mulinare J, Zhao P, Wong LYC, Grindler J, Hong SX, Correa A (1999) Prevention of neural tube defects with folic acid in China. *New England Journal of Medicine* 341(20):1485–1490.

Bouvier P, Breslow N, Doumbo O, Robert CF, Picquet M, Mauris A, Dolo A, Dembele HK, Delley V, and Rougemont A (1997) Seasonality, malaria, and impact of prophylaxis in a West African village, II: effect on birthweight. *American Journal of Tropical Medicine & Hygiene* 56:384–399.

Bray I, Wright DE, Davies C, Hook EB (1998) Joint estimation of Down Syndrome risk and ascertainment rates: a meta-analysis of nine published data sets. *Prenatal Diagnosis* 18:9–20.

Bronson F (1995) Seasonal variation in human reproduction—environmental factors. *Quarterly Review of Biology* 70:141–164.

Ceesay SM, Prentice AM, Cole TJ, Foord F, Weaver L., Poskitt EM, Whitehea, RG (1997) Effects on birth weight and perinatal mortality of maternal dietary supplements in rural Gambia: 5-year randomised controlled trial. *British Medical Journal* 315:786–790.

Challis J, Olson D (1988) Parturition. In E Knobil, J Neill (Eds) *The Physiology of Reproduction* (New York, Raven Press), 2177–2185.

Clifton VL, Challis JG (1997) Placental corticotropin releasing hormone function during human pregnancy. *Endocrinologist* 7:448–458.

Cuckle H (1995) Improved parameters for risk estimation in Down's Syndrome screening. *Prenatal Diagnosis* 15:1057–1065.

Czeizel AE, Timar L, Sarkozi A (1999) Dose-dependent effect of folic acid on the prevention of orofacial clefts. *Pediatrics* 104:E661–E667.

Dantzer R, Kelley K (1989) Stress and immunity: an integrated view of relationships between the brain and the immune system. *Life Science* 44:1995–2008.

Das Gupta M (1995) Life course perspectives on women's autonomy and health outcomes. *American Anthropologist* 97:481–491.

Denver R (1997) Environmental stress as a developmental cue: corticotropin-releasing hormone is a proximate mediator of adaptive phenotypic plasticity in amphibian metamorphosis. *Hormones and Behavior* 31:169–179.

Dodic, M, Peers A, Coghlan JP, Wintour M (1999) Can excess glucocorticoid, in utero, predispose to cardiovascular and metabolic disease in middle age? *Trends in Endocrinology and Metabolism* 10:86–91.

Drugan A, Yaron Y, Zamir R, Ebrahim SD, Johnson MP, Evans MI (1999) Differential effect of advanced maternal age on prenatal diagnosis of Trisomies 13, 18 and 21. *Fetal Diagnosis and Therapy* 14:181–184.

Dufour DL, Reina JC, Spurr GB (1999) Energy intake and expenditure of free-living, pregnant Columbian women in an urban setting. *American Journal of Clinical Nutrition* 70:269–276.

Ellison PT (1990) Human ovarian function and reproductive ecology: new hypotheses. *American Anthropologist* 92:933–952.

Ellison PT (1996) Developmental influences on adult ovarian hormonal function. *American Journal of Human Biology* 8:725–734.

Ellison PT, Lager C (1986) Moderate recreational running is associated with lowered salivary progesterone profiles in women. *American Journal of Obstetrics & Gynecology* 154:1000–1003.

Ellison PT, Panter-Brick C, Lipson SF, O'Rourke MT (1993) The ecological context of human ovarian function. *Human Reproduction* 8:2248–2258.

Erickson J (1978) Down Syndrome, paternal age, maternal age and birth order. *Annals of Human Genetics* 41:289–298.

Ferro-Luzzi A, Ashworth A, Martorell R, Scrimshaw N (1998) Report of the IDECG Working Group on effects of IUGR on infants, children and adolescents: immunocompetence, mortality, morbidity, body size, body composition, and physical performance. *European Journal of Clinical Nutrition* 52:s97–s99.

Fleagle J (1999) *Primate Evolution and Adaptation* (London, Academic Press).

Flinn M (1999) Family environment, stress, and health during childhood. In C Panter-Brick, C Worthman (Eds) *Hormones, Health, and Behavior: A Socio-ecologic and Lifespan Perspective* (Cambridge, Cambridge University Press), 105–138.

Foley RA (1993) The influence of seasonality on hominid behavior. In SJ Ulijaszek, SS Strickland (Eds) *Human Ecology and Seasonality* (Cambridge, Cambridge University Press) 17–37.

Forbes LS (1997) The evolutionary biology of spontaneous abortion in humans. *Trends in Ecology & Evolution* 12:446–450.

Fuchs F (1983) Endocrinology of parturition. In F Fuchs, A Klopper (Eds) *Endocrinology of Pregnancy* (Philadelphia, Harper & Row), 247–270.

Galdikas B, Wood J (1990) Birth spacing patterns in humans and apes. *American Journal of Physical Anthropology* 83:185–191.

Gennaro S, Fehder W (1996) Stress, immune function, and relationship to pregnancy outcome. *Nursing Clinics of North America* 31:293–303.

Gray SJ (1996) Ecology of weaning among nomadic Turkana pastoralists of Kenya: maternal thinking, maternal behavior, and human adaptive strategies. *Human Biology* 68:437–465.

Guerneri S, Bettio D, Simoni G, Brambati B, Lanzani A, Fraccaro M (1987) Prevalence and distribution of chromosome abnormalities in a sample of first trimester internal abortions. *Human Reproduction* 2:735–739.

Haig D (1993) Genetic conflicts of pregnancy. *Quarterly Review of Biology* 68:495–532.

Haig D (1999) Genetic conflicts of pregnancy and childhood. In S Stearns (Ed) *Evolution in Health and Disease* (Oxford, Oxford University Press), 77–90.

Haig D, Graham C (1991) Genomic imprinting and the strange case of the insulin-like Growth Factor-II receptor. *Cell* 64:1045–1046.

Hatch M, Levin B, Shu X, Susser M (1998) Maternal leisure time exercise and timely delivery. *American Journal of Public Health* 88:1528–1533.

Hediger M, Scholl T, Schall J, Miller L, Fischer R (1995) Fetal Growth and the Etiology of Preterm Delivery. *Obstetrics and Gynecology* 85:175–182.

Hurst LD (1997) Evolution of genomic imprinting. In W Reik, A Surani (Eds) *Frontiers in Molecular Biology: Genomic Imprinting* (Oxford, Oxford University Press), 211–237.

Hurst LD, McVean GT (1997) Growth effects of uniparental disomies and the conflict theory of genomic imprinting. *Trends in Genetics* 13:436–443.

Hurst LD, Atlan A, Bengtsson BO (1996) Genetic conflicts. *Quarterly Review of Biology* 71:317–364.

Huss-Ashmore R (1988) Seasonal patterns of birth and conception in rural highland Lesotho. *Human Biology* 60:493–506.

Innes KE, Marshall JA, Byers TE, Calonge N (1999) A woman's own birth weight and gestational age predict her later risk of developing preeclampsia, a precursor of chronic disease. *Epidemiology* 10:153–160.

Institute of Medicine (1990) *Nutrition during Pregnancy* (Washington DC, Institute of Medicine and National Academy of Sciences, National Academy Press).

Jelliffe D, Maddocks I (1964) Notes on ecological malnutrition in the New Guinea Highlands. *Clinics in Pediatrics* 3:432–438.

Jeong KH, Jacobson L, Widmaier EP, Majzoub JA (1999) Normal suppression of the reproductive axis following stress in corticotropin-releasing hormone-deficient mice. *Endocrinology* 140:1702–1708.

Kline J, Stein Z, Susser M (1989) *Conception to Birth: Epidemiology of Prenatal Development* (New York, Oxford University Press).

Kramer MS (1987) Determinants of low birth weight: methodological assessment and meta-analysis. *Bulletin of World Health Organization* 65:663–737.

Lawrence M, Whitehead R (1988) Physical activity and total energy expenditure of child-bearing Gambian village women. *European Journal of Clinical Nutrition* 42:1442–1450.

Leidy L (1996) Lifespan approach to the study of human biology: an introductory overview. *American Journal of Human Biology* 8:699–702.

Leslie PW, Fry PH (1989) Extreme seasonality of births among nomadic Turkana pastoralists. *American Journal of Physical Anthropology* 79:103–115.

Little M, Leslie P, Campbell K (1992) Energy reserves and parity of nomadic and settled Turkana women. *American Journal of Human Biology* 4:729–738.

Livingston R, Adams B, Bracha H (1993) Season of birth and neurodevelopmental disorders: summer birth is associated with dyslexia. *Journal of the American Academy of Child and Adolescent Psychiatry* 32:612–616.

Martin R (1990) *Primate Origins and Evolution: A Phylogenetic Reconstruction* (Princeton, Princeton University Press).

Martorell R (1995) Results and implications of the INCAP follow-up study. *Journal of Nutrition* 125:1127S–1138S.

McArdle HJ, Ashworth CJ (1999) Micronutrients in fetal growth and development. *British Medical Bulletin* 55:499–510.

McFalls JA, McFalls MH (1984) *Disease and Fertility* (New York, Academic Press).

McLean M, Smith R (1999) Corticotropin-releasing hormone in human pregnancy and parturition. *Trends in Endocrinology and Metabolism* 10:174–178.

McLean M, Bisits A, Davies J, Woods R, Lowry P, Smith R (1995) A placental clock controlling the length of human pregnancy. *Nature Medicine* 1:460–463.

Merchant K, Martorell R, Haas J (1990) Maternal and fetal responses to the stresses of lactation concurrent with pregnancy and of short recuperative intervals. *American Journal of Clinical Nutrition* 52:280–288.

Meuris S, Piko BB, Eerens P, Vanbellinghen AM, Dramaix M, Hennart P (1993) Gestational malaria: assessment of its consequences on fetal growth. *American Journal of Tropical Medicine & Hygiene* 48:603–609.

Moore LG, Niermeyer S, Zamudio S (1998) Human adaptation to high altitude: regional and life-cycle perspectives. *American Journal of Physical Anthropology* 27(suppl.):25–64.

Napier J, Napier P (1967) *A Handbook of Living Primates* (New York, Academic Press).

Nelson R, Drazen D (1999) Melatonin mediates seasonal adjustments in immune function. *Reproduction Nutrition Development* 39:383–398.

Paarlberg KM, Vingerhoets AJ, Passchier J, Dekker GA, Heinen AG, Van GH (1999) Psychosocial predictors of low birthweight: a prospective study. *British Journal of Obstetrics & Gynaecology* 106:834–841.

Panter-Brick C (1993) Seasonality of energy expenditure during pregnancy and lactation for rural Nepali women. *American Journal of Clinical Nutrition* 57:620–628.

Panter-Brick C (1996) Proximate determinants of birth seasonality and conception failure in Nepal. *Population Studies* 50:203–206.

Panter-Brick C, Lotstein DS, Ellison PT (1993) Seasonality of reproductive function and weight loss in rural Nepali women. *Human Reproduction* 8:684–690.

Peacock N (1991) An evolutionary perspective on the patterning of maternal investment in pregnancy. *Human Nature* 2:351–385.

Phillips D, Barker D (1997) Association between low birthweight and high resting pulse in adult life: is the sympathetic nervous system involved in programming of the Insulin Resistance Syndrome? *Diabetes Medicine* 14:673–677.

Phillips DW, Barker DP, Fall CD, Seckl JR, Whorwood CB, Wood PJ, Walker BR (1998) Elevated plasma cortisol concentrations: a link between low birth weight and the Insulin Resistance Syndrome? *Journal of Clinical Endocrinology and Metabolism* 83:757–760.

Pike IL (1999) Age, reproductive history, seasonality and maternal body composition during pregnancy for Turkana women of Kenya. *American Journal of Human Biology* 11:658–672.

Prentice AM, Spaaij C, Goldberg G, Poppitt S, van Raaij J, Totton M, Swann D, Black A (1996) Energy requirements of pregnant and lactating women. *European Journal of Clinical Nutrition* 50:s82-s111.

Rich KC, Fowler MG, Mofenson LM, Abboud R, Pitt J, Diaz C, Hanson IC, Cooper E, Mendez H (2000) Maternal and infant factors predicting disease progression in Human Immunodeficiency Virus Type 1-infected infants. *Pediatrics* 105:G7–H2.

Roberts C, Lowe C (1975) Where have all the conceptions gone? *Lancet* 1:498–499.

Roberts SB, Paul AA, Cole TJ, Whitehead RG (1982) Seasonal changes in activity, birth weight and lactational performance in rural Gambian women. *Transactions of the Royal Society of Tropical Medicine & Hygiene* 76:668–678.

Romero R, Mazor M (1988) Infection and preterm labor. *Clinical Obestetrics and Gynecology* 31:553.

Romero R, Mazor M, Munoz H, Gomez R, Galasso M, Sherer D (1994) The preterm labor syndrome. *Annals of the New York Academy of Science* 697:9–27.

Ronsmans C, Campbell O, Collumbien M (1999) Effect of supplementation with Vitamin A or Beta Carotene on mortality related to pregnancy: slight modifications in definitions could alter interpretation of results. *British Medical Journal* 319:1202–1203.

Ross C (1991) Life history patterns of New World primates. *International Journal of Primatology* 12:481–502.

Sachdev HP (1999) Effect of supplementation with Vitamin A or Beta Carotene on mortality related to pregnancy: no magic pills exist for reducing mortality related to pregnancy. *British Medical Journal* 319:1202–1203.

Samuelsson U, Johansson C, Ludvigsson J (1999) Month of birth and developing insulin dependent diabetes in southeast Sweden. *Archives of Disease in Childhood* 81:143–146.

Sandman CA, Wadhwa PD, Chicz-DeMet A, Dunkel-Schetter C, Porto M (1997) Maternal stress, HPA activity, and fetal/infant outcome. *Annals of the New York Academy of Sciences* 814:266–275.

Scholl TO, Hediger ML, Bendich A, Schall JI, Smith WK, Krueger PM (1997) Use of multivitamin/mineral prenatal supplements: influence on the outcome of pregnancy. *American Journal of Epidemiology* 146:134–141.

Scholl T, Hediger M, Schall J, Khoo C, Fischer R (1994) Maternal growth during pregnancy and the competition for nutrients. *American Journal of Clinical Nutrition* 60:183–188.

Senturia K (1997) A woman's work is never done: women's work and pregnancy outcome. *Medical Anthropology Quarterly* 1:375–395.

Shell-Duncan B (1995) Impact of seasonal variation in food availability and disease stress on the health status of nomadic Turkana children: a longitudinal analysis of morbidity, immunity, and nutritional status. *American Journal of Human Biology* 7:339–355.

Siega-Riz AM, Adair LS (1993) Biological determinants of pregnancy weight gain in a Filipino population. *American Journal of Clinical Nutrition* 57:365–372.

Spencer HG, Clark AG, Feldman MW (1999) Genetic conflicts and the evolutionary origin of genomic imprinting. *Trends in Ecology & Evolution* 14:197–201.

Stein AD, Ravelli ACJ, Masson GM (1995) Famine, third-trimester pregnancy weight gain, and intrauterine growth: the Dutch Famine birth cohort study. *Human Biology* 67:135–150.

Steketee RW, Wirima JJ, Slutsker L, Heymann DL, Breman JG (1996) The problem of malaria and malaria control in pregnancy in Sub-Saharan Africa. *American Journal of Tropical Medicine & Hygiene* 55:2–7.

Susser M (1991) Maternal weight gain, infant birth weight, and diet: causal sequences. *American Journal of Clinical Nutrition* 53:1384–1396.

Tejero E, Polo E, Pfeffer F, Meza C, Casanueva E(1994) Leukocyte ascorbic acid during pregnancy: seasonal variation in a tropical country. *Nutrition Research* 14:287–292.

Tomkins A (1993) Environment, season, and infection. In SJ Ulijaszek, SS Strickland (Eds) *Human Ecology and Seasonality* (Cambridge, Cambridge University Press), 123–133.

Tracer DP (1991) Fertility-related changes in maternal body composition among the Au of Papua New Guinea. *American Journal of Physical Anthropology* 85: p393–405.

Trivers R (1974) Parent-offspring conflict. *American Zoologist* 14:249–264.

Ulijaszek SJ (1995) *Human Energetics in Biological Anthropology* (Cambridge, Cambridge University Press).

Ulijaszek SJ, Strickland S (1993) Introduction. In SJ Ulijaszek, SS Strickland (Eds) *Human Ecology and Seasonality* (Cambridge, Cambridge University Press), 1–4.

Wadhwa P, Sandman C, Porto M, Dunkel-Schetter C, Garite T (1993) The association between prenatal stress and infant birth weight and gestational age at birth: a prospective investigation. *American Journal of Obstetrics and Gynecology* 169:858–865.

Wadhwa P, Porto M, Garite T, Chicz-DeMet A, Sandman C (1998) Maternal corticotropin-releasing hormone levels in the early third trimester predict length of gestation in human pregnancy. *American Journal of Obstetrics and Gynecology* 179:1079–1085.

West KP, Katz J, Khatry SK, LeClerq SC, Pradhan EK, Shrestha SR, Conner PB, Dali SR, Christian P, Pokhrel RP, Somme A (1999) Double blind, cluster randomised trial of low dose supplementation with Vitamin A or Beta Carotene on mortality related to pregnancy in Nepal. *British Medical Journal* 318:570–575.

Wilcox AJ, Weinberg CR, O'Connor JF, Baird DD, Schlatterer JP, Canfield RE, Armstrong EG, Nisula BC (1988) Incidence of early loss of pregnancy. *New England Journal of Medicine* 319:189–194.

Winkvist A, Rasmussen KM, Habicht JP (1992) A new definition of maternal depletion syndrome. *American Journal of Public Health* 82:691–694.

Wood JW (1994) *Dynamics of Human Reproduction: Biology, Biometry, Demography* (Hawthorne NY, Aldine de Gruyter).

3

Why Energy Expenditure Causes Reproductive Suppression in Women

An Evolutionary and Bioenergetic Perspective

GRAZYNA JASIENSKA

Low energy availability caused by inadequate caloric intake and high energy expenditure is a common feature of life of women from many traditional populations (Adams 1995; Benefice et al. 1996; Lawrence and Whitehead 1988; Panter-Brick 1993; Roberts et al. 1982). Moreover, it is likely that similar energetic stresses have been present throughout the course of human evolution (Leonard and Robertson 1997). Therefore, one may expect women to have evolved adaptive mechanisms which would allow them to cope with limited energy availability while promoting higher lifetime reproductive success. One such mechanism might be suppression of reproductive function during times when environmental conditions are poor and energy availability is low.

In this chapter, reproductive suppression is understood as any change in reproductive physiology that may lower the probability of a successful pregnancy during any given period of time. These changes can range from reduced production of ovarian steroid hormones (mainly estradiol and progesterone) to the lack of ovulation, and finally to the total absence of menstrual cycles (amenorrhea) (Ellison 1990). When menstrual cycles are anovulatory or absent, the probability of pregnancy is reduced to zero. However, it is important to emphasize that when cycles are ovulatory but characterized by reduced levels of circulating steroids, the probability of conception, of the successful implantation of an embryo, or of a successfully maintained pregnancy may also be diminished (Baulieu 1989; Dickey et al. 1993; Eissa et al. 1986; Liu et al. 1988; Maslar 1988; McNeely and Soules 1988; Stouffer 1988).

Reproductive suppression in women in response to energetic stress has been interpreted as an adaptive phenomenon and discussed within the framework of evolutionary theory and, especially, life history theory

(Ellison 1990, 1991, 1996; Peacock 1990, 1991; Vitzthum 1997). Most attention has been given to reproductive suppression associated with negative energy balance. When inadequate energy intake or excessive energy expenditures put a woman in a state of negative energy balance, temporary suppression of reproductive function may be expected. These predictions are well supported by evidence from the studies of both western women exposed to dieting and exercise as well as women from subsistence populations exposed to food shortages and increases in workload.

High levels of energy expenditure are associated with various degrees of ovarian suppression. This effect has been documented in many studies of sports activities (Elias and Wilson 1993; Henley and Vaitukaitis 1988; Howlett 1987; Loucks 1990; Noakes and van Gend 1988; Rosetta 1993) as well as a few studies of women from populations characterized by high levels of subsistence workload (Bailey et al. 1992; Bentley et al. 1990; Ellison et al. 1989; Jasienska 1996a; Jasienska and Ellison 1998; Panter-Brick and Ellison 1994; Panter-Brick et al. 1993). Sport participation, however, is usually associated with qualitatively different activities than is the subsistence work of agricultural or hunter-gatherer women. Sport also often involves intense but rather short-duration activity, as opposed to less intense, but much longer-lasting work typical of the harvest season in agricultural communities or of foraging trips in hunter-gatherer societies. Thus it is not clear whether responses to sport activities are generalizable to other forms of energy expenditure more typical of subsistence activities. In addition, since high levels of exercise are often associated with negative energy balance, it is not clear whether energy expenditure has an independent effect on female reproduction. In other words, will a woman who expends high levels of energy, but whose intake is high enough to maintain her energy balance, experience reproductive suppression?

I argue that ovarian suppression in response to increases in energy expenditure in women who are not in a state of negative energy balance may have adaptive significance. Two alternative evolutionary scenarios are suggested. The first (the "preemptive ovarian suppression" hypothesis) assumes that an increase in energy expenditure almost inevitably leads to a state of negative energy balance. Since reproductive function is designed to respond to changes in energy balance, increases in energy expenditure serve as an indicator of imminent changes in energetic status. The second scenario (the "constrained down-regulation" hypothesis) does not posit that energy expenditure necessarily leads to negative energy balance but explains ovarian suppression in the context of constraints on energy allocation. I consider, in particular, the effect of energy expenditure in increasing basal metabolic rate. Such an increase may be in conflict with energy-saving mechanisms which are often in use during pregnancy and lactation. In addition, I discuss topics relevant to both hypotheses, namely metabolic constraints on energy intake and an insufficiency of fat reserves for reproduction.

Reproductive function in human females is also known to be affected by factors other than energy expenditure—for example, dietary intake, temperature, possibly photoperiod and physiological stress (Bronson 1995; Hofman and Swaab 1992; Lam and Miron 1996; Pevet 1993; Roenneberg and Aschoff 1990; Rojansky et al. 1992; Spuy 1985; Stroud 1993; Vermeulen 1993). These factors are not considered within the framework of this chapter even though they may occur together with high levels of energy expenditure and confound its effects on reproductive function. Similarly, this paper does not attempt to discuss proximate mechanisms proposed to explain how, in the physiological sense, energy expenditure causes reproductive suppression (Cumming et al. 1994; Loucks 1990).

ENERGY EXPENDITURE AND REPRODUCTIVE
FUNCTION IN WOMEN

Severe menstrual disturbances (amenorrhea and oligomenorrhea) have been associated with participation in intense physical training in ballet dancers, rowers, marathon runners, swimmers, and gymnasts (Cumming 1993; Dale et al. 1979; Frisch et al. 1980; Schwartz et al. 1981; Veldhuis et al. 1985; Warren 1980; Zanker and Swaine 1998). More interestingly, significant changes in indices of ovarian function (including low levels of steroid hormones, disturbed follicular development, and shortened luteal phase) have been reported even in women who experience menstrual cycles of normal duration, but participate in recreational sports (Broocks et al. 1990; De Souza et al. 1998; Ellison and Lager 1986; Hoshi et al. 1989). These data show, some criticisms notwithstanding (Malina 1983), that even moderate levels of physical activity in untrained women have suppressive effects on reproductive function (for reviews of studies on exercise-related reproductive suppression see Elias and Wilson 1993; Henley and Vaitukaitis 1988; Howlett 1987; Loucks 1990; Noakes and van Gend 1988; Rosetta 1993). The importance of studies involving non-athletes lies in their ability to demonstrate that even moderate physical activity may cause changes in ovarian function, with potentially significant effects on reproductive performance. Furthermore, energy expenditure due to aerobic activities may influence ovarian function independently of changes in energy balance, as observed by Bullen (1985) and Ellison and Lager (1986) in women runners.

Studies of reproductive function of women involved in subsistence work have also shown compromised ovarian function associated with negative energy balance. Data come from two populations: Lese horticulturalists of the Ituri Forest in Zaire (Bailey et al. 1992; Bentley et al. 1990,

1998; Ellison et al. 1989) and Tamang agropastoralists of Nepal (Panter-Brick and Ellison 1994; Panter-Brick et al. 1993). Lese women experience seasonal changes in energy balance owing primarily to fluctuations in the availability of food, though workload varies seasonally as well. During the sustained periods of weight loss that usually precede the harvests each year, indices of menstrual and ovarian function decline steadily. After the hunger season, increases in progesterone levels and ovulatory frequency are observed in parallel with improved nutritional status (Bailey et al. 1992; Ellison et al. 1989). These seasonal changes in the levels of ovarian function in Lese are reflected in pronounced seasonality and interannual variation in births with successful conceptions less likely to occur during periods of low energy availability.

Ovarian suppression associated with negative energy balance was also detected among Tamang women in Nepal (Panter-Brick and Ellison 1994; Panter-Brick et al. 1993). In this case variation in energy balance results from seasonal changes in energy expenditure rather than energy intake. During times of increased energy expenditure, salivary progesterone levels were depressed in women who lost weight but not in women who gained weight. Consequently, when high energy expenditure causes negative energy balance, reduction in fecundity should be expected (Panter-Brick and Ellison 1994; Panter-Brick et al. 1993).

Polish farm women also show seasonal ovarian suppression in response to increases in workload (Jasienska 1996a, 1996b; Jasienska and Ellison 1993, 1998) despite relatively high nutritional status and stable weight. In addition, a significant negative relationship was detected between levels of energy expenditure and the severity of ovarian suppression. As indicated by path analyses, total daily energy expenditure was the only factor related to levels of ovarian progesterone. Body weight, body fat percentage, or changes in these indices showed no relationships with the levels of ovarian steroids. These findings remain in agreement with the theoretical predictions of Ellison (1990), who introduced a concept of the "graded continuum" of responses of ovarian function to energetic stresses. The severity of ovarian response should be related to the severity of energetic stress (Ellison 1990; Prior 1985), although individuals may vary in their sensitivity to energetically caused disturbances.

Some researchers have speculated on the adaptive significance of the response of human fertility to workload, yet no appropriate studies have been carried out to test the existence of such a response. Bentley (1985) has suggested that the extremely low fertility of the !Kung San might be explained by the existence of physiological mechanisms similar to those postulated in the exercise studies. Blurton-Jones and Sibley (1987) demonstrated that, given the practical constraints of the mobile hunter-gatherer lifestyle, traditional !Kung birth spacing ensures maximum reproductive success. The authors did not attempt to speculate, however, on the mechanisms responsible for the observed pattern of birth spacing. Peacock (1990) has suggested that variation in reproductive function among women can be at least partially explained by differences in workloads.

ENERGY BUDGETS AND COSTS OF REPRODUCTION

All available metabolic energy needs to be partitioned by the organism to support several main physiological functions (Sibly and Calow 1986). According to the models of dynamic allocation, available resources must be divided among competing demands in a way that maximizes fitness of the individual (Kozlowski and Wiegert 1986; Perrin and Sibly 1993). The following discussion will focus only on mature females since reproductive strategies and reproductive costs for males are likely to be outcomes of different evolutionary pressures.

In women of reproductive age, energy is divided to support two main functions: survival and reproduction. Energy devoted to survival is used to keep the organism alive and therefore is needed to support both metabolic maintenance and behavioral functions (e.g., finding and preparing food, building shelters). In bioenergetic terms, energy expenditure of a nonreproductive, nongrowing individual has three main components: resting energy expenditure, the thermic effect of food, and physical activity (Zemel et al. 1996). Resting energy expenditure includes energy used to maintain minimal body function in a fasted, alert, and rested state (Sibly and Calow 1986). Processes that must be supported include cardiac activity, nervous system activity, sodium and calcium pumping, and thermoregulation. The thermic effect of food includes the costs of digestion, absorption, metabolism, and storage of ingested food, amounting to about 10% of total energy intake (Ulijaszek 1996).

The portion of energy devoted to reproduction in females is used to maintain ovarian and uterine function, and especially to support pregnancy and lactation, and may also include costs associated with child care. Physiological events involved in the menstrual cycle are probably not very costly energetically. Small increases in resting metabolic rate occur during the luteal phase of the menstrual cycle, in comparison with menstrual or follicular phases (Howe et al. 1993; Meijer et al. 1992). Interestingly, there are significant increases in energy intake in women following ovulation (Johnson et al. 1994). This suggests that extra energy, beyond the regular maintenance metabolism, is indeed needed to support regular menstrual cycles (Cumming et al. 1994; Townsend and Calow 1981). It is unlikely, however, that ovarian suppression in women would occur because of the lack of energy to support production of hormones or endometrial development throughout the menstrual cycle. Rather, high energetic costs of pregnancy and lactation are the likely ultimate factors behind the phenomenon of reproductive suppression. Although it is true that being in the luteal phase of the menstrual cycle adds about 6% to the energetic costs of the regular maintenance metabolism (Howe et al. 1993; Meijer et al. 1992; Voland 1998), this extra expense lasts only for several days. In contrast, pregnancy involves increases in energetic costs from the beginning to term with, on average, an extra 250–300 kcal needed daily (Dewey 1997; Durnin 1991; Hytten and Leitch 1971) and may require up to 22% of additional energy over the pre-pregnant values during the last trimester (Butte et al. 1999; Hytten and Leitch 1971). The energy cost of lactation changes with the age of the child and frequency of feeding, but, on average, lactation requires additional 500 kcal/day (Dewey 1997; van Raaij et al. 1991) and may last several years. These estimates of the costs of reproduction, all based on data from well-nourished women from industrialized countries, have recently been criticized as possibly too high (Illingworth et al. 1986; Kopp-Hoolihan et al. 1999). Women from The Gambia, for example, seem to be able to support pregnancy and lactation with very limited energy intake (Prentice 1984). During the wet (hunger) season the average energy intake for a pregnant or lactating rural Gambian woman was only 1,299 kcal/day (Prentice 1984), while in comparison it was, on average, 1,980 kcal/day for pregnant and 2,293 kcal/day for lactating British women (Whitehead et al. 1981).

Women can reproduce when environmental conditions are unfavorable, but not without substantial risks. These risks include giving birth to premature, low-weight infants (Kusin et al. 1992; Lawrence, Coward et al. 1987; Lechtig et al. 1975; Matsuda et al. 1990; Mora et al. 1979; Roberts et al. 1982; Siniarska et al. 1992) and deterioration of maternal physiological condition (maternal depletion syndrome) (Little et al. 1992; Liu et al. 1988; Merchant and Martorell 1988; Miller et al. 1994; National Academy of Sciences 1989; Tracer 1991), including higher rates of parasitic infections suffered by pregnant women under poor nutritional conditions (Saowakontha et al. 1992). It is unlikely then that women who do not respond to a situation of low energy availability with a temporary suppression of reproductive function can achieve high lifetime reproductive success. Therefore, suppression of fecundity during periods of negative energy balance can be easily understood as an adaptive response (Ellison 1991, 1994; Ellison et al. 1993; Prior 1985; Spuy 1985; Ulijaszek 1996). Can we postulate an adaptive significance of reproductive suppression caused by energy expenditure when energy balance itself remains unchanged? Is the state of the negative energy balance a necessary or just a sufficient condition for reproductive suppression to occur?

THE "PREEMPTIVE OVARIAN SUPPRESSION" HYPOTHESIS

This hypothesis assumes that during human evolution an increase in workload was almost always associated with negative energy balance. Therefore, a physiological mechanism which tracks increases in the levels of energy expenditure and responds with reproductive suppression is likely to have evolved. In ancestral humans, increases in energy expenditure might have resulted from longer hours spent foraging, higher energetic demands of food-gathering (e.g., digging roots versus picking berries), or carrying heavier loads while on foraging trips. The question that must be asked is, in what situations would women sustain high levels of energy expenditure for longer periods of time, if this led to a state of negative energy balance? One would expect a reduction in the levels of physical activity in order to conserve energy. This situation may have been different for individuals with dependent offspring, however. A woman with one or two dependent children may, in some situations, be forced to increase her levels of physical activity in order to provide for children, even if this means falling herself into a state of negative energy balance. Since, according to the modern evolutionary paradigm, costs and benefits must be calculated for all involved (and genetically related) individuals, we can explain why women may have to increase levels of their physical activity despite a deterioration in their personal nutritional status.

The hypothesis discussed here has some serious problems. It is not clear, for example, why natural selection would design a mechanism that just tracks changes in energy expenditure without "waiting" for negative energy balance to result from this increased expenditure. What adaptive benefits could such a mechanism provide that would exceed the benefits of responding *after* the negative energy balance has occurred? This hypothesis also assumes that equally high or even higher energy intake rarely compensated for high energy expenditure, making the coupling between high energy expenditure and negative energy balance almost always inevitable. It is hard to put forward sound arguments in support of this assumption. In the following section I discuss an alternative hypothesis which does not require that energy expenditure must lead to negative energy balance for reproductive suppression to occur.

THE "CONSTRAINED DOWN-REGULATION" HYPOTHESIS

Jasienska and Ellison (1998) briefly outlined a hypothesis which attempts to explain why high energy expenditure alone may have a suppressive effect on reproductive function in women even when energy balance remains unchanged. Here I present a full argument underlying this view. I propose that constrained metabolic down-regulation is specific to situations in which energy expenditure is the main energetic stress. Other aspects of energy metabolism and allocation (e.g., metabolic ceilings, insufficient fat storage) must be taken into account to explain why patterns of energy reallocation are significantly constrained in women with high levels of energy expenditure and thus why more energy cannot simply be reallocated to support reproduction. These latter aspects are not specific to reproductive suppression resulting from to energy expenditure; they should also be considered when suppression results from food deprivation, weight loss, and negative energy balance.

Several hypothetical models of energy allocation in the states of positive, negative, and sustained energy balance are discussed first, followed by a discussion of constraints on energy allocation to reproductive processes. The latter discussion includes physiological constraints (e.g., metabolic ceilings) on increase in energy intake as well as limitations on redirecting energy flow to reproduction away from other energy-using processes.

Scenarios of Energy Allocation

As outlined earlier, in a typical model of energy allocation (Figure 3.1), energy obtained from food serves to support several main functions: maintenance metabolism (including heat production and renewal of tissues), physical activity, and reproduction (Sibly and Calow 1986; Van Zant 1992). Surplus energy can be stored as fat. The energy used for maintenance metabolism is typically expressed as basal metabolic rate (BMR) or resting metabolic rate (RMR).

Depending on environmental and physiological conditions, an individual can be either in a positive, negative, or sustained (neutral) energy balance (Blaxter 1989). In the state of a positive energy balance (Figure 3.2), energy intake (after digestion and absorption) is higher than the sum of energy expenditures in all categories. Therefore, that individual has enough energy to support maintenance, physical activity, reproduction, and energy storage. On the other hand, a state of negative energy balance (Figure 3.3) results when energy intake is lower than the sum of energy expenditures. When energy intake is very low, sufficient only to support BMR and low levels of physical activity, no energy is left for reproduction or fat storage.

Alternatively, very high levels of physical activity may result in a negative energy balance. Energy intake that would be sufficient for a moderately active individual becomes too low for an individual with increased

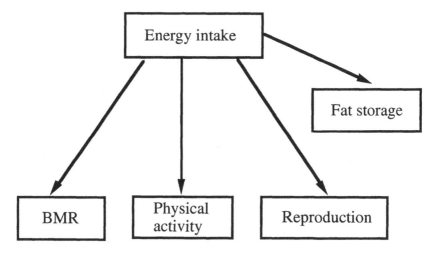

Figure 3.1. Allocation of energy by the individual. Energy from food is used to support BMR (which indicates energetic costs of the maintenance metabolism), physical activity, and reproduction. Surplus energy is stored as fat.

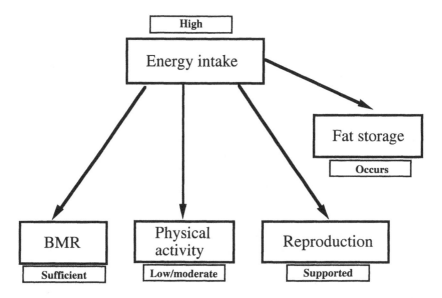

Figure 3.2. The state of positive energy balance. Energy intake is higher than the sum of energy expenditures. Levels of physical activity are low to moderate. Reproduction can be supported. Surplus energy is stored as fat.

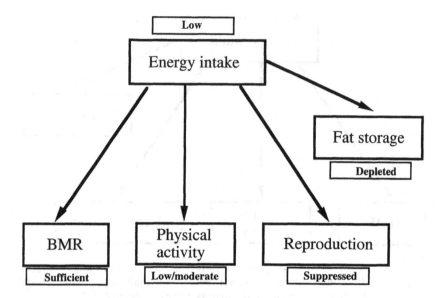

Figure 3.3.   The state of negative energy balance. Low energy intake is only sufficient to support BMR and low levels of physical activity. To support moderate
levels of activity, fat stores are used and increasingly depleted. Reproductive
function is suppressed.

levels of physical activity. In that case energy will be used to support BMR
and physical activity, but not reproduction or storage of fat. Negative
energy balance can also result from increased costs of reproduction in a
female who is pregnant and/or lactating and is not able to increase energy
intake, or decrease levels of physical activity. In this situation, energy will
be used to support physical activity, fetal growth and/or milk production,
and maternal BMR. Interestingly, the last element may be modified during
pregnancy and lactation (see the discussion below). In all situations, when
an individual is in a state of negative energy balance, energy stored previously as fat is used to help support costs of energy expenditure, and therefore fat stores gradually become depleted (Blaxter 1989).

A particularly interesting case is represented by sustained energy balance in which a constant body weight is maintained (Figure 3.4). Physiologists use this term to describe the situation in which metabolism of an
individual is fueled over a long period of time by food intake rather than
by transient depletion of energy reserves (Hammond and Diamond 1997;
Peterson et al. 1990). Sustained energy balance may represent a situation
in which both energy intake and energy expenditure are very high. Let us
consider two situations characterized by high energy intake, but different

levels of physical activity. In the first case, high energy intake is sufficient to support BMR and moderate levels of physical activity, and enough energy is left to support reproduction. This situation may be similar to the state of positive energy balance, but only if even more energy remains for fat storage.

In the second case of sustained energy balance, energy intake is equally high, but levels of physical activity significantly increase. Therefore, a higher fraction of energy intake has to be used to support physical activity. For simplicity, we will assume at first that the demands of BMR are the same. As a result, the fraction of energy which was earlier available for reproduction will be transferred to support physical activity. Therefore, despite high levels of energy intake, there may not be enough energy to devote to reproductive processes. When the sum of physical activity and BMR approximately equals energy intake, the individual can still have sustained energy balance, as long as energy intake remains high enough to facilitate these two functions. Therefore, it can be postulated that the suppression of reproductive function may occur not only in individuals who are in a state of negative energy balance but also in those who are in a state of sustained energy balance.

An explanation of why intense physical activity causes suppression of reproductive function must be based on the principle of energy allocation.

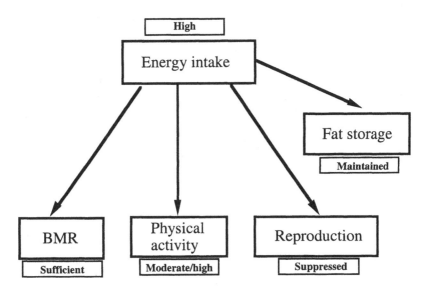

Figure 3.4. The state of sustained energy balance. High energy intake equals the sum of BMR and physical activity. No energy is left to allocate to reproduction. Fat storage remains unchanged.

When no energy is available to support all energy-requiring activities, some of them will have to be suppressed or receive less energy than they require. When work or exercise use a high fraction of energy intake, not enough energy may be left to support anticipated costs of reproduction. This explanation, however, must allow for the fact that women have the ability to use energy-saving mechanisms while pregnant or lactating (Poppitt et al. 1993; Prentice et al. 1989, 1995). Also, it is often believed that energy stores in humans are used to support reproduction (Caro and Sellen 1990; King et al. 1994; Little et al. 1992; Norgan 1997).

Another issue which needs to be addressed is why the pattern of energy allocation cannot be changed. Theoretically, an increase in energy intake, a decrease in physical activity, a decrease in BMR, or usage of stored energy may make more energy available for reproduction. Eating more and doing less are the most obvious solutions, but they may simply be impossible for many women in hunting and gathering or agricultural populations (Jenike 1996; King et al. 1994; Panter-Brick 1993; Prentice et al. 1996). Furthermore, increases in energy intake may be constrained by purely physiological limits (e.g., metabolic ceilings).

Metabolic Ceilings to Sustainable Energy Budgets

Environmental constraints on the energy budget of the individual have long been recognized and are well incorporated into life history theory. In particular, the effects of limited energy intake and negative energy balance on many life history characteristics can be supported by data from numerous species (Sibly and Calow 1986; Townsend and Calow 1981). However, the idea of physiological limits to the rate of food conversion into usable energy, and especially its implications for the optimal allocation of resources, is less commonly used in discussions of evolutionary strategies. An interesting debate continues in ecological physiology about "metabolic ceilings" to sustainable energy budgets (Hammond and Diamond 1994, 1997; Hammond et al. 1994, 1996; Konarzewski and Diamond 1994; Koteja 1995; Peterson et al. 1990; Saris et al. 1989; Weiner 1989, 1992). In all the studied species (including birds, eutherian mammals, and marsupials) the maximum sustainable metabolic rates (SusMR) are only a few times higher than the basal metabolic rates (BMR) (Hammond and Diamond 1997; Peterson et al. 1990). In general, this ratio (SusMR/BMR) was always less than 7. For human males, the most frequently reported values of SusMR/BMR are between 4.1 and 5.6 and come from measurements of Tour de France cyclists (Saris et al. 1989) who race for almost 4,000 km and cross 34 mountains in 22 days. Mean estimated total daily energy intake was 24.7 megajoules (MJ) and mean total daily energy expenditure 25.4 MJ, which is probably the highest level of prolonged energy expenditure ever reported for humans. In comparison, male soldiers expend between

13.5 and 21.0 MJ a day, and Antarctic explorers from 18.5 to 23.0 MJ a day (Peterson et al. 1990). It has been suggested that the Tour de France cyclists reach the upper limits to sustainable energy budgets—in other words, they would not be able to generate more energy even with additional increases in food consumption (Peterson et al. 1990).

How relevant to human ecophysiology is the discussion of the limits on sustainable energy budgets? Were these limits important constraints on energy allocation for our ancestors? It is unlikely that the levels of energy intake and expenditure characteristic of Tour de France cyclists were routinely experienced by our human ancestors. It is also possible that these extremely high ratios are only attainable in modern athletes owing to the high quality of food available only recently (Eissa et al. 1986). Food consumed by humans during the formative past might have permitted much lower maximum rates of energy assimilation. Among the !Kung San, who are commonly used as the model of human ancestral lifestyle, 60% to 80% of consumed energy is provided by plant food (Lee 1979). Similarly, Australian Aboriginal hunter-gatherers have diets characterized by low energy density (Maslar 1988). In several contemporary hunter-gatherer populations, consumption of dietary fiber is about 100 g per day, while in North America, by comparison, the average is about 15 g per day (Eaton et al. 1994). A diet high in fiber, low in fat, and low in simple carbohydrates was very likely associated with much lower rates of energy assimilation than the diet characteristic of modern industrial societies.

Thus, it is likely that sustainable energy budgets of human ancestors had much lower metabolic ceilings that those reported for modern athletes. This may imply that in the past there may have been effective limits to the degree to which increased energy intake could compensate for high expenditure. Even when the availability of food was sufficient, the maximum rate of energy assimilation may have acted as the limiting factor for sustainable energy budgets. Therefore, in women requiring high quantities of energy to support prolonged, intense physical activity, the pattern of energy allocation made energy unavailable for reproductive processes. Given the low quality of food, an increase in food consumption was not likely to increase energy intake significantly. In this situation, when an increase occurred in energy expenditure, even maximal energy intake was still not high enough to support allocation of energy to all energy-costly functions.

Physical Activity as a Constraint on Energy-Saving Mechanisms

When an individual has such high levels of physical activity that not enough energy is left for reproduction, some energy could in principle be regained by allocating less energy into other categories. For example, can the amount of energy used to support basal metabolism be reduced? I will show that high levels of physical activity usually require allocation of an even higher fraction of energy into basal metabolism. On the other hand, the evidence from a different area of research (human pregnancy and lactation) will be used to show that, in some situations, the reduction in basal metabolism may indeed be used as an energy-saving mechanism.

Basal metabolic rate (BMR) represents the fraction of energy that is used to support the maintenance metabolism. Maintenance metabolism is the sum of many physiological processes that serve to keep the individual alive. While some of these processes always have to operate at a high level since they are absolutely crucial for survival, other processes can be temporarily slowed down or even halted (King et al. 1994; Prentice and Whitehead 1987). However, a reduction in BMR may be associated with significant risks to the long-term condition of the individual. A low BMR may be achieved by a reduction in some components of maintenance metabolism (e.g., protein turnover), which may be detrimental to the individual, especially after a long period of time (Prentice and Whitehead 1987).

Responses of BMR to Physical Activity

The response of BMR to increased physical activity, especially exercise, has received much attention in sports medicine and research on obesity and weight control (Bingham et al. 1989; Broeder et al. 1992; Bullough et al. 1995; Burke et al. 1993; Lovelady et al. 1995; Poehlman and Horton 1989; Sjodin et al. 1996; Taaffle et al. 1995; Tremblay et al. 1997; Van Zant 1992; Westerterp 1998; Westerterp et al. 1991, 1994; Williamson and Kirwan 1997). The focus of these studies was to determine if physically active people have higher BMR than individuals with more sedentary lifestyles. Many studies reported that BMR increases as a result of prolonged sport participation (Burke et al. 1993; Dolezal and Potteiger 1998; Morio et al. 1998; Poehlman and Horton 1989; Sjodin et al. 1996; Tremblay et al. 1997; Van Zant 1992). Other studies, however, showed an increase in BMR only immediately after exercise without a long-lasting effect (Bingham et al. 1989). One study even reported a decrease in BMR owing to chronic exercise (Westerterp et al. 1994). It is possible that at least part of the disagreement in these results can be resolved when differences in research protocols are taken into account. The response of BMR to exercise may depend on the duration and intensity of single bouts of exercise, types of exercise, duration of the whole training session, pre-training condition of subjects, and, most important, changes in body composition with exercise. In general, longer-term physical training causes changes in body composition and, especially, increases in muscle mass. Muscle, as a metabolically active tissue, is energetically expensive.

Therefore, on average, the BMR of a more muscular person is expected to be higher than the BMR of a less muscular one. When a particular training regime does not produce changes in body composition, a change in BMR should not be expected. For example, after 15 weeks, neither low- nor high-intensity resistance exercise caused significant changes in body composition in women over age 65 (Taaffle et al. 1995). Not surprisingly, the BMR of those women remained at the pre-exercise level.

However, studies of endurance athletes, who usually have higher percentages of fat-free mass than less athletic people, and studies during which training caused changes in body composition often report positive effects of training on BMR. Increase in BMR with training was observed, for example, in women rowers (McCargar et al. 1993). Women who lost weight, as well as those who did not, showed significant increases in BMR. Changes in BMR appeared to reflect changes in fat-free mass in both groups of women. The BMR of elite endurance athletes was 16% higher than in a non-athletic control group (Sjodin et al. 1996). Significant increases in BMR after 10 weeks of training were reported in males engaged in resistance training, but not in males participating in endurance training (running and/or jogging) (Dolezal and Potteiger 1998).

Resting metabolic rate (RMR) was found to be greater in trained than in untrained men only when trained subjects had a high rate of energy flow—in other words, both high energy intake and high expenditure in physical activity (Bullough et al. 1995). Similar results were also reported for women (Burke et al. 1993). Women were divided into three groups depending on the level of aerobic fitness. Not only did women with the highest aerobic fitness have the highest RMR, but also a significant positive relationship between the rate of energy flow and RMR was shown. In conclusion, a prolonged regime of physical activity, especially when associated with changes in body composition, may induce a significant increase of BMR. Also, high rates of energy flow seem to contribute to increases in basal metabolic rate.

Responses of BMR to Pregnancy and Lactation

While physical activity causes an increase in BMR, pregnancy and lactation may require that a woman be able to decrease her BMR as a crucial energy-saving option (Peacock 1991; Prentice et al. 1989, 1995). Pregnancy adds additional energetic costs to the regular maintenance metabolism (Hytten and Chamberlain 1991). These costs are related to fetal growth, growth and maintenance of maternal supporting tissues, and maternal fat accumulation (Blackburn and Loper 1992). Lactation is associated with additional costs of milk synthesis and the maintenance of metabolically active mammary glands (Lunn 1994; Prentice and Prentice 1990; Thomson et al. 1970; Trayhurn 1989). Since BMR is an index integrating all metabolic activities, it would be expected to rise in women who are pregnant or nursing a child. Predictions have been made that BMR should increase during each of the four quarters of pregnancy respectively by about 3%, 7%, 11%, and 17% above pre-pregnant values (Hytten and Leitch 1971). During lactation, the increase in BMR should be on average about 12% above the non-pregnant, non-lactating state (Hytten and Leitch 1971). Empirical data, however, usually do not agree with these predictions (Durnin 1991, 1993; Lunn 1994; Prentice and Prentice 1990; Prentice and Whitehead 1987; Prentice et al. 1989, 1995, 1996). Swedish women in good nutritional status show increases in the BMR close to the predicted levels from the very beginning of pregnancy (Prentice and Whitehead 1987). In contrast, women from Scotland and The Gambia, in poorer nutritional condition, had very different responses: BMR showed a significant decrease from the beginning to about the twelfth week of pregnancy. After that time the BMR started to rise, but it was not until the twenty-second to twenty-sixth week that it reached pre-pregnancy levels, and even at term it was still much lower than the BMR of Swedish women (Prentice and Whitehead 1987). A marked variability in BMR responses during pregnancy among Nigerian women may also be explained by differences in nutritional status (Cole et al. 1989). Substantial variation related to initial body weight has been observed in the BMR changes in pregnancy even in well-nourished women (Prentice et al. 1989). The initial decrease in the BMR may be of crucial importance for women in poor nutritional condition, who often do not have additional energy intake while pregnant. Negative changes in the BMR not only considerably reduce energetic costs of pregnancy but also allow women to allocate some energy into fat storage which may be used during later pregnancy and lactation.

Similarly, during lactation BMR does not always respond as predicted. In lactating women, BMR may increase, decrease, or remain at pre-pregnant values (Forsum et al. 1992; Goldberg et al. 1991; Guillermo et al. 1992; Jiang and Ho 1992; Lawrence and Whitehead 1988; Madhavapeddi and Rao 1992; Piers et al. 1995). Again, some of the discrepancies between these findings may be explained by differences in the nutritional status of the women studied (Prentice and Prentice 1990). Gambian women showed a 5% decrease in the BMR compared with the pre-pregnant values during the first year of lactation (Lawrence and Whitehead 1988). Although this does not seem like a substantial reduction, it still saves about 500 kJ a day and represents savings of about 900 kJ a day in comparison with the predicted increase in energetic costs. The saved energy may be allocated into milk synthesis and help a mother with low energy intake to support a child. Since the average daily cost of milk production for Gambian women is about 2,000 kJ (Lunn 1994), the savings from the reduction of BMR is a relatively substantial contribution.

Fat stores may also be used to support the energy costs of milk production. However, in developing countries women often have very low fat reserves (Lawrence, Lawrence et al. 1987; Little et al. 1992; Panter-Brick 1996). If fat reserves were used to subsidize just 50% of the costs of lactation they would last only for 4 months in Gambian women (Prentice and Prentice 1990). In contrast, fat stores would last for 11 months in well-nourished western women. Therefore, it has been suggested that in the developing world the function of fat stores is to serve as an emergency resource for times when conditions become very hard, rather than to support milk production steadily (Lunn 1994; Prentice and Prentice 1990).

ENERGY EXPENDITURE AS A FECUNDITY REGULATOR: CONCLUSIONS

Reproduction in women who have poor nutritional status is characterized by marked decreases of BMR during pregnancy and lactation. Such changes in BMR serve as important energy-saving mechanisms, allowing the support of reproduction, especially in women who are not able to increase their food intake sufficiently while pregnant or lactating. On the other hand, intense physical activity forces individuals to have elevated levels of BMR in addition to the costs of the activity itself. Therefore, a hard-working woman may have a restricted ability to lower her BMR while pregnant or lactating. Reproductive suppression observed in hard-working women may be related to this constraint. If physical activity restricts the ability to obtain energy savings from reducing the BMR, fat storage at the beginning of pregnancy may not be possible. Without sufficient fat reserves and the flexibility to lower BMR during lactation, lactational performance may also suffer.

For reproductive suppression to occur one does not have to assume that the stress of intense physical activity will persist during the entire duration of pregnancy and lactation. Since humans most likely did not evolve in a predictable environment, natural selection could not predict how long-lasting this stress will be. Therefore, it is more advantageous to respond with suppression in order to prevent pregnancy, and remove suppression as soon as the stress relaxes. Consequently, one may expect that reproductive suppression is an evolved response ensuring survival of the woman and the maintenance of her future reproductive potential.

In conclusion, it is likely that reproductive suppression evolved as an adaptive response to high levels of physical activity in human females

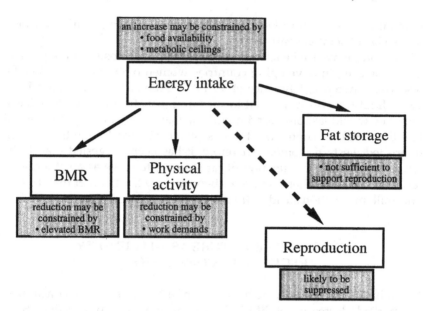

Figure 3.5. A model of energy allocation in hard-working women when constraints to energy flow to reproduction are present. Theoretically, when the
woman maintains a sustained energy balance, reproductive processes can be
supported by increases in energy intake, use of fat stores, or allocating the
energy from other energy-demanding functions. However, additional energy
intake may be constrained by both food availability and metabolic ceilings. A
decrease in physical activity may be constrained by work demands. Allocating
additional energy from BMR may be constrained by the BMR being elevated as
a consequence of increases in physical activity. Fat stores are not sufficient to
support the entire reproductive event. As a consequence, reproductive function
remains suppressed, as long as intense physical work continues.

(Figure 3.5). Energy intake is constrained not only by food availability but
also by metabolic ceilings to energy assimilation. However, the patterns of
energy allocation into energy-requiring functions have some degree of
flexibility, allowing for the prevention of reproductive failure in pregnant
and lactating females when environmental conditions are poor. Such flexibility, however, may have been substantially diminished in females who
at the same time had to sustain high levels of physical activity. Therefore,
high energy expenditure resulting from intense workloads might have
been used as a signal not only that not enough energy would be available
for reproduction, but also that it would be impossible to use the energy-
saving mechanisms normally mobilized during pregnancy and lactation.

This work greatly benefitted from suggestions by Peter Ellison and could have not been written without help and support from Michal Jasienski.

REFERENCES

Adams AM (1995) Seasonal variations in energy balance among agriculturalists in central Mali: compromise or adaptation? *European Journal of Clinical Nutrition* 49:809–823.

Bailey RC, Jenike MR, Ellison PT, Bentley GR, Harrigan AM, Peacock NR (1992) The ecology of birth seasonality among agriculturalist in central Africa. *Journal of Biosocial Science* 24:393–412.

Baulieu E (1989) Contragestion and other clinical applications of RU486, an antiprogesterone at the receptor. *Science* 245:1351–1357.

Benefice E, Simondon K, Malina RM (1996) Physical activity patterns and anthropometric changes in Senegalese women observed over a complete seasonal cycle. *American Journal of Human Biology* 8:251–261.

Bentley GR (1985) Hunter-gatherer energetics and fertility: a reassessment of the !Kung San. *Human Ecology* 13:79–109.

Bentley GR, Harrigan AM, Ellison PT (1990) Ovarian cycle length and days of menstruation of Lese horticulturalists. *American Journal of Physical Anthropology* 81:193–194.

Bentley GR, Harrigan AM, Ellison PT (1998) Dietary composition and ovarian function among Lese horticulturalist women of the Ituri Forest, Democratic Republic of Congo. *European Journal of Clinical Nutrition* 52:261–270.

Bingham SA, Goldberg GR, Coward WA, Prentice AM, Cummings JH (1989) The effect of exercise and improved physical fitness on basal metabolic rate. *British Journal of Nutrition* 61:155–174.

Blackburn S, Loper D (1992) *Maternal, Fetal, and Neonatal Physiology: A Clinical Perspective* (Philadelphis, W.B. Saunders).

Blaxter K (1989) *Energy Metabolism in Animals and Man* (Cambridge, Cambridge University Press).

Blurton-Jones N, Sibley RM (1987) Testing adaptiveness of culturally determined behaviour: do Bushmen women maximise their reproductive success by spacing births widely and foraging seldom? In *Human Behaviour and Adaptation* (London, Taylor and Francis), Society for the Study of Human Biology, Symposium 18, 135–157.

Broeder CE, Burrhus KA, Svanevik LS, Wilmore JH (1992) The effects of either high-intensity resistance or endurance training on resting metabolic rate. *American Journal of Clinical Nutrition* 55:802–810.

Bronson FH (1995) Seasonal variation in human reproduction: environmental factors. *Quarterly Review of Biology* 70:141–165.

Broocks A, Pirke KM, Schweiger U, Tuschl RJ, Laessle RG, Strowitzki T, Horl E, Horl T, Haas W, Jeschke D (1990) Cyclic ovarian function in recreational athletes. *Journal of Applied Physiology* 68:2083–2086.

Bullen BA, Skrinar GS, Beitins IZ, vonMering G, Turnbull BA, McArthur JW (1985) Induction of menstrual disorders by strenuous exercise in untrained women. *New England Journal of Medicine* 312:1349–1353.

Bullough RC, Gillette CA, Harris MA, Melby CL (1995) Interaction of acute changes in exercise energy expenditure and energy intake on resting metabolic rate. *American Journal of Clinical Nutrition* 61:473–481.

Burke CM, Bullough RC, Melby CL (1993) Resting metabolic rate and postprandial thermogenesis by level of aerobic fitness in young women. *European Journal of Clinical Nutrition* 47:575–585.

Butte NF, Hopkinson JM, Mehta N, Moon JK, Smith EO (1999) Adjustments in energy expenditure and substrate utilization during late pregnancy and lactation. *American Journal of Clinical Nutrition* 69:299–307.

Caro TM, Sellen DW (1990) The reproductive advantage of fat in women. *Ethology and Sociobiology* 11:51–66.

Cole AH, Ibeziako PA, Bamgboye EA (1989) Basal metabolic rate and energy expenditure of pregnant Nigerian women. *British Journal of Nutrition* 62:631–638.

Cumming DC (1993) The effects of exercise and nutrition on the menstrual cycle. In R Gray, H Leridon, A Spira (Eds) *Biomedical and Demographic Determinants of Reproduction* (Oxford, Clarendon Press), 132–156.

Cumming DC, Wheeler GD, Harber VJ (1994) Physical activity, nutrition, and reproduction. *Annals of the New York Academy of Sciences* 709:287–298.

Dale E, Gerlach DH, Wilhite AL (1979) Menstrual dysfunction in distance runners. *Obstetrics and Gynecology* 54:47–53.

De Souza MJ, Miller BE, Loucks AB, Luciano AA, Pescatello LS, Campbell CG, Lasley BL (1998) High frequency of luteal phase deficiency and anovulation in recreational women runners: blunted elevation in follicle-stimulating hormone observed during luteal-follicular transition. *Journal of Clinical Endocrinology and Metabolism* 83:4220–4232.

Dewey K (1997) Energy and protein requirements during lactation. *Annual Review of Nutrition* 17:19–36.

Dickey RP, Olar TT, Taylor SN, Curole DN, Matulich EM (1993) Relationship of endometrial thickness and pattern to fecundity in ovulation induction cycles: effect of clomiphene citrate alone and with human menopausal gonadotropin. *Fertility and Sterility* 59:756–760.

Dolezal BA, Potteiger JA (1998) Concurrent resistance and endurance training influence basal metabolic rate in non-dieting individuals. *Journal of Applied Physiology* 85:695–700.

Durnin JVGA (1991) Energy requirements of pregnancy. *Acta Paediatrica Scandinavica* 10(Suppl.):33–42.

Durnin JVGA (1993) Energy requirements in human pregnancy, in human nutrition and parasitic infection. *Parasitology* 107:S169–S175.

Eaton SB, Pike MC, Short RV, Lee NC, Trussell J, Hatcher RA, Wood JW, Worthman CM, Jones NG, Konner MJ (1994) Women's reproductive cancers in evolutionary context. *Quarterly Review of Biology* 69:353–367.

Eissa M, Obhrai M, Docker M, Lynch S, Sawers R, Newton R (1986) Follicular growth and endocrine profiles in spontaneous and induced conception cycles. *Fertility and Sterility* 45:191–195.

Elias AN, Wilson AF (1993) Exercise and gonadal function. *Human Reproduction* 8:1747–1761.

Ellison PT (1990) Human ovarian function and reproductive ecology: new hypotheses. *American Anthropologist* 92:933–952.

Ellison PT (1991) Reproductive ecology and human fertility. In GW Lasker, CGN Mascie-Taylor (Eds) *Applications of Biological Anthropology to Human Affairs* (Cambridge, Cambridge University Press), 14–54.

Ellison PT (1994) Advances in human reproductive ecology. *Annual Review of Anthropology* 23:255–275.

Ellison PT (1996) Developmental influences on adult ovarian hormonal function. *American Journal of Human Biology* 8:725–734.

Ellison PT, Lager C (1986) Moderate recreational running is associated with lowered salivary progesterone profiles in women. *American Journal of Obstetrics and Gynecology* 154:1000–1003.

Ellison PT, Panter BC, Lipson SF, O'Rourke MT (1993) The ecological context of human ovarian function. *Human Reproduction* 8:2248–2258.

Ellison PT, Peacock NR, Lager C (1989) Ecology and ovarian function among Lese women of Ituri Forest, Zaire. *American Journal of Physical Anthropology* 78:519–526.

Forsum E, Kabir N, Sadurskis A, Westerterp K (1992) Total energy expenditure of healthy Swedish women during pregnancy and lactation. *American Journal of Clinical Nutrition* 56:334–342.

Frisch RE, Wyshak G, Vincent L (1980) Delayed menarche and amenorrhea in ballet dancers. *New England Journal of Medicine* 303:17–19.

Goldberg GR, Prentice AM, Coward WA, Davies HL, Murgatroyd PR, Sawyer MB, Ashford J, Black AE (1991) Longitudinal assessment of the components of energy balance in well-nourished lactating women. *American Journal of Clinical Nutrition* 54:788–798.

Guillermo-Tuazon MA, Barba CV, van Raaij JM, Hautvast JG (1992) Energy intake, energy expenditure, and body composition of poor rural Philippine women throughout the first 6 mo of lactation. *American Journal of Clinical Nutrition* 56:874–880.

Hammond K, Diamond J (1994) Limits to dietary nutrient intake and intestinal nutrient uptake in lactating mice. *Physiological Zoology* 67:282–303.

Hammond KA, Diamond J (1997) Maximal sustained energy budgets in humans and animals. *Nature* 386:457–462.

Hammond KA, Konarzewski M, Torres RM, Diamond J (1994) Metabolic ceilings under a combination of peak energy demands. *Physiological Zoology* 67: 1479–1506.

Hammond KA, Lloyd KCK, Diamond J (1996) Is mammary output capacity limiting to lactational performance in mice? *Journal of Experimental Biology* 199: 337–349.

Henley K, Vaitukaitis JL (1988) Exercise-induced menstrual dysfunction. *Annual Review of Medicine* 39:443–451.

Hofman MA, Swaab DF (1992) The human hypothalamus: comparative morphometry and photoperiodic influences. *Progress in Brain Research* 93:133–147.

Hoshi A, Kita N, Arao T, Aoki K, Goto Y, Sugawara I, Yamada Y, Matsuda K, Tsutsumi T (1989) Hormonal status of menstrual cycles in female athletes. *Bulletin of the Physical Fitness Research Institute* 10:25–34.

Howe JC, Rumpler WV, Seale JL (1993) Energy expenditure by indirect calorimetry in premenopausal women: variation within one menstrual cycle. *Journal of Nutritional Biochemistry* 4:268–273.

Howlett TA (1987) Hormonal responses to exercise and training: a short review. *Clinical Endocrinology* 26:723–742.

Hytten F, Chamberlain G (1991) *Clinical Physiology in Obstetrics*, 2nd ed. (Oxford, Blackwell Scientific).

Hytten FE, Leitch I (1971) *The Physiology of Human Pregnancy*, 2nd ed. (Oxford, Blackwell Scientific).

Illingworth PJ, Jung RT, Howie PW, Leslie P, Isles TE (1986) Diminution in energy expenditure during lactation. *British Medical Journal* 292:437–441.

Jasienska G (1996a) *Energy Expenditure and Ovarian Function in Polish Rural Women* (PhD dissertation, Harvard University).

Jasienska G (1996b) Energy expenditure, but not caloric intake or body composition, correlates with ovarian progesterone in peasant women. *American Journal of Physical Anthropology* 22(Suppl):132.

Jasienska G, Ellison PT (1993) Heavy workload impairs ovarian function in Polish peasant women. *American Journal of Physical Anthropology* 16(Suppl):117–118.

Jasienska G, Ellison PT (1998) Physical work causes suppression of ovarian function in women. *Proceedings of the Royal Society of London* B 265:1847–1851.

Jenike MR (1996) Activity reduction as an adaptive response to seasonal hunger. *American Journal of Human Biology* 8:517–534.

Jiang Z, Ho Z (1992) Energy expenditure of lactating women in subtropic area. *Acta Nutrimenta Sinica* 14:270–275.

Johnson WG, Corrigan SA, Lemmon CR, Bergeron KB, Crusco AH (1994) Energy regulation over the menstrual cycle. *Physiology of Behavior* 56:523–527.

King JC, Butte NF, Bronstein MN, Koop LE, Lindquist SA (1994) Energy metabolism during pregnancy: influence of maternal energy status. *American Journal of Clinical Nutrition* 59(Suppl):S439–S445.

Konarzewski M, Diamond J (1994) Peak sustained metabolic rate and its individual variation in cold-stressed mice. *Physiological Zoology* 67:1186–1212.

Kopp-Hoolihan LE, van-Loan MD, Wong WW, King JC (1999) Longitudinal assessment of energy balance in well-nourished, pregnant women. *American Journal of Clinical Nutrition* 69:697–704.

Koteja P (1995) Maximum cold-induced energy assimilation in a rodent, *Apodemus flavicolis*. *Comparative Biochemistry and Physiology* A 112:479–485.

Kozlowski J, Wiegert RG (1986) Optimal allocation of energy to growth and reproduction. *Theoretical Population Biology* 29:16–37.

Kusin JA, Kardjati S, Renqvist U, Goei K (1992) Reproduction and maternal nutrition in Madura, Indonesia. *Tropical and Geographical Medicine* 44:248–255.

Lam DA, Miron JA (1996) The effects of temperature on human fertility. *Demography* 33:291–305.

Lawrence M, Whitehead R (1988) Physical activity and total energy expenditure in child-bearing Gambian women. *European Journal of Clinical Nutrition* 42:145–160.

Lawrence M, Coward WA, Lawrence F, Cole TJ, Whitehead RG (1987) Fat gain during pregnancy in rural African women: the effect of season and dietary status. *American Journal of Clinical Nutrition* 45:1442–1450.

Lawrence M, Lawrence F, Coward WA, Cole TJ, Whitehead RG (1987) Energy requirements of pregnancy in The Gambia. *Lancet* 2:1072–1076.

Lechtig A, Yarbrough C, Delgado H, Habicht JP, Martorell R, Klein RF (1975) Influence of maternal nutrition on birth weight. *American Journal of Clinical Nutrition* 28:1223–1233.

Lee RB (1979) *The !Kung San: Men, Women, and Work in a Foraging Society* (Cambridge, Cambridge University Press).

Leonard WR, Robertson ML (1997) Comparative primate energetics and hominid evolution. *American Journal of Physical Anthropology* 102:265–281.

Little MA, Leslie PW, Campbell KL (1992) Energy reserves and parity of nomadic and settled Turkana women. *American Journal of Human Biology* 4:729–738.

Liu H, Jones G, Jones H, Rosenwaks Z (1988) Mechanisms and factors of early pregnancy wastage in in vitro fertilization-embryo transfer patients. *Fertility and Sterility* 50:95–101.

Loucks AB (1990) Effects of exercise training on the menstrual cycle: existence and mechanisms. *Medicine and Science in Sports and Exercise* 22:275–280.

Lovelady CA, Nommsen RL, McCrory MA, Dewey KG (1995) Effects of exercise on plasma lipids and metabolism of lactating women. *Medicine and Science in Sports and Exercise* 27:22–28.

Lunn PG (1994) Lactation and other metabolic loads affecting human reproduction. *Annals of the New York Academy of Sciences* 709:77–85.

Madhavapeddi R, Rao BS (1992) Energy balance in lactating undernourished Indian women. *European Journal of Clinical Nutrition* 46:349–354.

Malina RM (1983) Menarche in athletes: a synthesis and hypothesis. *Annals of Human Biology* 10:1–24.

Maslar I (1988) The progestational endometrium. *Seminars in Reproductive Endocrinology* 6:115–128.

Matsuda S, Sone T, Doi T, Kahyo H (1990) [Analysis of factors associated with the occurrence of low birth weight infants]. *Sangyo Ika Daigaku Zasshi* 12:53–59.

McCargar L, Simmons D, Craton N, Taunton J, Birmingham C (1993) Physiological effects of weight cycling in female lightweight rowers. *Canadian Journal of Applied Physiology* 18:291–303.

McNeely MJ, Soules MR (1988) The diagnosis of luteal phase deficiency: a critical review. *Fertility and Sterility* 50:1–9.

Meijer GAL, Westerterp KR, Saris WHM, Ten HF (1992) Sleeping metabolic rate in relation to body composition and the menstrual cycle. *American Journal of Clinical Nutrition* 55:637–640.

Merchant KS, Martorell R (1988) Frequent reproductive cycling: does it lead to nutritional depletion of mothers? *Progress in Food and Nutrition Science* 12: 339–369.

Miller JE, Rodriguez G, Pebley AR (1994) Lactation, seasonality, and mother's postpartum weight change in Bangladesh: an analysis of maternal depletion. *American Journal of Human Biology* 6:511–524.

Mora JO, Paredes B, Wagner M, Navarro L, Suescun J, Christiansen N, Herrera M (1979) Nutritional supplementation and the outcome of pregnancy, 1: birth weight. *American Journal of Clinical Nutrition* 32:455–462.

Morio B, Montaurier C, Pickering G, Ritz P, Fellmann N, Coudert J, Beaufrere B, Vermorel M (1998) Effects of 14 weeks of progressive endurance training on energy expenditure in elderly people. *British Journal of Nutrition* 80:511–519.

National Academy of Sciences (1989) *Contraception and Reproduction: Health Consequences for Women and Children in the Developing World* (Washington DC, National Academy Press).

Noakes TD, van Gend M (1988) Menstrual dysfunction in female athletes. A review for clinicians. *South African Medical Journal* 73:350–355.

Norgan NG (1997) The beneficial effects of body fat and adipose tissue in humans. *International Journal of Obesity* 21:738–746.

Panter-Brick C (1993) Seasonality and levels of energy expenditure during pregnancy and lactation for rural Nepali women. *American Journal of Clinical Nutrition* 57:620–628.

Panter-Brick C (1996) Physical activity, energy stores, and seasonal energy balance among men and women in Nepali households. *American Journal of Human Biology* 8:263–274.

Panter-Brick C, Ellison P (1994) Seasonality of workloads and ovarian function in Nepali women. *Annals of the New York Academy of Sciences* 709:234–235.

Panter-Brick C, Lotstein DS, Ellison PT (1993) Seasonality of reproductive function and weight loss in rural Nepali women. *Human Reproduction* 8:684–690.

Peacock N (1990) Comparative and cross-cultural approaches to the study of human female reproductive failure. In CJ DeRousseau (Ed) *Primate Life History and Evolution* (New York, Wiley-Liss), 195–220.

Peacock N (1991) An evolutionary perspective on the patterning of maternal investment in pregnancy. *Human Nature* 2:351–385.

Perrin N, Sibly RM (1993) Dynamic models of energy allocation and investment. *Annual Review of Ecology and Systhematics* 24:379–410.

Peterson CC, Nagy KA, Diamond J (1990) Sustained metabolic scope. *Proceedings of the National Academy of Sciences* 87:2324–2328.

Pevet P (1993) Melatonin: present and future in the reproduction function among humans and animals. *Contraception Fertilité et Sexualité* 21:727–732.

Piers LS, Diggavi SN, Thangam S, Van RJMA, Shetty PS, Hautvast JGAJ (1995) Changes in energy expenditure, anthropometry, and energy intake during the course of pregnancy and lactation in well-nourished Indian women. *American Journal of Clinical Nutrition* 61:501–513.

Poehlman ET, Horton ES (1989) The impact of food intake and exercise on energy expenditure. *Nutrition Reviews* 47:129–137.

Poppitt SD, Prentice AM, Jequier E, Schutz Y, Whitehead RG (1993) Evidence of energy sparing in Gambian women during pregnancy: a longitudinal study using whole-body calorimetry. *American Journal of Clinical Nutrition* 57:353–364.

Prentice AM (1984) Adaptations to long-term low energy intake. In *Energy Intake and Activity* (New York, Alan R. Liss), 3–31.

Prentice AM, Prentice A (1990) Maternal energy requirements to support lactation. In SA Atkinson, LA Hanson, RK Chandra (Eds) *Breastfeeding, Nutrition, Infection and Infant Growth in Developed and Emerging Countries* (St. Johns, Newfoundland, ARTS), 69–86.

Prentice AM, Whitehead RG (1987) The energetics of human reproduction. *Symposia of the Zoological Society of London* 57:275–304.

Prentice AM, Goldberg GR, Davies HL, Murgatroyd PR, Scott W (1989) Energy-sparing adaptations in human pregnancy assessed by whole-body calorimetry. *British Journal of Nutrition* 62:5–22.

Prentice AM, Poppitt SD, Goldberg GR, Prentice A (1995) Adaptive strategies regulating energy balance in human pregnancy. *Human Reproduction Update* 1:149–161.

Prentice AM, Spaaij CJK, Goldberg GR, Poppitt SD, Van RJMA, Totton M, Swann D, Black AE (1996) Energy requirements of pregnant and lactating women. *European Journal of Clinical Nutrition* 50(Suppl):S82–S111.

Prior JC (1985) Luteal phase defects and anovulation: adaptive alterations occuring with conditioning exercise. *Seminars in Reproductive Endocrinology* 3:27–33.

Roberts SB, Paul AA, Cole TJ, Whitehead RG (1982) Seasonal changes in activity, birth weight and lactational performance in rural Gambian women. *Transactions of the Royal Society of Tropical Medicine and Hygiene* 76:668–678.

Roenneberg T, Aschoff J (1990) Annual rhythm of human reproduction, II: environmental correlations. *Journal of Biological Rhythms* 5:217–240.

Rojansky N, Brzezinski A, Schenker JG (1992) Seasonality in human reproduction: an update. *Human Reproduction* 7:735–745.

Rosetta L (1993) Female reproductive dysfunction and intense physical training. *Oxford Reviews of Reproductive Biology* 15:113–141.

Saowakontha S, Pongpaew P, Schelp FP, Rojsathaporn K, Intarakha C, Pipitgool V, Mahaweerawat U, Lumbiganon P, Sriboonlue P, et al. (1992) Pregnancy, nutrition and parasitic infection of rural and urban women in Northeast Thailand. *Nutrition Research* 12:929–942.

Saris WHM, Vanerpbaart MA, Brouns F, Westerterp KR, Tenhoor F (1989) Study on food intake and energy expenditure during extreme sustained exercise: the Tour de France. *International Journal of Sports Medicine* 10:S26–S31.

Schwartz B, Cumming DC, Riordan E, Selye M, Yen SSC, Rebar RW (1981) Exercise associated amenorrhea: a distinct entity? *American Journal of Obstetrics and Gynecology* 141:662–670.

Sibly R, Calow P (1986) Costs of living. In R Sibly, P Calow (Eds) *Physiological Ecology of Animals: An Evolutionary Approach* (Oxford, Blackwell Scientific), 44–65.

Siniarska A, Antoszewska A, Dziewiecki C (1992) Urbanization and industrialization versus biological status of human populations. *Studies of Human Ecology* 10:335–358.

Sjodin AM, Forslund AH, Westerterp KR, Andersson AB, Forslund JW, Hammbraeus LH (1996) The influence of physical activity on BMR. *Medicine and Science in Sports and Exercise* 28:85–91.

Spuy VD (1985) Nutrition and reproduction. *Clinical Obstetrics and Gynaecology* 12:579–604.

Stouffer RL (1988) Perspectives on the corpus luteum of the menstrual cycle and early pregnancy. *Seminars in Reproductive Endocrinology* 6:103–113.

Stroud MA (1993) Environmental temperature and physiological function. In SJ Ulijaszek, SS Strickland (Eds) *Seasonality and Human Ecology* (Cambridge, University Press), 38–54.

Taaffle D, Pruitt L, Reim J, Butterfield G, Marcus R (1995) Effect of sustained resistance training on basal metabolic rate in older women. *Journal of the American Gerontological Society* 43:465–471.

Thomson AM, Hytten FE, Billewicz WZ (1970) The energy cost of human lactation. *British Journal of Nutrition* 24:565–572.

Townsend C, Calow P (Eds) (1981) *Physiological Ecology: An Evolutionary Approach to Resource Use* (Sunderland MA, Sinauer Associates).

Tracer DP (1991) Fertility-related changes in maternal body composition among the Au of Papua New Guinea. *American Journal of Physical Anthropology* 85:393–406.

Trayhurn P (1989) Thermogenesis and the energetics of pregnancy and lactation. *Canadian Journal of Physiology and Pharmacology* 67:370–375.

Tremblay A, Poehlman ET, Despres JP, Theriault G, Danforth E, Bouchard C (1997) Endurance training with constant energy intake in identical twins: changes over time in energy expenditure and related hormones. *Clinical and Experimental Metabolism* 46:499–503.

Ulijaszek SJ (1996) Energetics, adaptation, and adaptability. *American Journal of Human Biology* 8:169–182.

van Raaij JM, Schonk C, Vermaat MS, Peek ME, Hautvast JG (1991) Energy cost of lactation, and energy balances of well-nourished Dutch lactating women: reappraisal of the extra energy requirements of lactation. *American Journal of Clinical Nutrition* 53:612–619.

Van Zant R (1992) Influence of diet and exercise on energy expenditure—a review. *International Journal of Sports Nutrition* 2:1–19.

Veldhuis JD, Evans WS, Demers LM, Thorner MO, Wakat D, Rogol AD (1985) Altered neuroendocrine regulation of gonadotropin secretion in women distance runners. *Journal of Clinical Endocrinology and Metabolism* 61:557–563.

Vermeulen A (1993) Environment, human reproduction, menopause, and andropause. *Environmental Health Perspectives* 2:91–100.

Vitzthum V (1997) Flexibility and paradox: the nature of adaptation in human reproduction. In M Morbeck, A Galloway, A Zihlman (Eds) *The Evolving Female: A Life-history Perspective* (Princeton, Princeton University Press), 242–258.

Voland E (1998) Evolutionary ecology of human reproduction. *Annual Review of Anthropology* 27:347–374.

Warren MP (1980) The effects of exercise on pubertal progression in reproductive function in girls. *Journal of Clinical and Endocrinological Metabolism* 51:1150–1157.

Weiner J (1989) Metabolic constraints to mammalian energy budgets. *Acta Theriologica* 34:3–36.

Weiner J (1992) Physiological limits to sustainable energy budgets in birds and mammals: ecological implications. *Trends in Ecology and Evolution* 7:384–388.

Westerterp KR (1998) Alterations in energy balance with exercise. *American Journal of Clinical Nutrition* 68:S970–S974.

Westerterp KR, Meijer GAL, Saris WHM, Soeters PB, Winants Y, Ten HF (1991) Physical activity and sleeping metabolic rate. *Medicine and Science in Sports and Exercise* 23:166–170.

Westerterp KR, Meijer GAL, Schoffelen P, Janssen EME (1994) Body mass, body composition and sleeping metabolic rate before, during and after endurance training. *European Journal of Applied Physiology and Occupational Physiology* 69:203–208.

Whitehead RG, Paul AA, Black AE, Wiles SJ (1981) Recommended dietary amounts of energy for pregnancy and lactation in the United Kingdom. *United Nations University Food and Nutrition Bulletin* 5(Suppl):259–265.

Williamson DL, Kirwan JP (1997) A single bout of concentric resistance exercise increases basal metabolic rate 48 hours after exercise in healthy 59- to 77-year-old men. *Journals of Gerontology* Series A, *Biological Sciences and Medicine* 52:M352–355.

Zanker CL, Swaine IL (1998) The relationship between serum oestradiol concentration and energy balance in young women distance runners. *International Journal of Sports Medicine* 19:104–108.

Zemel B, Ulijaszek S, Leonard W (1996) Energetics, lifestyles, and nutritional adaptation: an introduction. *American Journal of Human Biology* 8:141–142.

4

Lactation, Energetics, and Postpartum Fecundity

CLAUDIA R. VALEGGIA and PETER T. ELLISON

The last two decades of the twentieth century have witnessed a dramatic growth in the field of human reproductive ecology, resulting in a better understanding of variation in human fertility patterns related to changes in ecological context. The first, and perhaps most significant, advance in this area was the recognition of the suppressive effects of lactation on post-partum fecundity. It is now well established that lactation is the major determinant of the period of postpartum infecundity. As a result of this recognition, lactation plays a preponderant role in any discussion of variation in natural fertility patterns (Wood 1994). Many studies have shown the great variety of social and physical environments in which lactation occurs, as well as the variability in the response of female reproductive physiology. However, the proximate mechanisms underlying the phenomenon of lactational infecundity are still not clear. The aim of this chapter is to summarize the information available on lactation and postpartum fecundity and to present the current debate surrounding how the suppressive effects of lactation are mediated. After a brief introduction to the costs and benefits of breastfeeding, we concentrate on the links between lactation and postpartum fecundity. A historical overview describes the context in which the current ideas evolved and sets the stage for the presentation of the two leading hypotheses aimed at identifying the proximate causes of lactational infecundity. Although focused on mechanisms, these two hypotheses also have implications for the functional interpretation of lactational amenorrhea. We conclude with the presentation of data from our research of lactating Toba women of northern Argentina as a case study that allows us to confront the predictions of the two competing hypotheses.

THE ENERGETIC COSTS OF BREASTFEEDING

As with pregnancy, the lactating mother is, at least during the exclusive breastfeeding period, "metabolizing for two." In mammals, unlike other animals, the *direct* physiological investment of the female does not finish when the infant is born. The mother continues diverting certain amounts of her own available energy to her offspring until the moment of complete weaning. If we measure this investment in terms of calories it becomes clear that the process of lactation represents a considerable energetic burden. In human females, the average energy cost of the milk produced during the period of exclusive breastfeeding is approximately 500 kcal/day. Taking into account the efficiency of conversion of dietary energy to milk energy (approximately 80%), the total average cost can be estimated as 625 kcal/day (Dewey 1997). In cases of inadequate dietary intake this could represent as much as 50% of the mother's energy budget.

In order to meet the cost of milk production, a breastfeeding woman can increase the energy intake, mobilize fat reserves, reduce her energy expenditure, or any combination of these strategies. Well-nourished lactating mothers generally increase food consumption, particularly during the early postpartum period (Goldberg et al. 1991). However, for most populations in the developing world where inadequate diets are the norm, this option is not often feasible. Mobilization of fat reserves seems to be the most utilized mechanism for meeting the cost of lactation. Although there is substantial variability, on average, lactating women lose about 500 g/month of body weight. This weight loss could be taken as an indication that body fat reserves are indeed being mobilized to support lactation (Dewey 1997; Prentice et al. 1996). The third strategy would be to decrease the energy expenditure during the exclusive breastfeeding period. This could be achieved through reductions in basal metabolic rate (BMR), dietary-induced thermogenesis (DIT), or physical activity level (PAL). The basal metabolic rate seems to be unchanged or slightly increased during lactation (Goldberg et al. 1991; Singh et al. 1989). Studies examining changes in DIT during lactation have shown mixed results. Given that DIT contributes only about 10% of the total energy expenditure, even if there were changes in DIT they could only account for a minimal proportion of the total energy balance (Dewey 1997). There is a great variation in PALs during lactation depending on the ecological context of the woman. In affluent populations, PALs are slightly lower during the early postpartum period than during the non-pregnant/non-lactating period (Dewey 1997). In contrast, little difference in activity levels among women in different reproductive states has been found in developing world populations (Guillermo-Tuazón et al. 1992; Vinoy et al. 2000). Many times, lactating women cannot afford to cut back their level of activity and, hence, their contribution to family subsistence. In sum, women in different ecological contexts seem to use different strategies to balance the energy costs of lactation. These strategies are not mutually exclusive; they can be taken as complementary ways of saving energy. Even within the same population, there seems to be a significant variability in the type of energy-saving alternative utilized (Goldberg et al. 1991).

THE BENEFITS OF BREASTFEEDING

The contributions of lactation to infant survival and maternal health are manifold. Detailed accounts of the effects of breastfeeding on maternal health have been published by others (Heinig and Dewey 1997; Stuart-Macadam 1995) and are beyond the scope of this chapter. We will briefly describe three major contributions of breastfeeding to the mother's fitness (understood here as reproductive success). The most obvious is the nutritive function of breast milk. Breasts secrete a rich, dynamic substance capable of completely nourishing an infant for the first six to nine months of life. The energy density of breast milk depends mainly on its fat and lactose content. In well-nourished populations, fat contributes about 50% of the total milk energy; milk lactose adds 40% to 45%, whereas proteins contribute the rest (Dewey 1997). Although it is difficult to obtain an accurate estimate of the energy density of breast milk, the average gross energy content is generally reported to be about 0.68–0.74 kcal/g (Prentice et al. 1996). Milk fat or lactose concentrations vary very little during lactation, but they can be affected by maternal body composition. Field studies (Brown et al. 1986; Perez-Escamilla et al. 1995; Prentice et al. 1981) revealed a positive correlation between milk fat and estimations of total maternal body fat. In populations that practice on-demand breastfeeding, infants generally compensate for differences in energy density by consuming higher or lower volumes of milk (Perez-Escamilla et al. 1995).

The second major contribution of breastfeeding to the infant's survival is the immunological protection breast milk confers, mainly during the critical initial months. Throughout the world, breastfeeding is associated with significant prevention of infant mortality and morbidity (Cunningham 1995). The infant's own immune system is not fully developed and will not be for several months. The infant relies on its mother's supply of antibodies, transferred via colostrum and breast milk, to fight viruses, bacteria, and other parasites. In addition to this form of passive protection, breast milk is also rich in regulatory substances that stimulate the development of the infant's own secretory immune system. By reducing the exposure to external pathogens (microbial or allergenic) present in other fluids or foods, breastfeeding also lowers risk of gastrointestinal infections, respiratory illnesses, bacteremia, and meningitis (Cunningham et al. 1991). In rural or marginal populations this could be crucial since people often lack the opportunities to obtain uncontaminated water necessary to prepare powdered formula. Many studies point also to the benefits of breastfeeding for the long-term development and health of the infant. As an example, there is evidence for an association between early feeding practices and coronary pathologies, disorders of immune regulation, and psychomotor development (Cunningham 1995; Lucas 1998).

The fertility-reducing effects of lactation are beneficial for both the mother and her current and future offspring. In breastfeeding mothers the return to full postpartum fecundity is usually delayed several months. By extending the interbirth interval, lactation prolongs the period during which a given child benefits from breast milk, and lactation also contributes heavily to its survival and that of its siblings. It is now well established that closely spaced births, in other words, less than 2 years apart, lead to an increased rate of infant mortality, not only of the first born child in a sequence but also of the second (Mozumder et al. 2000). For example, Hobcraft et al. (1983) found that in 13 of 23 countries, a birth in the 2 years prior to the birth of the index child increases that child's risk of dying by more than 50%. In a study conducted in Guatemala, fetal asymmetric stunting or wasting was related to short interbirth intervals (Neel and Alvarez 1991).

In addition to the disadvantages for the offspring, the mother's energy supply may be severely affected by closely spaced births. A lactating woman who becomes pregnant while her infant is still young is burdened with the task of metabolizing for three, at least until the infant is completely weaned. Trying to meet those increased energy requirements will compromise her nutritional status and have a negative impact on her own health as well as her offspring's. The "maternal depletion syndrome" was first suggested by Jelliffe and Maddocks (1964). This syndrome is characterized by a progressive reduction in the female fat reserves and lean tissue with successive births and periods of lactation. If a woman consumes only the amount of protein recommended for non-pregnant/non-lactating women, she loses about 19% of her lean tissue (Dewey 1997). This syndrome is particularly notorious in developing countries where poor nutritional states and high female workloads are the norm. The Au women of Papua New Guinea, for example, show both a short-term decline in adiposity following childbirth and a long-term fertility-related decline (Tracer 1991). Low energy reserves can lead to low birth weights (Rodriguez et al. 1991; Tontisirin et al. 1986), intrauterine growth retardation (Bhatia et al. 1984), and premature labor (Khanna et al. 1977).

From an evolutionary perspective, we can say that female physiology has been shaped by natural selection to produce a fluid that both nourishes and protects her offspring. At the same time, by exerting its contraceptive effects, lactation helps to keep sufficient time between periods of increased metabolic requirements (gestation and lactation) and, hence, contributes greatly to the female's overall reproductive success.

LACTATION AND POSTPARTUM FECUNDITY

The fact that a lactating woman was less likely to be menstruating than a non-lactating one was commonly recognized from antiquity to the eighteenth century. However, the contraceptive effect of lactation was considered little more than an "old wives' tale" by western physicians in the late nineteenth and early twentieth centuries. Clinical studies demonstrated that there was indeed a period of amenorrhea following parturition, but it was not clear whether it was a refractory effect of gestation or a direct effect of lactation (Gioiosa 1955; McKeown and Gibson 1954; Sharman 1951).

In 1961, the French demographer Louis Henry published a seminal paper focused on the natural variation in human fertility and the proximate causes of that variation. An important hallmark of his work is that he turned attention away from *sociological* explanations and proposed *physiological* causes of variation in natural fertility. In his analysis, he found that the period of postpartum subfecundity was highly variable among populations, but that the current sociological explanations that implied postpartum sexual taboos in traditional societies could not account for that variability. He suggested that variation in the resumption of ovulation after childbirth might be the most important source of variation in interbirth intervals. The evidence available at that time indicated that women who lost a child at birth, and therefore never breast-fed, resumed menstruation earlier than those who did breast-feed. With that evidence in mind, Henry reckoned that the practice of lactation might be related, by some unknown mechanism, to the resumption of postpartum ovulation. However, he also recognized that the relationship between lactation and resumption of ovulation was not a simple one. He proposed that understanding the physiological factors that govern that relationship could "help us to understand why there exist among populations such variability in natural fertility" (Henry 1961).

The "Nursing Intensity" Hypothesis

Describing the proximate mechanisms that could account for the variation in the duration of lactational amenorrhea became a central problem for testing Henry's hypothesis. Reproductive biologists interested in solving this puzzle faced two different but intimately related problems: finding the neuroendocrine pathways that link the physiology of lactation with the physiology of reproduction, and finding what "observable" component of lactation was responsible for its suppressive effects on female fecundity. The first quest proved to be a difficult one, and to date a clear understanding of the neuroendocrine control of lactational infecundity remains elusive.

Early studies on the matter focused attention on *prolactin* as the primary hormone suppressing ovarian function. From clinical research, it was known that a pathological condition by which prolactin levels in blood are excessive was associated with ovarian dysfunction. Hyperprolactinemia is often treated with bromocriptine, a dopamine agonist that inhibits prolactin. This treatment causes a reduction in prolactin levels and a resumption of normal ovarian cycles (Robyn et al. 1976; Sartorio et al. 2000). Other studies with nursing women showed considerably high levels of prolactin throughout the period of amenorrhea and decreasing levels about the time of resumption of menses (Delvoye et al. 1976; Howie and McNeilly 1982; Wood et al. 1985). Tyson (1977) analyzed changes in prolactin levels in much more detail. Within minutes of the infant latching on to the nipple, prolactin levels increase dramatically. Then, soon after the infant stops nursing, prolactin levels slowly drop. Tyson's data suggested that the temporal pattern of suckling could be of importance in unmasking the link between lactation and ovarian function. A mother nursing her infant with sufficient frequency could maintain high levels of prolactin, which, in turn, could inhibit ovarian function.

The actual mechanism by which prolactin could suppress ovarian function remained unclear, despite the enthusiasm that this idea generated. In vitro studies performed by McNatty and colleagues (1974) indicated that high levels of prolactin in cultured granulosa cells were associated with a reduced ability of each cell to produce estradiol and with an inhibition in the secretion of progesterone. This study was strongly criticized, among other reasons, because prolactin receptors could not be found on granulosa cells (McNeilly et al. 1982). In recent years the contraceptive role of prolactin was called into question by several studies (McNeilly 1993; Schallenberger et al. 1981). As a result, it is now believed that prolactin is not directly involved in the system linking lactation and ovarian quiescence. Other mechanisms are being explored, most of them centered on the factors that might affect the pulsatile secretion of Gn-RH from the hypothalamus (Wood 1994). The current view of the neuroendocrine control of lactational infecundity is highly speculative, and more research is expected to settle some controversial relationships.

At another level of analysis, researchers began to investigate which aspects of the mechanics of lactation were associated with the period of amenorrhea. At the time when prolactin was the best candidate as suppressor of ovarian activity, Delvoye et al. (1977) presented data from a natural fertility population in Zaire providing evidence of the relationship between nursing frequency and prolactin levels. In their study, prolactin levels in mothers who nursed three times a day or less fell within the rage of values typical of non-pregnant, non-lactating women within six months. In contrast, prolactin levels in women who nursed six times a day or more were three times higher at six months. In 1980, Konner and Worthman published their study of nursing patterns and ovarian function among the!Kung San of the Kalahari Desert. !Kung San mothers nursed their infants very frequently, averaging 4 bouts per hour. Nursing bouts lasted, on average, 2 minutes, and they were separated by 13 minutes. This high frequency was maintained for the first two years of the infant's life. They inferred that such an intensive pattern would maintain high prolactin levels (although these were never measured), which in turn would exert a suppressive effect on the mother's fecundity, accounting for the 44-month interval between births. These results, coupled with Tyson's analysis, pointed to the centrality of the temporal arrangement of suckling events for modulating ovarian function.

So important appeared to be the choreography of nursing that it served as the basis for the postulation of a major hypothesis aimed at explaining the fertility-reducing effects of lactation. This hypothesis proposes that the "intensity" of nursing is a major controller of the duration of lactational infecundity. Although hard to operationalize initially, the intensity of nursing was then defined as a combined measure of suckling frequency, duration of the suckling bout, and total duration of nursing. The evidence suggested that either a high frequency of nursing or few nursing episodes of long duration were effective in preventing ovulation. Perhaps the most influential study that focused on this issue was the one conducted by McNeilly, Howie, and colleagues at the University of Edinburgh (Glasier et al. 1983; Howie et al. 1982a, 1982b; McNeilly et al. 1982). The researchers followed 27 breastfeeding mothers and 10 women who bottle-fed their infants from birth. Urine samples were collected weekly for estimation of estradiol and progesterone. Every two weeks, blood samples were collected for determination of prolactin levels. The results indicated that nursing behavior and ovarian function were indeed associated. Those mothers who resumed ovulation during the period of lactation (13 of 27) had reduced nursing frequency to less than 6 bouts/day, total nursing time to less than 60 minutes/day, and had introduced at least two supplementary feeds per day. The authors stressed the importance of the timing of introduction of supplementary feeds as starting point of the changes in nursing behavior and reproductive physiology. They argued that when supplements are introduced, women change their breastfeeding behavior to a pattern of less frequent, shorter nursing episodes. This, in turn, leads to decreasing levels of prolactin, which allowed the resumption of fecundity.

Data from many field studies of natural fertility populations around the world appeared to support the nursing intensity hypothesis (Jones 1989; Panter-Brick 1991; Vitzthum 1989; Wood et al. 1985). The idea was enthusiastically accepted by biological anthropologists and demographers alike, as it seemed to answer Henry's old question about the variation in fertility patterns. According to the nursing intensity hypothesis, variation in the duration of lactational infecundity can be interpreted to reflect the wide diversity in nursing behavior across populations: the more intensive the breastfeeding, the longer the impact on fertility. Women in the developing world, with patterns of on-demand breastfeeding, would have longer periods of lactational amenorrhea than women in industrialized societies where breastfeeding, if practiced at all, was much more structured, with long interbout intervals. The nursing intensity hypothesis seemed to make evolutionary as well as demographic sense. Short (1987) argued that, in our formative past, nursing patterns would have been very intensive. Infants would have nursed very frequently, until other foods were introduced. The reduction in nursing intensity as the baby fed on other foods would have been interpreted by the mother's body as a green light for resumption of ovarian activity: "your infant can survive on solids now, it is safe to get pregnant again." Lactation was favored by natural selection, among other things, as a mechanism to prevent dangerously close birth intervals.

The "Metabolic Load" Hypothesis

The nursing intensity hypothesis held strong until quite recently a number of contradictory results began to accumulate. The first assumption to be questioned was the validity of the physiological bases of that hypothesis. Prolactin per se cannot be considered the cause of reproductive suppression. Furthermore, recent data indicate that prolactin levels do not reflect nursing frequency as tightly as was previously thought. No clear correlation could be found between nursing bouts and prolactin profiles in a study that involved 24-hour video monitoring and blood sampling of nursing mothers housed in a clinical research unit (Tay et al. 1996). There is evidence that prolactin could be maintained at either relatively high (Stallings et al. 1996) or low (Tay et al. 1996) levels without acute response to nursing. Although these findings remove prolactin from its originally leading role, it is quite clear that it is indirectly associated with the period of lactational amenorrhea. Postpartum prolactin levels could be taken as a marker for a physiological state that leads to amenorrhea. Other field studies also pointed to problems with the nursing intensity hypothesis (Peng et al. 1998; Tracer 1991; Worthman et al. 1993). In these studies, the frequency or the duration of the nursing bout was not predictive of the duration of lactational amenorrhea. It was evident that the variation in the temporal pattern of nursing left a great part of the observed variation in the duration of lactational amenorrhea unaccounted for.

Several studies suggested that maternal condition might be associated with significant variation in the duration of lactational infecundity (for a review see Ellison 1995).[1] Huffman and colleagues (1987) reported the relationship among nutrition, breastfeeding, and postpartum amenorrhea in women of Matlab, Bangladesh. In their sample, women with poor nutritional status in the first months postpartum resume menses later (at 20.2 months) than those showing a better nutritional status (at 15.5 months). Data from another impressive longitudinal study conducted in The Gambia also suggested that maternal energetics play an important role in the resumption of postpartum fecundity (Lunn et al. 1984). In this study, maternal dietary supplementation during pregnancy and lactation, and during lactation alone, was associated with a decrease in the duration of lactational amenorrhea relative to that observed in mothers who did not receive dietary supplements.

In light of these findings, an alternative explanation for the great variation in the duration of lactational amenorrhea can be proposed (Lunn 1992; Ellison 1995, 2001). The argument behind this new hypothesis is that the intensity of suckling reflects the energetic stress that lactation represents for the mother. The attention is now shifted from the suckling stimulus per se to the *relative metabolic load* of lactation, in other words, the proportion of the mother's energy budget that is devoted to milk production. In this context, the variable effects of lactation on postpartum fertility may depend on the relative metabolic burden that lactation poses on the mother. The higher the relative metabolic load of lactation, the longer the period of lactational infecundity. Maternal condition would then contribute to the contraceptive effects of lactation. Lactation would represent a higher relative metabolic load for poorly nourished mothers than for well-nourished ones. Exclusively breastfeeding a young infant poses a higher metabolic stress than breastfeeding an older baby who had begun to be fed on semi-solids or solids.

Comparing Hypotheses

The metabolic load hypothesis explains the previous findings on the contraceptive role of lactation as well as the nursing intensity hypothesis. However, a problem soon becomes evident when one tries to differentiate the predictions of the two hypotheses. Under most circumstances, nursing

intensity is a strong predictor of relative metabolic load. Hence, the principal explanatory variables are often confounded. Available data come
mainly from two different settings: clinical studies and field studies. The
clinical studies provided information on the response of mainly well-
nourished women practicing some form of scheduled nursing (Diaz et al.
1988; Heinig et al. 1994). In these women, the mean duration of lactational
amenorrhea is relatively short (6.3 months). The explanation provided by
the nursing intensity hypothesis seems satisfactory: there is an early
resumption of ovarian activity because nursing frequency is low and/or
the intervals between nursing bouts are long. The metabolic load hypothesis would also be valid since the shorter period of amenorrhea might be
the result of a lesser energetic stress that lactation implies for women in
good nutritional status. Studies conducted among traditional societies (see
Ellison 1995 for a review) usually show the other extreme—the period of
lactational amenorrhea in poorly nourished women practicing intense
nursing is relatively long (mean = 20 months). Again, both hypotheses
explain the results equally well.

The vast majority of studies published to date focused on breastfeeding
women that were either (a) well-nourished with low nursing intensity
(clinical studies) or (b) undernourished with high nursing intensity (field
studies). In order to confront the predictions of the two hypotheses, we
would need to study women for whom both nursing intensity and energy
availability are high, or vice versa. We are currently working with one of
those populations. In 1997, we started the Toba Reproductive Ecology
Study in the province of Formosa, Argentina. The communities we are currently working with provide an excellent opportunity for evaluating the
factors affecting the duration of lactational amenorrhea.

LACTATIONAL AMENORRHEA AMONG TOBA WOMEN

The Toba are one of eight ethnic groups currently inhabiting the Argentine
Chaco (Braunstein and Miller 1999; Martinez Sarasola 1992). Originally
seminomadic hunter-gatherers, many groups moved to urban and periur-
ban environments during the past fifty years. These communities depend
mainly on the wage labor of men, but most aspects of their traditional life
remain deeply rooted.

We are conducting our studies in the village of Namqom, located 11 km
north of the city of Formosa (58° 12' W, 28° 10' S). Approximately 2,500
people are distributed in a 100-hectare area. Men are temporarily hired as
construction workers in Formosa city or by development programs in the
village. Women's activities include household chores, child caretaking,
and basket weaving. A few women are employed temporarily as cooks,

teaching assistants, or health agents. Some women go to the city once a week to sell their weavings or medicinal herbs door-to-door.

Namqom has relatively good access to health services, mainly provided by the local health center and the city's hospitals. Women receive free pre- and postnatal care and they are taken to the city hospital for delivery. Family-planning programs are not promoted in this area. Consequently, less than 5% of women use contraceptive methods (mainly oral contra- ceptives, when they are available at the health center). Complete family size for women in Namqom averages 7.8 (± 1.2), and the mean interbirth interval is 24.8 months (± 6.8). Infant mortality is high, with 14% of chil- dren born dying before their second birthday. Breastfeeding is almost uni- versal. Toba women breast-feed their children until they are 2–3 years of age, or until the next pregnancy. Cosleeping also allows for on-demand nighttime nursing.

We conducted an observational study of the nursing behavior of 32 mothers, whose babies ranged from 2 to 20 months of age (Valeggia and Ellison 1998). Each mother-infant pair was observed for two 4-hour peri- ods (one in the morning and another in the afternoon) separated by a month interval. Nursing activity was recorded to the nearest second. Although nursing practices can still be considered "on demand," we found a wide variation in the temporal arrangement of nursing periods. Overall, regardless of age of the infant and time of the day, the frequency of nursing events (periods when the infant was on the nipple) averaged 3.1 (± 1.9) per hour (Figure 4.1a). There was little variation in frequency of nursing during the first year of life; afterwards, it declined slowly. On average, the duration of nursing events did not change with age either (Figure 4.1b). The overall mean duration of nursing events was 2.3 (± 2.1) minutes. Note that these indices of nursing intensity are close to those

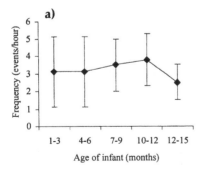
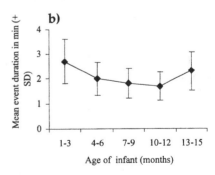

Figure 4.1. Mean frequency of nursing events (*a*) and mean duration of nursing events (*b*) for a sample of 70 lactating Toba women.

originally reported for the !Kung (Konner and Worthman 1980). Preliminary results of a follow-up study that involved 70 mother-infant pairs also
show an intense practice of nursing with high variability in the temporal
pattern among mother-infant pairs and little change in nursing frequency
during the first nine months of life.

Toba mothers offer semisolid supplements at 6 to 9 months of age. This
is a very gradual process—it generally starts with some broth or soup
given during the only structured meal of the day. They offer solid snacks
(bread, *torta frita*) only when the baby can sit by itself. The use of bottles
and commercial formula was uncommon until very recently.

Lactating Toba women in Namqom are in a state of high energy availability. The typical diet for Namqom villagers is quite monotonous. Early
in the morning they prepare *mate*, an herbal infusion typical of the region.
Later in the morning women and children may have a cup of sugared milk
with a roll of white bread or a round of *"torta frita,"* a flour patty fried in
oil or lard. The *"comida,"* the only structured meal of the day, typically con-
sists of a noodle or rice soup with onions, potatoes, manioc, and yams. In
higher income families the soup also contains beef and tomato sauce. During the afternoon and evening, they snack on pieces of bread or *torta frita*.
When they can afford it, they incorporate bananas, tangerines, and grape-
fruit. In general, this diet is highly caloric, very rich in complex carbohydrates and fat, and poor in proteins, iron, and essential micronutrients.

The energy expenditure of Toba women is low to moderate as suggested by behavioral observations of daily activity patterns of 70 lactating
women. Women spend most of the day in low energy activities; for example, 70% of daytime was spent sitting while washing clothes, breastfeeding, taking care of the infant, or simply chatting. Only 2% of their time was
spent in energetically demanding activities such as chopping wood, carrying loads of water or firewood, or walking long distances.

As a result of a relatively high calorie intake and low energy expenditure, women appear to be well nourished. Table 4.1 shows mean body
mass index (BMI = weight/height^2) by time postpartum for a group of lactating women. The values indicate that most women are heavy for their
height, according to international standards. Only two women in our
sample of 120 lactating mothers approached the value of 18.5 kg/m^2,
below which an adult is considered undernourished. The BMI values also
show that there is no change with time postpartum, which would indicate
drainage of maternal fat reserves. Measures of body fat, arm circumference, and skinfold thickness also follow the same trend, suggesting that
most of these women have high energy availability.

What would the current hypotheses predict for women in Namqom in
terms of the duration of lactational amenorrhea? Given the sustained,
intense pattern of nursing, the "nursing intensity" hypothesis would pre-

Table 4.1.   Body Mass Index of Toba Breastfeeding Women during the First 20 Months Postpartum

Month Postpartum	N	Mean BMI	s.d.	Range
0	35	26.3	3.0	19.0–32.5
1	57	26.0	3.6	18.8–33.8
2	60	26.0	3.7	18.0–33.0
3	66	25.6	3.6	17.7–33.2
4	62	25.6	4.1	17.7–37.5
5	59	25.1	4.1	17.8–37.8
6	68	25.4	4.5	17.6–37.6
7	60	25.5	4.0	17.8–35.0
8	73	25.5	4.3	17.5–35.3
9	54	26.1	4.5	17.5–36.3
10	63	25.4	4.5	18.0–36.8
11	51	25.6	4.5	18.2–36.6
12	54	25.9	4.4	18.8–36.9
13	40	25.6	4.8	16.9–37.0
14	42	26.6	5.0	18.9–37.9
15	32	26.2	4.3	18.6–37.3
16	29	26.2	3.8	20.2–35.1
17	24	26.1	4.4	18.9–36.3
18	18	26.3	4.5	19.8–37.1
19	13	25.6	5.3	19.0–37.3
20	32	25.0	4.7	18.3–37.4

dict a *long* period of lactational amenorrhea. According to the "metabolic load" hypothesis, however, given the high energy availability we should expect a *shorter* period of lactational amenorrhea. A survival analysis based on data from 120 women revealed a mean duration of lactational amenorrhea of 9.8 ± 4.0 months—from birth of an infant to the reported date of first postpartum menses (Figure 4.2). That is a relatively short period of lactational amenorrhea compared with most traditional populations practicing intensive breastfeeding. Furthermore, a preliminary analysis of the temporal pattern of nursing and the return to postpartum fecundity indicates that there is no association between these variables. Even within the same population, the effect of maternal condition on postpartum fecundity seems apparent. Older women, who also have higher parity, tend to have longer periods of amenorrhea than younger ones. Women who were 35 years old or more had an average period of lactational amenorrhea of 12.1 months (±5.4, $n = 12$). For the intermediate age category (20 to 34 years old) the mean was 9.7 months (±4.2, $n = 60$), while teenagers (14 to 19 years old) averaged 9.0 months (±3.9, $n = 36$).

In order to examine the hormonal milieu associated with the return to postpartum fecundity in these women, we are currently analyzing urine

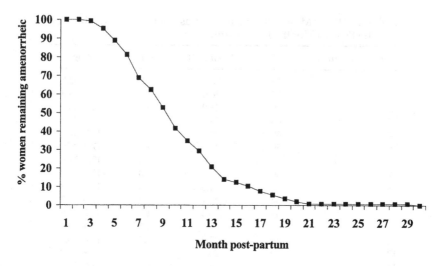

Figure 4.2. Survival curve representing percentage of breastfeeding women still amenorrheic by time postpartum.

samples collected weekly from 70 lactating Toba women. These samples are being analyzed for estrogen and progesterone metabolites (E1C and PdG, respectively), prolactin, and c-peptide (a metabolite of insulin). There is mounting evidence showing that insulin plays a crucial role in the integration between energy homeostasis and female reproductive physiology (Brüning et al. 2000; Burks et al. 2000). In addition to its well-known metabolic effects, insulin appears to modulate ovarian function (Franks et al. 1999; Wu et al. 2000) and has been shown to increase gonadotropin-stimulated gonadal steroid production (Poretsky et al. 1999). The association between insulin metabolism and the maturation of the HPO axis during human puberty has been well described (Caprio 1999; Moran et al. 1999). However, the postpartum changes in insulin levels that can be associated with the return to fecundity in women remain virtually unexplored.

Preliminary analyses of urine samples from 70 breastfeeding Toba women indicate that levels of urinary c-peptide increase steadily with time during the first year postpartum (Figure 4.3, $r = 0.94$). In addition, there seems to be a clear difference in insulin metabolism between women who resume menses early (3–6 months postpartum) and those who resume later (12–18 months postpartum). Women with short periods of lactational amenorrhea are characterized by lower c-peptide levels throughout lactation than are women who resume menstruation later. Women with longer periods of amenorrhea also display a drop in insulin values prior to resumption of menses, a pattern that is visible in a plot of aggregate data aligned on date of first postpartum menstruation (Figure 4.4). This pattern

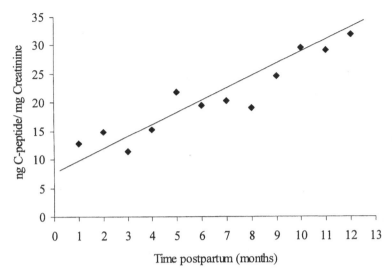

Figure 4.3. Concentration of urinary C-peptide (corrected by creatinine) during the first 12 months postpartum.

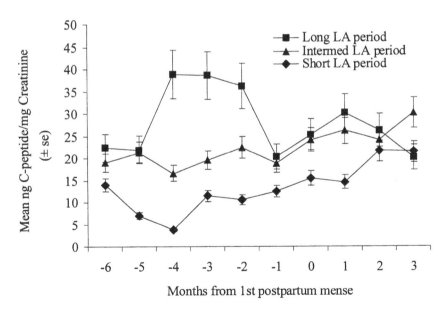

Figure 4.4. Mean concentration of urinary C-peptide (corrected by creatinine) aligned by date of first postpartum menstruation in women with relatively short (3–6 mo, *n* = 15), average (6–12 mo, *n* = 39), and long periods of lactational amenorrhea (12–18 mo, *n* = 16).

may reflect temporary insulin resistance among women with longer durations of amenorrhea, perhaps related to higher levels of prolactin (Bauman et al. 1982; Flint 1985; McNamara 1995). By combining an analysis of physiological markers of energy metabolism with indices of reproductive axis activity and behavioral observations of nursing behavior we hope to be in a position to evaluate the nursing intensity hypothesis and relative metabolic load hypothesis in the Toba context.

In sum, lactating women in Namqom represent one of the rarely reported cases of high nutritional status/intensive nursing populations that could serve to distinguish the intensity of nursing from the metabolic load hypothesis. For well-nourished Toba women, the metabolic cost of lactation represents less of a load than for women with low energy availability. Regardless of the intensity of the nursing pattern, these women can afford (in terms of energy) to shorten the period between lactation and the next gestation. Their physiology is responding to a local ecological context that allows them to meet (and even surpass) the energy requirements of lactation, gestation, and survival. Despite a nursing frequency nearly as high as that of the !Kung, they achieve fertility rates almost as high as those of the Hutterites (Eaton and Mayer 1953). Further analysis of energy metabolism in relation to the resumption of ovarian function, will provide insights into the mechanisms of fecundity regulation.

CONCLUSION

The proximate causes of the contraceptive effect of lactation are still a matter of productive debate. Although the metabolic load hypothesis is gaining increasing empirical support, the original appeal of the nursing intensity hypothesis seems to persist. Unfortunately, when two competing hypotheses get about equal support, they tend to be polarized. It should be stressed that the metabolic load hypothesis does not negate the importance of the suckling stimulus. Both hypotheses agree that lactation is the major determinant of the period of postpartum infecundity. In fact, when the breastfeeding woman's energetic budget is limited (for example, under malnutrition or under high energetic output), the intensity of lactation can be taken as a proxy for the relative cost of lactation for that woman.

From an evolutionary perspective, both hypotheses would agree that natural selection seems to have favored a mechanism (via lactation) to reduce the probability of dangerously close births. The nursing intensity hypothesis, as mentioned before, argues that in our formative past, infants had continuous access to the breast and breast-fed on demand day and night. The high frequency with which a young, unsupplemented baby would suckle would be the signal for suppressing the mother's reproductive system. As the baby becomes older, nursing frequency declines, which allows optimum birth intervals. The problem with this argument is that it rests on the assumption that there is no constraint on the feeding schedule of the infant. Populations differ widely in both the physical and the social environment in which lactation occurs. As a consequence, we find an enormous variation in nursing behavior depending on work schedules, presence of other children, social pressure to breast-feed or not, and individual maternal temperament. Temporal nursing patterns, then, may be a poor signal for the optimal resumption of postpartum fecundity. Not only might nursing intensity not be a simple reflection of infant demand, it would not reflect the relative burden on the mother of meeting that demand.

In contrast, a mechanism that relied on monitoring the energy available to the woman for resuming postpartum fecundity would make much more evolutionary sense. This mechanism would help to regulate the female's reproductive effort in the long term as well as the short term. We assume that natural selection would favor mechanisms that optimize the allocation of energy in reproductive effort. Given the costs of pregnancy and lactation, and for the many reasons iterated above, a female should not attempt to conceive again if her energy balance is poor. On the other hand, when her energy balance becomes positive, another reproductive attempt becomes feasible.

There is no longer any doubt that lactation exerts a powerful suppressing effect on postpartum fecundity and, consequently, on fertility in noncontracepting populations. A better understanding of the regulation of postpartum fecundity will come with further research into the interface between energy metabolism and reproductive physiology.

This work is supported by funds from The Nestlé Foundation, the National Institute of Child Health and Development, the David Rockefeller Center for Latin American Studies at Harvard University, the Wenner-Gren Foundation, and the National Scientific and Technological Research Council of Argentina (CONICET).

NOTE

1. Maternal condition is here taken as an umbrella term that reflects the energy available to the mother and generally involves such measures as maternal energy balance and nutritional status.

REFERENCES

Bauman DE, Eisenman JH, Currie WB (1982) Hormonal effects on partitioning of nutrients for tissue growth: role of growth hormone and prolactin. *Federation Proceedings* 41:2538–2544.

Bhatia BD, Agarwal KN, Jain NP, Bhargava V (1984) Growth pattern of intrauterine growth retarded (IUGR) babies in first nine months of life. *Acta Paediatrica Scandanavica* 73:189–196.

Braunstein JA, Miller E (1999) Ethnohistorical introduction. In E Miller (Ed) *Peoples of the Gran Chaco* (Westport CT, Bergin & Garvey).

Brown KH, Robertson AD, Akhtar HA, Ahmed MG (1986) Lactational capacity of marginally nourished mothers: relationships between maternal nutritional status and quantity and proximate composition of milk. *Pediatrics* 78:909–919.

Brüning JC, Gautam D, Burks D, Gillette J, Schubert M, Orban PC, Klein R, Krone W, Müller-Wieland D, Kahn C R (2000) Role of brain insulin receptor in control of body weight and reproduction. *Science* 289:2122–2125.

Burks D, Font de Mora J, Schubert M, Withers DJ, Myers MG, Towery HH, Altamuro SL, Flint CL, White, MF (2000) IRS-2 pathways integrate female reproduction and energy homeostasis. *Nature* 407:377–382.

Caprio, S (1999) Insulin: the other anabolic hormone of puberty. *Acta Paediatrica* (Suppl) 433:84–87.

Cunningham AS (1995) Adaptive behavior for child health and longevity In P Stuart-Macadam, KA Dettwyler (Eds) *Breastfeeding: Biocultural Perspectives* (New York, Aldine de Gruyter), 243–264.

Cunningham, AS, Jelliffe, DB, Jelliffe, EFP (1991) Breastfeding and health in the 1980s: a global epidemiologic review. *Journal of Paediatrics* 118:659–666.

Delvoye P, Delogne-Desnoeck J, Robyn C (1976) Serum prolactin in long-lasting amenorrhea. *Lancet* 2:288.

Delvoye P, Demaegd M, Delogne-Desnoeck J, Robyn C (1977) The influence of the frequency of nursing and of previous lactation experience on serum prolactin in lactating mothers. *Journal of Biosocial Science* 9:447–451.

Dewey, KG (1997) Energy and protein requirements during lactation. *Annual Review of Nutrition* 17:19–36.

Diaz S, Miranda P, Brandeis A, Cárdenas H, Croxatto HB (1988) A study on the feasibility of suppressing ovarian activity following the end of postpartum amenorrhea by increasing the frequency of suckling. *Clinical Endocrinology* 28:525–535.

Eaton SB, Mayer AJ (1953) The social biology of very high fertility among the Hutterites: the demography of a unique population. *Human Biology* 25:206–264.

Ellison PT (1995) Breastfeeding, fertility, and maternal condition. In P Stuart-Macadam, KA Dettwyler (Eds) *Breastfeeding: Biocultural Perspectives* (New York, Aldine de Gruyter), 305–345.

Ellison PT (2001) *On Fertile Ground* (Cambridge MA, Harvard University Press).

Flint DJ (1985) Role of insulin and the insulin receptor in nutrient partitioning between the mammary gland and adipose tissue. *Biochemical Society Transactions* 13:828–829.

Franks S, Gilling-Smith C, Watson H, Willis D (1999) Insulin action in the normal and polycystic ovary. *Endocrinology and Metabolism Clinics of North America* 28:361–368.

Gioiosa R (1955) Incidence of pregnancy during lactation in 500 cases. *American Journal of Obstetrics and Gynecology* 70:162–174.

Glasier A, McNeilly AS, Howie PW (1983) Fertility after childbirth: changes in serum gonadotrophin levels in bottle and breast feeding women. *Clinical Endocrinology* 19:493–501.

Goldberg GR, Prentice AM, Coward WA, Davies HL, Murgatroyd PR et al. (1991) Longitudinal assessment of the components of energy balance in well-nourished lactating women. *American Journal of Clinical Nutrition* 54:788–798.

Guillermo-Tuazón MA, Barba CV, van Raaij JM, Hautvast JG (1992) Energy intake, energy expenditure, and body composition of poor rural Philippine women throughout the first 6 mo of lactation. *American Journal of Clinical Nutrition* 56:874–880.

Henry L (1961) Some data on natural fertility. *Eugenics Quarterly* 8:81–91.

Heinig MJ, Dewey KG (1997) Health effects of breast feeding for mothers: a critical review. *Nutrition Research Reviews* 10:35–56.

Heinig MJ, Nommsen-Rivers LA, Peerson JM, Dewey K (1994) Factors related to duration of postpartum amenorrhoea among USA women with prolonged lactation. *Journal of Biosocial Science* 26:517–527.

Hobcraft J, McDonald JW, Rutstein S (1983) Child-spacing effects on infant and early child mortality. *Population Index* 49:585–618.

Howie PW, McNeilly AS (1982) Effect of breast feeding patterns on human birth intervals. *Journal of Reproduction and Fertility* 65:545–557.

Howie PW, McNeilly AS, Houston MJ, Cook A, Boyle H (1982a) Fertility after childbirth: infant feeding patterns, basal PRL levels and post-partum ovulation. *Clinical Endocrinology* 17:315–322.

Howie PW, McNeilly AS, Houston MJ, Cook A, Boyle H (1982b) Fertility after childbirth: post-partum ovulation and menstruation in bottle and breast feeding mothers. *Clinical Endocrinology* 17:323–332.

Huffmann SL, Chwodhury A, Allen H, Nahar L (1987) Suckling patterns and post-partum amenorrhea in Bangladesh. *Journal of Biosocial Science* 19:171–179.

Jelliffe DB, Maddocks I (1964) Notes on the ecologic malnutrition in the New Guinea highlands. *Clinical Pediatrics* 3:432–438.

Jones RE (1989) Breastfeeding and post-partum amenorrhea in Indonesia. *Journal of Biosocial Science* 21:83–100.

Khanna S, Agarwal KN, Murthy LS (1977) Placental histological changes in maternal undernutrition. *Indian Journal of Medical Research* 66:429–434.

Konner M, Worthman C (1980) Nursing frequency, gonadal function, and birth spacing among !Kung hunter-gatherers. *Science* 207:788–791.

Lucas A (1998) Programming by early nutrition: an experimental approach. *Journal of Nutrition* 128:S401–S406.

Lunn PG (1992) Breastfeeding patterns, maternal milk output and lactational infecundity. *Journal of Biosocial Science* 24:317–324.

Lunn PG, Austin S, Prentice AM, Whitehead RG (1984) The effect of improved nutrition on plasma prolactin concentrations and postpartum infertility in lactating Gambian women. *American Journal of Clinical Nutrition* 39:227–253.

Martinez Sarasola C (1992) *Nuestros paisanos los Indios: Vida, Historia y Destino de las comunidades indígenas en la Argentina* (Buenos Aires, Emecé Editores).

McKeown T, Gibson JR (1954) A note on the menstruation and conception during lactation. *Journal of Obstetrics and Gynaecology* 61:824–829.

McNamara JP (1995) Role and regulation of metabolism in adipose tissue during lactation. *Journal of Nutritional Biochemistry* 6:120–129.

McNatty KP, Sawers RS, McNeilly AS (1974) A possible role for prolactin in control of steroid secretion by the human Graafian follicle. *Nature* 250:653–655.

McNeilly AS (1993) Breastfeeding and fertility. In RH Gray, H Leirdon, A Spira (Eds) *Biomedical and Demographic Determinants of Reproduction* (Oxford, Clarendon Press).

McNeilly AS, Howie PW, Houston PJ, Cook A, Boyle H (1982) Fertility after childbirth: adequacy of postpartum luteal phases. *Clinical Endocrinology* 17:609–615.

Moran A, Jacobs DR, Steinberger J, Hong CP, Prineas R, Luepker R, Sinaiko AR (1999) Insulin resistance during puberty. *Diabetes* 48:2039–2044.

Mozumder AB, Barkat-E-Khuda, Kane TT, Levin A, Ahmed S (2000) The effect of birth interval on malnutrition in Bangladeshi infants and young children. *Journal of Biosocial Science* 32:289–300.

Neel NR, Alvarez JO (1991) Maternal risk factors for low birth weight and intrauterine growth retardation in a Guatemalan population. *Bulletin of the Pan-American Health Organization* 25:152–165.

Panter-Brick C (1991) Lactation, birth spacing and maternal work-loads among two castes in rural Nepal. *Journal of Biosocial Science* 23:137–154.

Peng YK, Hight-Laukaran V, Peterson AE, Perez-Escamilla R (1998) Maternal nutritional status is inversely associated with lactational amenorrhea in Sub-Saharan Africa: results from demographic and health surveys II and III. *Journal of Nutrition* 128:1672–1680.

Perez-Escamilla R, Cohen RJ, Brown KH, Landa Rivera L, Canahuati J, Dewey KG (1995) Maternal anthropometric status and lactation performance in a low-income Honduran population: evidence for the role of infants. *American Journal of Clinical Nutrition* 61:528–534.

Poretsky L, Cataldo NA, Rosenwaks Z, Giudice LC (1999) The insulin-related ovarian regulatory system in health and disease. *Endocrine Reviews* 20:535–582.

Prentice A, Prentice AM, Whitehead R G (1981) Breast-milk fat concentrations of rural African women, 2: long-term variations within a community. *British Journal of Nutrition* 45:495–503.

Prentice AM, Spaaij CJK, Goldberg GR, Poppitt SD, van Raaij JMA, Totton M, Swann D, Black AE (1996) Energy requirements of pregnant and lactating women. *European Journal of Clinical Nutrition* 50(Suppl 1):S82–S111.

Robyn C, Devoye C, Van Exter M, Vekemans A, Caufriez P, de Nayer J, Delogne-Desnoeck J, L'Hermite M (1976) Physiological and pharmacological factors influiencing prolactin secretion and their relation to human reproduction. In PG Crosignani, C Robyn (Eds), *Prolactin and Human Reproduction* (New York, Academic Press), 71–96.

Rodriguez OT, Szarfarc SC, Benicio MH (1991) Maternal anemia and malnutrition, and their relation to birth weight. *Revista Saude Publica* 25:193–197.

Sartorio A, Pizzocaro A, Liberati D, De Nicolao G, Veldhuis JD, Faglia G (2000) Abnormal LH pulsatility in women with hyperprolactinaemic amenorrhoea normalizes after bromocriptine treatment: deconvolution-based assessment. *Clinical Endocrinology* 52:703–712.

Schallenberger E, Richardson DW, Knobil E (1981) Role of prolactin in the lactational amenorrhea of the rhesus monkey *(Macaca mulatta)*. *Biology of Reproduction* 25:370–374.

Sharman A (1951) Menstruation after childbirth. *Journal of Obstetrics and Gynaecology* 58:440–445.

Short R (1987) The biological basis for the contraceptive effects of breastfeeding. *International Journal of Gynaecology and Obstetrics* 25(Suppl):207–217.

Singh J, Prentice AM, Diaz E, Coward WA, Ashford J, Sawyer M, Whitehead RG (1989) Energy expenditure of Gambian women during peak agricultural activity measured by the doubly-labelled water method. *British Journal of Nutrition* 62:315–329.

Stallings JF, Worthman CM, Panter-Brick C, Coates R J (1996) Prolactin response to suckling and maintenance of postpartum amenorrhea among intensively breastfeeding Nepali women. *Endocrine Research* 22:1–28.

Stuart-Macadam P (1995) Biocultural Perspectives on Breastfeeding. In P Stuart-Macadam, KA Dettwyler (Eds), *Breastfeeding: Biocultural Perspectives* (New York, Aldine de Gruyter), 75–99.

Tontisirin K, Booranasubkajorn U, Hongsumarn A, Thewtong D (1986) Formulation and evaluation of supplementary foods for Thai pregnant women. *American Journal of Clinical Nutrition* 43:931–939.

Tay CCK, Glasier AF, McNeilly AS (1996) Twenty-four hour patterns of prolactin secretion during lactation and the relationship to suckling an the resumption of fertility in breast-feeding women. *Human Reproduction* 11:950–955.

Tracer DP (1991) Fertility-related changes in maternal body composition among the Au of Papua New Guinea. *American Journal of Physical Anthropology* 85:393–405.

Tyson JE (1977) Neuroendocrine control of lactational infertility. *Journal of Biosocial Science* 4(Suppl):23–40.

Valeggia CR, Ellison PT (1998) Nursing patterns, maternal energetics, and postpartum fertility among Tobas of Formosa, Argentina. *American Journal of Physical Anthropology* 26(Suppl):54.

Vinoy S, Rosetta L, Mascie-Taylor CG (2000) Repeated measures of energy intake, energy expenditure and energy balance in lactating Bangladeshi women. *European Journal of Clinical Nutrition* 54:579–585.

Vitzthum VJ (1989) Nursing behavior and its relation to duration of postpartum amenorrhea in an Andean community. *Journal of Biosocial Science* 21(Suppl): 145–160.

Wood JW (1994) *Dynamics of Human Reproduction: Biology, Biometry, Demography* (New York, Aldine de Gruyter).

Wood JW, Lsi DL, Johnson PL, Campbell KL, Maslar IA (1985) Lactation and birth spacing in highland New Guinea. *Journal of Biosocial Science* 9(Suppl):159–173.

Worthman CM, Jenkins CL, Stallings JF, Lai D (1993) Attenuation of nursing-related ovarian suppression and high fertility in well-nourished, intensively breastfeeding Amele women of lowland Papua New Guinea. *Journal of Biosocial Science* 25:425–443.

Wu X, Sallinen K, Anttila L, Mäkinen M, Luo C, Pöllänen P, Erkkola R (2000) Expression of insulin-receptor substrate-1 and -2 in ovaries from women with insulin resistance and from control. *Fertility and Sterility* 74:564–572.

5

Reproductive Physiology of the Human Male
An Evolutionary and Life History Perspective

RICHARD G. BRIBIESCAS

Human reproductive ecology has traditionally focused on variation in female reproductive function in response to such factors as caloric intake, activity, and psychological stress (for review see Ellison 1994). Research on individual and interpopulation physiological variation, coupled with new hypotheses addressing the evolutionary significance of ovarian adaptability, has enhanced our understanding of the mechanisms and constraints which underlie important demographic and life history variables. However, our understanding of the range and evolutionary significance of male reproductive adaptability is less clear. Nonetheless, new studies and theoretical developments are guiding present research and providing clarity to clinical and anthropological data.

A central assumption guiding male reproductive ecology is the assertion that limitations on male fitness are distinct from those of females, resulting in energetic constraint differences that are reflected in their respective reproductive physiologies. Unlike females, mammalian males can reap large fitness benefits by maximizing mate access. This is not to say that increased mating opportunities for human females cannot result in fitness payoffs. Indeed, females can potentially enhance their fitness by increasing the number of mating partners through greater male provisioning or perhaps as a defense mechanism against infanticide (Hill and Kaplan 1988; Hrdy 1981; Smuts 1985). However, unlike in males, increased mate access cannot increase female reproductive output. In addition, males are not constrained by the reproductive costs of gestation and lactation, making reproductive investment energetically inexpensive and thereby permitting males to enhance their fitness by increasing mating opportunities. Consequently, male reproductive physiology exhibits sensitivities to energetic limitations dissimilar to that of females in regard to fecundity, somatic composition, and perhaps behavior (Bribiescas 1996, 1997).

This chapter provides an overview of male reproductive physiology as well as the environmental and constitutional factors that can alter reproductive function. In particular, the impact of energy intake and exertion will be discussed as well as the significance of micronutrients and aging. Population variation will also be discussed in light of clinical research and life history theory. Finally, several hypotheses regarding proximate constraints on male fitness are reviewed, culminating with a general theory of male reproductive ecology which attempts to reconcile clinical data with current anthropological research on nonwestern populations. Although male reproductive physiology will be shown to be relatively buffered against energetic constraints compared to that of females, males nonetheless face somatic trade-offs between survivorship and reproductive effort with the hypothalamic-pituitary-testicular (HPT) axis playing a central proximate role.

MALE REPRODUCTIVE PHYSIOLOGY

Reproductive Endocrinology

Male gonadal function is primarily controlled by the reproductive neuroendocrine system, which includes the hypothalamus, pituitary gland, and testes. It is important to remember, however, that the demarcation of the male neuroendocrine axis does not exclude the involvement of other endocrine factors, such as cortisol from the adrenal glands (Schaison et al. 1978), insulin from the pancreas (Semple et al. 1988), leptin from adipocytes (Garcia-Mayor et al. 1997), and thyroid hormone from the thyroid gland (Gordon et al. 1969) (to name just a few). All of these systems influence male reproductive endocrine function; however, the HPT axis is the central conduit of male reproductive function.

The influence of male-specific hormones is first evident during fetal development. Testes determining factor (TDF) (also known as Sry) is synthesized under the direction of genes such as Desert hedgehog (Dhh), located on the Y chromosome (Bitgood et al. 1996). TDF stimulates and promotes the growth of testicular tissue—specifically, Sertoli cells—around the eighth week of development (Koopman et al. 1991; Pelliniemi et al. 1993). Concurrently, Leydig cells within testicular tissue begin to secrete testosterone and, along with dihydrotestosterone (DHT), stimulate the formation of the external male genitalia. Müllerian inhibiting substance (MIS) is also produced around the eighth week of development, causing the degeneration of the Müllerian ducts and permitting the Wolffian ducts to develop into the internal reproductive tracts (vas deferens). Postpartum, testosterone levels rise to about half adult levels in response to a luteinizing hormone (LH) surge within the first six months (de Zegher et al. 1992), the significance of which remains unclear.

Hypothalamic-pituitary activity has been observed during infancy (Waldhauser et al. 1981), although childhood is generally characterized by hormonal quiescence, with the hypothalamus displaying extreme negative sensitivity to circulating steroids—in particular, testosterone, and to some extent estradiol. With the onset of puberty, hypothalamic sensitivity to androgen levels relaxes, allowing testosterone levels to rise. The mechanism for hypothalamic desensitization is unclear, although preadolescent changes in adrenal function, often referred to as *adrenarche,* may be a central catalyst. Subsequent to hypothalamic desensitization, nocturnal LH pulses appear, preceding full HPT maturation. Eventually, pulsatile release of gonadotropin releasing hormone (GnRH) is initiated by the hypothalamus, ultimately stimulating the anterior lobe of the pituitary gland to produce two primary gonadotropins, follicle stimulating hormone (FSH) and LH (Albertsson-Wikland et al. 1997). Composed of a common alpha but unique beta protein dimers, FSH and LH stimulate spermatogenesis in Sertoli cells and testosterone production in Leydig cells, respectively (Butler et al. 1989). Testosterone, estradiol, and inhibin, a peptide hormone produced by Sertoli cells, circulate back to the hypothalamus, thereby completing the negative feedback circuit.

Most circulating steroids are bound to sex-hormone-binding globulin (SHBG) or albumin, which inhibits cellular passage. Approximately 44% of circulating testosterone is bound to SHBG, 54% is bound to albumin and other proteins, with only about 2% occurring in free, cell-permeable unbound form. While SHBG has a thousandfold greater binding *affinity* to testosterone, albumin has a thousandfold binding *capacity,* which makes their contribution to steroid binding in serum more or less equal (Griffin 1996).

Spermatogenesis

Spermatogenesis involves the production of about 2×10^8 sperm/day. Approximately every seventy days, a cohort of maturing sperm enters the epididymis after having passed through various stages of development from primordial germ cell to spermatocyte, spermatid, and finally spermatozoa. The transit through the epididymis where development is completed and fluid from the seminal vesicles and prostate are added usually takes about twelve days (Griffin 1996).

Spermatogenesis also involves FSH, LH, and testosterone, with FSH acting as the primary agent responsible for stimulating sperm maturation within Sertoli cells in the testes. Aspermatogenesis in the human male as a result of pituitary removal can be reversed, however, with the

administration of human chorionic gonadotropin (hCG), a potent ana-
logue of LH, as well as human menopausal gonadotropin (hMG) which
contains FSH. Once spermatogenesis has been reestablished, sperm production can be maintained by hCG alone (Matsumoto et al. 1984). Indeed,
men who cannot produce FSH because of faulty gene transcription
nonetheless exhibit significant spermatogenesis and limited fertility
(Tapanainen et al. 1997). In addition, genetically engineered FSH knockout
mice that lack the necessary gene to produce FSH remain fertile and retain
the ability to father pups (Kumar et al. 1997). Although FSH, LH, and
testosterone all seem to be necessary for optimal sperm production (Griffin 1996; Matsumoto et al. 1986), spermatogenesis is a relatively robust
enterprise which tolerates a vast range of hormonal environments.

MALE REPRODUCTIVE FUNCTION AND
THE ENVIRONMENT

Caloric Deficiencies

Male reproductive physiology requires energy for proper functioning.
However, compared to those of females, male requirements are minimal,
with males exhibiting no significant changes in serum testosterone levels
in response to marginal negative energy balance (−15%) (Garrel et al.
1984). Nonetheless, males exhibit distinct responses to severe chronic and
acute caloric deficiencies. Ten-day fasts in obese men resulted in modest
decreases in testosterone and LH, with refeeding stimulating hormone
levels to pre-fast titers. Interestingly, a pronounced increase in urinary
FSH levels with no significant change in serum FSH suggests an escalation
of FSH production (Klibanski et al. 1981). Other studies have reported
decreases in male reproductive hormone function during acute fasts
although the results are confounded by obesity (Hoffer et al. 1986), dehy-
dration (Lee et al. 1977), and extreme psychological stress (Opstad 1992).

More controlled fasts result in consistent responses in male neuroendocrine function. For example, a 56-hour fast in healthy men was followed
by a significant decline in serum testosterone and LH levels, although FSH
remained unaffected. Subsequent GnRH administration stimulated a significantly higher LH and testosterone response in glucose-supplemented
individuals compared to fasting men (Röjdmark 1987a, 1987b). Forty-
eight-hour fasts have also been reported to alter testosterone production
by decreasing LH pulse frequency (Cameron et al. 1991) and decreasing
LH pulse amplitudes (Veldhuis et al. 1993).

Decreases in GnRH gene transcription may underlie fasting-induced
changes in the hypothalamus (Gruenewald and Matsumoto 1993). In rats,

four to six days of food deprivation decreased pituitary GnRH receptor levels by 50%, with serum and pituitary levels of LH and FSH declining 25–50%. Along with significant declines in testosterone levels, a 42% decrease in common alpha and beta subunit mRNA has also been observed in response to fasting in rats (Bergendahl et al. 1989). Administration of exogenous GnRH eliminates these differences, supporting the hypothesis that hypothalamic receptors are sensing and responding to energy-deficit cues (Bergendahl et al. 1991).

Peripheral hormonal responses to acute fasting can also affect male reproductive hormone function. Glucocorticoids have been shown to decrease testosterone levels, possibly through Leydig cell inhibition (Bambino and Hsueh 1981). Since fasting causes a significant rise in glucocorticoid levels and secretory burst mass (Bergendahl et al. 1996), glucocorticoids probably inflict some inhibitory function during periods of caloric deficiency.

Long-term fasting also compromises HPT function, although the locale of influence seems to lie within the testes and not the hypothalamus. For example, chronically undernourished Indian men exhibited lower testosterone and gonadotropin levels (Smith et al. 1975). Interestingly, this was not indicative of total gonadal arrest or significantly diminished fertility. After refeeding, testosterone levels were comparable to those of well-fed controls. Not surprisingly, injections of hCG, a potent LH analog, resulted in major testosterone rises in control males. Testosterone responses in Indian men were significantly muted, however, suggesting primary Leydig cell insensitivity to gonadotropin stimulation (Smith et al. 1975). Similar results were noted between urban Bolivian men living at sea level and high-altitude individuals, with urban men exhibiting a greater urinary testosterone response to hCG (Guerra-García et al. 1969). However, caloric intake was not monitored, and differences in urinary testosterone may not reflect circulating hormone levels since production and clearance rates can vary independently.

Declines in salivary testosterone levels among Lese horticultural men of central Zaire (now the Democratic Republic of Congo) have also been reported in association with a hunger season, although no increases were observed after the harvest when caloric intake increased. Bentley and colleagues suggest that the study may not have encompassed a sufficient period to observe any return in testosterone to pre-hunger levels; nonetheless, these results indicate that Lese male reproductive function is relatively insensitive to energy balance fluctuations (Bentley et al. 1993). Declines in salivary testosterone levels in Northern Ache men of Paraguay were noted, however, in association with declines in body mass index (BMI) in years of economic hardship compared with years of relative affluence (Bribiescas 1997). Nevertheless, Ñacunday Ache men from a relatively affluent community (though still quite poor by American standards) were not significantly different than their much poorer Northern Ache counterparts (Bribiescas 1994, 1997).

Although changes in male hormonal function in response to energetic intake are evident in males, there is no evidence to suggest any compromise in male fertility. These investigations imply that while human male reproductive endocrine function is responsive to energetic intake, fertility and gametogenesis are relatively unresponsive to caloric deficiencies compared to those of women, who exhibit significant declines in ovarian function and fecundity with even modest dietary restrictions (Lager and Ellison 1990; Lipson and Ellison 1996).

Lower Leydig cell sensitivity in chronically undernourished men may reflect permanent receptor priming prior or during adolescent development. In rats, acute fasting does not seem to alter pubertal development or adult male reproductive endocrine function (Bergendahl and Huhtaniemi 1993); however, chronic prepubertal energetic deficits do seem to modify HPT function permanently in mice (Jean-Faucher et al. 1982). The ramifications of this latter observation are important: energetic conditions during puberty may prime the HPT system, resulting in permanent sensitivity thresholds in Leydig cell receptors. Similar responses have been hypothesized to affect adult female reproductive endocrine function (Ellison 1997).

An example of this phenomenon is evident in males with Idiopathic Hypogonadotropic Hypogonadism (IHH) or Kallman's disease, a congenital absence of GnRH production. Males with IHH present differing phenotypes depending on the occurrence of some form of spontaneous pubertal development and exposure to endogenous sex steroids. Testicular volume differs significantly between IHH males with a history of some spontaneous pubertal development and those without (Spratt et al. 1987). In addition, GnRH therapy is augmented if males are given GnRH during adolescence compared with males who receive postadolescent treatment (Spratt and Crowley 1988). These studies provide compelling evidence for prepubertal hormonal priming and the implication that variation in the hormonal millieau in response to energetic circumstances during adolescence can have long-term effects on adult HPT function.

Micronutrients

Specific elements can affect spermatogenesis and male neuroendocrine function. For example, zinc deficiencies are associated with oligospermia and infertility, and zinc supplementation is sometimes used to treat suspected male infertility (Hartoma et al. 1977). The elimination of dietary zinc reduces sperm counts and gonadotropin levels but is reversed by zinc replacement (Abbasi et al. 1980). Testosterone levels have also been reported to be affected, but results have been inconsistent (Hunt et al. 1992). Ten days of zinc supplementation in Ache men did not result in any significant changes in gonadotropin or salivary testosterone titers (Bribiescas, unpublished data). Population differences in mean testosterone levels have also been associated with varying fat intake (Hamalainen et al. 1984), although in another study the association with diet is unclear (Howie and Schultz 1985). The role of micronutrient availability in the evolution of male reproductive physiology is uncertain, although the effects of micronutrients are probably area-specific.

Energetic Expenditure

Unlike in women, only the most strenuous exercise regimens impact male reproductive function. In a comparison of marathon runners and sedentary men, with the exception of bioactive LH levels there were no significant differences in LH, FSH, free and total testosterone, or sperm count (Bagatell and Bremner 1990). Although declines in reproductive function have been noted in marathon runners, androgen levels and sperm counts remained well within the range of clinical acceptability (Ayers et al. 1985; Roberts et al. 1993). Indeed, exercise-induced declines in testosterone and sperm counts are sometimes associated with elevated cortisol levels (Roberts et al. 1993).

In contrast, short-term, anabolic exercise can increase testosterone levels (Cumming et al. 1986), with nutritional supplementation augmenting this effect (Chandler et al. 1994). However, very little information on the effects of activity is available from nonwestern populations. Worthman and Konner report small but significant declines in nocturnal serum testosterone levels in !Kung hunter-gatherer men during a week-long hunt. The patterns observed were similar to the responses of western men during prolonged exercise (Worthman and Konner 1987), although salivary testosterone responses to short-term exercise in Ache men of Paraguay were inconclusive (Bribiescas 1997).

Social Context

Libido. Testosterone is associated with libido, although there is no direct correlation between androgen levels within the common range of variation and changes in behavioral parameters associated with libido. Exogenous testosterone administration within the common range does not result in any significant changes in libidinous behavior (Buena et al. 1993). Testosterone administration in hypogonadal men does result in apparent dose-dependent responses, however, as evident in elevated erection, masturbation, and ejaculatory frequencies (Davidson et al. 1978).

A classic study reflecting the interaction of androgens and mating opportunities involved a lone male conducting research on a remote island. The subject/researcher weighed his daily beard clippings as a gross androgen bioassay in response to mating opportunities. On days immediately prior to leaving the island for female companionship his beard growth increased significantly, and it slowed again during subsequent periods of isolation (Anonymous 1970). Moreover, salivary testosterone levels declined in response to abstinence in two anthropologists conducting remote field research. Testosterone levels rebounded with the arrival of the subjects' spouses and the resumption of sexual activity (Bribiescas, unpublished data).

Aggression.   Testosterone is often associated with aggressive behavior. However, clear associations between androgen levels and behavior considered to be aggressive have been elusive. Correlations between testosterone and aggression vary, depending on the variable used to define aggression. Nonetheless, investigators have reported relationships between androgens and aggressive behavior (Dabbs 1996). There is no evidence, however, to suggest that short-term changes in testosterone levels correlate with increased levels of aggression (Albert et al. 1993).

Competition.   Salivary testosterone levels respond to competitive interactions in males (Booth et al. 1989). Collegiate wrestlers exhibit a significant pre-competition rise within one hour of a match. Afterwards, the loser exhibits a sharp decline in salivary testosterone levels while the winner maintains his pre-match levels (Elias 1981). This phenomenon has been replicated under nonphysical competitive conditions (Mazur et al. 1997). No changes in androgen levels have been noted during competitive interactions between females, possibly belying the role of Leydig cell production (Mazur et al. 1997). Dominance relationships have been suggested to underlie testosterone variation (Mazur and Booth 1998), although variation between individuals and between populations is not taken into consideration (Bribiescas 1998; Spratt et al. 1988).

It must be kept in mind that statistical significance is not the same as biological significance (Lewontin 1974). Changes in salivary testosterone levels have been assumed to have behavioral significance, although evidence linking short-term testosterone changes to behavioral modification is minimal. Indeed, short-term changes in testosterone levels may involve the mobilization of energy in muscle cells. Muscle cells in vitro exhibit a 25% increase in metabolic rate within one minute of exposure to testosterone. Moreover, cell metabolism remains higher for a period of hours. If these results represent effects in vivo, short-term fluctuations in association with competition may involve glucose mobilization and increased muscle metabolism (Tsai and Sapolsky 1996).

Psychological stress. Salivary testosterone levels are inversely related to glucocorticoid levels in response to acute stresses such as skydiving (Chatterton et al. 1997), suggesting that cortisol increases may underlie HPT suppression in stressed males (Bambino and Hsueh 1981). However, naloxone treatment reverses stress-induced LH suppression in male rhesus monkeys, suggesting that endogenous opioids may also play a role in stress-induced hypothalamic reproductive suppression in primates (Gilbeau and Smith 1985).

VARIATION IN MALE REPRODUCTIVE FUNCTION

Individual Variation

Reproductive endocrine function. American males exhibit an extremely broad range of variability in HPT function (Spratt et al. 1988). Moreover, reproductive hormone variation is not associated with any obvious anthropometric characteristics (Knussmann and Sperwien 1988). A frequent sampling assessment of testosterone, estradiol, and gonadotropins revealed tremendous (and previously unsuspected) daily variation in hormone levels and pulsatility patterns. Some males showed little or no diurnal variation, while several individuals exhibited hormonal declines that would be considered clinically hypogonadal (Spratt et al. 1988). The source of interindividual variation is still unclear, although diet, activity patterns, and even exposure to exogenous steroids in the environment have been suggested to underlie this variation.

Studies of monozygotic twins suggest that serum free and total testosterone levels are the result of some measure of heritability, although spermatogenesis heritability is equivocal (Handelsman 1997). Genetic inheritance accounts for approximately 40–50% of testosterone and DHT variability (Meikle et al. 1988), while a study of monozygotic twins showed that serum testosterone levels are under significant environmental control, with diet—in particular, fat intake—being highly correlated with testosterone and LH levels (Bishop et al. 1988).

Sperm count. Males from industrialized countries exhibit a broad range of sperm count and quality (Cooper et al. 1991). Sperm counts range from 1 to 120 million/ml, with counts greater than 20 million being considered clinically acceptable for full fecundity (Glass 1991). However, there is significant disagreement surrounding the minimum clinically acceptable sperm count. Proposed lower limits have ranged from 60 to 10 million/ml, although 20 million has been the most commonly accepted limit (Glass 1991). Sources of variation in sperm count and quality are unclear, although temperature, photoperiodicity (Levine et al. 1992), and ejaculation frequency (Cooper et al. 1993) are potentially important.

Within clinically acceptable parameters, variation in sperm count and quality seems to contribute minimally to a couple's fertility. An examination of sperm count and quality in 210 men coupled with women with clinically acceptable fertility showed that none of the parameters commonly associated with male fecundity was correlated with subsequent conceptions (Polansky and Lamb 1988). Even the most advanced semen analysis has met with limited success in predicting future male fertility (Krause 1995).

Sperm count: seasonality. Increases in birth rates and ovarian function are associated with seasonal variation in energy availability (Bailey et al. 1992). However, seasonal variation due to photoperiodicity is less evident (Bronson 1995). Modest seasonality in sperm counts has been reported in urban human males (Levine 1994), some in association with reproductive endocrine variation (Meriggiola et al. 1996). However, the effects are mild and unlikely to contribute to variation in fecundity. Theoretically, given the likelihood of the emergence of hominids and modern humans from equatorial Africa, there is little reason to expect photoperiod-driven seasonality except as an epiphenomenon of mammalian physiology.

Declines in sperm count? The reported decline in sperm counts within the twentieth century has received a significant amount of press (Becker and Berhane 1997). Upon further analysis, sampling biases (Fisch and Goluboff 1996), changes in the definition of clinical norms (Bromwich et al. 1994), and inappropriate statistical analyses (Olsen et al. 1995) may underlie many of the reported differences. In addition, there is no reason to believe that according to clinical standards, any compromise in male fecundity has occurred. Nonetheless, it has been suggested that environmental steroids or phytoestrogens may underlie these observations (Sharpe and Skakkebaek 1993). If so, testosterone levels in American males would be some of the lowest, not the highest in the world (Bribiescas 1996)! The reported temporal variation in sperm count could easily be due to differences in quantitative methods (Emanuel et al. 1998).

Population Variation

Medical literature focuses primarily on the physiology of individuals from industrial nations. This is especially true in endocrinology since hormone measurements have typically involved costly tests that require careful treatment of perishable samples. However, recent advances in sample storage techniques and the advent of robust and more sensitive assays have resulted in significant growth in our knowledge of reproductive hormone physiology in nonwestern populations who are more representative of humans around the globe (Ellison 1994).

The earliest endocrinological studies of male reproductive function consistently suggested that interpopulation variation may be related to ecological factors. In the 1940s, Africans were reported to exhibit what was then called "estrinization," that is, elevated levels of estrogens (Davies 1949). Other researchers echoed these results, suggesting that indigenous Africans had higher levels of estrogens than did Europeans (Bersohn and Oelofse 1957). However, no explanatory mechanism was ever found.

With the advent of salivary steroid assays, data from remote populations grew steadily (Figure 5.1). The ability to store salivary samples at ambient

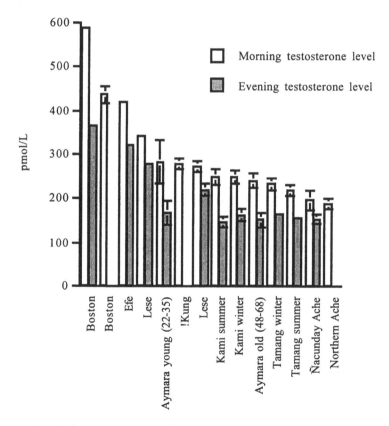

Figure 5.1. Salivary testosterone (Tsal) exhibits significant population variation. Data are derived from Ellison and Panter-Brick 1996 (Kami and Tamang of Nepal); Ellison et al. 1989a (Boston 1, Efe, Lese 1); Bribiescas 1997 (Boston 2, Ñacunday Ache); Beall et al. 1992 (Aymara); Christiansen 1991b (!Kung); Bentley et al. 1993 (Lese 2); Bribiescas 1996 (Northern Ache).

temperatures without refrigeration as well as the reflection of only free bioactive steroid in circulation makes this methodology ideal for biological anthropologists (Ellison 1988; Lipson and Ellison 1989). In addition to finding significantly lower progesterone levels in Lese women (Ellison et al. 1989b), researchers note that Efe and Lese men exhibit significantly lower salivary testosterone levels compared to Boston men (Bentley et al. 1993; Ellison et al. 1989a). Other African populations such as the !Kung (Christiansen 1991b) and Namibians (Christiansen 1991a) presented salivary testosterone levels significantly lower than western samples. Interestingly, Turkana males of Kenya exhibit testosterone levels that are not different from those of western populations despite their extreme leanness (Campbell et al. 1995).

Other nonwestern populations also exhibited significant variation. Urinary testosterone levels were shown to differ between Bolivian men living at high altitude and men at sea level (Guerra-García et al. 1969). Moreover, undernourished Indian men exhibited blunted testosterone responses to hCG stimulation, suggesting that developmental processes underlie adult Leydig cell insensitivity (Smith et al. 1975). Among New World populations presenting lower salivary testosterone levels compared with those of American males are the Ache of Paraguay (Bribiescas 1996, 1997) and the Aymara of Bolivia (Beall et al. 1992), although there is no evidence to suggest that low salivary testosterone levels among these populations are indicative of subfecundity (Galard et al. 1987). The Gainj of New Guinea manifest high FSH levels in otherwise healthy men, a reflection of possible Sertoli cell insensitivity. The investigators suggest that this may indicate male subfecundity, although sperm counts were not available (Campbell 1994).

Salivary testosterone measurements of healthy urban men in Venezuela, Poland, Zimbabwe, and Japan have shown that the distinction between American and non-American populations is even more profound than previously suspected. Salivary testosterone levels from these urban populations, with the exception of Polish men, were lower than those for Americans. Moreover, modest age-related declines in salivary testosterone were noted relative to Americans (Campbell et al. 2000; Ellison et al. 1998).

It is unlikely that population differences in reproductive endocrine function are the result of genetic polymorphisms. With the exception of extremely rare gonadotropin transcription mutations that may be inherent to specific communities (Tapanainen et al. 1997), and perhaps testosterone hormone binding globulin (TeBG) (Larrea et al. 1995), there is little evidence to suggest that genetic population differences in gonadotropin production or transcription underlie population variation (Jameson 1996). Genetic differences in receptor affinities are a possibility, but evidence is lacking. Most likely, chronic dietary intake and activity patterns during development are at the core of population variation. For example, poor urban youths in Kenya revealed significantly lower FSH levels in urinary gonadotropins compared with economically privileged Kenyan adolescents (Kulin et al. 1984).

Sperm count. Sperm counts have been reported to vary between populations (Fisch et al. 1996), although the differences do not suggest any differences in fecundability (Cooper et al. 1991). Longitudinal studies of nonwestern populations are few; however, available evidence does not indicate any significant temporal changes in sperm counts or semen quality (Seo et al. 2000; Tortolero et al. 1999).

Prostate cancer risk. Steroid-sensitive cancers vary significantly across populations (Rose et al. 1986). Although caution is merited when attempting to examine the etiology of disease by race owing to the ambiguous and often misleading nature of this classification (Lewontin 1972), certain communities do exhibit differential rates of prostate disease. African-American males have a twofold higher risk of contracting prostate cancer compared with non-African-American males and present significantly higher androgen levels (Ross et al. 1986). Given the central role of androgens in promoting prostate carcinomas (Henderson et al. 1982), differences in community steroid levels are noteworthy, although the relationship between individual lifetime androgen levels and prostate cancer risk remains unclear (Carter et al. 1995).

Environmental factors such as diet and activity patterns warrant close attention because of their impact on the neuroendocrine system (Key 1995). Nigerian males exhibit less aggressive bouts of prostate cancer as well as lower androgen levels than do urban African-American males, suggesting that lifestyle differences before and after adolescence, such as diet, stress, and activity, may influence population risk (Jackson et al. 1977; Shimizu et al. 1991).

Data from nonwestern populations as well as ethnic differences in prostate cancer risk imply that population variation in testosterone levels reflects hormonal release in American populations rather than hormonal suppression among nonwestern populations. Ethnic differences in cancer risk and androgen levels also underscore the importance of developing an increased awareness of population variation in neuroendocrine function as well as the central role of environmental factors such as diet, activity, and stress. As suggested in reference to female reproductive endocrine function (Ellison 1994), clinical research on American male populations must be viewed as representative of the extreme range of human variability and not the common or "healthiest" representation of *Homo sapiens*.

MALE NEUROENDOCRINE FUNCTION AND AGING

Women undergo an abrupt and complete cessation of ovulatory function during menopause, resulting in diminished and ultimately zero fecundity. Men do not undergo menopause; however, there are subtle changes which characterize aging of the HPT axis. In American males over the age of forty, testosterone levels tend to decrease by about 1.2% per year, with sex-hormone-binding globulin increasing at a rate of 1.4% per year, suggesting that changes in free versus bound testosterone ratios may account for some age-related changes in male endocrine function (Gray et al. 1991). A slight elevation in FSH and LH levels also suggests some degree of age-related testicular insensitivity (Gray et al. 1991). Older males also lose the diurnal patterns of testosterone secretion that are common in younger men (Bremner et al. 1983), although the physiological significance is unknown. Age-related changes in male neuroendocrine function do not seem to affect fecundity, although decreases in skeletal muscle mass and increased fat deposition are common (Campbell et al. 2000).

The association between aging and HPT function in nonwestern populations is sparse, although an attenuated decline with age compared to American men is apparent (Bribiescas 1997; Ellison et al. 1998). Among Ache hunter-gatherers of eastern Paraguay, a significant increase in FSH was noted with age, although no change was noted in LH (Bribiescas 2000).

MALE REPRODUCTIVE ECOLOGY:
A THEORETICAL SYNTHESIS

The relationship between energetic allocation and ovarian function in women is clear, with energy balance exhibiting an explicit effect on reproductive function and subsequent fecundity. However, there is scant evidence to suggest an analogous relationship between energy balance and male fecundity. Nonetheless, testicular function is sensitive to energy balance. Is this relationship evolutionarily significant or a metaphenomenon with no adaptive significance? Given basic mammalian constraints and life history trade-offs regarding male reproduction—in particular, reproductive effort and survivorship (Stearns 1992)—are there any insights to be gained in regard to the male reproductive physiology? Several perspectives have emerged which attempt to reconcile physiological observations with evolutionary and life history theory.

The Challenge Hypothesis

To explain variation in seasonal testosterone fluctuations in some birds, Wingfield and colleagues have suggested that testosterone levels respond to physical and territorial challenges of rival males. Experimental testosterone implantation of males and observations of subsequent territorial and mating behaviors demonstrate that a significant survivorship cost accompanies testosterone-augmented reproductive effort (Wingfield et al. 1990). Testosterone implants lose weight and suffer higher mortality rates than controls (Ketterson et al. 1992). Similar effects have been noted in other vertebrates (Marler and Moore 1988).

The contribution of this hypothesis to our understanding of male reproductive ecology has been to demonstrate the central role of testosterone in delineating life history trade-offs between survivorship and reproductive effort. Although the relationship between testosterone and behavior is more subtle in humans than in birds, the somatic effect of androgens is a commonality that may aid in our understanding of individual and population differences in human male reproductive physiology.

Ejaculates as Units

While energy balance does not seem to affect sperm count in a manner that would imply compromised fertility, it has been suggested that sperm count may not be the appropriate unit of analysis when analyzing variation in male reproductive potential. Dewsbury (1982) has suggested that since sperm are delivered in packets as ejaculates, the number and quality of ejaculates should be the unit of analysis since they are limited over time and accompanied by declines in sperm count with repeated ejaculations. Because of the perceived limitations imposed by ejaculate quantity and quality, Dewsbury suggests that contrary to traditional biological thought, mammalian males should be somewhat discriminate of potential mates and that ejaculates may be a limiting factor in male reproductive effort (Dewsbury 1982).

This is an intriguing idea since energetic investment in ejaculates or other forms of sperm delivery is quite significant in some organisms, especially some insects. Not surprisingly these species can be very discriminate about their potential mates. However, no mammals invest so much in ejaculates. In addition, there is little evidence to suggest that mammalian males limit reproductive effort in the presence of novel females. Indeed the "Coolidge Effect" among mammals notes that refractory periods between ejaculations diminishes with the presentation of novel receptive females (Beamer et al. 1969). Also, frequent ejaculations have only modest effects on human sperm counts, quality, and fecundity (Cooper et al. 1993).

Testosterone and Somatic Energy Allocation

It has been suggested that human male reproductive physiology reflects central life history trade-offs between survivorship and reproductive effort and that testosterone is an important mechanism regulating somatic investment allocation decisions (Bribiescas 1996, 1997, 2000). Such life history trade-offs are reflected by the effect of the availability of potential mates in *Drosophila* and *C. elegans* (Gems and Riddle 1996; Partridge and Farquhar 1981). Indeed, metabolic investment in spermatogenesis alone decreases survivability in *C. elegans* (Van Voorhies 1992). Spermatogenesis in mammals involves a trivial amount of metabolic investment, however, accounting for less than 1% of basal metabolic rate (BMR) in human males (Elia 1992). The minor metabolic cost of spermatogenesis is clearly evident by the robustness of sperm production in humans, even under the most taxing circumstances. In contrast, many vertebrates exhibit an important metabolic trade-off between sexually dimorphic muscle mass, a reflection of somatic investment in reproductive effort, and somatic investment indicative of survivorship, such as adipocyte deposition or increased immune competence (Figure 5.2). It must be noted that phenotypic correlations can confound somatic investment trade-offs between survivorship and reproductive effort, particularly in organisms that exhibit high paternal investment in offspring. Under these conditions, fat deposition can be viewed as contributing to both survivorship and reproductive effort if paternal survivorship is predictive of offspring survivorship (Fowler et al. 1994).

Seasonal changes in sexually dimorphic muscle mass in association with distinct increases in testosterone are well-documented in seasonally breeding mammals (Field et al. 1985; Forger and Breedlove 1987). Often

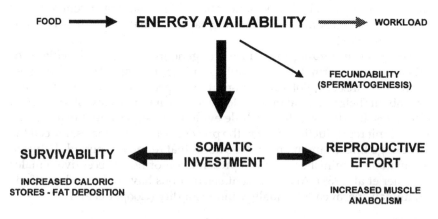

Figure 5.2.   A model of male energy allocation based on premises derived from life history theory. Energetic resources are allocated between reproductive effort and survivorship, with testosterone acting as a primary regulator of metabolism and anabolism.

these changes are coupled with decreased caloric intake resulting from rises in mating effort (McMillin et al. 1980). Since a significant portion of male metabolic investment is in sexually dimorphic muscle tissue, variation between human male populations may involve the modulation of muscle anabolism and metabolism in response to energy availability (Bribiescas 1996, 1997, 2000).

In human males, approximately 20% of male basal metabolic rate (BMR) involves skeletal muscle tissue (Elia 1992). Other tissues, including the brain, also contribute about 20% to BMR; however, unlike skeletal muscle, neural tissue cannot fluctuate during periods of energy deficiencies. Skeletal muscle tissue undergoes significant atrophy during periods of negative energy balance. Glucocorticoids play a significant role in muscle catabolism during periods of acute energy stress, decreasing metabolic costs and perhaps liberating amino acids for increased energy availability (Crowley and Matt 1996). More important for male somatic investment trade-offs, testosterone is a key hormone agent which regulates muscle anabolism and metabolism. Acute and chronic patterns of testosterone variation may reflect an adaptive mechanism to attenuate somatic investment between reproductive effort and survivability in human males (Bribiescas 1996, 1997).

The effects of testosterone on somatic composition in humans are well-documented. Testosterone administration stimulates fat catabolism, adipose tissue redistribution (Marin et al. 1992), as well as increased protein synthesis and glucose uptake in muscle (Bardin 1996; Bhasin et al. 1996; Griggs et al. 1989; Longcope et al. 1976; Powers and Florini 1975). In addition, testosterone stimulates metabolic rates in muscle cells in vitro (Tsai and Sapolsky 1996), and overall BMR in men. For example, three months of testosterone administration (3 mg/kg of weight per week) to men with muscular dystrophy (MD) as well as controls resulted in significant increases in BMR in both groups (13% and 7%, respectively), with BMR remaining elevated after twelve months in muscular dystrophy patients. The primary cause of the hypermetabolic effect of testosterone was attributed to the significant increase in lean body mass in both groups (10% in MD men; 11% in controls) (Welle et al. 1992).

The population differences in reproductive endocrine function as well as the acute response of the HPT system to negative energy balance seem to reflect an adaptive mechanism that decreases metabolic costs in light of energy deficits. It has been suggested that alterations in muscle metabolism during periods of energetic stress are an adaptive response that decreases metabolic costs in order to increase survivability (Henriksson 1992). Although the hypermetabolic effects of testosterone on survivorship in human males have not been studied, data from other vertebrates suggest that testosterone induces changes in somatic composition that are associated with increases in reproductive effort and compromised survivorship (Ketterson and Nolan 1992; Ketterson et al. 1992).

For example, testosterone implants in male desert lizards (*Sceloporus jarrori*) were associated with increased male mortality. Males with implants spent a significantly greater amount of time in courtship display and aggressive territoriality than sham-treated males did. Although it was initially believed that increased predation risk was the source of higher mortality among implanted males, higher metabolic costs incurred by testosterone implantation may have been the primary source of mortality (Marler and Moore 1988). Similar results have been noted in avian species (Ketterson et al. 1992). The mosaic impression implied by these varied studies of humans and other animals suggests that male reproductive endocrine responses, both chronic and acute, represent an adaptive response to reconcile reproductive effort with survivorship needs (Figures 5.3a and 3b).

CONCLUSION

The emerging picture of male reproductive ecology suggests that men are indeed quite different from their female counterparts. Spermatogenesis is relatively insensitive and is buffered from energetic stresses, although androgen physiology reflects selection for optimizing somatic energy allocations while maintaining adequate hormonal support for spermatogenesis during periods of energetic stress. The broad spectrum of population and individual variation implies that environmental and ecological factors are key players in male reproductive physiology, a crucial reaction norm for understanding the evolution and life history of male reproduction. Furthermore, the range of population variation has important ramifications for male reproductive health and what is considered clinically "normal." Indeed, evolutionary and life history theory can make substantial contributions to our understanding of contemporary male health issues and reproductive ecology.

I would especially like to thank Peter Ellison and all of the members of the Reproductive Ecology Laboratory at Harvard University for years of collaborative and intellectual support. In addition, Kim Hill, A. Magdelena Hurtado, Martin Achipurangi, Roberto Achipurangi, Angel Tatunambiangi, Bjarne and Rosalba Fostervold, as well as the Ache communities of Chupa Pou, Arroyo Bandera, and Puerto Barra have been most gracious collaborators. Countless conversations with colleagues have provided the intellectual stimulus necessary for this synthesis. These individuals include Ben Campbell, William F. Crowley, Jr., Terry Deacon, Irven DeVore, Stephanie Firos, Judith Flynn, Jamie Jones, Cheryl Knott, Greg Laden, Susan Lipson, Bill Lukas, Michael Muehlenbein, Mary O'Rourke, Nadine Peacock, Diana Sherry, and Richard Wrangham.

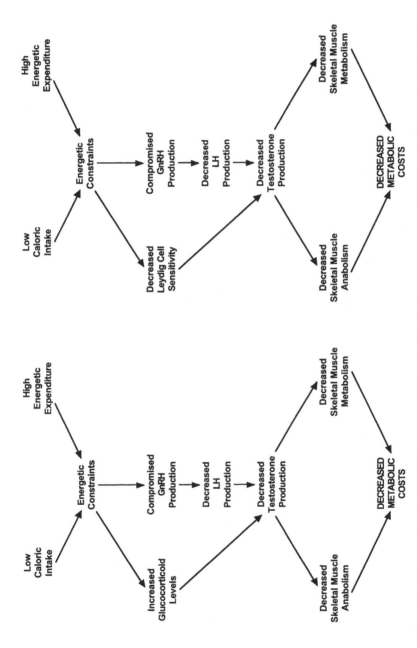

Figure 5.3. Diagrams showing the HPT response and the potential adaptive consequences to (*right*) short-term or acute energetic stress and (*left*) long-term or chronic energetic stress.

REFERENCES CITED

Abbasi AA, Prasad AS, Rabbani P, DuMouchelle E (1980) Experimental zinc deficiency in man: effect on testicular function. *Journal of Laboratory and Clinical Medicine* 96:544–550.

Albert DJ, Walsh ML, Jonik RH (1993) Aggression in humans: what is its biological foundation? *Neuroscience and Biobehavioral Reviews* 17:405–425.

Albertsson-Wikland K, Rosberg S, Lannering B, Dunkel L, Selstam G, Norjavaara E (1997) Twenty-four-hour profiles of luteinizing hormone, follicle-stimulating hormone, testosterone, and estradiol levels: a semilongitudinal study throughout puberty in healthy boys. *Journal of Clinical Endocrinology and Metabolism* 82:541–549.

Anonymous (1970) Effects of sexual activity on beard growth in man. *Nature* 226:869–870.

Ayers JW, Komesu Y, Romani T, Ansbacher R (1985) Anthropomorphic, hormonal, and psychologic correlates of semen quality in endurance-trained male athletes. *Fertility and Sterility* 43:917–921.

Bagatell CJ, Bremner WJ (1990) Sperm counts and reproductive hormones in male marathoners and lean controls. *Fertility and Sterility* 53:688–692.

Bailey RC, Jenike MR, Ellison PT, Bentley GR, Harrigan AM, Peacock NR (1992) The ecology of birth seasonality among agriculturalists in central Africa. *Journal of Biosocial Science* 24:393–412.

Bambino TH, Hsueh AJ (1981) Direct inhibitory effect of glucocorticoids upon testicular luteinizing hormone receptor and steroidogenesis in vivo and in vitro. *Endocrinology* 108:2142–2148.

Bardin CW (1996) The anabolic action of testosterone. *New England Journal of Medicine* 335:52–53.

Beall CM, Worthman CM, Stallings J, Strohl KP, Brittenham GM, Barragan M (1992) Salivary testosterone concentration of Aymara men native to 3600 m. *Annals of Human Biology* 19:67–78.

Beamer W, Bermant G, Clegg M (1969) Copulatory behavior in the ram, *Ovis aries*, II: factors affecting copulatory satiety. *Animal Behavior* 17:706–711.

Becker S, Berhane K (1997) A meta-analysis of 61 sperm count studies revisited. *Fertility and Sterility* 67:1103–1108.

Bentley GR, Harrigan AM, Campbell B, Ellison PT (1993) Seasonal effects on salivary testosterone levels among Lese males of the Ituri Forest, Zaire. *American Journal of Human Biology* 5:711–717.

Bergendahl M, Huhtaniemi I (1993) Acute fasting is ineffective in suppressing pituitary-gonadal function of pubertal male rats. *American Journal of Physiology* 264:E717–722.

Bergendahl M, Perheentupa A, Huhtaniemi I (1989) Effect of short-term starvation on reproductive hormone gene expression, secretion and receptor levels in male rats. *Journal of Endocrinology* 121:409–417.

Bergendahl M, Perheentupa A, Huhtaniemi I (1991) Starvation-induced suppression of pituitary-testicular function in rats is reversed by pulsatile gonadotropin-releasing hormone substitution. *Biology of Reproduction* 44: 413–419.

Bergendahl M, Vance ML, Iranmanesh A, Thorner MO, Veldhuis JD (1996) Fasting as a metabolic stress paradigm selectively amplifies cortisol secretory burst mass and delays the time of maximal nyctohemeral cortisol concentrations in healthy men. *Journal of Clinical Endocrinology and Metabolism* 81:692–699.

Bersohn I, Oelofse PJ (1957) A comparison of urinary oestrogen levels in normal male South African Bantu and European subjects. *South African Medical Journal* 31:1172–1174.

Bhasin S, Storer TW, Berman N, Callegari C, Clevenger B, Phillips J, Bunnell TJ, Tricker R, Shirazi A, Casaburi R (1996) The effects of supraphysiologic doses of testosterone on muscle size and strength in normal men. *New England Journal of Medicine* 335:1–7.

Bishop DT, Meikle AW, Slattery ML, Stringham JD, Ford MH, West DW (1988) The effect of nutritional factors on sex hormone levels in male twins. *Genetic Epidemiology* 5:43–59.

Bitgood MJ, Shen L, McMahon AP (1996) Sertoli cell signaling by Desert hedgehog regulates the male germline. *Current Biology* 6:298–304.

Booth AG, Shelley A, Mazur G, Tharp G, Kittock R (1989) Testosterone and winning and losing in human competition. *Hormones and Behavior* 23:556–571.

Bremner WJ, Vitiello MV, Prinz PN (1983) Loss of circadian rhythmicity in blood testosterone levels with aging in normal men. *Journal of Clinical Endocrinology and Metabolism* 56:1278–1281.

Bribiescas RG (1994) Salivary testosterone levels in a population of Aché agriculturalists in eastern Paraguay. *American Journal of Physical Anthropology* (Suppl 18):59.

Bribiescas RG (1996) Testosterone levels among Aché hunter-gatherer men: a functional interpretation of population variation among adult males. *Human Nature* 7:163–188.

Bribiescas RG (1997) *Testosterone as a Proximate Determinant of Somatic Energy Allocation in Human Males: Evidence from Ache Men of Eastern Paraguay* (PhD dissertation, Harvard University).

Bribiescas RG (1998) Testosterone and dominance: between-population variance and male energetics. *Brain and Behavioral Sciences* 21:364–365.

Bribiescas RG (2000) Male reproductive ecology: development and life history. *American Journal of Physical Anthropology* (Suppl 30):111.

Bromwich P, Cohen J, Stewart I, Walker A (1994) Decline in sperm counts: an artefact of changed reference range of "normal"? *British Medical Journal* 309:19–22.

Bronson FH (1995) Seasonal variation in human reproduction: environmental factors. *Quarterly Review of Biology* 70:141–165.

Buena F, Swerdloff RS, Steiner BS, Lutchmansingh P, Peterson MA, Pandian MR, Galmarini M, Bhasin S (1993) Sexual function does not change when serum testosterone levels are pharmacologically varied within the normal male range. *Fertility and Sterility* 59:1118–1123.

Butler GE, Walker RF, Walker RV, Teague P, Riad-Fahmy D, Ratcliffe SG (1989) Salivary testosterone levels and the progress of puberty in the normal boy. *Clinical Endocrinology* 30:587–596.

Cameron JL, Weltzin TE, McConaha C, Helmreich DL, Kaye WH (1991) Slowing of pulsatile luteinizing hormone secretion in men after forty-eight hours of fasting. *Journal of Clinical Endocrinology and Metabolism* 73:35–41.

Campbell B, Leslie P, Quigley J, Campbell K (1995) Hormonal assessment of reproductive function among males in Turkana, Kenya: LH and FSH. *American Journal of Physical Anthropology* (Suppl 20):72.

Campbell BC, Ellison PT, Lipson S, O'Rourke M, Bribiescas RG, Uchida A, Jasienska G (2000) Population variation in age-related decline of salivary testosterone and its relationship to body composition. *American Journal of Physical Anthropology* (Suppl 30):117.

Campbell KL (1994) Blood, urine, saliva, and dip-sticks: experiences in Africa, New Guinea, and Boston. *Annals of the New York Academy of Science* 709:312–330.

Carter HB, Pearson JD, Metter EJ, Chan DW, Andres R, Fozard JL, Rosner W, Walsh PC (1995) Longitudinal evaluation of serum androgen levels in men with and without prostate cancer. *Prostate* 27:25–31.

Chandler RM, Byrne HK, Patterson JG, Ivy JL (1994) Dietary supplements affect the anabolic hormones after weight-training exercise. *Journal of Applied Physiology* 76:839–845.

Chatterton R Jr, Vogelsong KM, Lu YC, Hudgens GA (1997) Hormonal responses to psychological stress in men preparing for skydiving. *Journal of Clinical Endocrinology and Metabolism* 82:2503–2509.

Christiansen KH (1991a) Sex hormone levels, diet and alcohol consumption in Namibian Kavango men. *Homo* 42:43–62.

Christiansen KH (1991b) Serum and saliva sex hormone levels in !Kung San men. *American Journal of Physical Anthropology* 86:37–44.

Cooper TG, Jockenhovel F, Nieschlag E (1991) Variations in semen parameters from fathers. *Human Reproduction* 6:859–866.

Cooper TG, Keck C, Oberdieck U, Nieschlag E (1993) Effects of multiple ejaculations after extended periods of sexual abstinence on total, motile and normal sperm numbers, as well as accessory gland secretions, from healthy normal and oligozoospermic men. *Human Reproduction* 8:1251–1258.

Crowley MA, Matt KS (1996) Hormonal regulation of skeletal muscle hypertrophy in rats: the testosterone to cortisol ratio. *European Journal of Applied Physiology* 73:66–72.

Cumming DC, Brunsting LA III, Strich G, Ries AL, Rebar RW (1986) Reproductive hormone increases in response to acute exercise in men. *Medicine and Science in Sports and Exercise* 18:369–373.

Dabbs JM Jr (1996) Testosterone, aggression, and delinquency. In S Bhasin, HL Gabelnick, JM Spieler, RS Swerdloff, C Wang, C Kelly (Eds) *Pharmacology, Biology, and Clinical Applications of Androgens* (New York, Wiley-Liss), 179–190.

Davidson JM, Camargo CA, Smith ER (1978) Effects of androgen on sexual behavior in hypogonadal men. *Journal of Clinical Endocrinology and Metabolism* 48:955–958.

Davies JNP (1949) Sex hormone upset in Africans. *British Medical Journal* 2:676.

de Zegher F, Devlieger H, Veldhuis JD (1992) Pulsatile and sexually dimorphic secretion of luteinizing hormone in the human infant on the day of birth. *Pediatric Research* 32:605–607.

Dewsbury DA (1982) Ejaculate cost and male choice. *American Naturalist* 119: 601–610.

Elia M (1992) Organ and tissue contribution to metabolic rate. In JM Kinney, HN Tucker (Eds) *Energy Metabolism: Tissue Determinants and Cellular Corollaries* (New York, Raven Press), 61–79.

Elias M (1981) Serum cortisol, testosterone, and testosterone-binding globulin responses to competitive fighting in human males. *Aggressive Behavior* 7:215–224.

Ellison PT (1988) Human salivary steroids: methodological considerations and applications in physical anthropology. *Yearbook of Physical Anthropology* 31: 115–142.

Ellison PT (1994) Advances in human reproductive ecology. *Annual Review of Anthropology* 23:255–275.

Ellison PT (1997) Developmental influences on adult ovarian hormonal function. *American Journal of Human Biology* 8:725–734.

Ellison PT, Panter-Brick C (1996) Salivary testosterone levels among Tamang and Kami males of central Nepal. *Human Biology* 68:955–965.

Ellison PT, Lipson SF, Bribiescas RG, Bentley GR, Campbell BC, Panter-Brick C (1998) Inter- and intra-population variation in the pattern of male testosterone by age. *American Journal of Physical Anthropology* 105:26.

Ellison PT, Lipson SF, Meredith MD (1989a) Salivary testosterone levels in males from the Ituri Forest of Zaire. *American Journal of Human Biology* 1:21–24.

Ellison PT, Peacock NR, Lager C (1989b) Ecology and ovarian function among Lese women of the Ituri Forest, Zaire. *American Journal of Physical Anthropology* 78:519–526.

Emanuel ER, Goluboff ET, Fisch H (1998) MacLeod revisited: sperm count distributions in 374 fertile men from 1971 to 1994. *Urology* 51:86–88.

Field RA, Young OA, Asher GW, Foote DM (1985) Characteristics of male fallow deer muscle at a time of sex-related muscle growth. *Growth* 49:190–201.

Fisch H, Goluboff ET (1996) Geographic variations in sperm counts: a potential cause of bias in studies of semen quality. *Fertility and Sterility* 65:1044–1046.

Fisch H, Ikeguchi EF, Goluboff ET (1996) Worldwide variations in sperm counts. *Urology* 48:909–911.

Forger NG, Breedlove M (1987) Seasonal variation in mammalian striated muscle mass and motoneuron morphology. *Journal of Neurobiology* 18:155–165.

Fowler GS, Wingfield JC, Boersma PD, Sosa RA (1994) Reproductive endocrinology and weight change in relation to reproductive success in the magellanic penguin *(Spheniscus magellanicus). General and Comparative Endocrinology* 94:305–315.

Galard R, Antolin M, Catalan R, Magana P, Schwartz S, Castellanos JM (1987) Salivary testosterone levels in infertile men. *International Journal of Andrology* 10:597–601.

Garcia-Mayor RV, Andrade MA, Rios M, Lage M, Dieguez C, Casanueva FF (1997) Serum leptin levels in normal children: relationship to age, gender, body mass index, pituitary-gonadal hormones, and pubertal stage. *Journal of Clinical Endocrinology and Metabolism* 82:2849–2855.

Garrel DR, Todd KS, Pugeat MM, Calloway DH (1984) Hormonal changes in normal men under marginally negative energy balance. *American Journal of Clinical Nutrition* 39:930–936.

Gems D, Riddle DL (1996) Longevity in *Caenorhabditis elegans* reduced by mating but not gamete production. *Nature* 379:723–725.

Gilbeau PM, Smith CG (1985) Naloxone reversal of stress-induced reproductive effects in the male rhesus monkey. *Neuropeptides* 5:335–338.

Glass RH (1991) Infertility. In S Samuel, C Yen, RB Jaffe (Eds) *Reproductive Endocrinology: Physiology, Pathophysiology, and Clinical Management* (Philadelphia, WB Saunders), 689–709.

Gordon GG, Southren AL, Tochimoto S, Rand JJ, Olivo J (1969) Effect of hyperthyroidism and hypothyroidism on the metabolism of testosterone and androstenedione in man. *Journal of Clinical Endocrinology and Metabolism* 29:164–170.

Gray A, Feldman HA, McKinlay JB, Longcope C (1991) Age, disease, and changing sex hormone levels in middle-aged men: results of the Massachusetts Male Aging Study. *Journal of Clinical Endocrinology and Metabolism* 73:1016–1025.

Griffin JE (1996) Male reproductive function. In JE Griffin, SR Ojeda (Eds) *Textbook of Endocrinology* (Oxford, Oxford University Press), 201–222.

Griggs RC, Kingston W, Jozefowicz RF, Herr BE, Forbes G, Halliday D (1989) Effect of testosterone on muscle mass and muscle protein synthesis. *Journal of Applied Physiology* 66:498–503.

Gruenewald DA, Matsumoto AM (1993) Reduced gonadotropin-releasing hormone gene expression with fasting in the male rat brain. *Endocrinology* 132:480–482.

Guerra-García R, Velásquez A, Coyotupa J (1969) A test of endocrine gonadal function in men: urinary testosterone after the injection of HCG, II: a different response of the high altitude native. *Journal of Clinical Endocrinology* 29:179–182.

Hamalainen E, Adlercreutz H, Puska P, Pietinen P (1984) Diet and serum sex hormones in healthy men. *Journal of Steroid Biochemistry* 20:459–464.

Handelsman DJ (1997) Estimating familial and genetic contributions to variability in human testicular function: a pilot twin study. *International Journal of Andrology* 20:215–221.

Hartoma TR, Nahoul K, Netter A (1977) Zinc, plasma androgens and male sterility. *Lancet* 1:125–126.

Henderson BE, Ross RK, Pike MC, Casagrande JT (1982) Endogenous hormones as a major factor in human cancer. *Cancer Research* 42:3232–3239.

Henriksson J (1992) Energy metabolism in muscle: its possible role in the adaptation to energy deficiency. In JM Kinney, HN Tucker (Eds) *Energy Metabolism: Tissue Determinants and Cellular Corollaries* (New York, Raven Press), 345–365.

Hill K, Kaplan H (1988) Tradeoffs in male and female reproductive strategies among the Ache, part 2. In L Betzig, M Borgerhoff Mulder, P Turke (Eds) *Human Reproductive Behaviour: A Darwinian Perspective* (Oxford, Oxford University Press), 291–305.

Hoffer LJ, Beitins IZ, Kyung NH, Bistrian BR (1986) Effects of severe dietary restriction on male reproductive hormones. *Journal of Clinical Endocrinology and Metabolism* 62:288–292.

Howie BJ, Schultz TD (1985) Dietary and hormonal interrelationships among vegetarian Seventh-Day Adventists and nonvegetarian men. *American Journal of Clinical Nutrition* 42:127–134.

Hrdy S (1981) *The Woman That Never Evolved* (Cambridge, Harvard University Press).

Hunt C, Johnson PE, Herbel J, Mullen LK (1992) Effects of dietary zinc depletion on seminal volume and zinc loss, serum testosterone concentrations, and sperm morphology in young men. *American Journal of Clinical Nutrition* 56:148–157.

Jackson MA, Ahluwalia BS, Herson J, Heshmat MY, Jackson AG, Jones GW, Kapoor, SK, Kennedy J, Kovi J, Lucas AO, Nkposong EO, Olisa E, Williams AO (1977) Characterization of prostatic carcinoma among blacks: a continuation report. *Cancer Treatment Reports* 61:167–172.

Jameson JL (1996) Inherited disorders of the gonadotropin hormones. *Molecular and Cellular Endocrinology* 125:143–149.

Jean-Faucher C, Berger M, de Turckheim M, Veyssiere G, Jean C (1982) The effect of preweaning undernutrition upon the sexual development of male mice. *Biology of the Neonate* 41:45–51.

Ketterson ED, Nolan V Jr (1992) Hormones and life histories: an integrative approach. *American Naturalist* 140:S33–S62.

Ketterson ED, Nolan V Jr, Wolf L, Ziegenfus C (1992) Testosterone and avian life histories: effects of experimentally elevated testosterone on behavior and correlates of fitness in the dark-eyed junco *(Junco hyemalis)*. *American Naturalist* 140:980–999.

Key T (1995) Risk factors for prostate cancer. *Cancer Surveys* 23:63–77.

Klibanski A, Beitins IZ, Badger T, Little R, McArthur JW (1981) Reproductive function during fasting in men. *Journal of Clinical Endocrinology and Metabolism* 53:258–263.

Knussmann R, Sperwien A (1988) Relations between anthropometric characteristics and androgen hormone levels in healthy young men. *Annals of Human Biology* 15:131–142.

Koopman P, Gubbay J, Vivian P, Goodfellow R, Lovell-Badge R (1991) Male development of chromosomally female mice transgenic for Sry. *Nature* 351:117–121.

Krause W (1995) Computer-assisted semen analysis systems: comparison with routine evaluation and prognostic value in male fertility and assisted reproduction. *Human Reproduction* 1:60–66.

Kulin HE, Bwibo N, Mutie D, Santner SJ (1984) Gonadotropin excretion during puberty in malnourished children. *Journal of Pediatrics* 105:325–328.

Kumar TR, Wang Y, Lu N, Matzuk MM (1997) Follicle stimulating hormone is required for ovarian follicle maturation but not male fertility. *Nature Genetics* 15:201–204.

Lager C, Ellison PT (1990) Effect of moderate weight loss on ovarian function assessed by salivary progesterone measurements. *American Journal of Human Biology* 2:303–312.

Larrea F, Carino C, Hardy DO, Musto NA, Catterall JF (1995) Genetic variations in human testosterone-estradiol binding globulin. *Journal of Steroid Biochemistry and Molecular Biology* 53:553–559.

Lee PA, Wallin JD, Kaplowitz N, Burkhartsmeier GL, Kane JP, Lewis SB (1977) Endocrine and metabolic alterations with food and water deprivation. *American Journal of Clinical Nutrition* 30:1953–1962.

Levine RJ (1994) Male factors contributing to the seasonality of human reproduction. In KL Campbell, JW Wood (Eds) *Human Reproductive Ecology: Interactions of Environment, Fertility, and Behavior* (New York, New York Academy of Sciences), 29–35.

Levine RJ, Brown MH, Bell M, Shue F, Greenberg GN, Bordson BL (1992) Air-conditioned environments do not prevent deterioration of human semen quality during the summer. *Fertility and Sterility* 57:1075–1083.

Lewontin RC (1972) The apportionment of human diversity. *Evolutionary Biology* 6:381–398.

Lewontin RC (1974) Annotation: the analysis of variance and the analysis of causes. *American Journal of Human Genetics* 26:400–411.

Lipson SF, Ellison PT (1989) Development of the protocols for the applicaton of salivary steroid analyses to field conditions. *American Journal of Human Biology* 1:249–255.

Lipson SF, Ellison PT (1996) Comparison of salivary steroid profiles in naturally occurring conception and non-conception cycles. *Human Reproduction* 11:2090–2096.

Longcope C, Pratt JH, Schneider SH, Fineberg SE (1976) The in vivo metabolism of androgens by muscle and adipose tissue of normal men. *Steroids* 28:521–533.

Marin P, Krotkiewski M, Bjorntorp P (1992) Androgen treatment of middle-aged, obese men: effects on metabolism, muscle and adipose tissues. *European Journal of Medicine* 1:329–336.

Marler CA, Moore MC (1988) Evolutionary costs of aggression revealed by testosterone manipulations in free-living lizards. *Behavioral Ecology and Sociobiology* 23:21–26.

Matsumoto AM, Karpas AE, Bremner WJ (1986) Chronic human chorionic gonadotropin administration in normal men: evidence that follice-stimulating hormone is necessary for the maintenance of quantitatively normal spermato-genesis in man. *Journal of Clinical Endocrinology and Metabolism* 62:1184–1192.

Matsumoto AM, Paulsen CA, Bremner WJ (1984) Stimulation of sperm production by human luteinizing hormone in gonadotropin-suppressed normal men. *Journal of Clinical Endocrinology and Metabolism* 59:882–887.

Mazur A, Booth A (1998) Testosterone and dominance in men. *Behavioral and Brain Sciences* 21:353–364.

Mazur A, Susman E, Edelbrock S (1997) Sex difference in testosterone response to a video game contest. *Evolution and Human Behavior* 18:317–326.

McMillin JM, Seal US, Karns PD (1980) Hormonal correlates of hypophagia in white-tailed deer. *Federation Proceedings* 39:2964–2968 (Federation of American Societies for Experimental Biology).

Meikle AW, Stringham JD, Bishop DT, West DW (1988) Quantitating genetic and nongenetic factors influencing androgen production and clearance rates in men. *Journal of Clinical Endocrinology and Metabolism* 67:104–109.

Meriggiola MC, Noonan EA, Paulsen CA, Bremner WJ (1996) Annual patterns of luteinizing hormone, follicle stimulating hormone, testosterone and inhibin in normal men. *Human Reproduction* 11:248–252.

Olsen GW, Bodner KM, Ramlow JM, Ross CE, Lipshultz LI (1995) Have sperm counts been reduced 50 percent in 50 years? A statistical model revisited. *Fertility and Sterility* 63:887–893.

Opstad PK (1992) Androgenic hormones during prolonged physical stress, sleep, and energy deficiency. *Journal of Clinical Endocrinology and Metabolism* 74: 1176–1183.

Partridge L, Farquhar M (1981) Sexual activity reduces lifespan of male fruitflies. *Nature* 294:580–582.

Pelliniemi LJ, Fröjdman K, Paranko J (1993) Embryological and prenatal develop-ment and function of Sertoli cells. In LD Russell, MD Griswold (Eds) *The Ser-toli Cell* (Clearwater, Florida, Cache River Press), 87–113.

Polansky FF, Lamb EJ (1988) Do the results of semen analysis predict future fertil-ity? A survival analysis study. *Fertility and Sterility* 49:1059–1065.

Powers ML, Florini JR (1975) A direct effect of testosterone on muscle cells in tissue culture. *Endocrinology* 97:1043–1047.

Roberts AC, McClure RD, Weiner RI, Brooks GA (1993) Overtraining affects male reproductive status. *Fertility and Sterility* 60:686–692.

Röjdmark S (1987a) Increased gonadotropin responsiveness to gonadotropin-releasing hormone during fasting in normal subjects. *Metabolism* 36:21–26.

Röjdmark S (1987b) Influence of short-term fasting on the pituitary-testicular axis in normal men. *Hormone Research* 25:140–146.

Rose DP, Boyar AP, Wynder EL (1986) International comparisons of mortality rates for cancer of the breast, ovary, prostate, and colon, and per capita food con-sumption. *Cancer* 58:2363–2371.

Ross R, Bernstein L, Judd H, Hanisch R, Pike M, Henderson B (1986) Serum testos-terone levels in healthy young black and white men. *Journal of the National Cancer Institute* 76:45–48.

Schaison G, Durand F, Mowszowicz I (1978) Effect of glucocorticoids on plasma testosterone in men. *Acta Endocrinologica* 89:126–131.

Semple CG, Gray CE, Beastall GH (1988) Androgen levels in men with diabetes mellitus. *Diabetic Medicine* 5:122–125.

Seo JT, Rha KH, Park YS, Lee MS (2000) Semen quality over a 10-year period in 22,249 men in Korea. *International Journal of Andrology* 23:194–198.

Sharpe RM, Skakkebaek NE (1993) Are oestrogens involved in falling sperm counts and disorders of the male reproductive tract? *Lancet* 341:1392–1395.

Shimizu H, Ross RK, Bernstein L, Yatani R, Henderson BE, Mack TM (1991) Cancers of the prostate and breast among Japanese and white immigrants in Los Angeles County. *British Journal of Cancer* 63:963–966.

Smith SR, Chhetri MK, Johanson J, Radfar N, Migeon CJ (1975) The pituitary-gonadal axis in men with protein-calorie malnutrition. *Journal of Clinical Endocrinology and Metabolism* 41:60–69.

Smuts B (1985) *Sex and Friendship in Baboons.* (Hawthorne, New York, Aldine).

Spratt DI, Crowley W Jr (1988) Pituitary and gonadal responsiveness is enhanced during GnRH-induced puberty. *American Journal of Physiology* 254:E652–657.

Spratt DI, Carr DB, Merriam GR, Scully RE, Rao PN, Crowley W Jr (1987) The spectrum of abnormal patterns of gonadotropin-releasing hormone secretion in men with idiopathic hypogonadotropic hypogonadism: clinical and laboratory correlations. *Journal of Clinical Endocrinology and Metabolism* 64:283–291.

Spratt DI, O'Dea LS, Schoenfeld D, Butler J, Rao PN, Crowley W Jr (1988) Neuroendocrine-gonadal axis in men: frequent sampling of LH, FSH, and testosterone. *American Journal of Physiology* 254:E658–666.

Stearns SC (1992) *The Evolution of Life Histories* (Oxford, Oxford University Press).

Tapanainen JS, Aittomaki K, Min J, Vaskivuo T, Huhtaniemi IT (1997) Men homozygous for an inactivating mutation of the follicle-stimulating hormone (FSH) receptor gene present variable suppression of spermatogenesis and fertility. *Nature Genetics* 15:205–206.

Tortolero I, Bellabarba AG, Lozano R, Bellabarba C, Cruz I, Osuna JA (1999) Semen analysis in men from Merida, Venezuela, over a 15-year period. *Archives of Andrology* 42:29–34.

Tsai LW, Sapolsky RM (1996) Rapid stimulatory effects of testosterone upon myotubule metabolism and sugar transport, as assessed by silicon microphysiometry. *Aggressive Behavior* 22:357–364.

Van Voorhies WA (1992) Production of sperm reduces nematode lifespan. *Nature* 360:456–458.

Veldhuis JD, Iranmanesh A, Evans WS, Lizarralde G, Thorner MO, Vance ML (1993) Amplitude suppression of the pulsatile mode of immunoradiometric luteinizing hormone release in fasting-induced hypoandrogenemia in normal men. *Journal of Clinical Endocrinology and Metabolism* 76:587–593.

Waldhauser F, Weissenbacher G, Frisch H, Pollak A (1981) Pulsatile secretion of gonadotropins in early infancy. *European Journal of Pediatrics* 137:71–74.

Welle S, Jozefowicz R, Forbes G, Griggs RC (1992) Effect of testosterone on metabolic rate and body composition in normal men and men with muscular dystrophy. *Journal of Clinical Endocrinology and Metabolism* 74:332–335.

Wingfield JC, Hegner RE, Dufty AM Jr, Ball GF (1990) The "Challenge Hypothesis": theoretical implications for patterns of testosterone secretion, mating systems, and breeding strategies. *American Naturalist* 136:829–846.

Worthman CM, Konner MJ (1987) Testosterone levels change with subsistence hunting effort in !Kung San men. *Psychoneuroendocrinology* 12:449–458.

Part II

ECOLOGICAL CONTEXT

6

Reproductive Filtering and the Social Environment

SAMUEL K. WASSER and NED J. PLACE

In evolutionary terms, successful reproduction ultimately means producing offspring that are themselves successful at reproducing. Proximately, this requires integration of many complex systems. Appreciating the complexities of these proximate mechanisms gives one a better understanding of the magnitude of selection pressures that have shaped them. This is important because those same selection pressures also shaped physiological responses to the environment—mechanisms that maximize future reproductive opportunities by minimizing costly reproductive effort when environmental conditions for reproduction are temporarily poor. This paper describes the role of the environment, and especially the social environment, in shaping reproductive processes, and it emphasizes the importance of reproductive failure as a means to control the timing of reproduction. We begin by summarizing some of the proximate mechanisms that must be integrated to produce successful offspring in an attempt to illustrate the magnitude of selection pressures that shaped them. We then describe how and why these same proximate and ultimate mechanisms promote reproductive failure in a manner that ultimately maximizes reproductive success. Our final message concerns the need to address the role of the social environment in clinical approaches to human reproduction and infertility.

A BRIEF SUMMARY OF PROXIMATE MECHANISMS REQUIRED FOR SUCCESSFUL REPRODUCTION

The neuroendocrine system directs the endocrine system through a series of positive and negative feedback loops starting with the central nervous system (CNS) and proceeding through the hypothalamic-pituitary-ovarian (HPO) axis. The amplitude and pulse of Gn-RH from the female's hypothalamus stimulates the release of follicle stimulating hormone (FSH) and luteinizing hormone (LH), respectively. These hormones must be released at the right times and concentrations to produce the proper amounts of estrogens, androgens, and progesterone. These combined processes, in turn, orchestrate follicular development, including selection of the dominant follicle and subsequent inhibition of any other developing follicles; induce ovulation; condition the cervical mucus to promote fertilization; support production and maturation of the endometrial lining required for successful implantation; impact gonadal hormone receptor densities, and more. Any one of these events can result in reproductive failure if the amount and proportion of the hormones that promote it are not just right. In this regard, it is noteworthy that the pre-ovulatory LH surge is dependent on a positive feedback loop, whereby the dominant ovarian follicle must maintain elevated estradiol plasma levels for at least 36 hours. Positive feedback systems are rare in nature because of their inherent instability; this one in particular must be fairly exact or else ovulation will fail to occur (Norris 1997; Young and Jaffe 1976).

The conceptus facilitates implantation by signaling its presence long before implantation actually takes place on day 9 postovulation (Hearn et al. 1991; Wasser 1996). The otherwise short-lived corpus luteum is then rescued by the stimulatory effects of human chorionic gonadotropin (hCG), produced by the synciotrophoblast of the conceptus. This relationship between the embryo and the ovary must be maintained through the ninth gestational week, as the placenta cannot secrete sufficient quantities of progesterone to maintain the pregnancy until then (Csapo et al. 1973).

Other mechanisms are also important. The maternal immune system must carefully monitor sperm, egg, and embryo to facilitate implantation and prevent her immune system from destroying the embryo once implanted (Harbour and Blalock 1989). Meiosis and mitosis must progress according to plan (Battaglia et al. 1996). The gametes of two very different individuals must merge, while avoiding production of aneuploidy or tetraploidy conceptions (Ayme and Lippman-Hand 1982). The maternal autonomic nervous system must properly balance sympathetic and parasympathetic tone to insure motility of gametes and the blastocyst through the oviduct and into the uterus, as well as delivery of nutrients to the placenta. Many other systems are involved as well, but a complete review is beyond the scope of this chapter.

After parturition, another complex suite of hormones, from numerous endocrine glands (hypothalamic-pituitary-gonadal axis, pancreas, adrenal gland), is required for the initiation and maintenance of lactation. Hormones such as oxytocin, vasopressin, and prolactin promote mother-newborn and father-newborn bonding (Insel 1997; Insel et al. 1998). The newborn has physical features that elicit its attractiveness to its parents

(Lorenz 1952). And, in primates, the milk is very low in fat and protein (Ben Shaul 1962), creating the need for young to suckle frequently and therefore remain close to the mother, in the safe learning environment this provides. Lactation is, in fact, the most energetically expensive activity in which a mammal ever engages (Millar 1977). It is also arguably the most costly event to survivorship and future reproductive success of the mother (Clutton-Brock et al. 1989).

When you think about all the complex physiological processes that must be integrated to reproduce successfully, it is truly a miracle that this can actually result in the production of a live human being that can in time produce its own offspring. But this is not a divine miracle; rather, it is a miracle of millions of years of evolution.

SELECTION PRESSURES SHAPING REPRODUCTIVE PROCESSES, INCLUDING REPRODUCTIVE FAILURE

What drives the evolution of a trait is the degree to which it impacts the host's ability to produce reproductively successful offspring. Offspring need to be healthy, attractive to their parents and mates, intelligent, and eventually able to fend for themselves and compete in their natural world. That takes at least one and a half decades of parental investment for our own species. It is the need to safeguard this extensive parental investment that has created the strong selection pressures that fine-tuned the orchestration of the above-mentioned reproductive processes. The considerable environmental variation that may be expressed at any time during these reproductive events has also selected for other important mechanisms to conserve parental investment, aptly termed "product rejection" (Roberts and Lowe 1975). After observing the high rate of malformation among abortuses, Roberts and Lowe noted that "in the world of early embryos, malformation may be the norm rather than the exception." Accordingly, "product rejection by way of implantation failure and spontaneous abortion is (Nature's) principal method of quality control" (Roberts and Lowe 1975:498). Essentially, the high likelihood of developmental errors when the embryo is formed has selected for physiological mechanisms to filter out those embryos whose probability of survival is relatively poor. These events are not trivial. Fifty to seventy-five percent of all human conceptions spontaneously abort during the first trimester(Roberts and Lowe 1975), reflecting the importance of safeguarding the enormous reproductive effort that is required to produce successful offspring. From an energetic and evolutionary perspective, zygotes are cheap (Kozlowski and Stearns 1989). Thus, production of excess zygotes can be explained if the mother can identify variation in fitness expectations among early-stage offspring. The filtering out of suboptimal reproductive efforts can be achieved fairly easily by simply preventing implantation, or even delaying implantation beyond 10 days postovulation (Wilcox et al. 1999).

THE REPRODUCTIVE FILTERING MODEL

Generally speaking, factors influencing the female's probability of reproductive success can vary enormously during attempts to produce an offspring. Such factors include a number of internal events as well as a host of external environmental conditions—ranging from weather to resource availability, predation risk, and psychosocial stress—that can impact the health of the mother, embryo, or fetus. High variation in these reproductive conditions, combined with the considerable parental investment required to rear reproductively successful offspring, has selected for sophisticated *reproductive filtering mechanisms* that can be activated at all stages of reproduction, and these mechanisms are equally vital to ensuring lifetime reproductive success. Specifically, females should conserve reproductive investment by suppressing reproduction whenever conditions for reproductive success are poor *and* likely to substantially improve in the foreseeable future (Koslowski and Stearns 1989; Wasser and Barash 1983). As a general rule, reproductive filtering should be more readily triggered earlier in maternal life since, all else being equal, future reproductive opportunities decrease with advancing age. Reproductive filtering should also be more readily triggered early in a given reproductive event because the amount of parental investment that would be wasted is relatively low.

REPRODUCTIVE FILTERING AND DEVELOPMENT

The entire reproductive system appears to be designed as a reproductive filtering system that starts when the mother is herself a fetus. Thus, ovarian differentiation is well underway in the female fetus by 6 weeks postconception, marked by rapid mitotic multiplication of the primordial germ cells. By the time the female fetus is 20 weeks, her newly formed ovaries contain 6–7 million oogonia; yet, all of these 6–7 million follicles will be depleted by the time the female reaches menopause, and this may well be the result of the selection process attempting to choose the best material to put forward. The most rapid rate of follicular atresia in the female fetus occurs between her twentieth week of development and birth. The newborn ovaries contain ~2 million follicles, an 80% loss from the initial allotment. The rate of atresia then slows, but during the 10–16 years before the female's first ovulation at puberty, the follicular number has fallen to

300,000 (Yeh and Adashi 1999). The menarche (onset of first menstrual bleeding) results from increasing estrogen levels and is associated with anovulatory cycles. It may take several years before the hypothalamic-pituitary-gonadal (HPG) axis matures and ovulatory cycles ensue; atresia continues throughout this period. The timing of cyclicity is also very much determined by the environment, as prematurely entering the costly process of reproduction can have severe negative impacts on the female's future reproductive success (Williams 1966).

Once cyclicity begins, many follicles are recruited during each menstrual cycle. The dominant follicle inhibits further growth of these other follicles—a survival of the fittest (see Gore et al. 1997). It is also the case that the more follicles present during any follicular phase, the higher the circulating levels of estrogen, the more healthy the dominant follicle and subsequent corpus luteum, lowering the probability of luteal phase deficiency (LPD)—insufficient amounts of progesterone during the luteal phase to mature endometrial cells adequately for implantation (Miller and Soules 1998).

Heavy filtering continues from prior to implantation (Wilcox et al. 1999) through the entire first trimester (Roberts and Lowe 1975). But much more is going on than simply cleaning up developmental errors. Other aspects of the "reproductive" environment also trigger reproductive filtering here, and at all other stages of reproduction (Chrousos et al. 1998; Wasser 1990; Wasser and Barash 1983). Reproductive filtering slows during mid-pregnancy and increases somewhat in late pregnancy, especially in the form of premature births (Berkowitz and Papiemik 1993; Erhardt 1963; Taylor 1964; prior to the advent of modern medicine, the majority of premature births would have resulted in reproductive failure). Presumably, this temporarily lowered "reproductive failure" rate during mid-pregnancy occurs because the infection risk of an incomplete mid-pregnancy abortion following in utero mortality is greater than the risk of prematurely delivering an offspring with a higher probability of mortality during late pregnancy. Reproductive filtering has also been reported in response to harsh environmental conditions following birth, in the form of abandonment and infanticide, particularly among aboriginal groups (Hausfater and Hrdy 1984; see also Daly and Wilson 1984, 1988; Glass 1999).

TEMPORAL PREDICTORS OF REPRODUCTIVE FAILURE, BASED ON THE RFM

While low food availability is a common correlate of neonatal loss (Bongaarts 1980; Clutton-Brock 1988), the RFM predicts that reproductive failure will more commonly occur early in the reproductive event in response to temporally varying food shortages (Wasser 1990; Wasser and Barash 1983). In fact, this was the basis for the pioneering work of Frisch and McArthur (1974), describing amenorrhea in response to low body fat among contemporary women. This same model explains amenorrhea in response to increased energetic expenditures and associated low body fat in dancers and runners (Loucks and Horvath 1985).

There are also conditions in which nutritionally induced reproductive failure should not occur early in the reproductive event, based on the RFM, and these temporal differences illustrate a key assumption of this model: Reproduction should only be suppressed under poor conditions *when those conditions are likely to improve in the foreseeable future.* If females suppressed reproduction under poor conditions that were unlikely to improve, they would never produce any offspring. Women experiencing chronic malnutrition in developing countries provide a case in point. Their poor conditions are unlikely to improve, based on their long-term past. They accordingly should and do experience relatively low rates of ovulatory failure and spontaneous abortion; most reproductive loss results from mortality in the neonatal stage. By contrast, poor conditions should be relatively likely to improve in the foreseeable future—in other words, return to their long-term norm—among women experiencing acute malnutrition in developed countries. As expected, these women exhibit relatively high levels of amenorrhea and spontaneous abortion, with considerably lower rates of neonatal mortality (Bongaarts 1980).

The RFM also predicts that reproductive filtering will become relaxed as women approach the age of menopause because their future reproductive opportunities are quickly diminishing. Data on the increased prevalence for women of advancing age to produce children with chromosomal abnormalities such as Down's syndrome (trisomy 21) appear to be consistent with these expectations. Sved and Sandler (1981) postulated that women approaching menopause become less likely to abort Down's children, based on the observation that this age-related event in women occurs regardless of whether the man or woman contributed the extra chromosome. This hypothesis was further evaluated by Ayme and Lippman-Hand (1982). They analyzed pooled data from three large epidemiological studies on rates of spontaneous abortions and live births with autosomal as well as XXX and XXY trisomies among women over the age of 29. Both the overall tendency towards spontaneous abortion and the tendency to conceive aneuploidies increased with advancing reproductive age of the woman. However, two thirds of the variance in live-birth trisomies were explained by the decline in spontaneous abortion of these trisomies among women 30–39 years of age. In short, reproductive filtering appears to have diminished as future reproductive opportunities declined among women nearing the end of their reproductive lifetime, increasing the proportion of trisomy births. This same argument may additionally explain the increased rate of twinning that occurs with advancing age in women (Rassaque et al. 1990).

Environmental conditions likely to hasten the occurrence of age-related sterility should also result in relaxation of reproductive filtering according to the RFM. This may explain the prevalence of teenage pregnancies among girls at high risk for sexually transmitted diseases (STDs). STDs have undoubtedly been around throughout evolutionary history and have been closely associated with high-risk sexual behavior. STDs do not typically cause tubal infertility with the first infection; rather, rates of tubal infertility usually increase rapidly after two or more infections (Westron and Eschenbach 1992). This implies that future reproductive opportunities diminish quickly in young girls practicing high-risk sex, making pregnancies at an early age the most likely means to maximize their lifetime reproductive success (see also Geronimus 1996, 1997).

A COMPARATIVE PERSPECTIVE

A central theme of this chapter is that natural selection has caused the environment to have a powerful impact on human reproductive processes, especially on the occurrence of reproductive failure. Key to this is an appreciation that timing reproduction in response to environmental cues is critical to assuring reproductive success among most animals.

The timing of reproduction in relation to environmental conditions has historically been the single biggest factor affecting a female's reproductive success (Austin and Short 1985:24–61; Clutton-Brock 1988). This is why the vast majority of plants and animals reproduce seasonally. Extreme variation in reproductive conditions occurs in a highly predictable manner among strict seasonal breeders, producing strong selection pressure for mechanisms that suppress reproduction at suboptimal times. The divergent role played by melatonin as a function of gestation length in seasonally reproducing mammals in temperate environments provides a case in point (Follett 1985). Melatonin is secreted at night; thus, concentrations are highest when days are shortest, making it an ideal neuroendocrine marker of season. Yet, strong selection pressures for most temperate species to give birth in the spring/summer, when offspring survival is greatest, have resulted in melatonin producing diametrically opposed physiological effects in species with short versus long gestations. Melatonin promotes reproduction in the spring and inhibits reproduction in the fall among species whose gestation length is less than 6 months. By contrast, melatonin has the opposite effect in species whose gestation length is greater than 6 months.

While most species are seasonal breeders, some species, including our own, live in an environment that permits or even requires a more extended breeding season. Sometimes, this results from a highly unpredictable environment, as in Australian deserts, where some of the most elaborate reproductive onset and suppression mechanisms have evolved. The highly unpredictable rainfall in these deserts require animals to be maximally opportunistic, capable of reproducing as soon as good conditions arise (Low 1978). The reproductive strategy of the eastern gray kangaroo illustrates just how opportunistic a mammal can be. It has a one-month gestation length, followed by 11 months of lactation with the joey nursing in the pouch. By the joey spending most of its early development in the pouch, the mother is afforded the opportunity to dispose of her nursing young easily, as necessary to conserve her future reproductive success. Lactational anestrus usually prevents new conceptions from occurring when an offspring is in the pouch, but this can be overridden when food is particularly abundant. In this case, conception is followed by facultative embryonic diapause, whereby further development is arrested by the nursing joey in the pouch. If the joey dies or is abandoned, embryonic development will begin anew. Moreover, this facultative embryonic diapause can also be overridden when food is scarce because of the high likelihood that pouch young will be abandoned. Lastly, cold weather can also produce seasonal diapause, delaying fetal development so young are not born under these harsh conditions. These proximate mechanisms for delaying reproductive effort may appear to be redundant, but they are vital to maximizing reproductive opportunities in this highly unpredictable environment (Follett 1985).

Other species, such as baboons, rely on their intelligence and associated behavioral plasticity to cope with seasonal hardships, enabling them to reproduce successfully throughout the year. Humans do this as well. However, despite year-round breeding, most baboon births still tend to occur during the ecologically optimal time of year. Early humans also probably had seasonal birth peaks, as these still persist among modern-day humans (Bronson 1995; Warren et al. 1986).

Baboons in Mikumi National Park, Tanzania, appear to vary the timing of births in response to seasonal and social pressures. Although females mate year-round, conception is more likely to occur during the early wet season. This results in a birth peak during the early dry season, enabling females to begin weaning their young during the subsequent early wet season when weaning foods are most available (Wasser and Norton 1993). Females who implant during the early wet season appear to be able to do so with lower concentrations of luteal phase progesterone than females who implant during the early dry season. A similar pattern occurs with respect to female dominance rank. Timing reproduction in response to social conditions is important to the reproductive success of low-ranking females, whereas high-ranking females are somewhat buffered from these impacts. High-ranking females are, accordingly, able to implant a conceptus successfully with lower concentrations of luteal phase progesterone than are low-ranking females. Indirect evidence suggests that luteal phase progesterone receptor densities are higher in dominant females and are generally higher in the early wet season. This enables females to implant with lower concentrations of progesterone under these optimal conditions (Wasser 1995, 1996). By contrast, lower luteal phase progesterone receptor densities in low-ranking females or in suboptimal seasons make implantation more difficult among females conceiving under harsh conditions (low rank or poor season). This increases the likelihood of luteal phase deficiency (LPD) if not compensated by relatively high levels of progesterone secretion in these females. In this way, only females who are "healthy" enough to produce sufficiently high progesterone concentrations, despite these typically suboptimal conditions, appear to be able to implant their conceptions. These tend to be females who are experiencing sufficiently good conditions to rear offspring successfully despite the suboptimal season or their low rank. In the case of low-ranking females, for example, reduced exposure to social stress around the time of conception is probably the most reliable cue that it is "safe" to proceed with reproduction. These conditions would also promote relatively high progesterone levels at this time. This filtering mechanism seems particularly effective because preventing implantation is probably the least risky method of suppressing reproduction. Unlike inducing ovulatory failure, luteal phase deficiency will not increase the likelihood of the female becoming anovulatory, nor would she run the risk of experiencing unopposed estrogen and associated endometrial hyperplasia. Implantation failure should also enable the female to return to a state of reproductive readiness rapidly once conditions improve. In this regard, it is interesting that LPD is reportedly the most common disorder of the menstrual cycle among women (Soules 1993) and also is frequently associated with social stress (e.g., Wasser et al. 1993).

REPRODUCTIVE FAILURE IN RESPONSE
TO SOCIAL STRESS

Social stressors are perhaps the most studied and pervasive of the stressors triggering reproductive failure among social mammals, for a good reason. The salience of social stress as a reproductive suppresser probably results from the importance of social support among these species. Social species need each other around, but this proximity inevitably results in competition (Alexander 1974). Social stress is an important correlate of this conflict. Its impact is great because, by nature, the health of our social environment has been vital to survival and successful reproduction throughout the development and evolutionary history of virtually all social species, including our own. Yet, because social partners are essentially always present, social stress is probably among the most persistent chronic stressors that animals experience—one that also leads to reproductive suppression (see review by Wasser and Barash 1983). In fact, the dichotomy of social support and social stress is evident early in life among even the most asocial eutherian mammals. Humans are no exception to this rule (Wasser 1990; Wasser et al. 1993).

Every species of eutherian mammal, including humans, gestates and delivers live-born young. The umbilical cord represents the lifeline of the fetus through which the mother provides total support. But, given that mother and fetus are genetically distinct beings traveling within a single vessel, conflicts arise and they arise early. The nausea and vomiting associated with the first trimester of human pregnancy has been ascribed to genetic conflict (Haig 1993). Social support and conflict continue throughout gestation. The mother supports her fetus by supplying fuel in the form of glucose which must course through the maternal circulation and reach the fetus via the uterus and placenta. When the maternal supply fails to keep up with fetal demand, Haig (1993) suggests the genetic conflict might be expressed clinically as gestational diabetes or pregnancy-induced hypertension.

Lactation, by definition, is a social event, but here again social support and conflict go hand-in-hand. Lactational amenorrhea (anovulation) plays a critical role in establishing the interbirth interval. Mother and suckling young benefit as future reproductive effort is delayed, saving the mother from additional energetic demands, while the young avoids sibling rivalry. The social dyad of mother and child reaches another point of conflict at the time of weaning (Trivers 1974). For example, weaning in baboons may last for weeks or months even though loud cries from the infant place both mother and infant at risk of predator attack. Both must decide whether or not persisting in their respective behaviors—the mother trying to terminate lactation while her baby tries to prolong it—is ultimately worth the risk (DeVore 1963).

Once weaned, a young female's next reproductive milestone is puberty, when menses and ovulatory cycles begin. In some species, puberty and/or first reproduction may be delayed for years owing to social pressures (e.g., tamarins, marmosets, wolves). In fact, social suppression can delay reproduction for the female's entire lifetime in some communal breeders (e.g., naked mole rats; Wasser and Barash 1983). Delayed puberty also appears to be an extreme form of socially mediated reproductive suppression among humans. (Bentley et al. 1999; Ellison et al. 1993). Competitive pressures may contribute to the common occurrence of delayed puberty among female athletes (Loucks and Horvath 1985; Nattiv et al. 1997). Anorexia nervosa provides one of the most extreme examples of psychosocially mediated pubertal delay and/or anovulatory conditions in young women. This disorder is primarily associated with low body fat but also includes considerable psychosocial maladjustment. Females presenting with anorexia often stop ovulating before their body fat levels reach critically low proportions. In addition, ovulatory cycles are often relatively slow to resume once these women have returned to a normal weight, as compared to other anovulatory weight loss conditions (Cerutti et al. 1979; Frick et al. 1978; Schindler et al. 1978, 1979; Warren et al. 1975). Several authors describe this potentially life threatening condition as being triggered by female-female competition and early sexual advances of men. Delaying puberty and adult body image reduces both of these pressures (Anderson and Crawford 1992; Surbey 1987; Voland and Voland 1989; Wasser and Barash 1983). Sadly, anorexia nervosa also exemplifies how potentially adaptive mechanisms can be taken to a maladaptive, pathological extreme. This makes an important clinical point. The prevalence of socially and nutritionally mediated suppression mechanisms that have resulted from natural selection also provided the substrate for these mechanisms to become pathologically exaggerated.

Numerous examples of reproductive failure in response to social conditions among sexually mature individuals exist throughout the animal and human literature (reviewed in Wasser 1990; Wasser and Barash 1983; Wasser and Isenberg 1986). This has also been tied to social competition in hunter-gatherers. Hunter-gatherers have historically been resource-limited, and individuals appear to have regulated their reproduction, and hence population growth, in response to resource limitation (Cohen et al. 1980; Lee 1980; Schrimshaw 1984; Wagley 1977). In a study of stress-related infertility among contemporary women, Wasser et al. (1993) found that the most salient stressors likely to result in infertility were social stressors (including amount and quality of social support, conflict with father, support from best friend, conflict with second best friend, hostility, and social anxiety). The temporal patterns of social stress leading to reproductive failure are also consistent with expectations from the RFM. For example, Ilsley (1955) conducted an epidemiological study of birth outcomes among 3,911 women in England, based on the social class (occupation) of both their husband and father. Women who rose substantially in social class as a result of their marriage (i.e., were experiencing relatively improved socioeconomic conditions) exhibited a dramatic decline in reproductive failure rates (prematurity and obstetric death rates) compared with those who remained in their same social class. By contrast, women who declined substantially in socioeconomic class as a result of their marriage (experiencing relatively poor socioeconomic conditions)

exhibited a dramatic rise in prematurity and obstetric death rates compared with women who remained in their socioeconomic class (Ilsley
1955). These differences persisted despite improvements in the delivery of
prenatal care to individuals of low socioeconomic class (see also Easterlin
1980; Kasarda et al. 1986).

Conscious decisions to contracept, or terminate reproduction using therapeutic abortion, similarly appear to be consistent with temporal expectations from the RFM. Women whose long-term socioeconomic histories, as
well as those of their mates, provide little hope for future improvement are
also those who most often use contraceptives ineffectively. In addition,
while these women may initially opt for therapeutic abortion, they are also
the ones most likely to change their minds and continue with the pregnancies. By contrast, women whose socioeconomic futures hold considerably
better promise for successful reproductive opportunities compared with
the present are those who use contraception most effectively, and who most
quickly obtain therapeutic abortions of unwanted pregnancies (David and
Johnson 1977; Mindick et al. 1977; Wasser and Isenberg 1986). If conscious
decisions to opt for therapeutic abortion tend to be truly adaptive, one
would predict that reproductive outcomes should have improved immediately after therapeutic abortion became legal. This was indeed the case.
Lanman et al. (1974) reported that rates of spontaneous abortion and premature deliveries decreased by 20% and 30%, respectively, in one carefully
monitored hospital in New York. Rates of spontaneous abortion decreased
by 70% in a well-monitored Seattle hospital during this same time period
(Shepard and Fantel 1979; see also Joyce 1987).

Data also suggest that women who desire but are denied a therapeutic
abortion often have poorer reproductive outcomes, including spontaneous
abortion, premature births, and increased neonatal morbidity and mortality. In a prospective study of 8,000 women who conceived between 1960
and 1966, prior to legalization of abortion, women with a negative attitude
about their pregnancy had significantly higher rates of perinatal death,
congenital anomalies, and postpartum infection and hemorrhage (Laukaran and van den Berg 1980). Matejcek et al. (1978) found higher rates of
minimal brain dysfunction, acute illness, and a tendency to be slightly
overweight among 220 unwanted children born in Czechoslovakia to
mothers twice denied an elective abortion, compared with controls. Moreover, these differences persisted until age 16, when monitoring ceased.

CLINICAL IMPLICATIONS

Taken together, a wide body of evidence suggests that the reproductive
system of female mammals, including women, evolved to suppress repro-

duction in response to environmental pressures. Thus, a significant portion of reproductive failure in women may have an environmental component, and especially a psychosocial stress component (Chrousos et al. 1998). Yet, the majority of physicians and patients appear reluctant to address these potentially causal environmental pressures as part of their treatment regime. There are probably several reasons for this reluctance, not the least of which is the difficulty of proving the existence of stress effects on reproductive outcome among contemporary humans.

Recall the numerous mechanisms described above that have to be integrated to insure successful reproduction. Environmentally mediated reproductive suppression could in theory occur by disrupting any number of these mechanisms. In fact, there is good reason to suspect that this is exactly what happens. Stress affects the neuroendocrine system, the autonomic nervous system, the central nervous system, and the immune system (Sapolsky 1998). If selection pressures for reproductive filtering have been as pervasive as we've proposed, this could promote mechanisms involving any combination of these systems to induce reproductive failure under relatively harsh conditions. This makes it particularly difficult to tease apart the role of stress in reproductive failure because such failure can, and does, result from these pressures via any number of different routes (Wasser and Isenberg 1986). Additionally, the efficacy, or even existence, of reproductive filtering can come into question whenever a child is born with a major chromosomal or congenital abnormality. However, these filtering mechanisms do not have to work perfectly; they merely need to lead to better outcomes, on average, than nothing at all.

Documenting the effects of stress on infertility has been further complicated by experimental designs that tend to lump all forms of infertility when looking for sequelae of stress. This dilutes the overall observed stress effects since some of these disorders are unlikely to be caused by stress. Specifically, anatomic causes of infertility (e.g., proximal and distal tubal obstructions, pelvic adhesions, severe endometriosis, anatomic disorders of the cervix and uterus) are relatively unlikely to be caused by stress; these disorders can only be corrected through surgery. By contrast, neuroendocrine and immune-related disorders are more likely to be caused by stress; these are the same kinds of disorders that appear to mediate environmentally induced reproductive failure among mammals in general (Arck et al. 1996; Bronson 1989; Chrousos et al. 1998; Markert et al. 1997).

These problems are complicated further because the extreme stressfulness of experiencing reproductive failure in humans, regardless of its cause, makes it difficult to determine whether stress caused the reproductive failure or vice versa. Prospective studies could help address this problem, but they are largely prohibitive because of time, cost, and subject availability constraints. Wasser et al. (1993) conducted a pilot study of stress and infertility designed to address each of the above problems. Women from infertile couples were divided into three groups: women with anatomic causes of their infertility; women with functional (neuroendocrine and immune) causes; and intermediates (those who had both functional and anatomic causes or an etiology that was difficult to classify as either functional or anatomic—e.g., polycystic ovarian disease, PCO). Controls included women with disorders similar to those in the functional infertility group but who did not wish to become pregnant; hence, controls did not have the stress of being infertile. Wasser et al. (1993) predicted that if stress causes infertility, infertile women with functional infertility disorders should report higher levels of psychosocial stress than infertile women with anatomic or intermediate disorders, even though all three infertility groups share the stress of being infertile. Moreover, if psychosocial stress is a significant cause of functional disorders, controls should also report higher levels of stress than do women with anatomic or intermediate fertility disorders. Women with functional causes of their infertility, as well as controls, did, in fact, report higher levels of psychosocial stress than women with anatomic and, secondarily, intermediate causes of their infertility, supporting the role of psychosocial stress as a cause of some forms of infertility.

A parallel study conducted by Giles and Berga (1993) reported similar results. They compared women with functional amenorrhea to matched eumenorrheic controls as well as to women with organic amenorrhea. In this study they found that the women with functional amenorrhea were characterized by dysfunctional attitudes, a decreased ability to cope, and a greater dependence as compared with one or both of the other groups.

The Wasser et al. (1993) study is presently being replicated with a much larger sample size. However, 94% of the 600 patients who declined to participate in this new study stated their reason for decline as being "too stressed out" to participate (Wasser, unpublished data). This further emphasizes the difficulty of conducting social stress and infertility studies. Lack of well-controlled studies also led Istvan (1986) to conclude that there is no clear-cut support for the role of psychosocial factors in relation to birth outcomes in women. Yet in the same paper he states that stress effects on birth outcomes are clear from the animal literature. Effects include decreased litter size, reduced birth weights, and lower neonatal survival. Intergenerational effects on the reproductive capacity of the offspring have also been reported in rats (Pollard 1984) and humans (Sever and Emanuel 1981). Istvan's conclusions are also in direct contrast to those of other investigators who report significant psychosocial stress effects on pregnancy outcomes (Nuckolls et al. 1972; Norbeck and Tilden 1983; Rizzardo 1985).

Additional problems exist as well. Bergant et al. (1997) used a design based on the Wasser et al. (1993) study to investigate stress as a cause of spontaneous abortion (SAB). However, this recent paper illustrates how an erroneous conclusion can be reached about the role of psychosocial stress in fertility disorders simply by making the wrong assumptions. They divided patients who previously had more than two SABs into those with physical causes and those with idiopathic causes (assuming the latter group to parallel the functional infertility group in the Wasser et al. 1993 study). They predicted a higher subsequent SAB rate in the idiopathic versus physical SAB group, but found the reverse. This led them to conclude that psychosocial stress does not play a significant causal role in recurrent SAB. However, their study defined physical causes of SAB as any documented cause. By this definition, the most common physical cause (6/16) in their SAB group was luteal phase deficiency (LPD). LPD was among the reproductive disorders most likely to be caused by stress in the Wasser et al. study, as well as in other human and mammal studies (Wasser 1990, 1995, 1996). Moreover, because of its neuroendocrine origin (see above), LPD was placed in the functional (versus "physical") infertility group in the Wasser et al. (1993) study. The Bergant et al. (1997) paper appeared in *Human Reproduction*—one of the leading reproductive medicine journals in Europe. Undoubtedly, many physicians will read this paper and be reassured that they are justified in failing to consider psychosocial stress reduction as a part of the treatment for recurrent SAB. This is unfortunate as some earlier studies have demonstrated pregnancy success rates of 81% to 86% among prior habitual aborters following prenatal counseling and psychosocial support ("tender loving care") (Grimm 1962 and Stray-Pedersen and Stray-Pedersen 1984, respectively). Again, these latter studies have been questioned because they did not include control groups. However, their overwhelming success rates warrant further study and possible implementation of psychosocial treatments.

In short, the difficulties of studying impacts of social stress on reproductive failure should not be taken to imply a lack of an effect. The contrary appears to hold true, and, as argued below, it is time for physicians to start paying greater attention to this in their diagnosis and treatment of these reproductive "problems." Indeed, failure to do so could result in far more serious complications at later stages of a given reproductive event (Wasser 1990). Likewise, it is time for health insurance companies and HMOs to start covering psychosocial interventions in the treatment of reproductive failure.

CONCLUDING REMARKS

Patients experiencing reproductive failure, and especially infertility, are some of the most anxious patients a physician is likely to encounter.

Moreover, these patients rarely want to do the personal work required to resolve their stresses as long as they believe they can rely on biomedical treatments to solve their fertility problems. This puts enormous pressure on physicians to use the biomedical treatments at their finger tips to treat these disorders. In the competitive biomedical environment that now exists, patients will simply go elsewhere if physicians fail to meet their demands. The problem is made worse by the media, who characterize the assisted reproductive technologies as the gold standard for treating these disorders when, in reality, they simply don't work very well (Collins et al. 1983). To make matters worse, when they do work, many infertility treatments significantly increase the risk of multiple pregnancies (Jansen 1982), potentially producing a whole new set of stresses on an already stressed couple.

If stress causes reproductive failure and reproductive failure causes stress, it may also be the case that prior history or even fear of reproductive failure can increase its prevalence, regardless of the initial etiology. Evidence for this comes from Domar et al. (1990, 1998). Of 185 infertility patients, randomly assigned to either a cognitive-behavioral therapy group, a support group, or a routine care control group, 76% of the cognitive-behavioral and 68% of the support group members had viable pregnancies compared with 28% of controls ($p < 0.02$). These results point to the importance of reducing the stress associated with reproductive failure in all patients undergoing treatment. This will only come about when physicians begin to appreciate the pervasive role social stress can play as a cause of reproductive failure.

In summary, despite multiple historical problems associated with the study of stress and reproductive failure, we believe that there are now ample theoretical, natural history, and controlled experimental-design studies to conclude that the environment, and especially one's social environment, plays a significant role in mediating all forms of reproductive failure among women. It is, accordingly, time for our health care system to start taking this problem more seriously. Current demographic trends make this need even more pressing. There are now greater demands on women to work and reproduce as double incomes become increasingly essential to maintain a middle-class status. We also tend to operate on significantly less sleep. These factors greatly increase opportunities for social stress. At the same time, women are delaying their first birth, increasing both their likelihood of being infertile and their urgency to conceive. These pressures will likely increase the stress of infertility, feeding back to suppress fertility even further. Given the above, we can only conclude that psychosocial stress evaluation should become an integral part of the diagnosis and treatment of persistent reproductive failure. Potential mothers and their future children are in desperate need of this help, and clinicians have a responsibility to provide it for them.

REFERENCES

Alexander RD (1974) The evolution of social behavior. *Annual Review of Ecology and Systematics* 5:325–383.

Anderson JL, Crawford CB (1992) Modeling costs and benefits of adolescent weight control as a mechanism for reproductive suppression. *Human Nature* 3:299–334.

Arck PC, Merali F, Chaouat G, Clark DA (1996) Inhibition of immunoprotective CD8(+) T cells as a basis for stress-triggered substance P-mediated abortion in mice. *Cellular Immunology* 171:226–230.

Austin CR, Short RV (Eds) (1985) *Reproduction in Mammals,* book 4 (Cambridge, Cambridge University Press).

Ayme S, Lippman-Hand A (1982) Maternal-age effect in aneuploidy: does altered embryonic selection play a role? *American Journal of Human Genetics* 34:558–565.

Battaglia DE, Goodwin P, Klein NA, Soules MR (1996) Influence of maternal age on meiotic spindle assembly in oocytes from naturally cycling women. *Human Reproduction* 11:2217–2222.

Ben Shaul DM (1962) The composition of the milk of wild animals. *International Zoo Yearbook* 4:333–342.

Bentley GR, Aunger R, Harrigan AM, Jenike M, Bailey RC, Ellison PT (1999) *Social Science and Medicine* 48:149–162.

Bergant AM, Reinstadler K, Moncayo HE, Solder E, Heim K, Ulmer H, Hinterhuber H, Dapunt O (1997) Spontaneous abortion and psychosomatics. A prospective study on the impact of psychological factors as a cause for recurrent spontaneous abortion. *Human Reproduction* 12:1106–1110.

Berkowitz GS, Papiemik E (1993) Epidemiology of pre-term birth. *Epidemiology Reviews* 15:414–443.

Bongaarts J (1980) Does malnutrition affect fecundity? A summary of evidence. *Science* 208:564–569.

Bronson FH (1989) *Mammalian Reproductive Biology* (Chicago, University of Chicago Press).

Bronson FH (1995) Seasonal variation in human reproduction: environmental factors. *Quarterly Review of Biology* 70:141–164.

Cerutti R, Foresti G, Ferraro M, Crema MG, Grazioli EA (1979) Juvenile dysmenorrhea, personality profiles and therapeutic approach with autogenic training. *Emotions and Reproduction* 20:165–167.

Check JH (1978) Emotional aspects of menstrual dysfunction. *Psychosomatic Medicine* 19:178–184.

Chrousos GP, Torpy DJ, Gold PW (1998) Interactions between the hypothalamic-pituitary-adrenal axis and the female reproductive system: clinical implications. *Annals of Internal Medicine* 120:229–240.

Clutton-Brock TH (Ed) (1988) *Reproductive Success: Studies of Individual Variation in Contrasting Breeding Systems* (Chicago, University of Chicago Press).

Clutton-Brock TH, Albon SD, Guinness FE (1989) Fitness costs of gestation and lactation in wild mammals. *Nature* 337:260–262.

Cohen MN, Malpas RS, Klein HG (Eds) (1980) *Biosocial Mehcanisms of Population Regulation* (New Haven, Yale University Press).

Collins JA, Wrixton W, Janes LB, Wilson EH (1983) Treatment-independent pregnancy among infertile couples. *New England Journal of Medicine* 309:1201–1206.

Csapo AI, Pulkkinen MO, Weist WG (1973) Effects of luteoectomy and progesterone replacement in early pregnant patients. *American Journal of Obstetrics and Gynecology* 115:759–765.

Daly M, Wilson M (1984) A sociobiological analysis of human infanticide. In G Hausfater, S Hrdy (Eds) *Infantificide: Comparative and Evolutionary Perspectives* (New York, Aldine), 487–502.

Daly M,Wilson M (1988) *Homicide* (New York, Aldine de Gruyter).

David H, Johnson RL (1977) Fertility regulation in child bearing years: psychosocial and psychoeconomic aspects. *Preventative Medicine* 6:52–64.

DeVore I (1963) Mother-infant relations in free-ranging baboons. In H Reingold (Ed) *Maternal Behavior in Mammals* (New York, Wiley), 305–335.

Domar AD, Freizinger M, Clapp D, Slawsby E, Mortola J, Kessel B, Friedman R (1998) The impact of group psychological interventions on pregnancy rates in infertile women. *Fertility and Sterility* 70(Suppl 1):S30.

Domar AD, Seibel MM, Benson H (1990) The mind/body program for infertility: a new behavioral treatment approach for women with infertility. *Fertility and Sterility* 53:246–249.

Easterlin RA (1980) *Birth and Fortune* (New York, Basic Books).

Ellison PT, Panter-Brick C, Lipson SF, O'Rourke MT (1993) The ecological context of human ovarian function. *Human Reproduction* 8:2248–2258.

Erhardt CL (1963) Pregnancy losses in New York City, 1960. *Journal of Public Health* 53:1337–1352.

Follett BK (1985) The environment and reproduction. In Austin CR, Short RV (Eds) *Reproduction in Mammals,* book 4 (Cambridge, Cambridge University Press), 103–132.

Frick V, Lubke R, Sommer K, Schindler AE (1978) Psychological evaluation in anorexia nervosa and anorectic reaction. *Clinical Psychneuroendocrinology of Reproduction* 22:295–300.

Frisch RE, McArthur JW (1974) Menstrual cycles: fatness as a determinant of minimum weight for height necessary for their maintenance or onset. *Science* 185:548–556.

Geronimus AT (1996) What teen mothers know. *Human Nature* 7:323–52.

Geronimus AT (1997) Teenage childbearing and personal responsibility: an alternative view. *Political Science Quarterly* 112:405–430.

Giles DE, Berga SL (1993) Cognitive and psychiatric correlates of functional hypothalamic amenorrhea: a controlled comparison. *Fertility and Sterility* 60: 486–492.

Glass N (1999) Infanticide in Hungary faces stiffer penalties. *Lancet* 353:570.

Gore MA, Nayudu PL, Vlaisavlejevic V (1997) Attaining dominance in vivo: distinguishing dominant from challenger follicles in humans. *Human Reproduction* 12:2741–2747.

Grimm ER (1962) Psychological investigation of habitual abortion. *Psychosomatic Medicine* 24:369–378.

Haig D (1993) Genetic conflicts in human pregnancy. *Quarterly Review of Biology* 68:495–533.

Harbour DV, Blalock JE (1989) Lymphocytes and lymphocytic hormones in pregnancy. *Psychoneuroendocrinimmunology* 2:55–63.

Hausfater G, Hrdy S (Eds) (1984) *Infanticide: Comparative and Evolutionary Perspectives* (New York, Aldine).

Hearn JP, Webley GE, Gidley-Baird AA (1991) Chorionic gonadotrophin and embryonic-maternal recognition during the peri-implantation period in primates. *Journal of Reproduction and Fertility* 92:497–509.

Ilsley R (1955) Social class selection and class differences in relation to stillbirths and infant deaths. *British Medical Journal* (Dec 24):1520–1524.

Insel TR (1997) A neurobiological basis of social attachment. *American Journal of Psychiatry* 154:726–735.

Insel TR, Winslow JT, Wang Z, Young LJ (1998) Oxytocin, vasopressin, and the neuroendocrine basis of pair bond formation. *Advances in Experimental Medicine and Biology* 449:215–224.

Istvan J (1986) Stress, anxiety, and birth outcomes: a critical review of the evidence. *Psychological Bulletin* 100:331–348.

Jansen RPS (1982) Spontaneous abortion incidence in the treatment of infertility. *American Journal of Obstetrics and Gynecology* 143:451.

Joyce T (1987) The impact of induced abortion on black and white birth outcomes in the United States. *Demography* 24:229–244.

Kasarda JD, Billy JOG, West K (1986) *Status Enhancement and Fertility: Reproductive Responses to Social Mobility and Educational Opportunity* (New York, Academic Press).

Kozlowski J, Stearns SC (1989) Hypothesis for the production of excess zygotes: models of bet-hedging and selective abortion. *Evolution* 43:1369–1377.

Lanman JT, Kohl SG, Bedell JH (1974) Changes in pregnancy outcome after liberalization of the New York State abortion law. *American Journal of Obstetrics and Gynecology* 118:485.

Laukaran VH, van den Berg BJ (1980) The relationship of maternal attidtude to pregnancy outcomes and obstetric complications: a cohort study of unwanted pregnancy. *American Journal of Obstetrics and Gynecology* 136:374–379.

Lee RB (1980) Lactation, ovulation, infanticide, and women's work: a study of hunter-gatherer population regulation. In Cohen MN, Malpas RS, Klein HG (Eds) *Biosocial Mechanisms of Population Regulation* (New Haven, Yale University Press), 321–348.

Loucks AB, Horvath SM (1985) Athletic amenorrhea: a review. *Medicine and Science in Sports and Exercise* 17:56–72.

Lorenz K (1952) *King Solomon's Rings: New Light on Animal Ways*. (New York, Crowell).

Low BS (1978) Environmental uncertainty and the parental stratetgies of marsupials and placentals. *American Naturalist* 112:197–213.

Markert UR, Arck PC, McBey BA, Manuel J, Croy BA, Marshall JS, Chaouat G, Clark DA (1997) Stress-triggered abortions are associated with alterations of granulated cells into the decidua. *American Journal of Reproductive Immunology* 37:94–100.

Matejcek Z, Dytrych Z, Schuller V (1978) Children from unwanted pregnancies. *Acta Psychiatrica Scandinavica* 57:67–90.

Millar JS (1977) Adaptive features of mammalian reproduction. *Evolution* 31: 370–386.

Miller PB, Soules MR (1998) Luteal phase deficiency—pathophysiology, diagnosis, and treatment. In JJ Sciarra (Ed) *Gynecology and Obstetrics*, vol. 5 (Philadelphia, Lippincott-Raven), 1–29.

Mindick B, Oskamp S, Berge DE Jr (1977) Prediction of success or failure in birth planning: an approach to prevention of individual and family stress. *American Journal of Community Psychology* 5:447–459.

Nattiv A, Puffer JC, Green GA (1997) Lifestyles and health risk of collegiate athletes: a multi-center study. *Clinical Journal of Sports Medicine* 7:262–272.

Norbeck JS, Tilden VP (1983) Life stress, social support, and emotional disequilibrium in complications of pregnancy: a prospective, multivariate study. *Journal of Health and Social Behavior* 24:30–46.

Norris DO (1997) *Vertebrate Endocrinology*, 3rd ed. (San Diego, Academic Press).

Nuckolls KB, Cassel J, Kaplan BH (1972) Psychosocial assets, life crises and the prognosis of pregnancy. *American Journal of Epidemiology* 95:431–441.

Pollard I (1984) Effects of stress administered during pregnancy on reproductive capacity and subsequent development of the offspring of rats. Prolonged effects on the litters of a second pregnancy. *Journal of Endocrinology* 100:301–306.

Rakoff AE (1962) Psychogenic factors in anovulatory women. *Fertility and Sterility* 13:1–10.

Rassaque A, Ahmed K, Wai L (1990) Twinning rates in a rural area of Bangladesh. *Human Biology* 62:505–514.

Rizzardo R, Magni G, Andreoli C, Merlin G, Andreoli F, Fabbris L, Martinotti G, Cosentino M (1985) Psychosocial aspects during pregnancy and obstetrical complications. *Journal of Psychosomatic Obstetrics and Gynecology* 4:11–22.

Roberts CJ, Lowe CR (1975) Where have all the conceptions gone? *Lancet* 1:498–499.

Sapolsky RM (1998) *Why Zebras Don't Get Ulcers* (San Francisco, WH Freeman).

Schindler AE, Shier I, Frick V, Gundling F, Goser R, Keller E (1978) Psychogenic amenorrhea: endocrine evaluation and follow-up. *Clinical Psychoneuroendocrinology of Reproduction* 22:281–293.

Schindler AE, Frick V, Goser R, Keller E (1979) The endocrine profile of psychogenic amenorrhea: correlates of homronal and psychosomoatic findings and effect of therapy. *Emotions and Reproduction* 20:169–172.

Schrimshaw SCM (1984) Infanticide in human populations: social and individual concerns. In G Hausfater, S Hrdy (Eds) *Infanticide: Comparative and Evolutionary Perspectives* (New York, Aldine), 439–462.

Sever LE, Emanuel I (1981) Intergenerational factors in the etiology of anencephalus and spina bifida. *Developmental Medicine and Child Neurology* 23:151–154.

Shepard TH, Fantel AG (1979) Embryonic and early fetal loss. *Clinics in Perinatology* 6:219–243.

Soules MR (1993) Luteal dysfunction. In EY Adashi, PCK Leung (Eds) *The Ovary* (New York, Raven Press), 607–627.

Stray-Pedersen B, Stray-Pedersen S (1984) Etiologic factors and subsequent reproductive performance in 195 couples with prior history of habitual abortion. *American Journal of Obstetrics and Gynecology* 148:140–146.

Surbey MK (1987) Anorexia nervosa, amenorrhea and adaptation. *Ethology and Sociobiology* 8 (Supplement):47–61.

Sved JA, Sandler L (1981) Relation of maternal age effect in Down's Syndrome to nondisjunction. In FF De la Cruz, PS Gerald (Eds) *Trisomy 21 (Down Syndrome): Research Prospectives* (Baltimore, University Park Press), 95–98.

Taylor WF (1964) On the methodology of measuring the probability of fetal death in a prospective study. *Human Biology* 36:86–103.

Trivers RL (1974) Parent-offspring conflict. *American Zoologist* 14:249–264.

Voland E, Voland R (1989) Evolutionary biology and psychiatry: the case of anorexia nervosa. *Ethology and Sociobiology* 10:223–240.

Wagley C (1977) *Welcome of Tears: The Tapirape Indians of Central Brazil* (New York, Oxford University Press).

Warren CW, Gwinn ML, Rubin GL (1986) Seasonal variation in concepttion and various pregnancy outcomes. *Social Biology* 33:116–126.

Warren MP, Jewelewicz R, Dyrenfurth I, Ans R, Khalaf S, Van de Wiele RL (1975) The significance of weight loss in the evaluation of pituitary response to LH-RH in women with secondary amenorrhea. *Journal of Clinical Endocrinology and Metabolism* 40:601.

Wasser SK (1990) Infertility, abortion and biotechnology: When it's not nice to fool Mother Nature. *Human Nature* 1:3–25.

Wasser SK (1995) Costs of conception in baboons. *Nature* 376:219–220.

Wasser SK (1996) Reproductive control in wild baboons measured by fecal steroids. *Biology of Reproduction* 55:393–399.

Wasser SK, Barash DP (1983) Reproduction suppression among female mammals: implication for biomedicine and sexual selection theory. *Quarterly Review of Biology* 58:513–538.

Wasser SK, Isenberg DY (1986) Reproductive suppression: pathology or adaptation. *Journal of Psychosomatic Obstetrics and Gynecology* 5:153–175.

Wasser SK, Norton GW (1993) Baboons adjust secondary sex ratio in response to predictors of sex-specific offspring survival. *Behavioral Ecology and Sociobiology* 32:273–281.

Wasser SK, Sewall G, Soules MR (1993) Psychosocial stress as a cause of infertility. *Fertility and Sterility* 59:685–689.

Westrom L, Eschenbach D (1992) Pelvic inflamatory disease and infertility. A cohort study of 1884 women with laparoscopically verified disease and 657 control women with normal laproscopic findings. *Sexually Transmitted Disease* 19:185.

Wilcox AJ, Baird DD, Weinberg CR (1999) Time of implantation of the conceptus and loss of pregnancy. *New England Journal of Medicine* 340:1796–1799.

Williams GC (1966) Natural selection, the costs of reproduction, and a refinement of Lack's principle. *American Naturalist* 100:687–690.

Yeh J, Adashi EY (1999) The ovarian life cycle. In SSC Yen, RB Jaffe, RL Barbieri (Eds) *Reproductive Endocrinology: Physiology, Pathophysiology, and Clinical Management*, 4th ed. (Philadelphia, WB Saunders), 155.

Young JR, Jaffe RB (1976) Strength-duration characterisitics of estrogen effects on gonadotropin response to gonadotropin releasing hormone in women. *Journal of Clinical Endocrinology and Metabolism* 42:432–442.

7

Reproductive Ecology of Male Immune Function and Gonadal Function

BENJAMIN C. CAMPBELL, WILLIAM D. LUKAS,
and KENNETH L. CAMPBELL

Although immunity and reproductive function are often considered as if they were entirely separate physiological systems, a moment's consideration makes their deep and intimate relationship clear. The production of both ova and sperm results in genetically distinct haploid cells, necessitating special measures to prevent attack by the immune system (Hilgarth et al. 1997). Similarly, the fetus is a genetically foreign body, requiring modulation of immune function to maintain pregnancy (Grossman 1984; Roberts et al. 1996). More importantly for reproductive ecologists, at a somatic level immune function and reproductive function are balanced against one another as trade-offs under organismic energetic constraints (Hill 1993).

Recently, anthropologists have begun investigation of immune function and reproductive function in nonwestern subsistence populations (Flinn and England 1997; McDade and Worthman 1999; Shell-Duncan 1997), where energetic constraints are likely to make such trade-offs more pronounced. Such work is still in its infancy, however, and relating immunity in all its complexity to reproduction, with equal complexity, is a daunting task. In women, the high energetic demands on pregnancy and lactation add an additional factor that may overshadow the interaction of immune and reproductive function. On the other hand, males bear no direct costs of conception, and the energetic costs of sperm are relatively minor. The major portion of reproductive function involved in trade-offs with immunity among males should be its labile somatic component, which is critical to work capacity and sexual selection—namely, skeletal muscle.

In this chapter we restrict our focus to the interaction of immune function and reproductive function among males. Our initial goal is to determine the possibility of a demonstrable impact of testosterone on health status among males in a nonwestern population. We start by outlining differences in immunocompetence between males and females, suggesting that testosterone is a significant cause of increased male susceptibility to disease. Next, we discuss how this greater susceptibility is related to trade-offs between the immune and muscle systems of the male soma. We then detail specific mechanisms by which testosterone, the key male hormone, may suppress immune function in males. In the succeeding section we review evidence from animal studies demonstrating that testosterone has an impact on the immune response to malaria and helminthic infections. Finally, we explore the possibility that under conditions of energetic constraints or chronic undernutrition testosterone may be related to health status using data from the Turkana, a group of pastoral nomads from northwest Kenya.

MALE-FEMALE DIFFERENCES IN IMMUNOCOMPETENCE

Both naturalistic studies and laboratory experiments demonstrate that male mammals are more vulnerable to infectious disease than females. Male mammals have both higher prevalence and greater intensity of infection with nematode helminths (Poulin 1996). Evidence from field studies include higher intensity of fly larvae infestation in male reindeer (Folstad et al. 1989) and higher probability of death from infectious disease in male macaques (Fedigan and Zohar 1997). Male atypical-species hosts show a higher intensity of infections with nematode infections, which indicates that macrophage-based defenses against the infective stage of parasites are less effective in males (Tiuria et al. 1995).

Sex differences in parasite infection are apparent in adult mammals, but not juveniles, implicating a role for sex steroids (Schalk and Forbes 1997). Experimental evidence implicates testosterone as the major cause of sex differences in disease resistance. Male-female differences in immune function are *increased* under controlled conditions. Contrary to the hypothesis that immune dimorphism is mainly due to differences in exposure, castration of laboratory rodents produces increased spleen weight, lymphocyte count, cellular and humoral immunity, and graft rejection, while testosterone administration reverses these effects (Zuk and McKean 1996). Testosterone administration reduces expulsion of gut nematodes in rats (Tiuria et al. 1995) and promotes tapeworm egg production (Folstad and Karter 1992).

Humans are no exception to the mammalian pattern of sexual dimorphism in susceptibility to infection and disease burdens. In the United States, the age-adjusted death rates from both infectious and noninfectious diseases are higher in men (Zopf 1992). Men have a higher rate of a wide spectrum of infections and are more likely to serve as disease carriers

(Otten 1985). Men also exhibit high rates of nearly all categories of noninfectious disease, including cardiovascular, nephritic, and hepatic disease and neoplasms. The growing evidence for viral involvement in various forms of cancer (Rakowicz et al. 1998; Storey et al. 1998) suggests that, in addition to lifestyle factors, differential resistance to infection may play a role in the epidemiological pattern of these diseases. The only diseases to which men are less susceptible than women are autoimmune diseases and sex-specific diseases such as ovarian cancer and those associated with pregnancy (Otten 1985).

Sexual dimorphism in immunocompetence is consistent with the sex-differentiated epidemiological pattern; for example, women have higher immunoglobin levels than men (Otten 1985), especially of IgM (Kacprzak-Bergman 1994).

REPRODUCTION AND IMMUNITY IN
LIFE HISTORY TRADE-OFFS

The major compartments of energetic allocation are maintenance, growth, storage, and reproduction (Hill 1993). The first three can be categorized under enhancement of survival, reducing the primary life history trade-off to one of reproduction versus survival. For males, the cost of gametes and their delivery systems is only a small part of the physiological cost of reproduction. For example, the testes account for just 0.06% of the body mass of human males (Harcourt et al. 1981); the prostate weighs only 20 grams (Tanagho 1995). Instead, the greatest bulk of resource expenditure differentiating males from females is in somatic maintenance, including higher skeletal muscle mass, bone density, red blood cells, and metabolic rate. For example, while on average males age 20–29 have 23% more body mass than females, they have 46% more total protein and 27% more bone mineral (Groff et al. 1995). Higher skeletal mass, bone density, red blood cells, and metabolic rate are all components more highly related to the musculoskeletal system than to the reproductive system per se. However, each of these traits is promoted by testosterone and serves to enhance all aspects of male survival and reproduction, including work capacity, male-male competition, and mate choice.

Thus for the purposes of our argument here, we consider the fundamental physiological burden of reproduction and maintenance for adult males to be a trade-off between immunity and musculoskeletal maintenance. This trade-off can be categorized in terms of the four major costs of immune response: (1) increased metabolic rate, (2) catabolism of muscle and fat, (3) increased risk of autoimmunity, and (4) oxidative stress. The former two may be considered energetic/resource trade-offs between immunity and other physiological compartments, while the latter two represent trade-offs between disease resistance and immunopathology.

An effective immune response requires the rapid utilization of body stores for both fuel and protein substrate. When mounting an immune defense, especially when fever is produced by inflammatory cytokines, the energetic cost of the immune system is dramatically elevated. Human metabolic rate increases by 13% for each degree Celsius body temperature is raised (Elia 1992).

In addition to its energetic costs, an immune response also results in fat being catabolized by cytokines for use by the immune system. The cytokine TNF prevents the uptake of lipids by cells by its inhibition of the enzyme lipoprotein lipase, resulting in increased circulatory lipids available as a substrate for immune response (Zuk 1996). The immune response also relies on rapid protein metabolism. The amino acid glutamine is one link between skeletal muscle and the immune system (Newsholme et al. 1992). More than 60% of free amino acid in skeletal muscle is in the form of glutamine (Young et al. 1992), which is also an important fuel for macrophage activity and lymphocyte proliferation. The cytokines TNF and IL-1 catabolize skeletal muscle in response to both injury and infection to free up amino acids required for the immune response and tissue repair (Young et al. 1992).

Besides a trade-off of energy and proteins between compartments, immunocompetence also presents a trade-off between disease resistance and immunopathology (Raberg et al. 1998). During physiological stress, muscle damage and expression of heat-shock proteins may result in a change in the self-antigen repertoire and stimulation of the immune response, causing autoimmunity (Raberg et al. 1998). In addition, free radicals secreted by immune cells to attack pathogens result in oxidative damage to cells and tissues (Owens 1999).

As well as modulating the allocation of nutrients to somatic tissues, the suppression of immune activity by testosterone may also serve the function of reducing autoimmune destruction of antigenic haploid sperm (Folstad and Skarstein 1997; Hillgarth et al. 1997). The testis is relatively immunoprivileged, but not wholly so, since leukocytes perform the function of removing abnormal sperm.

Variation between individuals in allocation decisions in the immunity vs. reproduction trade-off may depend, at least in part, on genetic variation. For example, MHC genotype is strongly associated with susceptibility to autoimmune diseases and allergies, and resistance to several infectious diseases, including leprosy (Weiss 1993), malaria, and hepatitis B (Edwards and Hedrick 1998). Testosterone levels in humans are associated with MHC genotype (Finch and Rose 1995), leading to the hypothesis that males with greater innate disease resistance are able to maintain higher testosterone levels, *all other things being equal*. It has also been suggested that males with greater specific antigen recognition will be able to suppress overall immune function with less costs to parasite resistance, so they are also able to maintain ejaculate quality (and other male phenotypic traits) at lower costs than less resistant males (Folstad and Skarstein 1997).

Finally, the role of testosterone in promoting male secondary sexual characteristics means that male phenotypic traits may function as a bioassay of both immunocompetence and gonadal function for prospective mates. The close relationship between immunity and spermatogenesis means that females may be able to evaluate male disease resistance and fertility status simultaneously by observing the expression of male phenotypic traits (Hillgarth et al. 1997). Thus the interaction of testosterone and immune function operates at multiple levels: gamete production, organismic allocation between tissues, and social signaling as an aspect of reproductive behavior.

DIET, TESTOSTERONE, AND IMMUNITY

Physiological systems involved in both the immune and reproductive systems should be responsive to messages about somatic stores, since the size of the somatic energy pool must be ascertained before it is divided. The roles of energetic status and immune function are well-known. The immune response relies on stores of energy and protein to build immunoglobins. Protein-energy malnutrition results in reduced cell-mediated immunity, complement defense (Ulijaszek 1990), and atrophy of the thymus and lymph nodes (Frisancho 1993). Reduced secretory IgA occurs even in cases of moderate malnutrition, while severe malnutrition causes inhibition of other immunoglobin classes as well (Frisancho 1993).

Male reproductive function, on the other hand, appears less sensitive to energetic status (Campbell and Leslie 1995; DeSouza et al. 1994; Ellison and Panter-Brick 1996) and more responsive to dietary quality. This is particularly the case in regard to protein, which is critical for building the most expensive type of male reproductive tissue, skeletal muscle. The inclusion of protein in calorically insufficient diets helps to maintain testosterone levels during weight loss (Hoffer et al. 1986) Among hospitalized patients testosterone levels are related to mid upper arm circumference, implicating the importance of protein reserves (Lado-Abeal et al. 1999). In addition, studies of subsistence populations, including both the Kung and the Kavango, indicate that a diet low in protein is associated with lower testosterone levels (Christiansen 1991a, 1991b).

The specific physiological mechanisms that coordinate changes in immune and gonadal systems with energy balance are just beginning to be characterized. Leptin, which acts as a peripheral signal from adipocytes probably via the hypothalamus (Ahima et al. 1996), has a strong modulatory role in immunity (Wislon et al. 1997) as well as in the gonadal and thyroid axes (Ahima et al. 1996), all of which have energy-consuming downstream effects. Experimental treatments indicate that the decline in leptin levels produced by starvation causes suppression of cell-mediated immunity (Lord et al. 1998), as well as suppression of testosterone and thyroxine production (Ahima et al. 1996), which would normally increase muscle glucose uptake and metabolic activity, respectively. When this apparent negative feedback relationship is extended, testosterone appears to have a downregulating effect on leptins and may be responsible for men having lower leptin levels than women (Behre et al. 1997).

EFFECTS OF TESTOSTERONE ON THE IMMUNE SYSTEM

Although the impact of testosterone on immune function has generally been construed as suppressive (Folstad and Karter 1992; Grossman 1984), some field studies in animals report that testosterone enhances specific components of immune function (Klein and Nelson 1998; Ros et al. 1997). Braude and colleagues (1999) propose that the effects of testosterone are better described as "immunoredistribution," referring to the reallocation of components within the immune system, rather than "immunosuppression," which implies the depression of a unitary system. It may be that such distinctions are related to the acute versus long-term effects of testosterone. We will use the term *immunosuppression* when discussing the inhibitory actions of testosterone on the immune system and *immunomodulation* in reference to the general relationship of testosterone to immunity. Although the effects of testosterone and other steroids on immunity are part of a highly complex network, here we focus on the inhibitory actions of testosterone.

Testosterone's main inhibitory effects on the immune system fall into three main categories: (1) inhibition of lymphopoiesis, (2) biasing T cell populations in favor of CD8 antigen presenting cells, and (3) inhibition of cytokines. At the most global level, testosterone causes atrophy of the tissues that promote lymphocyte production and maturation, as well as the inhibition of lymphopoiesis itself. Androgens have a suppressive effect on the growth and activity of the thymus, the spleen, and lymph nodes (Grossman 1984). After a peak mass twice that of adult levels, lymphoid tissue rapidly regresses with the rise of immunosuppressive sex steroids at puberty (Katchadourian 1977; McCruden and Stimson 1995). Androgens also reduce B cell lymphopoiesis (Olsen and Kovacs 1996).

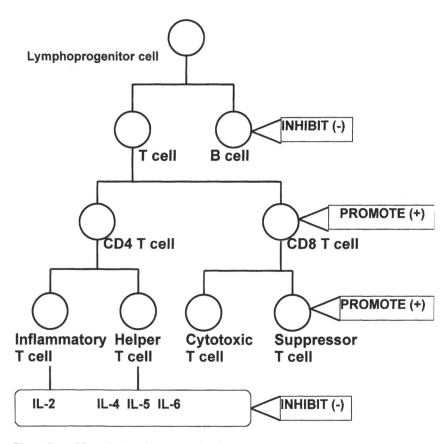

Figure 7.1. Hypothesized actions of testosterone on immunity.

Testosterone has effects on several levels of the immune cascade (summarized in Figure 1). At the cell population level testosterone alters the CD4/CD8 T cell ratio in favor of CD8 cells (Olsen et al. 1991; Weinstein and Bercovich 1981). CD4 T cells bind to HLA Class II molecules and are represented mainly by helper and inflammatory T cells, while CD8 T cells, which are mostly cytotoxic and suppressor T cells, bind to HLA class I molecules (Janeway and Travers 1996). Increases in the population of suppressor T cells may be a major means through which testosterone depresses immunity. In a study of a Japanese population, men had relatively higher levels of CD8 cells, whereas women had relatively higher levels of CD4 cells (Lee et al. 1996). This difference is consistent with the sex difference in autoimmune disease, with men having higher MHC I and women having a higher prevalence of MHC II type diseases (Grossman et al. 1991).

Testosterone also inhibits the activity of cytokines IL-1 (Lin et al. 1996), IL-2 (Grossman 1994), and IL-6 (Smithson et al. 1998), and its more active form, dihydrotestosterone (DHT), inhibits the secretion of IL-4, IL-5, and gamma IFN (Daynes and Araneo 1991) by T cells. IL-2 is an inflammatory cytokine secreted by inflammatory and cytotoxic T cells that promotes B cell and natural killer cell activity. In addition to inhibiting cytokines, testosterone also inhibits some hormones secreted by the thymus. IL-6 promotes lymphocyte maturation and osteoclast activity. Testosterone suppresses immunoglobin-stimulating thymic fraction 5 (TF5) (Catanzano et al. 1992) and the thymosins beta 4 and alpha 1 (Wise 1992). IL-1 has a reciprocal effect on the gonadal axis, inhibiting testosterone synthesis through several pathways (Ogilvie et al. 1999; Rivier 1990).

Estrogens have some effects on immunity that are similar to those of testosterone. Like testosterone, estrogen suppresses B cell lymphopoiesis in the bone marrow (Smithson et al. 1998). However, though estrogen inhibits cell-mediated immunity, unlike testosterone it enhances humoral immunity (Grossman 1984). Estrogen promotes secretion of Igm and IgG in concert with TF5 (Erbach and Bahr 1991). In addition, the activity of suppressor T cells is inhibited by estradiol, an effect opposite to that of testosterone. This results in increased maturation and immunoglobin secretion by B cells (Grossman 1984).

TESTOSTERONE EFFECTS ON MALARIA, HELMINTHIC INFECTION, AND TUBERCULOSIS

In addition to in vitro studies demonstrating testosterone's suppressive effects on the immune system, studies with animal models indicate that testosterone can play a role in susceptibility to specific diseases. Among the most important of these are malaria and helminth infections. Testosterone reduces resistance to the malarial parasite *Plasmodium chabaudi* in mice; this vulnerability can be transferred between individuals through splenic T cells. Vulnerability is associated with testosterone-induced changes in immune parameters, including increased proportion of CD8 T cells and decreased immunoglobins (Benten et al. 1997).

Helminth infections in the gut stimulate a CD4 T cell–based response. T cells induce secretion in B cells of IgE, which bind to the worms, targeting them for eosinophils. Inflammation of the gut causes diarrhea and shedding of the worms (Noble et al. 1989). Testosterone administered to female soft-furred rats infected with the nematode *Nipostrongylus brasilnesis* caused suppressed goblet cell proliferation and reduced helminth expulsion (Hadid et al. 1995).

In contrast, there is no direct evidence that testosterone plays a role in male disease burdens in nonwestern subsistence populations where disease burdens are likely to be high and nutritional status is poor. However, although animal studies cannot replicate the complex variables that determine susceptibility to infectious disease in humans, they do demonstrate that testosterone does increase vulnerability to infections prevalent in many subsistence populations. In addition, testosterone's effect on CD4/CD8 ratios suggests an important pathway that may play a role not only in malaria and helminth infections but in other important infections of human populations as well. These include tuberculosis, which is both widely prevalent and sensitive to nutritional status (Mims et al. 1995) and for which the first line of immune response is based on CD4+ cells (Janeway and Travers 1996). Thus in the next section we explore the relationship of testosterone to symptoms related directly to these important diseases using data from the Turkana of Kenya.

TURKANA

The Turkana are a group of pastoral nomads in the Turkana district of northeastern Kenya. Work by members of the South Turkana Ecosystems Project (STEP) over the past 15 years has done much to elucidate their ecology and human biology. Here we give only a very brief account of those aspects directly relevant for this paper. (For a more comprehensive description, see Little and Leslie 1999.)

The climate of the Turkana region is semi-arid with a highly seasonal pattern of rainfall. The Turkana depend largely on their animals, including goats, sheep, cattle, and camels, for subsistence. Their diet is based primarily on animal products—milk, blood, and meat—with up to 80% of calories in the wet season consumed in the form of milk. During the dry season, consumption of grains, particulary maize, substitutes for lower consumption of milk. Total caloric intake is limited, with dietary estimates of approximately 1,300 kcal/day, but protein intake is quite high, with estimates indicating more than twice the USDA requirements (Galvin and Little 1999).

In terms of overall physique, the Turkana are tall and lean, with average adult stature equal to that of U.S. standards, but average weight at about the lowest fifth percentile. Birthweights are above the U.S. mean, but infant weights fall behind U.S. standards quickly and continue to lag throughout childhood. Prolonged growth into the early twenties and late age at reproductive maturation are consistent with chronic undernutrition (Little et al. 1999).

Along with experiencing chronic undernutrition, the Turkana are thought to carry a relatively high disease burden, in part because of close association with their herds (Majok and Schwabe 1996). Important diseases associated with their animals include hydatid cysts and tuberculosis, the latter of which is thought to be transmitted through untreated milk, leading to potential universal exposure of the population. In addition, malaria is considered holoendemic, and reports of diarrheal disease and ARI (acute respiratory infection) are common. Assessment of cellular immune reactivity among children using DTH (delayed-type hypersensitivity) suggests suppressed immune function, which has been related to chronic undernutrition (Shell-Duncan 1997; Shell-Duncan et al. 1999).

In addition to the nomadic groups, there are also sedentary Turkana. While some of these settlements are indigenous, many more are the result of recent events. Morelum, from which the settlement data provided here were obtained, is an agricultural scheme run by World Vision, an NGO. The settlement dates from the 1960s as a result of loss of animals to drought or raiding. Unfortunately, we have much less evidence documenting the specific conditions in Morulem, though there is evidence for less consumption of meat, and most likely greater exposure to malaria (B. Campbell et al. 1999). Thus Morelum represents a subpopulation of individuals who share a close history with the nomads but differ in terms of their current diet and disease exposure (Barkey et al. 2001).

The evidence for undernutrition and immunosuppression combined with the existence of two closely related subpopulations make the Turkana an appropriate group with which to investigate the potential role of testosterone on immuno-suppression and health status in a naturalistic setting. Here we use data collected as part of a larger study of Turkana male reproductive ecology carried out between 1992 and 1995 to explore the relationship of nutritional status, testosterone, and health complaints. Nomadic males were sampled in June/July of 1992, settled males in March/April of 1993. Standard anthropometric measurements, 48-hour dietary recall, self-reported local (Turkana) health complaints, and finger-prick blood spots and urine samples were taken for the determination of hormonal measures. Assays of testosterone (T) from blood spots and estrone-3-glucuronide (E-3-G) were done in Kenneth L. Campbell's laboratory at the University of Massachusetts at Boston (Campbell 1994; Campbell et al. n.d.)

Table 7.1 shows the 11 Turkana disease categories used in our study along with their English translation, based on Shelley's (1985) study of Turkana ethnomedicine. These categories represent a cultural interpretation of the subjective experience of illness. They are not clinical diagnoses, but rather can be considered as self-reports of pain or symptoms. Such self-

Table 7.1.   Turkana Disease Categories and English Equivalents

Turkana Term	English Equivalent
Etid	Discomfort or sharp pains in left abdomen—spleen
Loriwo	Abdominal pain or swelling, liver-related
Lokou	Serious headache, often with sweating and dizziness
Akurut	Diarrhea
Eguru	Backache
Erarum	Chest pains, lasting at least five days; cough and fever
Arukum	Common cold of a few days duration, with cough
Lomeskin	Swelling of the joints, and jaundice
Angakonyen	Literally "eyes"; refers to all eye problems: irritation, infection, etc.
Ngipeeli	Tapeworm or threadworm
Loku	"Whooping cough"

(adapted from Shelley 1985)

reports are not without their own biases, but they should be considered against the background of the Turkana's extensive experience of their own bodies, and the body's relationship to health and well-being.

The three categories of particular interest here are *erarum, etid,* and *ngipeeli,* all symptoms of widely prevalent conditions with serious potential health impacts. *Erarum* is translated as 'chest infection' or 'chest pain' and is thought to be related to TB and pneumonias, both prevalent in the population. It is distinguished from *arukum,* which refers to a cold, and also from *lokud,* which is translated as a whooping cough. *Etid* is translated as 'spleen pain.' Shelley (1985) was able to show that reports of spleen pain are significantly associated with actual splenomegaly, which is one of the classic symptoms of malarial infection. Finally, *ngipeeli* refers explicitly to the presence of threadworms in feces. This category is most likely to be biased, as our informants told us that people did not like to report the presence of worms, an intuitively understandable social problem. Reported rates were very low (see Table 7.1) and we did not use them in further analyses.

Table 7.2 compares the two subpopulations in terms of the basic reports of health complaints, nutritional status, and hormone levels. BMI is quite low in both subpopulations, while testosterone levels are within the normal range based on western standards. Settled males have higher rates of complaints of chest infection as well as higher BMI, but lower T levels. Therefore, higher rates of disease complaints among the settled group cannot be directly related to either poorer nutritional status, as indicated by BMI, or higher T levels, but may represent greater exposure to pathogens (B. Campbell et al. 1999).

Table 7.2.   Comparison of Male Characteristics in the Two
             Turkana Subpopulations

Variable	Subpopulation	
	Nomadic	Settled
N	155	129
Age (yrs)	40.5 ± 17.2	40.3 ± 18.8
Testosterone (nM)	33.9 ± 16.1	25.1 ± 19.3
BMI (kg/m2)	17.0 ± 1.8	17.6 ± 2.1
Fat-free mass (kg)	47.8 ± 8.0	46.1 ± 8.4
Erarum (% reporting)	22	49
Ngipeeli (% reporting)	04	9.8
Etid (% reporting)	38	.31

Fat-free mass is based on weight and % body fat derived
   from skinfolds using the equations of Durnin and
   Wormsely (1974). Reports of health complaints are
   based on current status.

At the same time however, estimates of caloric intake (1,800 kcal/day for the settled and 700 kcal/day for the nomads; Muehlenbein 1998) suggest that males in the two subpopulations are experiencing two very different short-term energetic states: acute undernutrition in the nomads and overall positive energy balance in the settled group. Thus by comparing the relationship between T levels and disease symptoms in the two groups, we can examine our basic hypothesis that under conditions of limited energetic availability a relationship between testosterone levels and disease symptoms will be more evident. We make three specific predictions: (1) Higher levels of T will be associated with presence of health complaints, but only when nutritional status, as reflected in BMI, is controlled. (2) The impact of T on disease complaints will be greater in the nomadic population, because poorer nutrition means a more limited energy budget. (3) Protein stores, as reflected in fat-free mass, will have an effect on the relationship between testosterone and disease complaints separate from that of total energy stores.

Table 7.3 shows the results of logistic analyses for nomadic and settled males predicting the presence/absence of current complaints of chest infection and spleen complaints. Among the nomads, T is a marginally significant predictor for complaints of erarum (chest infection) when both a BMI of less than 18.5 and age are controlled. Similar results are obtained for settled males. T is a significant predictor for complaints of erarum in that group even when controlling for age and BMI. We tested to see if the impact of T was different in the two populations, but the interaction term between subpopulation and T was not significant. In addition, because the

Table 7.3. Testosterone and Nutritional Status as Predictors of
Erarum and *Etid*

Erarum			Settled	
	Nomads			
χ^2	15.7		12.3	
N	91		64	
Variable	β	p	β	p
Age	.05	.002	.021	.155
Testosterone	2.01	.086	1.88	.036
Low BMI	.83	.239	−1.00	.121

Etid				
	Nomads		Settled	
χ^2	.55		4.4	
N	91		64	
Variable	β	p	β	p
Age	−.006	.643	.002	.155
Testosterone	.310	.731	1.66	.060
Low BMI	.195	.722	.683	.121

Note: Testosterone represents the log of blood spot values. BMI is a
binary variable with BMI < 18.5 coded as 0. While BMI < 18.5 is
generally thought to represent the cutoff for chronic energy deficiency (Ferro-Luzzi et al. 1992), it may be a bit arbitrary in the case
of Turkana because of the body proportions associated with a tall,
lean physique. However, similar results are achieved with both
unlogged testosterone values and BMI as a continuous variable.

impact of BMI and testosterone on health complaints may be confounded
by developmental changes during adolescence, we also tested models
with a dummy term for adolescence versus adults but found no interaction between T and adult status.

In contrast to the findings for chest infection, T is a marginally significant predictor of spleen complaints among the settled population, but the
association is not significant among the nomads. Similar results are
obtained when fat-free mass is used instead of BMI.

These admittedly very simple analyses suggest some impact of testosterone on the health status of Turkana males. We failed to find a relationship with spleen complaints, a symptom of malaria, which is both widely
prevalent among the Turkana and related to testosterone-mediated
immunosuppression in animal models. However, we did find an association between higher testosterone and the existence of complaints of chest
infection in both subpopulations.

Careful consideration of these two diseases suggests that the results may not be simple artifacts. Failure to find an association with spleen complaints is perhaps more problematic but may be explained by the episodic nature of malarial symptoms and the fact that anthropometric markers of nutritional status show little relationship to malarial morbidity (Tonglet et al. 1999) or parasitaemia (Ghosh et al. 1995). On the other hand, to the extent that chest infection is related to TB, it may represent the conditions most directly related to our original hypothesis, in which suppression of immune function by T allows the expression of a chronic disease. As noted earlier, raw milk consumption means tuberculosis exposure is probably universal from a young age. Approximately one-third of Turkana children show evidence of exposure to tuberculin antigens (Shell-Duncan et al. 1999). Early exposure to TB is generally never resolved, and it remains a chronic, lifelong infection.

However, the simple fact of a significant relationship between T and complaints of *erarum* does not by itself support the interpretation that chest infection is related to testosterone immunosuppression. Testosterone has many different physiological effects in men, including behavior. Men with higher T exhibit more dominant personalities (Gray et al. 1991). In addition, Granger et al. (2000) have reported a positive, albeit weak, relationship between T, aggression, and CD4 cells in a sample of U.S. men. Thus Turkana men with higher T might both complain more and have higher levels of CD4 cells. If a positive relationship between T, aggression, and immune function was important in accounting for the results reported here, we might expect to find a relationship between T and a substantial number of the 11 disease categories. However, none of the nine other disease categories showed any relationship with T (analyses not shown).

The use of local disease categories as health complaints obviously adds an additional level of interpretation to the analysis. Self-reports of disease are biased by individual interpretation. In addition, differences in reports of symptoms between settled and nomadic populations may be related to differences in access to local health clinics, or perhaps there is a tendency for members of the settled population to complain more. Nonetheless, all of these factors would presumably obscure any relationship between T and disease complaints rather than create it.

Our results fail to indicate a stronger effect of testosterone on disease complaints among the nomads, despite poorer nutritional status compared with the settled males, nor do they suggest that variation in nutritional status within either subpopulation mediates the relationship of testosterone to health complaints. These caveats notwithstanding, our results taken at face value suggest that individual differences in testosterone levels among Turkana males may play a role in TB infections independent of nutritional status, whether measured in terms of BMI or fat-free mass, even under conditions of pronounced undernutrition. Thus, these findings do not provide support for a simple trade-off between testosterone-mediated somatic and immune function (whether mediated by total energy or protein stores).

However, the extremely lean physique of Turkana males may limit the possibility of a direct trade-off between muscle and immune function. Instead, there may be a trade-off in the balance between disease resistance and immunopathology. In this case, maintaining T levels would suppress the initial immune response to pathogens and lead to reliance on cell-mediated immunity as a potentially more damaging second line of defense. More specifically, complaints of chest infection may represent a relationship between the immune response to pathogens in the lungs and the associated damage it can cause. Testosterone-mediated bias in CD4/CD8 cell ratios would result in a reduction of the initial CD4+ response to mycobacterium, allowing the infection to spread and leading to the formulation of granulomas and tissue necrosis that represent the pathological effects of chronic TB infection (Haas and DesPrez 1995).

If we are correct in our interpretation of the relationship of T and complaints of "chest infection," Turkana males with elevated testosterone levels may be at risk for higher levels of immunopathology, leading to greater cumulative damage to their lungs and greater susceptibility to other respiratory infections as well. If so, testosterone may have important implications for male life history. In a population where reproduction among males has a late onset and extends to late ages (Leslie et al. 1999), survivorship may play a significant role in differential reproduction. The costs of testosterone-mediated immunosuppression may be evident in its long-term effects on health and mortality. Whether such costs are balanced by reproductive benefits of testosterone related to mating or paternal behavior is unknown at this point (cf. Wingfield et al. 1990).

SUMMARY

One of the costs of testosterone in males is widely acknowledged to be higher rates of disease relative to females, which are thought to result, in part, from the suppression of immune function by testosterone. We have argued here that such suppression may impact any one of several aspects of immunity, including energetic costs such as increased metabolic rate and the catabolism of muscle and fat, and immunopathologies such as an increased risk of autoimmunity and oxidative stress. In addition we have suggested that such trade-offs might be evident in nonwestern subsistence populations with limited energy budgets.

Our own analysis of nutritional status, testosterone levels, and disease complaints from Turkana males does indicate a limited impact of testosterone on disease complaints, specifically chest complaints thought to be associated with TB. However, our rather simple results fail to support a trade-off between testosterone and immunity based on the physiological compartments including total energy (BMI) and protein (fat-free mass). Turkana males may simply be sufficiently energetically limited that trade-offs between physiological compartments have given way to less favorable trade-offs between disease resistance and immunopathology or the cost of maintaining an immune response with poor nutritional status. Whether such a situation is specific to pastoral nomadic populations like the Turkana with close association with animals and zoonotic diseases, lean physiques, and a high protein diet or is more generally applicable to other populations requires further research including direct measures of male immune function.

REFERENCES

Ahima RS, Prabakaran D, Mantzoros C, Qu D, Lowel B, Maratos-Flier E, Flier JS (1996) Role of leptin in the neuroendocrine response to fasting. *Nature* 382:250–252.

Barkey NL, Campbell BC, Leslie PW (2001) Differential disease complaints among nomadic and settled Turkana males. *Medical Anthropology* 15:391–408.

Behre HM, Simoni M, Nieschlag E (1997) Strong association between serum levels of leptin and testosterone in men. *Clinical Endocrinology* 47:237–240.

Benten WPM, Ulrich P, Kuhn-Velten WN, Vohr H-W, Wunderlich F (1997) Testosterone-induced susceptibility to *Plasmodium chabaudi* malaria: persistence after withdrawal of testosterone. *Journal of Endocrinology* 153:275–281.

Braude S, Tang-Martinez Z, Taylor GT (1999) Stress, testosterone, and the the immunoredistribution hypothesis. *Behavioral Ecology* 10:354–350.

Campbell BC, Leslie PW, Little MA, Brainard JM, DeLuca MA (1999) Settled Turkana. In MA Little, PW Leslie (Eds) *Turkana Herders of the Dry Savanna: Ecology and Biobehavioral Response of Nomads to an Uncertain Environment* (Oxford, Oxford University Press), 333–354.

Campbell BC, PW Leslie (1995) Reproductive ecology of human males. *Yearbook of Physical Anthropology* 38:1–26.

Campbell KL (1994) Blood, urine, saliva, and dipsticks: experiences in Africa, New Guinea and Boston. *Annals of the New York Academy of Sciences* 709:313–331.

Campbell KL, Dookhran L, Evindar A (n.d.) Blood or urine dried on paper: cellulase digestion of paper affects few clinical assays and permits use of suboptimal samples. Unpublished manuscript in the authors' possession.

Catanzano P, Troutaud D, Ardaill D, Deschaux PA (1992) Testosterone inhibits the immunostimulant effect of thymosin fraction 5 on secondary immune response in mice. *International Journal of Immunology* 14:263–268.

Christiansen KH (1991a) Serum and saliva sex hormones levels in !Kung San men. *American Journal of Physical Anthropology* 86:37–44.

Christiansen KH (1991b) Sex hormone levels, diet, and alcohol consumption in Namibian Kavango men. *Homo* 42:43–62.

Daynes RA, Araneo BA (1991) Regulation of T-cell function by steroid hormones. In MS Meltzer, A Mantovani (Eds) *Cellular and Cytokine Networks in Tissue Immunity* (New York, Wiley-Liss), 77–82.

DeSouza MJ, Arce JC, Pescatello LS, Scherzer HS, Luciano AA (1994) Gonadal hormones and semen quality in male runners. A volume threshold effect of endurance training. *International Journal of Sports Medicine* 15:383–391.

Durnin JVA, Wormsely JW (1974) Body fat assessed from total body density and its estimation from skinfold thickness: measurement on 481 men aged from 16-72 years. *British Journal of Nutrition* 32:77–97.

Edwards SV, Hedrick PW (1998) Evolution and ecology of MHC molecules: from genomics to sexual selection. *Trends in Evolution and Ecology* 13:305–311.

Elia M (1992) Organ and tissue contribution to metabolic rate. In JM McKinney, HN Tucker (Eds) *Energy Metabolism: Tissue Determinants and Cellular Corollaries* (New York, Raven Press), 61–80.

Ellison PT, Panter-Brick C (1996) Salivary testosterone levels among Tamang and Kami males from central Nepal. *Human Biology* 68:955–965.

Erbach GT, Bahr JM (1991) Enhancement of *in vivo* humoral immunity by estrogen permissive effect of a thymic factor. *Endocrinology* 128:1352–1358.

Fedigan LM, Zohar S (1997) Sex differences in mortality of Japanese macaques. *American Journal of Physical Anthropology* 102:161–175.

Ferro-Luzzi A, Sette S, Franklin M, James WP (1992) A simplified approach of assessing adult chronic energy deficiency. *European Journal of Clinical Nutrition* 46:173–186.

Finch CE, Rose MR (1995) Hormones and the physiological ecology of life history evolution. *Quarterly Review of Biology* 70:1–52.

Flinn MV, England BG (1997) Social economics of childhood glucocorticoid stress response. *American Journal of Physical Anthropology* 102:33–53.

Folstad I, Karter AJ (1992) Parasites, bright males, and the immunocompetence handicap. *American Naturalist* 139:603–622.

Folstad IA, Nilssen C, Halvorsen O, Andersen J (1989) Why do male reindeer *(Rangifer t. tarandus)* have higher abundance of second and third instar larvae of *Hypoderma tarandi* than females? *Oikos* 55:87–92.

Folstad I, Skarstein F (1997) Is male germ line control creating avenues for female choice? *Behavioral Ecology* 8:109–112.

Frisancho AR (1993) *Human Adaptation and Accommodation* (Ann Arbor, University of Michigan Press).

Galvin KA, Little MA (1999) Dietary intake and nutritional status. In MA Little, PW Leslie (Eds) *Turkana Herders of the Dry Savanna: Ecology and Biobehavioral Response of Nomads to an Uncertain Environment* (Oxford, Oxford University Press), 125–146.

Ghosh SK, Yadav S, Das BS, Sharma VP (1995) Influence of nutritional and haemoglobin status on malaria infection in children. *Indian Journal of Pediatrics* 62: 321–326.

Granger DA, Booth A, Johnson DR (2000) Human aggression and enumerative measures of immunity. *Psychosomatic Medicine* 62:583–590.

Gray A, Jackson DN, McKinley JB (1991) The relationship between dominance, anger, and hormones in the normally aging male. *Pyschosomatic Medicine* 53:375–385.

Groff JL, Gropper SS, Hunt SM (1995) *Advanced Nutrition and Human Metabolism,* second ed. (New York, West).

Grossman CJ (1984) Regulation of the immune system by sex steroids. *Endocrine Reviews* 5:435–455.

Grossman CJ (1994) The role of sex steroids in immune system regulation. In CJ Grossman (Ed) *Bilateral Communication between the Endocrine and Immune System* (New York, Springer-Verlag), pp. 1–11.

Grossman CJ, Roselle GA, Mendenhall CL (1991) Sex steroid regulation of autoimmunity. *Journal of Steroid Biochemistry and Molecular Biology* 40:649–659.

Haas DW, DesPrez RM (1995) Mycobateria Tuberculosis. In CL Mandell, JF Bennett, R Doln (Eds) *Mandell, Douglas and Bennett's Principles and Practices of Infectious Diseases*, fourth ed. (New York, Churchill Livingstone), 2213–2242.

Hadid R, Spinedi E, Daneva T, Grau G, Gaillard RC (1995) Repeated endotoxin treatment decreases immune and hypothalamic-pituitary-adrenal axis response: effects of orchidectomy and testosterone therapy. *Neuroendocrinology* 62:348–355.

Harcourt AH, Harvey PH, Larson SG, Short RV (1981) Testis weight and breeding system in primates. *Nature* 293:55–57.

Hill K (1993) Life history theory and evolutionary anthropology. *Evolutionary Anthropology* 2:78–88.

Hillgarth N, Ramenofsky M, Wingfield J (1997) Testosterone and sexual selection. *Behavioral Ecology* 8:108–109.

Hoffer LJ, Beitins IZ, Kyung NH, Bistrain BR (1986) Effects of severe dietary restriction on male reproductive hormones. *Journal of Clinical Endocrinology and Metabolism* 62:288–292.

Janeway CA, Travers P (1996) *Immunobiology: The Immune System in Health and Disease*, second ed. (New York, Garland).

Kacprzak-Bergman I (1994) Sexual dimorphism of heritability of immunoglobin levels. *Annals of Human Biology* 21:563–569.

Katchadourian H (1977) *The Biology of Adolescence* (San Francisco, WH Freeman).

Klein S, Nelson R (1998) Adaptive immune responses of arvicoline rodents. *American Naturalist* 151:59–67.

Lado-Abeal J, Prieto D, Lorenzo M, Lojo S, Febrero M, Camarero E, Cabezas-Cerrato J (1999) Differences between men and women as regards the effects of protein-energy malnutrition on the hypothalamic-pituitary-gonadal axis. *Nutrition* 15:351–358.

Lee BW, Yap HK, Chew FT, Quah TC, Prabhakaran K, Chan GSH, Wong SC, Seah CC (1996) Age- and sex-related changes in lymphocyte subpopulations of healthy Asian subjects: from birth to adulthood. *Cytokine* 26:8–15.

Leslie PW, Campbell KL, Campbell BC, Kigondu CS, Kirumbi LH (1999) Fecundity and fertility. In MA Little, PW Leslie (Eds) *Turkana Herders of the Dry Savanna: Ecology and Biobehavioral Response of Nomads to an Uncertain Environment* (Oxford, Oxford University Press), 249–280.

Little MA, Gray SJ, Pike IL, Mugambi M (1999) Infant, child and adolescent growth, and adult physical status. In MA Little, PW Leslie (Eds) *Turkana Herders of the Dry Savanna: Ecology and Biobehavioral Response of Nomads to an Uncertain Environment* (Oxford, Oxford University Press), 187–206.

Little MA, Leslie PW (Eds) (1999) *Turkana Herders of the Dry Savanna: Ecology and Biobehavioral Response of Nomads to an Uncertain Environment* (Oxford, Oxford University Press).

Lord GM, Matarese G, Howard JK, Baker RJ, Blooms SR, Lechler RI (1998) Leptin modulates the T-cell immune response and reverses starvation-induced immunosuppression. *Nature* 394:897–901.

Majok AA, Schwabe CW (1996) *Development among Africa's Migratory Pastoralists* (Westport, CT, Bergin and Garvey).

McCruden AB, Stimson WH (1994) Effects of androgens/estrogens on the immune response. In CJ Grossman (Ed) *Bilateral Communication in the Endocrine and Immune Systems* (New York, Springer Verlag), 36–50.

McDade T, Worthman CM (1999) Evolutionary process and ecology of human immune function. *American Journal of Human Biology* 11:705–717.

Mims C, Dimmock N, Nash A, Stephen J (1995) *Mims' Pathogenesis of Infectious Disease*, fourth ed. (New York, Academic Press).

Muehlenbein MP (1998) The Ngisonyka of Turkana: Environment, Nutrition, and Disease in Northwest Kenya. Senior Honors Thesis, Department of Environmental Science, Northwestern University.

Newsholme EA, Crabtree B, Parry-Billinge M (1992) The energetic cost of regulation: an analysis based on the principles of metabolic-control-logic. In JM Kinney, HN Tucker (Eds) *Energy Metabolism: Tissue Determinants and Cellular Corollaries* (New York, Raven Press), 467–493.

Noble ER, Noble GA, Schad GA, MacInnes AJ (1989) *Parasitology: The Biology of Animal Parasites*, sixth ed. (Philadelphia, Lea and Febiger).

Ogilvie KM, Hales KH, Roberts ME, Hales DB, Rivier C (1999) The inhibitory effect of intracerebroventricularly injected interleukin-1 beta on testosterone secretion in the rat: role of steroidogenic acute regulatory protein. *Biology of Reproduction* 60:527–533.

Olsen NJ, Kovacs WJ (1996) Gonadal steroids and immunity. *Endocrine Reviews* 17:369–384.

Olsen NJ, Watson MB, Henderson GS, Kovacs WJ (1991) Androgen deprivation induces phenotypic and functional changes in the thymus of adult male mice. *Endocrinology* 129:2471–2476.

Otten CM (1985) Genetic effects on male and female development and on the sex ratio. In RL Hall (Ed) *Male-Female Differences: A Bio-Cultural Perspective* (New York, Praeger), 155–217.

Owens IPF (1999) Immunocompetence: a neglected life history trait or red herring? *Trends in Evolution and Ecology* 14:170–172.

Poulin R (1996) Sexual inequalities in helminth infections: a cost of being a male? *American Naturalist* 147:287–295.

Raberg L, Grahn M, Hasselquist D, Svensson E (1998) On the adaptive significance of stress-induced immunosuppression. *Proceedings of the Royal Society of London*, B 265:1637–1641.

Rakowicz SE, Jackson B, Szulczynska AM, Smith M (1998) Human immunodeficiency virus type 1-like DNA sequences and immunoreactive virtal particles with unique association with breast cancer. *Clinical and Diagnostic Laboratory Immunology* 5:645–653.

Rivier C (1990) Role of endotoxin and interleukin-1 in modulating ACTH, LH, and sex steroid secretion. In JC Porter, D Jezova (Eds) *Circulating Regulatory Factors and Neuroendocrine Factors* (New York, Plenum Press), 295–301.

Roberts CW, Satoskar A, Alexander J (1996) Sex steroids, pregnancy-associated hormones and immunity to parasitic infection. *Parasitology Today* 12:382–388.

Ros AFH, Groothius TGG, Apanius V (1997) The relation among gonadal steroids, immunocompetence, body mass, and behavior in young black-headed gulls *(Larus ridibundus)*. *American Naturalist* 150:201–219.

Schalk G, Forbes MR (1997) Male biases in parasitism of mammals. *Oikos* 78:67–74.

Shell-Duncan B (1997) Evaluation of infection and nutritional status as determinants of cellular immunosuppression. *American Journal of Human Biology* 9: 381–390.

Shell-Duncan B, Shelley JK, Leslie PW (1999) Health and morbidity: ethnomedical and epidemiological perspectives. In MA Little, PW Leslie (Eds) *Turkana Herders of the Dry Savanna: Ecology and Biobehavioral Response of Nomads to an Uncertain Environment* (Oxford, Oxford University Press), 207–230.

Shelley JK (1985) Medicines for misfortune: diagnosis and health among southern Turkana pastoralists of Kenya. Ph.D. dissertation. Department of Anthropology, University of North Carolina, Chapel Hill.

Smithson G, Couse JF, Lubahn BB, Korach KS, Kincaid PW (1998) The role of estrogen receptors and androgen receptors in sex steroid regulation of B lymphopoeisis. *Journal of Immunology* 16:27–34.

Storey A, Thomas M, Kalita A, Harwood C (1998) Role of p53 polymorphism in the development of human pailloma-virus-associated cancer. *Nature* 393:229–245.

Tanagho EE (1995) Anatomy of the genitourinary tract. In EA Tanagho, JW McAninch (Eds) *Smith's General Urology*, fourteenth ed. (Norwood, CT, Appleton and Lange), 1–16.

Tiuria R, Hrii Y, Makimura S, Ishikawa N, Tsuchiya K, Nawa Y (1995) Effect of testosterone on the mucosal defense against intestinal helminths in soft-furred rats, *Millardia meltada*, with reference to goblet and mast cell responses. *Parasite Immunology* 17:479–484.

Tonglet R, Mahangaiko Lembo E, Zihindula PM, Wodon A, Dramaix M, Hennart P (1999) How useful are anthropometric, clinical and dietary measurements of nutritional status as predictors of morbidity of young children in central Africa? *Tropical Medicine and International Health* 4:120–130.

Ulijaszek SJ (1990) Nutritional status and infectious disease. In GA Harrison, JC Waterlow (Eds) *Diet and Disease in Traditional Communities* (Cambridge, UK, Bath Press), 137–154.

Weinstein Y, Bercovich Z (1981) Testosterone effects on bone marrow, thymus and suppressor T cells in the (NZB x NZW) F1 mice: its relevance to autoimmunity. *Journal of Immunology* 126:998–1002.

Weiss KM (1993) *Genetic Variation and Human Disease* (Cambridge, Cambridge University Press).

Wilson CA, Bekele G, Nicols M, Ravess E, Pratley RE (1997) Relationship of the white cell count to body fat: role of leptin. *British Journal of Haematology* 99: 447–451.

Wingfield JC, Hegner RE, Dufty AM, Ball GF (1990) The "challenge hypothesis": theoretical implications for patterns of testosterone secretion, mating systems, and breeding strategies. *American Naturalist* 136:829–846.

Wise TH (1992) Developmental changes of serum thymosin alpha 1 and beta 4 in male and male castrated pigs: modulation by testosterone and human chorionic gonadotropin. *Biology of Reproduction* 46:892–897.

Young VR, Yu Y, Fukagawa NK (1992) Energy and protein turnover. In JM McKinney, HN Tucker (Eds) *Energy Metabolism: Tissue Determinants and Cellular Corollaries* (New York, Raven Press), 439–466.

Zopf PE (1992) *Mortality Patterns and Trends in the United States* (Westport, CT, Greenwood Press).

Zuk, M (1996) Disease, endocrine-immune interactions, and sexual selection. *Ecology* 77:1037–1042.

Zuk M, McKean KA (1996) Sex differences in parasite infections: patterns and processes. *International Journal for Parasitology* 26:1009–1024.

8

Why Not So Great Is Still Good Enough

Flexible Responsiveness in Human Reproductive Functioning

VIRGINIA J. VITZTHUM

The intriguing debate regarding the role of nutrition and workload in human reproductive functioning has drawn considerable attention (NYAS Conference 1993). On the one hand, it has been observed that women of marginal nutritional status engaged in long days of arduous activities often average seven or eight pregnancies and may have as many as twelve or thirteen. In an evaluation of data from populations worldwide, Bongaarts (1980) concluded that, except in cases of famine, nutritional factors play a very minor role in the fertility levels of women in developing countries. In general, the work of human demographers lends support to this position (e.g., Bongaarts and Potter 1983; Menken et al. 1981).

In contrast, clinical studies of American women indicate a sensitivity of ovarian function to even moderate amounts of nutritional and work stress (Lager and Ellison 1990; Pirke et al. 1985, 1989; Schweiger et al. 1987). Exercise-associated menstrual disruption among athletes is the most extreme response to high activity levels; however, conditions far less demanding than athletic training have been demonstrated to have a negative effect on ovarian function in healthy women. These clinical findings are consistent with research, both in laboratories and field settings, that the reproductive functioning of mammals in general is affected by the intake and expenditure of energy, that is, energy balance (Bronson 1989). For example, in studies of rhesus monkeys (Cameron 1989a), reproductive functioning is suppressed by daily vigorous exercise and restored by an increase in caloric intake.

From the perspective of evolutionary ecology, it is to be expected that energy balance has consequences for reproductive functioning since all organisms must partition energy intake into growth, survival (maintenance), and reproduction. This central tenet of evolutionary ecology is supported by a wealth of empirical evidence for numerous species (Pianka

1974, 1988). As humans are subject to the same selective processes as any other mammal, it would be extraordinary if the human reproductive system did not respond to energetic constraints.

How is it then that the findings of demographic and physiological studies appear to be at such variance? Why might reproductive functioning actually be more sensitive in some cases than in others to environmental stressors (whether nutritional, activity, or pyschosocial)? A reconciliation, at least in part, of this seeming paradox may be achieved by incorporating an evolutionary approach to human reproductive functioning. This perspective, while not ignoring pathology, considers the possibility that a change in ovarian function may be an adaptive response to environmental conditions. Hence, a significant proportion of variation in ovarian function within and between individuals is normal, the result of natural selection, and potentially adaptive. The role of adaptation in explaining variation in human reproductive functioning has been suggested by several investigators (e.g., Borgerhoff Mulder 1992; Ellison 1990; Frisch 1978; Gage et al. 1989; Hill and Hurtado 1996; Leslie and Fry 1989; Leslie and Gage 1989; Peacock 1990; Prior 1985; Tracer 1996; Vitzthum 1990; Wasser and Barash 1983; Worthman 1990). While differences in perspectives have led to alternative models, all incorporate this fundamental concept of evolutionary ecology.

In addition, just as the functioning of the reproductive system has an evolutionary history, an organism has an individual life history that is also integral to explanations of reproductive processes. Physiological responses at any moment are a reflection of the history of interactions between the genotype and the environment; evaluations of these responses must include an evaluation of these interactions. It is this component of evolutionary ecology that has been the most neglected, yet it may be the most significant factor in unraveling inexplicable variation and seeming paradoxes.

The model developed here is a set of working hypotheses that provides an adaptive explanation for variable responsiveness among women to seemingly identical conditions. As such, this approach integrates the sometimes contradictory information regarding human reproductive functioning with the paradigms and research pertaining to life history strategies, developmental biology, and human adaptability. Although diverse in methodology and focus, these subfields grapple with a common set of questions in evolutionary biology. At their intersection lies a fuller comprehension of individual variation and evolutionary processes. Integrating known attributes of mammalian physiology and the changing probabilities of successful reproduction in different conditions, I propose a Flexible Response Model (FRM) that considers the specific conditions under which a reduction in reproductive effort decreases or increases Darwinian fitness, delineates the evolution and attributes of a reproductive system that can flexibly respond to ecological conditions, incorporates the role of individual life history, and offers predictions regarding the life history parameters and econiche characteristics of species that have evolved a flexibly responsive reproductive system.

A MODEL OF FLEXIBLE RESPONSIVENESS

Axioms of Human Reproductive Functioning

At the foundation of the Flexible Response Model are four supportable givens regarding human reproductive functioning.

1.   There is considerable variation in ovarian function among women and among populations.
Substantial intrapopulational variation in ovarian function (due to differences in age, differences among same-aged individuals, and differences among an individual's cycles) has been demonstrated for numerous populations (Chiazze et al. 1968; Lipson and Ellison 1992; Riad-Fahmy et al. 1982; Treolar et al. 1967; Vollman 1977; Walker et al. 1984).

Until recently, normal interpopulational variation in ovarian function was often assumed to be negligible (cf. Bongaarts and Potter 1983). However, several studies have demonstrated significant differences among populations in a variety of settings (Ellison et al. 1989; Jasienska and Ellison 1998; Johnson et al. 1987; Panter-Brick et al. 1993; Seaton and Riad-Fahmy 1980; van der Walt et al. 1978; Vitzthum et al. 1994, 2000).

2.   Human physiology, in general, is flexible and responsive to environmental cues.
This *phenotypic plasticity*, characteristic of organisms in general, is one of two sources of variation (the other being genetic) among individuals (see Stearns 1989 and West-Eberhard 1989 for the history and development of this concept). *Reaction norm* refers to the production by genetically identical organisms of phenotypes that vary as a continuous function of some environmental signal (Woltereck 1909). As described by Stearns (1989:436), "a reaction norm is a mirror that reflects environmental effects into phenotypes." Reaction norms can be either inflexible (i.e., permanent once determined) or flexible. Life history traits, such as age at maturity, are often inflexible; physiological processes are often flexible. Genetically variable reaction norms are capable of evolving. As Wright (1931:147) notes, "Individual adaptability . . . is itself perhaps the chief object of selection."

3.   Human adult physiology reflects a particularly lengthy developmental period.
Developmental stages are believed to be the important periods during which reaction norms translate environmental effects into phenotypes

(Stearns 1989; West-Eberhard 1989). Schmalhausen (1949) called this relationship *dependent development* and Levins (1968) hypothesized the existence of developmental switches, which have been observed for such characteristics as environmental sex determination in crocodiles and turtles, caste determination in social insects, and a host of behavioral repertoires in several species (Stearns 1989; West-Eberhard 1989).

There is evidence that physiological functioning in the human adult reflects environmental conditions experienced during pre-adult stages (Baker 1975, 1988; Frisancho and Greksa 1989; Lasker 1969; Little 1982). For example, relative to individuals raised at sea level, respiratory physiology among individuals raised at high altitude is superior, allowing them to tolerate hypoxic conditions more effectively (Baker and Little 1976; Frisancho and Greksa 1989; Greksa 1991). The lengthy developmental period in humans allows ample opportunity for the environment to influence physiological reaction norms and to generate marked phenotypic variation.

4. *Human reproductive systems must be subject to natural selection.*

It is to be expected that all evolutionary processes (e.g., drift) have played some role in shaping reproductive functioning. However, as the essence of evolution comprises the causes and consequences of differential fertility, it cannot be easily argued that the very physiological/morphological system for translating current selective advantage into a larger share of the next generation's gene pool is not itself significantly shaped by natural selection. To cite the wealth of support for this viewpoint is frankly impossible. Perhaps it suffices to note that "the reproductive system [is] eminently susceptible to changes in the conditions of life" (Darwin 1859).

Obligates vs. Delayers

In light of these axioms, what pattern of ovarian function, under what conditions, is the most adaptive; that is, which would lead to the relatively greatest number of total offspring surviving to adulthood in a lifetime?[1] More specifically, under what conditions does it make sense to ovulate no matter what sort of environmental conditions exist? (that is, a phenotype of obligate reproductive investment at every opportunity). Or, when is it better to adjust functioning according to the quality of the environment? And what sort of adjustment is best? In other words, when would a delayer have the selective advantage over obligates?

As an initial step in addressing these questions I have been exploring the implications of a set of concepts and equations (Vitzthum 1990) that seeks to elucidate the advantages and disadvantages of different patterns of ovarian response to environmental stressors. In this model, ovarian function reflects two sets of probabilities: first, the probability of successful reproduction (that is, conceiving and giving birth to a viable infant) in a given set of conditions; second, the probability of conditions changing (for better or worse) within some finite time limit.

Under "optimal" conditions—that is, the best conditions that exist in that environment for that population—the probability of bringing a fetus to term is at its maximum for that population. This statement is analogous, in population genetics theory, to setting the fitness of the relatively most successful phenotype, irrespective of actual reproductive output, at 1 (Cavalli-Sforza and Bodmer 1971). As discussed below, the concept of optimal does not refer to ideal, but rather to that set (or sets) of conditions most likely to produce the outcome (in this model as developed thus far, a successful birth). For example, in comparing two sets of conditions, if greater energy availability in one set does not translate into a greater probability of reproductive success, then the conditions are equivalent with respect to this variable. "Conditions" includes, but is not limited to, energy balance.

If a change from population-specific optimal conditions reduces fecundity, this may be seen as an adaptive response if the probability of successful reproduction is reduced under the new suboptimal conditions. If these conditions are short term—*and* current investment risks future investment— selection is expected to favor those who wait until improved conditions occur; that is, delayers have the selective advantage over obligates.[2] However, although necessary, suboptimal conditions alone are not sufficient to confer a selective advantage to delayed reproduction. Rather, obligate reproduction has the advantage, even if current conditions are relatively poor, when there is no cost (i.e., lost future opportunity) in attempting and/or succeeding at reproduction in the current suboptimal conditions—that is, when current investment does not risk future success.

Future success may be put at risk through two primary avenues. First, maternal survival may be compromised because of a divergence of energy from the support of maternal life into reproductive effort and/or because of a high (or increased) risk of parturition mortality. Second, the hormonal conditions and/or energy demands associated with current investment in gestation and lactation can prevent or curtail future investment. For example, pregnancy prevents ovulation in most cases; milk production diverts energy from fetal development. Current investment under suboptimal conditions is increasingly costly, either as a result of a reduction in the probability of maternal survival or in the prevention of future successful reproduction, when offspring require extended postpartum investment.

Thus, when the costs of current attempts at reproduction are relatively inconsequential, every reproductive opportunity will be tried, and there is no evolution of delaying mechanisms. But if current effort in suboptimal conditions sufficiently risks future success, then delayers can be at an advantage. Note that up to now delayers are depicted as all-or-nothing investors; this point will be modified later.

Delayers vs. Detectors

Obligate reproduction may risk future success, but delaying also carries a risk, specifically because future conditions are unknown. If there is some non-zero probability that future conditions will be worse than current conditions, then delaying may be disadvantageous and selection would act against these individuals. Thus, we must also consider the second set of probabilities regulating ovarian function; that is, the probabilities of better and equal-or-worse conditions occurring at the next reproductive opportunity. Different relative values of these probabilities represent different environmental patterns, some of which may not be advantageous for delayers.

If the probability of conditions getting worse is equal to that of conditions getting better, then on average there would be no selection for delay mechanisms. Given a simple environment having two states, optimal and suboptimal, occurring in equal frequency, delayers do have the selective advantage (because given either state, the probability of change is always greater than the probability of no change).

However, in increasingly complex environments, delayers do not clearly have the advantage. If conditions vary over time, but an organism cannot correctly detect the direction of change, then there is no stable selection in favor of delaying mechanisms. However, when an organism can more-often-than-not detect the direction of change, then delayers are favored. Thus, detectors have a clear advantage over mere delayers in complex environments.

Detection mechanisms need not be accurate sooths of the distant future to be selectively advantageous. Although measures of successful reproduction (i.e., fitness) theoretically encompass offspring lifespan until reproductive maturity, selection differentials are not constant throughout this time. With respect to ovarian function, the most significant period of natural selection is probably during gestation (and secondarily, lactation), when maternal maintenance/survival is at greatest risk and reproductive investment in additional offspring is impossible (or at least curtailed). Thus, an organism "evaluating" the probabilities of successful reproduction and/or changing conditions cannot and need not "assess" all those conditions the organism and progeny might face till offspring maturity. Detection that encompasses current conditions and possible conditions at the next reproductive opportunity can garner substantial information, particularly because of temporal autocorrelation (i.e., in reality, conditions do not occur randomly). Further, the advantage brought by even a short delay in reproduction need not be large (selection differentials are notoriously small) to be of evolutionary significance.

Detection mechanisms are likely to be most accurate when the environment is regular and predictable, but the advantage of detectors over simple delayers is mitigated. And in turn, the advantage of either over obligates is lessened. Where the environment is more erratic, detection mechanisms are likely to be less accurate in predicting the future, but the advantage of detectors over simple delayers and obligates is greater. Thus, delay mechanisms, when present, are very likely to be accompanied by detection mechanisms, albeit imperfect ones. Detection mechanisms may assess environmental conditions indirectly (e.g., sensing photoperiod as an proxy for seasonally available energy) or more directly (e.g., caloric intake). Although largely speculative, it is likely that there are a variety of detection mechanisms (Bronson 1989). Regarding human reproduction, Frisch (1978, 1988) has argued that proportion of body fat regulates fecundity and hypothesized that this dependency is an evolved signal to prevent reproductive investment having a low probability of success. A substantial body of evidence now argues against a "critical fat threshold"; however, the core of Frisch's hypothesis, that nutrition has consequences for human fecundity, has merit.

Perhaps the clearest case of a detection mechanism operating in humans as well as other mammals is the body of evidence that links changes in reproductive function to weight loss and gain (Bronson 1989; Cameron 1989a; Cameron and Nosbisch 1991). For example, rhesus monkeys show a decrease in the frequency of pulsatile LH secretion when fed calorically restricted diets, and the magnitude of recovery is linearly related to the calorie content of subsequent feeds (Parfitt et al. 1991). In humans, decreasing weight is associated with progressive ovarian suppression (Ellison 1990; Lager and Ellison 1990; Pirke et al. 1985, 1989; Schweiger et al. 1987). Further, in both humans and other mammals, the relation between energy balance and reproductive function holds even for those of normal weight for height. Apparently, this putative detection mechanism is tuned to signals regarding a change in conditions rather than to some absolute level of energy stores (Cameron 1989a; Ellison 1990). In a similar manner, most proposed detection mechanisms in the set-point theory of body weight regulation (see discussion below) are not geared to weight per se (Keesey and Powley 1986).

The Cost of Detection-Delay and Compensating Mechanisms

Up to this point, only the benefits of detection-delay have been considered. Counterselection derives from the cost in lost reproductive opportunities—both current and future—through three avenues: (1) lost current opportunity is not offset by sufficiently high gains at future opportunities; (2) imperfect detection; (3) death before reproductive senescence.

These costs can be offset by compensating mechanisms, thereby enhancing the advantage of detection-delay. Specifically: (1) increase the number of opportunities, thereby reducing the opportunity cost for each delay; (2) adjust to reproduce even when conditions are not optimal.

Increasing the number of reproductive opportunities is perhaps the most reliable set of compensating mechanisms for reducing the potential cost of delay-detection mechanisms. This can be done in a number of ways: (1) increase the reproductive lifespan (by accelerating menarche, postponing menopause, and/or increasing longevity); (2) increase the number of cycles per year; (3) increase coital frequency (by increasing female receptivity and/or increasing male availability).

Increases in female receptivity and male availability are often noted in monogamous species (although this is not the only mating structure in which these features may be present); it is generally argued that increased female receptivity is a female ploy to ensure male investment in offspring. This model demonstrates that an additional (or alternative) advantage to increased female receptivity is that it increases the probability that reproductive opportunities under favorable conditions will not be lost. Males as well as females clearly benefit in this case, even when male investment in offspring is low, because males are ensured of inseminating a female with a high probability of success.

The second set of compensating mechanisms, adjustment to reproduce even when conditions are not optimal, can be engaged in two ways. First, in the context of a current opportunity—having detected that conditions are less than optimal but expected to improve at the next opportunity—it is better to reduce but not eliminate effort at reproduction (as was initially presented in the discussion above). As outlined before, under these conditions delaying is advantageous over obligate investment, which incurs a cost in lost future opportunity even when not successful. More importantly, a reduced but non-zero response is advantageous over forgoing the opportunity entirely when (1) there is some chance that conditions will improve very soon (within the time frame in which the current reproductive opportunity can be pursued) or (2) conditions at the next opportunity will be, in fact, worse. In other words, a non-zero response reduces the number of lost opportunities and mitigates mistaken detection regarding future conditions. This feature of the model parallels the empirically supported hypotheses of other workers (Cameron 1989b; Ellison 1990; Parfitt et al. 1991; Prior 1985) that ovarian function is graded to the magnitude of stress. As argued here, a graded response is advantageous over an all-or-nothing (threshold) approach to reproductive effort when conditions are less than optimal.

Second, adjustment can also be engaged in the context of successive, equally poor reproductive opportunities. When suboptimal conditions persist, and the probability of successful reproduction is greater than 0, then selection will favor those whose physiology adjusts to reproduce under these conditions. Such an adjustment is advantageous because, over a lifetime, a phenotype that never ovulates is at an obvious disadvantage relative to one that tries to reproduce, even if the chances for success are not very high. The process of adjusting to new conditions and the resumption of normal functioning, usually referred to as acclimatization, is known to occur for numerous physiological processes (Baker 1988; Fields et al. 1993; Little and Haas 1989). Clearly, acclimatization is facilitated when physiological responses are graded according to the magnitude of the stressor. The importance of acclimatization as a compensating mechanism may be the greatest advantage afforded by the graded responsiveness observed in ovarian functioning.

Adjustment compensating mechanisms (i.e., adjustment to reproduce under less than optimal conditions) can be likened to a poker game with a finite number of hands. If the dealer calls a game you don't like, you bow out and wait till the next dealer's call, hoping it will be better (zero-investment delayers). You've lost an opportunity to win, but you still have your stake for the next game. But if the next call is equally or more distasteful, your gambit was wasted; if you never play, in the reproductive game you lose. Clearly, it's worth the ante to get in the game. But if you bet your entire stake (obligates) and lose, you can't play the next hand. Over the long haul, the one who plays the game, but adjusts her bets to the cards, is the winner. In the language of life history theory, such variability in reproductive investment is termed "bet-hedging," a buffer in the face of environmental variation (Chisholm 1993; Seger and Brockmann 1987).

Obviously, there are limits to an organism's ability to adjust to less than ideal conditions. The probability of successful reproduction would be 0, for example, if there is less than the minimum energy necessary for the development of the fetus and the maintenance of maternal life. However, owing to differences in newborn and maternal body size, and possibly basal metabolic rate, the minimum energy requirements will vary among individuals and among populations, a factor that further compounds heterogeneity in reproductive function.

Adjustment compensating mechanisms may be more fallible (i.e., less certain to consistently yield an advantage) than those compensating mechanisms that increase reproductive opportunities; hence stable equilibria are less likely and the population will display relatively higher variation. For example, amongst 30-year-old normally cycling women there is relatively little specieswide variation in the number of cycles per year (about 13); in contrast, the ability to acclimatize varies greatly. However, adjustment mechanisms are likely to be as important as those that increase opportunities when (1) the environment is particularly risky, especially for extended periods; (2) investment in offspring is particularly extended; and (3) reproductive opportunities cannot be further increased. In humans, the second and third conditions are well met, suggesting acclimatization is a particularly significant compensating mechanism.

What's Optimal?

A key component of this model is the concept of population-specific environmental conditions. As outlined here, organisms are expected to adjust reproductive investment depending upon current conditions relative to "optimal" conditions. However, as previously noted, optimal does not equate with ideal. Rather, the best environmental conditions experienced by one population, and hence "optimal" in that case, may be conditions that are uncommon and relatively poor in a different locale. Selection operates on the phenotypes within a population with respect to the environmental context of that population; more desirable conditions (for example, greater energy availability) elsewhere are irrelevant. Differences among individuals in developmental experiences would also contribute to intrapopulational variation in reproductive functioning. However, as previously noted, there is some lower boundary beyond which the best conditions that obtain are still not sufficient for successful reproduction. Adaptation and acclimatization cannot occur in such inadequate conditions.[3]

Given sufficient, if not ideal, conditions, how can the adult organism judge what constitutes "optimal"? As noted earlier, developmental stages are believed to be the important periods during which reaction norms translate environmental effects into phenotypes. Thus, response patterns in the adult are calibrated according to conditions experienced during the pre-adult developmental period. It is likely that adult responsiveness in ovarian function to environmental conditions is mediated along the hypothalmo–hypophyseal–adrenal cortical–gonadal axis (Cameron 1989b).

Since conditions experienced during the developmental period are not identical for all individuals across all populations, what are the consequences for adult function of differing magnitudes of stress during development? Based on our understanding of acclimatization in other physiological systems (Baker 1988; Little and Haas 1989), tentative predictions can be made regarding ovarian response to stress, given different developmental conditions.

Before outlining these predictions, it may be helpful to describe what is known of adjustment processes for some physiological functions other than reproduction. A substantial body of data (Harris 1990; Keesey and

Powley 1986) is supportive of the hypothesis, generally known as "set-point theory," that body weight (or some aspect of body mass and/or composition) is internally regulated by complex and not-well-understood mechanisms such that deviations in energy intake are partially countered by changes in resting metabolism and other avenues of energy expenditure. This response is seen in individuals irrespective of starting weight, though not in all individuals, suggesting that the internal "scales" (detectors) have been calibrated to some homeostatic value (that need not be ideal for optimal health as defined by a biomedical paradigm). Apparently this calibration can be adjusted, though not easily, through changes in activity and possibly dietary composition. Interestingly, many of the posited detectors do not appear to sense energy as such, an observation relevant to the earlier discussion of putative detection mechanisms in reproductive functioning. Keesey and Powley (1986) compare this proposed body weight regulatory system to what is known of blood pressure regulation, another physiological function known to defend against perturbation, even when levels are too high for optimal health.

Respiratory functioning at high altitude (Baker and Little 1976; Greksa 1991) illustrates other aspects of physiological acclimatization. Environments at 4,000 m are hypoxic and cold. Adults raised at sea level initially have difficulty tolerating these conditions, but over time most can acclimatize and function normally. Adults raised at 4,000 m not only tolerate these conditions well because of prior exposure during development but can more easily tolerate even higher altitudes than those from sea level. However, there is a limit. There is a minimal oxygen requirement for growth and development; if not met, the organism cannot survive, much less function normally.

How might adult ovarian function be expected to respond to stress? As part of the set of hypotheses developed here, it is proposed that under conditions of light short-term stress during the subadult developmental period, adult physiological functioning is easily perturbed but will acclimatize with continued exposure to the stressor. Such relatively easy perturbation is seen, for example, among healthy American women (Lager and Ellison 1990; Pirke et al. 1985, 1989; Schweiger et al. 1987), although there is as yet no study of sufficient length to determine if acclimatization does occur. I suggest that having experienced an "energy-rich" environment during development, the system is accustomed to these conditions and "expects" relatively poorer conditions to improve shortly. Thus ovarian functioning is initially perturbed by moderate environmental stress. However, if the moderate stress persists, over time normal functioning is expected to return (that is, acclimatization will occur and homeostasis will be achieved) since the probability of successful reproduction is still greater than 0.

From the vantage point of energy sufficiency, the seemingly "senseless" response of healthy well-fed women to moderate stress now becomes comprehensible. During its evolutionary history, the human (and mammalian) reproductive system must have rarely encountered conditions of excessive plenty; rather, reproduction under less-than-ideal conditions was (and, for most, still is) the norm. Thus, in these samples of American women, it is not the response of the reproductive system to perturbation that is inexplicable; rather, it is the unusual living conditions that are aberrant. A similar case has been made regarding the current consequences (obesity and diabetes) of the previously advantageous "thrifty gene" (Neel 1962).

As has been argued with respect to a variety of issues (for example, considerable controversy surrounds standards for stature, weight, and nutrient intake), it is merely an assumption that North American samples represent a human norm against which others may be appropriately compared. With respect to reproductive function, it is more likely that Americans represent an extreme in ovarian function (Ellison et al. 1993). Nonetheless, this extreme may still be explicable in terms of specieswide reproductive adaptations.

Under conditions of moderate stress during the subadult developmental period, the Flexible Response Model hypothesizes that adult physiology is relatively insensitive to lighter stress but is perturbed by moderate to heavy stress and is expected to acclimatize with continued exposure. This is the situation that likely prevails in most populations, particularly in the "developing world." Reproduction under conditions that appear arduous is to be expected if these are the conditions experienced during the individual's developmental period; though difficult, these conditions are normal in that population. In the evolutionary foot race, one must have at least some reproductive output. This hypothesis accords well with the findings of demographic studies that nutritional factors, other than starvation, play a minor role in the fertility levels of women in developing countries (Bongaarts 1980; Bongaarts and Potter 1983; Menken et al. 1981).

The FRM predicts that under conditions of extreme stress during the subadult developmental period, the adult is expected to be sensitive to even light stress and unlikely to acclimate easily. Given such marginal conditions, the probability of successful reproduction is too low (because maternal life and/or fetal development is severely compromised) and is outweighed by the combined probabilities of a return to better conditions and successful reproduction under those conditions. This may be the process operating in populations experiencing very marginal conditions over the long term, such as the !Kung (van der Walt et al. 1978), the Lese (Ellison et al. 1989), and the Gainj (Wood et al. 1985).

Light, moderate, and extreme are classes of conditions that cannot be easily assigned some absolute value. Among the many factors that can stress an organism, those that are amenable to quantification—and hence may provide boundaries to these categories—are the caloric demands of (1) basal metabolic rate, (2) those activities necessary to the continuance of maternal life, and (3) fetal development. Analyses of other energetically constrained processes may yield additional insight. For example, Ellison (1990) has hypothesized that developmental rates may act as a "bioassay" of environmental conditions. This is an attractive suggestion as it is known that development is affected by psychosocial factors as well as energy variables; hence, developmental rates provide a common pathway for several aspects of environmental "conditions" (Chisholm, personal communication)

Here, "moderate" is heuristically defined as conditions that are within the organism's ability to respond to without marked, extended loss of well-being. "Light" is less than that experienced during the developmental period, and "extreme" is that beyond which the organism can respond to effectively (i.e., achieve homeostasis) or that which creates significant loss of well-being. Stressors which markedly reduce well-being are likely to reveal the limits of acclimatization as determined by the genes and developmental calibration.

Positing that adult response is calibrated according to developmental optima in the manner proposed here links several intriguing aspects of ovarian function. In particular, these hypotheses simultaneously explain why some women with substantial energy (fat) reserves may easily experience ovarian dysfunction while other women under arduous conditions appear to be less affected by energetic constraints. In other words, substantial heterogeneity in ovarian response to stress is to be expected.

Furthermore, this model offers a new perspective on the advantages of acclimatization and the importance of a graded response in this adjustment process. Within this framework, acclimatization does not simply serve to return the organism to some previously ordained or desirous homeostatic condition; rather, adjustment to reproduce in the face of persistent suboptimal conditions is an important compensating mechanism that mitigates the potential costs of detection-delay mechanisms, thereby enhancing the overall advantages of a flexibly responsive reproductive system.

Predictions

This model leads to several predictions regarding the life history parameters that are expected to have coevolved with detection-delay mechanisms, and the kind of environment in which this set of attributes is expected to be most advantageous.

Detection-delay mechanisms are not clearly advantageous when:

1.   current investment incurs no cost in lost future opportunity
2.   there is relatively high early adult mortality
3.   there are few reproductive opportunities
4.   there is no opportunity to calibrate detection mechanisms; i.e., a short developmental period
5.   the environment is stable and/or very predictable

The enhanced flexibility afforded by detection-delay mechanisms are increasingly advantageous when:

1.   there is relatively high reproductive investment owing to
     a.   high parturition mortality and/or the compromising of maternal life
     b.   extended offspring care
2.   there are multiple potential reproductive opportunities
3.   there is relatively low young-adult mortality
4.   there is an extended developmental period
5.   the environment is variable and/or relatively unpredictable

Clearly, detection-delay mechanisms do not suddenly appear and rapidly spread through the population when any or all of these conditions are met; rather, variable responsiveness coevolves in a species in concert with these life history parameters.

Additional Models

There is a long-standing interest among ecologists in how organisms might go about allocating energy among competing demands over the course of their reproductive lifespan. Though sometimes prompted by different questions and developed independently, several of the models have many features in common—as might be expected given that they are all guided by the evolutionary paradigm—and are not necessarily mutually exclusive.

Both Wasser and Barash (1983) and Peacock (1990, 1991) have sought to explain observations of widespread reproductive wastage in humans and many other animals, arguing that curtailment of current reproductive investment may be an adaptive strategy to increase total lifetime reproductive success. In both models, which recognize that some minimal caloric need must be met to ensure successful gestation and subsequent maturity of the offspring, detection of insufficient energy availability would be one reason for "cutting one's current losses" in favor of some future and hopefully better opportunity. In the formulation of their Reproductive Suppression Model (RSM), Wasser and Barash (1983) also elaborate on the contribution of social factors to "decisions" of reproductive investment and on the possibility that suppression of another's reproductive effort may be a strategy to improve one's own relative reproductive output. (For more discussion of these issues, see Holman and Wood, chapter 1; Pike, chapter 2; and Wasser and Place, chapter 6, this volume.)

Seeking to explain significant interpopulational variation in progesterone (Ellison et al. 1989; Jasienska and Ellison 1998; Panter-Brick et al. 1993; Vitzthum et al. 1994, 2000) and coupled with studies of the causes of ovarian suppression within women from industrialized populations (Lager and Ellison 1990; Pirke et al. 1985, 1989; Schweiger et al. 1987), Ellison (1990, 1996) has proposed a Developmental Model (DM) that links adult levels of ovarian hormonal function with the tempo of childhood and adolescent growth and maturation. A slower tempo is known to be associated with less resources and hence may act as a "bioassay" of environmental conditions, such an assessment being essential to maintaining long-term energy balance in a woman of reproductive age. Thus, in the face of constrained resources, a slower rate of reproductive output is selectively advantageous. In support of its intuitive plausibility, Ellison outlines physiological mechanisms by which this assessment of the environment may occur (see also Jasienska, chapter 3; Lipson, chapter 10).

The Flexible Response Model (Vitzthum 1990, 1992, 1997) was initially prompted by the observation of a paradox: why is ovarian function easily perturbed in women from industrialized populations, while women working in arduous conditions typically have seven or eight pregnancies and some as many as a dozen or more (Vitzthum and Smith 1989)? The FRM provides at least a partial resolution of this paradox by hypothesizing that a current reproductive "decision" is dependent on both the *absolute quality* of current conditions and the *relative quality* of these conditions compared to prior conditions and predicted future conditions. Thus, the FRM proposes that ovarian function in adult women is dependent upon conditions experienced during pre-adult development such that some women are better able to tolerate environmental stressors because of prior exposure to these conditions. That is, specific magnitudes of responsiveness in ovarian function to energetic and other factors are dependent upon temporal patterns in environmental conditions as well as some absolute measure of the quality of those conditions. Within limits, human reproductive physiology is expected to be able to acclimatize to initially stressful conditions, a flexibility that has been shaped by natural selection.

Upon careful reflection it is apparent that these models, and perhaps others not considered here, are not so much alternatives as nuances on solutions of the fundamental ecological dilemma. How can an organism most successfully apportion its resources into the demands of growth, maintenance (survival), and reproduction? Clearly, these demands also are not mutually exclusive. To reproduce, one must survive; yet maximizing the probability of survival is meaningless (in an evolutionary sense) if one has not reproduced. The Reproductive Suppression Model takes a closer look at what would be the selective advantages of curtailing current reproductive investment for future investment, noting that current investment would be a poor choice if maternal survival is at risk. The Developmental Model examines the selective advantages of favoring long-term maternal survival over more rapid reproductive output (in effect, delaying a new investment for a longer period of time than one might under more favorable conditions).

The Flexible Response Model explicitly comprises both "strategies" in addition to other strategic options (e.g., increasing female receptivity) for increasing total lifetime reproductive success relative to others within one's population. The FRM also argues that compensating mechanisms offset the potential cost of inevitably imperfect predictions of future conditions. In this view, acclimatization of the reproductive system to less-than-ideal conditions is not solely a mechanism for returning an organism to homeostasis but rather a strategy for reproductive success under conditions of chronic stress. In addition, the FRM outlines those ecological and life history features that would most favor the evolution of detection-delay/compensating mechanisms. Several of these are well known to characterize humans—most notably, high maternal investment and a long developmental period.

TESTING MODELS

Empirical testing of the Flexible Response Model as well as the DM, the RSM, and other models formulated elsewhere is no simple task, particularly in humans. Longitudinal data from several populations having different environmental characteristics would be ideal, but collection of such data is clearly a daunting prospect. Several investigators have, however, begun to lay such a foundation. Field and laboratory studies of other mammals as well as computer simulations will also help to refine our understanding of variation in human reproductive functioning

Wasser and Barash (1983) present a substantial body of evidence from the literature to support the hypothesis that reproductive suppression does occur in a wide variety of species, though there are few data for humans, and it is difficult to confirm that such suppression leads to relatively greater reproductive success. Peacock (1990:213) suggests an experiment to test the hypothesized advantage of "responders" (i.e., delayers) over "nonresponders" (i.e., obligates) in which the two groups are subjected to alternating periods of food deprivation and adequate food supply to see if the delayers had higher or lower reproductive success than the obligates. "In other words, do individuals that conceive at the 'right time' [delayers] . . . successfully raise more offspring than those conceiving at the 'wrong time' [obligates]?" Naturally, such an experiment cannot be constructed for humans, though it may be possible to seek out "natural experiments" that can provide the necessary comparisons.

In support of a link between the tempo of maturation and adult ovarian function, Ellison (1996) notes that within populations of Swedish (Apter and Vihko 1983), Italian (Venturoli et al. 1987), and North American (Gardner 1983) women, those who matured later had relatively greater impaired ovarian function as adults than early maturers. The difficulty is in knowing whether the intrapopulational variation in age at menarche in these industrialized populations reflects variation in resources and hence is a bioassay of environmental conditions, or whether some individual attribute is responsible for both late maturation and adult ovarian impairment.

Evaluating interpopulational differences in average menarcheal age and measures of average ovarian function is even more challenging. Upon first inspection, it appears that there is a negative relationship between average adult mid-luteal progesterone levels and average menarcheal age in five populations (Boston, Poland, Bolivia, Zaire, and Nepal) for which data are available (Ellison 1996). However, this relationship is less definitive if we restrict comparisons to data for which intrapopulational seasonal variations in ovarian function have been controlled. For example, during seasons of relative energy abundance, mid-luteal progesterone levels for women 25–35 years old are nearly identical in the Bolivia and Nepal samples (respectively, 251 pmol/L [Vitzthum et al. 2000] and 253 pmol/L [but 124 pmol/L in the energy-deficient monsoon season; Panter-Brick et al. 1993]) even though the average menarcheal age is 3 years earlier in the former. In addition to the difficulties faced from inferring the cause of interpopulational variation based on knowledge of the causes of intrapopulational variation (the so-called ecological fallacy), our comparisons may also be confounding the effects of acute stressors with those of chronic stressors. A conundrum, to say the least.

The Flexible Response Model originally derived from an effort to understand the bases of varying responsiveness among women to similar stressors; hence perhaps the most profitable first approach for testing the model lies in evaluating its predictions about response to stress among different groups of women. It is important to emphasize that the FRM does *not* predict a specific level of ovarian functioning or reproductive output for a given level of stress. Nor does it predict that all populations will have the same level of ovarian function and reproductive output as a result of differing abilities to adjust to environmental stressors because of varying developmental conditions. Nor does the FRM predict the same level of fertility will obtain in a chronically stressed population as would obtain in the same population if the stress did not exist.

Rather, the arguments presented here explain variation in response to a given stress level, both within and between populations. Hence, the FRM resolves, at least partially, the paradox that the ovarian function of women from industrialized settings is easily perturbed while women in chronically stressed environments continue to reproduce in the face of greater assaults. Further, the model explains why the same fertility level can exist, though it may not necessarily exist, when various measures of ovarian function appear to differ. It is noteworthy that, to date, no clinical or subclinical studies have demonstrated a functional threshold of salivary progesterone, or discontinuity in salivary progesterone levels, that distinguishes ovulatory and anovulatory cycles (Lipson et al. 1991). Hence, some populations in less than ideal circumstances, particularly with respect to a relatively extreme standard such as healthy North American women, may be able to tolerate stress more effectively than those seemingly more robust individuals. The FRM also predicts acclimatization to initially stressful conditions, and also that there are boundaries of stress below which reproduction will not occur. In other words, the "choice" is made to allocate all resources to survival, regardless of the probability of improved or not improved future conditions.

In collaboration with colleagues in Bolivia and the United States, Project REPA (Reproduction and Ecology in Provincia Aroma) was designed to test predictions of the Flexible Response Model as well as address several other issues in reproductive ecology and health (Vitzthum et al. 1998a). While earlier studies had found significantly lower progesterone (P) levels in nonindustrialized populations (Ellison et al. 1989; Jasienska and Ellison 1998; Panter-Brick et al.1993; Vitzthum et al. 1994, 2000), their cross-sectional designs and other methodological difficulties limited interpretations of these data. Further, it was unknown if ovulations and conceptions occurred at the lower P levels. The Flexible Response Model predicts that conceptions should occur at the low P levels observed in this chronically stressed population. REPA enrolled 316 women of reproductive age and collected serial samples of saliva, to be assayed for progesterone and estradiol, throughout sequential menstrual cycles while simultaneously collecting urine samples during the late luteal phase to detect hCG, indicative of a conception. As predicted, the average P levels in this population are lower than in comparative samples from industrialized countries, and conceptions do occur at these lower levels (Vitzthum et al. 1998a). Furthermore, these conceptions are also successfully maintained throughout gestation at relatively lower levels of P (1998b). It must be noted that while these findings are consistent with the predictions of the FRM, they do not "prove" the FRM in its entirety, nor are they necessarily inconsistent with the predictions of other models. Rather, the data from REPA failed to disprove specific hypotheses of the FRM, suggesting that the model deserves further testing.

CLOSING

"a riddle wrapped in a mystery inside an enigma"
(attributed to Winston Churchill)

The Flexible Response Model presented here is but a starting point for further exploration. I expect it may be modified and perhaps, eventually, even discarded once having generated, through careful investigations, enough rope to hang itself. However we may come to model human reproduction, there is currently sufficient data to argue that the variable responsiveness of human ovarian functioning among women and among populations is not necessarily pathological nor paradoxical. Rather, modern humans reflect a long and successful evolution during which selection shaped a species characterized by flexibility, opportunism, longevity, and high offspring investment. Detection-delay mechanisms, in concert with cost-mitigating compensation mechanisms, particularly acclimatization, are highly flexible reproductive adaptations appropriate to a range of mammalian niches. This set of adaptations is particularly advantageous in the exploitation of otherwise unavailable (relatively risky) niches, and in offsetting the costs of extended offspring investment.

These ideas have benefited substantially by the generous input of several colleagues. My sincere appreciation to G. Bentley, M. Borgerhoff Mulder, J. Chisholm, K. Dettwyler, P. Ellison, G. Estabrook, A.G. Fix, K. Hill, N. Peacock, and C. Worthman. This work was supported by the Hewlett Foundation, NICHD (T32-HD07339), the University of California, and NSF SBR 9506107.

NOTES

1. Lifetime reproductive success (LRS) is neither the only nor, perhaps, the best measure of fitness (cf. Burns 1992; Chisholm 1993; Endler 1986; Sober 1984). This common definition is used here as a starting point for exploring these hypotheses regarding reproductive function; however, alternative fitness definitions may prove more appropriate and will be considered as this work progresses. For example, if selection favors traits that minimize the intergenerational variance in offspring number (see Chisholm 1993; Seger and Brockmann 1987), then delayed reproduction may have selective advantages that are not apparent when only LRS is considered.

2. The hypothesis that delayed reproduction is advantageous has received considerable attention in evolutionary ecology (Boyce 1988; Holliday 1989; Pianka

1974, 1988; Seger and Brockmann 1987) but has rarely been applied to human reproduction. Notable exceptions are the discussion of reproductive "failure" by Wasser and Barash (1983) and Peacock (1990), and Ellison's (1990) proposals regarding ovarian function.

3.   As Peacock (1990:214) suggests, it can prove useful to distinguish "between responses that are the result of physiological limitations to reproduction [versus an] adaptive response to environmental cues or predictors." This view helps to explain how it is that weight change rather than weight status is associated with changes in ovarian function. On the other hand, in some cases such a distinction may be methodologically intractable and, from the standpoint of natural selection, moot. The long-term cessation of ovarian function in the face of inadequate resources (that is, an absence of acclimatization) may be seen as both a response to the physiological limitations of reproduction and an adaptive response to preserve maternal survival until such time as resources are adequate.

REFERENCES

Apter D, Vihko R (1983) Early menarche, a risk factor for breast cancer, indicates early onset of ovulatory cycles. *Journal of Clinical Endocrinology and Metabolism* 57:82–86.

Baker PT (1975) The place of physiological studies in anthropology. In A Damon (Ed) *Physiological Anthropology* (New York, Oxford University Press), 3–12.

Baker PT (1988) Human adaptability. In GA Harrison, JM Tanner, DR Pilbeam, PT Baker (Eds) *Human Biology*, third ed. (New York, Oxford University Press), 439–447.

Baker PT, Little ML (Eds) (1976) *Man in the Andes: A Multidisciplinary Study of High-Altitude Quechua* (Stroudsburg, PA, Dowden, Hutchinson and Ross).

Bongaarts J (1980) Does malnutrition affect fecundity? A summary of the evidence. *Science* 208:564–569.

Bongaarts J, Potter RG (1983) *Fertility, Biology and Behavior* (New York, Academic Press).

Borgerhoff Mulder M (1992) Reproductive decisions. In EA Smith, B Winterhalder (Eds) *Evolutionary Ecology and Human Behavior* (New York, Aldine de Gruyter), 339–374.

Boyce MS (Ed) (1988) *Evolution of Life Histories of Mammals: Theory and Pattern* (New Haven, Yale University Press).

Bronson FH (1989) *Mammalian Reproductive Biology* (Chicago, University of Chicago Press).

Burns TP (1992) Adaptedness, evolution, and a hierarchical concept of fitness. *Journal of Theoretical Biology* 154:219–237.

Cameron JL (1989a) Nutritional and metabolic determinants of GNRH secretion in primate species. In HA Delemarre-van de Waal, et al. (Eds) *Control of the Onset of Puberty*, III (New York, Elsevier Science), 275–284.

Cameron JL (1989b) Influence of nutrition on the hypothalamic-pituitary-gonadal axis in primates. In *Influence of Nutrition, Exercise and Neurotransmitters* (Berlin, Springer-Verlag), 66–78.

Cameron JL, Nosbisch C (1991) Suppression of pulsatile LH and testosterone secretion during short-term food restriction in the adult male rhesus monkey (*Macaca mulatta*). *Endocrinology* 128:1532–1540.

Cavalli-Sforza LL, Bodmer WF (1971) *The Genetics of Human Populations* (San Francisco, WH Freeman).

Chiazze L, Brayer FT, Macisco JJ, Parker MP, Duffy BJ (1968) The length and variability of the human menstrual cycle. *Journal of the American Medical Association* 203:377–380.

Chisholm JS (1993) Death, hope, and sex: life-history theory and the development of reproductive strategies. *Current Anthropology* 34:1–24.

Darwin C. (1859) *The Origin of Species* (1968 paperback edition) (New York, Penguin Books).

Ellison PT (1990) Human ovarian function and reproductive ecology: new hypotheses. *American Anthropology* 92:933–952.

Ellison PT (1996) Developmental influences on adult ovarian function. *American Journal of Human Biology* 8:725–734.

Ellison PT, Peacock NR, Lager C (1989) Ecology and ovarian function among Lese women of the Ituri Forest, Zaire. *American Journal of Physical Anthropology* 78:519–526.

Ellison PT, Lipson SF, O'Rourke MT, Bentley GR, Harrigan AM, Panter-Brick C, Vitzthum VJ (1993) Population variation in ovarian function. *Lancet* 342: 433–434.

Endler JA (1986) *Natural Selection in the Wild* (Princeton, Princeton University Press).

Fields, RD, Guthrie PB, Russell JT, Kater SB, Malhotra BS, Nelson PG (1993) Accommodation of mouse DRG growth cones to electrically induced collapse: kinetic analysis of calcium transients and set-point theory. *Journal of Neurobiology* 24:1080–1098.

Frisancho AR, Greksa LP (1989) Developmental responses in the acquisition of functional adaptation to high altitude. In MA Little, JD Haas (Eds) *Human Population Biology: A Transdisciplinary Science* (New York, Oxford University Press), 203–221.

Frisch RE (1978) Population, food intake, and fertility. *Science* 199:22–30.

Frisch RE (1988) Fatness and fertility. *Scientific American* 258:88–95.

Gage TB, McCullough JM, Weitz CA, Dutt JS, Abelson A (1989) Demographic studies and human population biology. In MA Little, JD Haas (Eds) *Human Population Biology: A Transdisciplinary Science* (New York, Oxford University Press), 45–65.

Gardner J (1983) Adolescent menstrual characteristics as predictors of gynœcological health. *Annals of Human Biology* 10:31–40.

Greksa LP (1991) Human physiological adaptation to high-altitude environments. In CGN Mascie-Taylor, GW Lasker (Eds) *Applications of Biological Anthropology to Human Affairs* (Cambridge, Cambridge University Press), 117–142.

Harris RBS (1990) Role of set-point theory in regulation of body weight. *FASEB Journal* 4:3310–3318.

Holliday R (1989) Food, reproduction and longevity: is the extended lifespan of calorie-restricted animals an evolutionary adaptation? *Bioessays* 10:125–127.

Hill K, Hurtado AM (1996) *Ache Life History: The Ecology and Demography of a Foraging People* (New York, Aldine de Gruyter).

Jasienska G, Ellison PT (1998) Physical work causes suppression of ovarian function in women. *Proceedings of the Royal Society of London*, B 265:1847–1851.

Johnson PL, Wood JW, Campbell KL, Maslar IA (1987) Long ovarian cycles in women of highland New Guinea. *Human Biology* 59:837–845.

Keesey R, Powley TL (1986) The regulation of body weight. *Annual Review of Psychology* 37:109–133.

Lager C, Ellison PT (1990) Effect of moderate weight loss on ovarian function assessed by salivary progesterone measurements. *American Journal of Human Biology* 2:303–312.

Lasker GW (1969) Human biological adaptability. *Science* 166:1480–1486.

Leslie PW, Fry PH (1989) Extreme seasonality of births among nomadic Turkana pastoralists. *American Journal of Physical Anthropology* 27:103–115.

Leslie PW, Gage TB (1989) Demography and human population biology: problems and progress. In MA Little, JD Haas (Eds) *Human Population Biology: A Transdisciplinary Science* (New York, Oxford University Press), 15–44.

Levins R (1968) *Evolution in Changing Environments* (Princeton, Princeton University Press).

Lipson SF, Ellison PT (1992) Normative study of age variation in salivary progesterone profiles. *Journal of Biosocial Science* 24:233–244.

Lipson SF, O'Rourke MT, Ellison PT (1991) Salivary progesterone profiles: reference data for anthropological studies of reproductive function. *American Journal of Physical Anthropology* (Suppl 12):115–116.

Little M (1982) The development of ideas about human ecology and adaptation. In F Spencer (Ed) *A History of American Physical Anthropology* (New York, Academic Press), 405–434.

Little MA, Haas JD (Eds) (1989) *Human Population Biology: A Transdisciplinary Science* (New York, Oxford University Press).

Menken J, Trussell J, Watkins S (1981) The nutrition fertility link: an evaluation of the evidence. *Journal of Interdisciplinary Histology* 11:425–441.

Neel JV (1962) Diabetes mellitus: a thrifty genotype rendered detrimental by progress. *American Journal of Human Genetics* 14:353–360.

NYAS Conference (1993) Human Reproductive Ecology: Interactions of Environment, Fertility and Behavior, May 21–24 (Research Triangle Park, North Carolina).

Panter-Brick C, Lotstein DS, Ellison PT (1993) Seasonality of reproductive function and weight loss in rural Nepali women. *Human Reproduction* 8:684–690.

Parfitt DB, Church KR, Cameron JL (1991) Restoration of pulsatile LH secretion after fasting in rhesus monkeys *(Macaca mulatta):* dependence on size of the refeed meal. *Endocrinology* 129:749–756.

Peacock N (1990) Comparative and cross-cultural approaches to the study of human female reproductive failure. In CJ DeRousseau (Ed) *Primate Life History and Evolution* (New York, John Wiley), 195–220.

Peacock, N (1991) An evolutionary perspective on the patterning of maternal investment in pregnancy. *Human Nature* 2:351–385.

Pianka ER (1974) *Evolutionary Ecology*, first ed. (New York, Harper and Row).

Pianka ER (1988) *Evolutionary Ecology*, fourth ed. (New York, Harper and Row).

Pirke KM, Schweiger U, Lemmel W, Krieg JC, Berger M (1985) The influence of dieting on the menstrual cycle of healthy young women. *Journal of Clinical Endocrinology and Metabolism* 60:1174–1179.

Pirke KM, Wuttke W, Schweiger U (Eds) (1989) *The Menstrual Cycle and Its Disorders: Influences of Nutrition, Exercise and Neurotransmitters* (Berlin, Springer-Verlag).

Prior JC (1985) Hormonal mechanisms of reproductive function and hypothalamic adaptation to endurance training. In J Puhl (Ed) *The Menstrual Cycle and Physical Activity* (Champaign, Illinois, Human Kinetics), 63–75.

Riad-Fahmy D, Read GF, Walker RF, Griffiths K (1982) Steroids in saliva for assessing endocrine function. *Endocrinology Reviews* 3:367–395.

Schmalhausen II (1949) *Factors of Evolution: The Theory of Stabilizing Selection* (Philadelphia, Blakiston).

Schweiger U, Laessle R, Pfister H, Hoehl C, Schwingenschloegel MM, Schweiger M, Pirke KM (1987) Diet-induced menstrual irregularities: effects of age and weight loss. *Fertility and Sterility* 48:746.

Seaton B, Riad-Fahmy D (1980) Use of salivary progesterone assays to monitor menstrual cycles in Bangladeshi women. *Journal of Endocrinology* 87:27P.

Seger J, Brockmann J (1987) What is bet-hedging? In P Harvey, L Partridge (Eds) *Oxford Surveys in Evolutionary Biology*, vol. 4 (Oxford, Oxford University Press), 182–211.

Sober E (Ed) (1984) *Conceptual Issues in Evolutionary Biology: An Anthology* (Cambridge, MIT Press).

Stearns SC (1989) The evolutionary significance of phenotypic plasticity. *BioScience* 39:436–445.

Tracer D (1996) Lactation, nutrition, and post-partum amenorrhea in lowland Papua New Guinea. *Human Biology* 68:277–292.

Treolar AE, Boynton RE, Behn BG, Brown BW (1967) Variation of the human menstrual cycle through reproductive life. *International Journal of Fertility* 12:77–126.

van der Walt LA, Wilmsen EH, Jenkins T (1978) Unusual sex hormone patterns among desert-dwelling hunter-gatherers. *Journal of Clinical Endocrinology and Metabolism* 46:658–663.

Venturoli S, Porcu E, Fabbri R, Magrini O, Paradisi R, Pallotti G, Gammi L, Famigni C (1987) Post menarcheal evolution of endocrine pattern and ovarian aspects in adolescents with menstrual irregularities. *Fertility and Sterility* 48:78–85.

Vitzthum VJ (1990) *An Adaptational Model of Ovarian Function.* Population Studies Center Research Report No. 90-200 (Ann Arbor, University of Michigan).

Vitzthum VJ (1992) The physiological basis of developmental calibration. *Abstracts of the 91st Annual Meeting* (Washington DC, American Anthropological Association), 334.

Vitzthum VJ (1997) Flexibility and paradox: the nature of adaptation in human reproduction. In A Zihlman, A Galloway, ME Morbeck (Eds) *The Evolving Female: A Life History Perspective* (Princeton, Princeton University Press), 242–258.

Vitzthum VJ, Smith SL (1989) Evaluation of data on menstrual status and activity: an evolutionary perspective (abstract). *American Journal of Physical Anthropology* 78:318–319.

Vitzthum VJ, Ellison PT, Sukalich S (1994) Salivary progesterone profiles of indigenous Andean women (abstract). *American Journal of Physical Anthropology* (Suppl 18):201–202.

Vitzthum VJ, Bentley GR, Spielvogel H, Chatterton RT (1998a) Fecundity in nutritionally stressed Bolivian women (abstract). Annual Meeting of the Population Association of America, Chicago.

Vitzthum VJ, Bentley GR, Caceres E, Spielvogel H, Crone K, May L, Chatterton RT (1998b) Correlates of conception in high altitude Aymara women (abstract). *FASEB Journal* 12:A726.

Vitzthum VJ, Ellison PT, Sukalich S, Caceres E, Spielvogel H (2000) Does hypoxia impair ovarian function in Bolivian women indigenous to high altitude? *High Altitude Medicine and Biology* 1:39–49.

Vollman RF (1977) *The Menstrual Cycle* (Philadelphia, WB Saunders).

Walker SM, Walker RF, Riad-Fahmy D (1984) Longitudinal studies of luteal function by salivary progesterone determinations. *Hormone Research* 20:231–240.

Wasser SK, Barash DP 91983) Reproductive suppression among female mammals: implications for biomedicine and sexual selection theory. *Quarterly Review of Biology* 58:513–538.

West-Eberhard MJ (1989) Phenotypic plasticity and the origins of diversity. *Annual Review of Ecology and Systematics* 20:249–278.

Woltereck R (1909) Weitere experimentelle Untersuchungen uber Artveranderung, speziell uber das Wesen quantitativer Artunterschiede bei Daphniden. *Verhandlingen des Deutsch-Tschechischen Zoologischen Gesellschaft* 1909:110–172 (cited in Stearns 1989).

Wood JW, Johnson PL, Campbell KL (1985) Demographic and endocrinological aspects of low natural fertility in highland New Guinea. *Journal of Biosocial Science* 17:57–79.

Worthman CM (1990) Socioendocrinology: key to a fundamental synergy. In TE Ziegler, FB Bercovitch (Eds) *Socioendocrinology of Primate Reproduction* (New York, Wiley-Liss), 187–212.

Wright S (1931) Evolution in Mendelian populations. *Genetics* 16:97–159.

9

Fertility Changes with the Prehistoric Transition to Agriculture

Perspectives from Reproductive Ecology and Paleodemography

GILLIAN R. BENTLEY, RICHARD R. PAINE,
and JESPER L. BOLDSEN

Since the last Ice Age, agriculture has essentially replaced foraging as the human means of subsistence. At the end of the Pleistocene all humans were foragers. Today, foragers represent such a small proportion of the human population as to be essentially nonexistent. In geological terms this replacement was rapid, although for most groups it was a slow, incremental process. Population issues have been central to debate surrounding the agricultural transition (Cohen 1977, 1989; Cohen and Armelagos 1984; Cowgill 1975; Hassan 1981; Rafferty 1985; Wood et al. 1992). One particularly controversial issue has been the relative importance of changes in fertility and mortality in the long-term demographic growth that followed the adoption of agriculture (Buikstra and Konigsberg 1985; Cohen 1989; Pennington 1996). Specifically, what was the relative importance of increases in fertility and/or decreases in mortality for human population growth that followed the transition to agriculture?

Demographic studies of contemporary foragers and transitional groups have not been particularly informative on this issue. Population studies of contemporary foraging societies are limited by their scarcity and typically small size. There are also questions about how representative contemporary groups are of prehistoric foragers. Contemporary foragers tend to live in more marginal environments and are affected, to varying degrees, by contact with non-foraging peoples. Important outside factors include sexually transmitted diseases (STDs), health care, and agriculturally based foods.

There are also divergent conclusions on the relationship between subsistence mode and fertility, although the majority of the small number of studies point towards higher fertility among farming communities compared with foragers. For example, Hewlett (1991) compiled data from 57 hunter-gatherer, horticulturalist, and pastoralist groups (but not sedentary agriculturalists). The latter two groups combined had slightly higher fertility than hunter-gatherers, but this was not statistically significant. In their meta-analyses of contemporary foraging and agricultural populations, Campbell and Wood (1988) and Bentley and colleagues (1993a, 1993b) demonstrate the challenges inherent to the demography of such groups. These two separate studies compared the total fertility rates (TFRs) of contemporary ethnographic groups by subsistence strategies and attempted to see whether agriculturalists had higher fertility rates than foragers. Bentley and colleagues (1993a, 1993b) found evidence of higher fertility among agriculturalists; Campbell and Wood (1988) could find no significant effect of subsistence on fertility rates.[1]

More recently, Sellen and Mace (1997) undertook a phylogenetic analysis of subsistence modes and fertility enlarging the samples used by Campbell and Wood and by Bentley and colleagues to control for cultural associations within their sample. They used the World Ethnographic Sample (WES) to code subsistence strategies for the populations. WES uses a system that assesses the proportional dependence on foraging, fishing, agriculture, and so forth, and is therefore more accurate than a categorical division into an agricultural or nonagricultural society. Sellen and Mace (1997) found that increases in fertility rates were strongly associated with a higher dependence on agriculture, such that a 10% increase in dependence on agriculture resulted in an increase of 0.2 live births per woman.

In contrast, Pennington (1996) has argued that population increases attributed to agriculture could be maintained with small improvements in early childhood survival, even if fertility remained unchanged and overall life expectancy decreased. She has used the ethnographic record to show that survival among young children (1–5 years) often improves as foraging groups become more sedentary and more dependent on agricultural products. Again, using a phylogenetic analysis, Sellen and Mace (1999) also demonstrate that child mortality (in this case 1–15 years) is higher among groups with a greater reliance on foraging and hunting. Sellen and Mace note two possibilities that might influence their findings. In contrast to horticultural or agricultural groups, contemporary hunter-gatherers: (1) may have been more susceptible to disease following contact and, (2) because of their continued mobility, may have had little or no access to health care that could have improved mortality rates.

There has been a tendency in the literature to view demographic changes that took place with advent of agriculture in either/or terms: either fertility increased or mortality decreased. But, as can be seen from the review of recent studies on fertility and mortality provided above, these two positions are far from mutually exclusive and may even have been complementary.

This chapter explores the question of fertility increase after the transition to agriculture, combining data from reproductive ecology and paleodemography. Our focus is on women and their children. We emphasize women's fertility for two reasons: (1) women have a greater (and more quantifiable) biological investment in their offspring, resulting from their exclusive role in the gestation and lactation processes; and (2) male fertility is more difficult to measure. We consider various ecological issues that arise from this subsistence transition, such as changes in nutrition, maternal and child health, child care, lactational practices, sedentism, workloads, and so forth, and discuss how these might affect life history parameters of prehistoric individuals. We then present paleodemographic data from Europe and discuss, briefly, some issues of reconstructing past population dynamics from skeletal series. We use these data, which span the Mesolithic period through the Iron Age, to explore how the shape of childhood mortality and female reproductive mortality may have changed with the advent of food production. Finally, we discuss what the paleodemographic and reproductive ecology data presented here contribute to the debate over whether fertility increase was an important factor in post-transition population growth.

REPRODUCTIVE ECOLOGY AND SUBSISTENCE TRANSITIONS

There is substantial evidence of dramatic ecological changes that occurred for human populations during the transition to agriculture. Any one of these changes, and certainly a combination of such changes, would be expected to impact on human life history and reproductive ecology. This section reviews the kinds of effects that might be expected to affect reproductive function following this transition.

Nutritional Changes

The advent of agriculture introduced major dietary changes, although the archaeological record attests to their gradual nature (e.g., Hutchinson et al. 1998; Katzenberg et al. 1995; Szuter and Bayham 1989; Whittle 1996). There is wide variation in the diets of recent and contemporary hunter-gatherer societies depending on the diversity of their environments (Jenike 2001; Kelly 1995). Given the higher energy yield of animal and fish resources per hour of foraging where these are readily available (Layton et al. 1991), we might expect that foragers would concentrate on these protein-rich food items where possible. Ethnographic evidence certainly supports the notion that meat is a preferred food among hunter-gatherers (Kelly 1995). In general, foragers enjoy a variety of food items, whereas horticulturalists typically have a less varied diet, often focused on a few staple crops and/or animals. Hunting and gathering would, however, undoubtedly have supplemented food production during the initial transition to agriculture, much as it does today for many swidden horticulturalists. Domesticated plants and animals also vary significantly in macronutrient, energy, and fiber content compared with their wild counterparts.

Both foraging and horticultural societies suffer from seasonal fluctuations in food resources (Bailey and Peacock 1988; Bailey et al. 1992; Hill et al. 1984; Hurtado and Hill 1990; Huss-Ashmore et al. 1989; Jenike 1995, 2001; Pagezy 1982; Ulijaszek and Strickland 1993). These seasonal fluctuations as well as the possibility of chronic undernutrition among some groups would be expected to affect reproductive function and, ultimately, fertility. Nutritional stress has been shown to alter gonadal function among women who experience insufficient energy intake, whether from intentional dietary restrictions or otherwise (Bates et al. 1982; Cumming et al. 1994; Warren 1983). The effects on reproduction include alteration of menstrual patterns, a reduction in reproductive hormone levels, an increase in the proportion of anovulatory cycles, and sometimes complete loss of menstrual cyclicity. Jasienska provides greater detail about the effects of nutrition on reproductive function in chapter 3 of this volume.

Clinical studies among western women link low energy intakes with suppression of reproductive capacity. For example, Kurzer and Calloway (1986) report that, while there was no change in levels of progesterone or estradiol in ovulatory cycles among women who reduced their energy intake for one month, the thinnest women failed to ovulate. Similarly, Dorgan et al. (1996) observed a high correlation between energy intake in the diet and the probability of a rise in progesterone levels during the luteal phase of the menstrual cycle. Green et al. (1988) found a 4.6% increase in the risk of infertility with associated ovulatory abnormalities among underweight women (85% of ideal body weight) who were attempting to conceive. Likewise, Bates et al. (1982) examined 26 underweight women with unexplained infertility who participated in a weight-gain program. Of these, 19 (73%) conceived spontaneously following a return to normal weight.

Among more traditional populations, a similar relationship has been found between poor energy intake and reproductive function. The Lese of the Ituri Forest, Democratic Republic of Congo, experience seasonal nutritional stress when energy intake is insufficient (Bailey et al. 1992; Bentley et al. 1998a; Ellison et al. 1986, 1989). During these times, women who suffer from weight loss have altered menstrual patterns and lower reproductive hormone levels. The chances of conception are also lower during these stressful periods, and higher during periods of greatest food availability. This suppression of reproductive function is interpreted as an adaptation to poor environmental conditions, where potential conception, gestation, and lactation might endanger the health and survival of mothers (Bentley 1985; Ellison 1990, 1991, 1994; Vitzthum 1990, 1992). If prehistoric agriculturalists suffered from periodic food shortages through crop failure or other factors, then reproductive function could be expected to decline during these times of stress.

The relationship between *chronic* energy stress and gonadal function in women is not as well understood as the effects of short-term nutritional stress. But, many researchers are now looking at how chronically low energy intake might affect the reproductive development of individuals during childhood and adolescence. We do know that women in populations characterized by markedly different lifestyles and subsistence bases vary in their reproductive hormone levels, with those from industrialized and less active populations having the highest (Ellison et al. 1993). Ellison (1996) associates adult variation in reproductive hormone levels with differences in the rates of childhood and adolescent growth, suggesting that such variation may function to sensitize adult female reproductive function to potentially suboptimal conditions for reproductive investment. Under suboptimal conditions, Ellison theorizes that women would have a reduced probability of ovulation, fertilization, implantation, and conception. In contrast, Vitzthum (1990, 1992, 1997) argues that the response of the reproductive system to environmental perturbations such as low energy availability is more flexible and, within limits, can be expected to adapt over time to chronic stress. Her model predicts both differences in reproductive hormone levels among populations experiencing different levels of energetic stress and conceptions at these low levels. Data from rural Aymara women, who conceive at significantly lower levels of salivary progesterone than women from the U.S. and U.K. (Bentley et al. 1998b; Vitzthum et al. 1998), but at levels of estradiol that are comparable to those of western women (Bentley et al. 2000), may shed light on the relationship between low hormone levels and fecundity. For further discussion of these issues see Lipson (chapter 10) and Vitzthum (chapter 8) in this volume.

Dietary composition is another factor that can affect ovarian function and steroid hormone levels. A higher ratio of carbohydrate to protein can lower levels of progesterone and estradiol by reducing the concentrations of binding globulins (cortisol-binding globulin and sex-hormone-binding globulin) that transport reproductive steroids (Anderson et al. 1987). The advent of cereal food crops such as wheat, corn, and rice, which became staples for Neolithic and later agriculturalists, increased the ratio of carbohydrates to protein (Larsen 1995) and thus might have lowered the available levels of reproductive hormones. Dietary composition is also known to affect metabolic clearance rates and measurable levels of reproductive steroids. For example, vegetarian diets, which usually have a lower fat content and higher amounts of fiber, can lead to an increase in the metabolism and excretion of reproductive steroid hormones with less available hormone for reproductive purposes (Adlercreutz and Martin 1980; Goldin et al. 1981, 1982; Longcope 1990). Bentley et al. (1998a) have already suggested that the primarily vegetarian diet of Lese women may lower their reproductive steroid levels. The advent of agriculture and sedentism may have reduced the amount of meat available for dietary intake from hunting or herding, resulting in a primarily vegetarian diet. The ratio of vegetables to meat in the diet, as well as the kinds of plants depended on by either foragers or horticulturalists, would also potentially affect their intake of phytoestrogens. Phytoestrogens are known to affect circulating levels of estrogens and consequently reproductive function in humans and other animals (Bentley 2000; Kaldas and Hughes 1989; Whitten 1999).

Changes in nutritional status could also affect maternal status and in particular the occurrence and severity of maternal depletion syndrome, where women's energy reserves are diminished by the demands of repeated gestation and lactation (Little et al. 1992; Miller et al. 1994; Tracer 1991; Winkvist et al. 1992). Energy invested in pregnancy and lactation cannot be used for somatic maintenance or repair, resulting in weight loss among women for whom adequate supplies of energy are unavailable. Mothers with poor energy balance have longer periods of lactational amenorrhea (and hence longer interbirth intervals) partly because of their own poor nutritional status but also because of more intense suckling by the infant in their efforts to acquire sufficient milk (Delgado et al. 1978; Howie and McNeilly 1982; Huffman et al. 1987a, 1987b; Lunn et al. 1980; Paul et al. 1979; Vitzthum 1994; Wenlock and Wenlock 1981). Valeggia and Ellison discuss the interaction between lactation, energetics, and postpartum fecundity in greater detail in chapter 4 of this volume. By analyzing anthropometric data and information on socioeconomic status in Bangladesh and Papua, New Guinea, respectively, both Miller et al. (1994) and Tracer (1991) have found that the severity of weight loss among pregnant and/or lactating women is related to the amount of energy available to women. Campbell and Wood (1988), using a sensitivity analysis, found that the duration of postpartum lactational infecundability was the most important factor contributing to the length of interbirth intervals and hence the potential fertility of women in noncontracepting societies.

The potential importance of nutrition and its effects on lactation in different human societies has been underscored by studies in The Gambia.

Lunn and his coworkers (1984) investigated the effects of nutritional sup-plementation on lactation in a longitudinal analysis of rural Gambian women. Over a period of four years, the length of postpartum amenorrhea was recorded for lactating women, some of whom received nutritional supplementation. The latter experienced significantly shorter periods of postpartum amenorrhea. Women who received supplements only during postpartum lactation resumed menstrual cycles 21 months earlier than women who were not supplemented postpartum, while women who received supplements during both pregnancy and lactation experienced a 35-week reduction in postpartum amenorrhea. The factors responsible for these dramatic differences are probably related to differences in milk vol-ume and infant suckling, since the actual nutritional composition of the mothers' milk did not differ between supplemented and unsupplemented periods of lactation.

Nutrition is not just important for a lactating mother; it is also impor-tant for her infant. An agricultural diet generally provides better weaning foods for infants, such as milk from other animals, grains that produce eas-ily digestible gruels, and so forth. Ceramic pots, usually associated with the introduction of sedentism and agriculture, allow food to be boiled for long periods. A number of authors have associated this technological inno-vation with the use of cereal gruels suitable as weaning foods (Buikstra et al. 1986; Haaland 1995; Mølleson 1995). Age at weaning, or the age when weaning foods were introduced, has been reconstructed for a number of different archaeological populations. Several methods have been used, including bone chemistry analyses, paleonutritional information, paleo-pathological patterns of morbidity and mortality, and ceramic data (Buik-stra et al. 1986; Herring et al. 1998; Katzenberg et al. 1996; Schurr 1997; Stuart-Macadam 1995; Wright and Schwarcz 1998).

For example, Wright and Schwarcz (1998) examined stable carbon and oxygen isotopes in dental enamel to reconstruct the age of weaning using 35 skeletons from Middle Preclassic to Late Postclassic Kaminaljuyú in Guatemala (ca. 700 B.C. to A.D. 1500). Results from these analyses suggest that maize was introduced as a weaning food before the age of two years, though breast milk continued to be an important part of the diet until much later, possibly as late as six years. Similarly, Herring et al. (1998), using stable nitrogen isotopes, suggest that solid foods were introduced at about five months, with weaning occurring by 14 months, in a nineteenth-century skeletal population from Canada. Perhaps the most important aspect of these studies is the emphasis on weaning as a process rather than a single event.

Earlier weaning and the potential reduction of nursing periods would tend to shorten interbirth intervals and potentially increase fertility levels.

An earlier introduction of weaning foods could, however, also increase infants' exposure to pathogens, thus elevating their risk of morbidity and mortality. Higher early childhood mortality would return mothers to a state of fecundity earlier, again shortening interbirth intervals, though the actual number of surviving children would not necessarily increase.

In a recent ethnographic analysis of the relationship between weaning age, types of weaning foods, and subsistence strategies, Sellen and Smay (2001) found a significant difference in the earliest reported age at which lactation was terminated, with agriculturalists weaning a higher proportion of children early. This might seem to support the notion that food-producers have better weaning foods available to them. However, Sellen and Smay found no significant difference between subsistence groups in the age at which supplementary foods were first introduced to infants, the age at which breastfeeding was stopped, or the average duration of breastfeeding. In fact, foraging populations were more likely to introduce supplemental foods earlier than agriculturalists, even though the duration of breastfeeding was longer.

The occurrence of earlier weaning does not, therefore, necessarily appear to be linked to the availability of foods based on agricultural produce as was previously thought. We do not know, however, if children weaned on to such foods may have been better off nutritionally compared to foraging children who would not have had such foods available to them.

Changes in Energy Expenditure

The kinds of activities women perform, as either foragers or agriculturalists, is crucial given the relationship between women's energetic output and gonadal function. Clinical data from sports medicine, as well as a more limited literature on the energetics of women in traditional rural societies where activity levels are high, reveal that a heavy expenditure of energy alters reproductive function. Again Jasienska (chapter 3, this volume) covers many of these issues in greater detail than is possible here. High energy outputs can change menstrual patterns, lower reproductive hormone levels, and affect the ability to conceive (Cumming et al. 1994; De Souza et al. 1998). The causal mechanisms of this gonadal suppression are not fully understood but are ultimately thought to operate through alteration of hypothalamic signaling, which controls the secretion of gonadotropin-releasing hormone. However, the relationship between high energy outputs and ultimate fertility is clear. For example, Green et al. (1986) found a 4.7% increased risk of infertility among women who exercised more than one hour a day. Jasienska and Ellison (1998) found that salivary progesterone levels were lowered in rural Polish women during the heaviest agricultural season of the year.

One of the most important issues associated with the adoption of agriculture relates to the levels of mobility required for subsistence activities and their associated energetic cost. Mobility refers to both long-term migrations that foraging societies follow in search of wild foods and also to the daily foraging range that women would typically cover in the course of their search for food items. Although many scholars have assumed that mobility generally declined for populations once more permanent habitations were constructed at the transition to agriculture, the evidence from archaeology and ethnography is equivocal (e.g., Dufour 1984; Hard and Merrill 1992; Kelly 1992; Kent 1989; Lieberman 1993; Panter-Brick and Pollard 1999; Price and Brown 1985; Rocek 1995; Rosenberg 1998). In fact, mobility varies considerably among hunter-gatherers and horticulturalists (Kelly 1995:112–115, Table 4-1). One of the constraints on residential mobility for horticulturalists is the location and relative permanence of their gardens and associated settlements. Paradoxically, this permanence often results in longer daily trips for women in search of supplementary wild foods, essential firewood, and to reach their garden plots. In contrast, foragers are more likely and willing to move their camps closer to new resources as older ones decline in abundance (Kelly 1995:133–141). As Kelly (1995:149) states, "sedentism does not save energy, but it does reorganize it."

Kelly (1995) provides comparative data for residential migrations among foraging groups, and complementary data from time-allocation studies shed light on distances covered for daily foraging activities in contrast to habitation shifts. Lee (1979) estimated that Dobe !Kung women covered approximately 2,400 km each year in their food quest in the Kalahari Desert (a range from between 3 and 20 km for each foraging trip). If we estimate that !Kung women walked at a slow pace of 5 km/hr, given the burdens they had to carry, then on an average day women would walk for approximately 1.3 hours. Efe women from the Ituri Forest were estimated to spend 0.8 hours/day in foraging activities and a further 0.7 hours in traveling between camps and settled villages of neighboring Lese horticulturalists each day (Peacock 1985). Ache women in Paraguay were calculated to spend 1.9 hours/day walking during foraging trips, often carrying heavy loads of game and gathered produce (Hurtado et al. 1985). Hadza women of reproductive age spent 3.94 hours/day in food acquisition activities, a figure that includes food processing as well as travel times (Hawkes et al. 1997).

The ethnographic data on time allocation efforts by horticulturalist women are more limited. Dufour (1984) calculated that Yapú women, in the tropical rainforests of Colombia, spent 1.88 hours traveling to their food acquisition areas. Most of these were accessible by foot, but 14% were only accessible by canoe. More than half of the pedestrian trips (63%)

involved carrying loads. The distance between garden sites also varied considerably for individual women, ranging from a 15- minute distance to as much as two and a half hours. Given these data, it appears that mobility is just as great for horticulturalist women as it is for foragers, and that they are frequently required to carry heavy burdens.

Time-allocation data cannot tell us how much energy expenditure is involved in the respective activities of foraging or horticulturalist women. But, it is unlikely that food-processing activities are less arduous for horticulturalists than for foragers. In fact, garden work, such as hoeing, weeding, and harvesting as well as processing agricultural produce are frequently repetitive, labor-intensive tasks. The seasonal nature of such activities are probably also matched by the seasonal variation in available food items in foraging societies (Jenike 2001). A great deal of data on physical activity levels (PAL) has been compiled for contemporary foraging, horticulturalist, and agricultural societies, which helps to interpret the energy expended in various tasks. PAL is calculated as 24-hour energy expenditure divided by the basal metabolic rate and corrected for age, sex, and body weight (Jenike 2001; Panter-Brick and Pollard 1999; Sackett 1996).

There is clearly a wide range of variation among foraging groups depending on their local ecology. PAL estimates range from 1.5 (defined as "light") for the !Kung to 1.9 (defined as "heavy") for the Ache (Jenike 2001; Panter-Brick and Pollard 1999:Table 5.1). Similar ranges exist for horticulturalists, whereas women involved in agricultural labor in temperate climates usually have high PALs. Sackett (1996:Table 11.7) calculated a mean PAL for women in foraging (1.72), horticulturalist (1.79), and agricultural (2.31) societies, reinforcing the idea that the energy expenditure of women in foraging and horticulturalist groups is very similar, but it increases for sedentary agricultural communities.

The data summarized here all point to the complex relationship between subsistence base and energy expenditure. They suggest that the transition to agriculture did not necessarily decrease workloads for women, but rather changed the kinds of activities that were required. This supposition is supported by archaeological and paleopathological data. Bridges (1985), for example, found that female skeletons from the Mississippian period in north Alabama, when horticulture based on maize, beans, and squash was already well-established, were characterized by greater long bone size and strength in comparison with Archaic foraging females. Bridges linked these skeletal changes among the horticulturalist women to their subsistence activities, such as gardening, food preparation and cooking, hauling of firewood and water, ceramic and leather manufacture, and a variety of other tasks. Among these, the use of pestles and mortars to pound corn would have been particularly onerous.

Similarly, Bridges et al. (2000) examined changes in long bone diaphyseal strength from skeletal series spanning the Middle Woodland through Mississippian periods in west-central Illinois—a period spanning the intensification of hoe horticulture and the introduction of more intensive agricultural techniques. Female skeletons showed greater changes than those of males, with significant increases in the strength of the lower limbs particularly during the transition from the Middle to early Late Woodland period when horticultural techniques were intensified, but before the introduction of more intensive maize agriculture. There was also a decline in arm strength during the Mississippian. These latter data support the idea that the transition from a foraging subsistence base to a horticulturalist one may have involved more hard labor for women than the transition to intensive agriculture.

Hard repetitive activities might be expected to leave their mark on the skeleton in the form of osteoarthritis, but paleopathological data are conflicting about whether arthritis becomes more or less prevalent in skeletal populations in response to agricultural technologies. Most of these data come from North American skeletal series (Bridges 1992; Larsen 1995). Buikstra et al. (1986) found an increase in arthritis among west-central Illinois female skeletons from the Late Woodland and Mississippian periods compared with their earlier counterparts and connected this difference to a change in subsistence activities. In contrast, Larsen (1984) found a decrease in the prevalence of osteoarthritis with the introduction of agriculture using skeletal series from Georgia. What does appear less equivocal is that there is a greater degree of sexual dimorphism in the occurrence of osteoarthritis following the introduction of agriculture. Males show a higher incidence than females; this may be related to changes in the division of labor (Bridges 1992).

A combination of stressors such as high energy output and poor energy intake is known to intensify the effects on ovarian function. Women exposed to both kinds of stressors would, therefore, have a higher degree of reproductive impairment. This was made clear in a study by Bullen et al. (1985; Beitins et al. 1991) when untrained women volunteered to participate in a running program. Half of these women were also placed in a weight-reducing program. The latter experienced more menstrual and ovulatory problems than the women who merely ran, while both groups had more problems than sedentary controls. These acute effects on reproductive function are readily reversible, however, resulting in a relatively rapid return to fecundity when conditions improve.

Finally, women's workloads heavily influence breastfeeding schedules in terms of both the duration of each feed and the interval between them. Maternal work patterns are therefore likely to affect the timing of lactational supplements to infants, the age at which total weaning occurs (Sellen and Smay 2001), and the resumption of postpartum fecundity (Panter-Brick 1991; Vitzthum, 1994).

Disease Loads

This is not the place to write at length about the interaction of disease and fertility in prehistoric and historic times. The outstanding issues of interest here are the origin of diseases known to affect fertility, and their likely prevalence in pre-agricultural and later agricultural communities. Unfortunately, other than for sexually transmitted diseases, very little new work documenting the effects of disease on fertility has been undertaken since the publication of the extensive volume by McFalls and McFalls (1984). However, Froment (2001) includes a useful discussion of the epidemiology of contemporary hunter-gatherers and the prevalence of specific diseases in their societies. He stresses some of the major factors in foraging societies, such as their low density and limited contacts with other societies, that protect them from the spread of certain pathogens. At the same time, contact with wild animals may lead to a higher risk of exposure to certain rare viruses.

McFalls and McFalls (1984) list a number of non-sexually-transmitted diseases that can affect fertility, including tuberculosis (TB), malaria, filariasis, schistosomiasis, sleeping sickness, and Chagas' disease. STDs—not including the recent emergence of HIV/AIDS—that can affect fertility include gonorrhea, pelvic inflammatory disease (PID), syphilis, genital herpes, mycoplasmas, and chlamydia.

Many of the diseases listed above leave little or no trace on skeletal remains, and thus there is scant evidence with which to document their existence or effects in prehistoric times. These "invisible" diseases include (among the non-STDs) filariasis, schistosomiasis, sleeping sickness, and Chagas' disease, and for the STDs—gonorrhea, PID, genital herpes, mycoplasmas, and chlamydia. Diseases such as syphilis and TB leave skeletal traces only when in their advanced forms. Another problem is trying to reconstruct the impact of these diseases on fertility. The fact that syphilis can be congenital in form already argues that fertility is not always impaired by this disease, although fecundability may be lower (McFalls and McFalls 1984). If sufficiently debilitating, most diseases are, in any case, likely to affect fecundability by reducing coital rates (individuals may either have insufficient energy for coitus, or may be rendered unattractive to potential mates by their illness).

Even clear identification of specific diseases in individual skeletons cannot inform us about the prevalence of this condition on a population level. For example, skeletal lesions develop in only about 10–20% of individuals suffering from syphilis (Steinbok 1976), and the corresponding proportion of skeletons one would expect to exhibit such lesions from archaeological populations would be significantly lower (Baker and Armelagos 1988). The ability to survive disease episodes is largely dependent on the general health as well as underlying frailty of the population at risk. As outlined further below, the interpretation of paleopathological data is at best equivocal (Cohen and Armelagos 1984; Wood et al. 1992). As Wood et al. (1992) point out, evidence of morbidity is more likely to be visible in skeletal remains from healthier populations.

There does appear to be sufficient evidence supporting the existence of treponemal infections (possibly syphilis) in prehistoric times in the Americas, with some specimens dated as early as the fourth millennium B.C. (Baker and Armelagos 1988). The existence of treponemal antigens in Pleistocene bear remains dated to 11, 500 B.P. suggests a zoonotic origin for this suite of infections in humans, although the validity of this finding is under debate (Buikstra, personal communication 2000). It is quite possible then that other STDs manifested themselves in humans prior to agriculture. Many scholars would argue that a high prevalence of STDs is unlikely prior to large aggregations of human populations more typical of agricultural communities. But Pennington (2001) disputes this assertion. She argues that many diseases, even if characterized by long infection periods, can be endemic in small populations. Furthermore, if extremely low rates of population growth in prehistory are an accurate reconstruction, they cannot be easily explained from other causes.

Although TB probably originated in prehistoric times, it is generally a disease associated with relatively high population densities and hence is more likely to be associated with agricultural populations. Given its zoonotic origins, it is likely to have originated in the Old World following the domestication of cattle (Roberts and Manchester 1995). The disease can easily be contracted by drinking milk from infected cows, and children may thus have been particularly vulnerable to infection. One of the earliest European skeletons exhibiting the destructive lesions typical of advanced tuberculosis dates to fourth millennium B.C. Italy. In the New World, tubercular bacilli have been found in buffalo, elk, moose, and deer, from which animals the disease may have spread to human groups. It was identified in 15.8% of skeletons in one precolumbian Peruvian skeletal series (Buikstra and Williams 1991). One of the earliest example from the New World dates to around 800 B.C. (Roberts and Manchester 1995).

Sterility due to TB is usually associated with the genital form of the disease, and 55% of affected women may be infertile (McFalls and McFalls 1984:84). It is difficult to estimate the proportion of individuals afflicted with TB who are likely to develop genital manifestations, but the younger the age when the disease is contracted, the more likely that genital TB will develop (McFalls and McFalls 1984). Given that children would be more likely than adults to drink the milk of infected animals, it is possible that many young individuals in the Old World would have been exposed to TB and develop the genital form. Women may also be more susceptible (McFalls and McFalls 1984).

The diagnosis of malaria from skeletal remains must be made inferentially through recognition of anemic conditions related to thalassemia and/or sickle-cell anemias (e.g., Angel 1964). These conditions are thought to have become more prevalent as selective pressures for adaptations conferring protection against malaria increased (Friedman and Trager 1981; Frisancho 1993). Diagnosis is thus problematic since anemias can be related to a range of different morbid factors, including nutritional deficiencies. Like TB, malaria is more likely to have reached endemic proportions once human groups aggregated in densely packed settlements. Infertility associated with malaria is mostly associated with fetal loss resulting from the high fevers, anemia, and placental parasitization associated with the disease (McFalls and McFalls 1984).

In conclusion, the emergence of agriculture and increasing density of settlements probably exacerbated susceptibility to specific diseases, such as TB and malaria, that are known to reduce fertility. If, as many argue, nutritional stress increased with agriculture, individuals would also have become more vulnerable to pathologies. In addition, infection with one pathology can increase the risk of contracting others. This has become evident in the association between prior exposure to STDs and the increased individual risk of contracting HIV/AIDS (Caldwell and Caldwell 2000). However, until more research on fertility and diseases is undertaken, any reconstructions for prehistory must remain highly conjectural.

PALEODEMOGRAPHY

Reproductive ecology identifies several factors that could lead to higher fertility after the agricultural transition. However, it cannot demonstrate that these factors led to actual fertility increases in prehistory, nor does the contemporary record provide any clear trend toward higher fertility among agricultural groups. Paleodemography has the potential to identify selective pressures that might affect life history and to supply physical evidence of fertility increase in prehistory.

Paleodemographic data present a number of obstacles to analysis. Chief among these are (1) the under-representation of infants; (2) potential age-related bias in morphological sex markers, especially those of the cranium (Walker 1995); (3) accuracy and bias in age estimators (Bocquet-Appel and Masset 1982, 1996; Konigsberg and Frankenberg 1992; Konigsberg et al.

1997; Meindl et al. 1985; Paine and Harpending 1998); (4) the influence of population growth, which is usually unknown, on the population at risk (Sattenspiel and Harpending 1983); and (5) the question of unobserved population heterogeneity and selective mortality (Wood et al. 1992). The results of paleodemographic studies must be viewed with these issues in mind (for more detailed discussion see Buikstra 1997; Paine 1997; Wood et al. 1992).

Relationships between agriculture and urbanism, human health, and demography have long been a central theme in paleopathology and paleodemography (e.g., Acsádi and Nemeskéri 1970; Boldsen 1984; Buikstra et al. 1986; Cohen 1977, 1989; Cohen and Armelagos 1984; Konigsberg and Frankenberg 1994; Larsen 1995; Pennington 1996; Wood et al. 1992). Numerous osteological studies have documented paleopathological changes following the adoption of agriculture (e.g., Acsádi and Nemeskéri 1970; Angel 1984; Buikstra and Williams 1991; Cohen and Armelagos 1984; Cook 1984; Larsen 1987, 1995; Meiklejohn et al. 1984, 1997; Milner 1991; Rose et al. 1984; Ubelaker 1984). These include a lower mean age at death, reduced stature, increases in the frequency of both specific and nonspecific lesions (e.g., cribra orbitalia, porotic hyperostosis, periosteal reactions), and increases in frequencies of stress markers (e.g., Harris lines, enamel hypoplasias). The correct interpretation of lesion frequencies is unclear. The most widespread interpretation has been that these changes reflect general increases in the level of infection and declines in overall health with the advent of densely settled agricultural communities (e.g., Cohen 1989; Cohen and Armelagos 1984; Larsen 1987, 1995). However, as Wood and colleagues (1992) have demonstrated, the link between lesion frequencies in skeletal samples and health conditions in living populations is uncertain. Higher lesion frequencies may reflect increased survivorship through disease episodes rather than increased rates of disease, indicating improving (vs. declining) health conditions. Given current questions about paleodemographic reconstructions, what can the paleodemographic record tell us about the relationship between agriculture and fertility?

Using data from the Historical Perspectives on Human Demography (HPHD) database, Paine and Boldsen (in press) examined the structure of childhood mortality after the end of the last Ice Age.[2] The HPHD database combines data from 105 published and unpublished skeletal series from central and northern Europe. The database includes approximately 23,000 individuals and covers the period from the Mesolithic to the Middle Ages (approximately 8,000 B.C. to A.D. 1400). Paine and Boldsen used broad age brackets (2–5 years for younger children and 5–18 years for older children) to summarize childhood mortality patterns. Children under 2 years were not included in the study because of problems estimating infant underrepresentation.

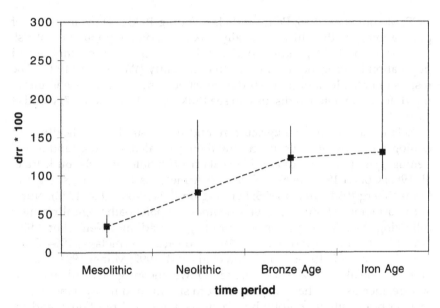

Figure 9.1. Death rate ratio (drr) tracked from Mesolithic Period through Iron Age. Lower values indicate greater concentration of risk of death in early childhood (ages 2–5 years) compared with later childhood (ages 5–18 years). Vertical lines represent bootstrapped 95% confidence intervals.

The shape of childhood mortality, as described by the death rate ratio (drr),[3] changes in the first few millennia after the adoption of agriculture (Figure 9.1). In central and northern Europe, the trend toward increased proportions of older childhood death (aged 5–18) lasts from the Mesolithic through the Iron Age. This change could represent either improvement in early child survival (<5 years) or an overall increase in the frequency of age-independent mortality, possibly caused by increases in the frequency of epidemic events (Paine and Boldsen in press).

The inability to estimate the population-at-risk reliably makes it problematic to assess the impact of changes on the drr in younger versus older child survivorship. Either improvements in younger child survival or declines in older child survival could produce the observed pattern (Paine and Boldsen in press). Pennington (1996) has argued that population increases attributed to agriculture could be maintained with small improvements in early childhood survival, even if fertility remained unchanged and overall life expectancy decreased. She has used the ethnographic record to show that early child survival (1–5 years) often improves when foraging groups become more sedentary and more dependent on agricultural products. The model she presents creates age-at-death distributions that are closer to those found in the HPHD than to those from model life tables commonly used by paleodemographers (e.g., the Coale and Demeny 1983 or Brass 1971 models), especially at older ages. If changes in the drr observed in the HPHD data can be attributed to improvements in early child survival, this would tend to support Pennington's hypothesis.

Although the bones do not permit us to distinguish the cause(s) of the changes in the drr directly, computer models allow a more detailed examination of hypotheses. Paine and Boldsen (in press; see also Paine 2000) tested the epidemic frequency hypothesis using a series of population projections. They created a model stable living population, based on the Brass (1971) standard model life tables (Standard, $\alpha = .65$, $\beta = .95$), designed to conform to general estimates of preindustrial, agrarian populations. The population was characterized by a TFR of 6.15 consistent with natural fertility populations (Bentley et al. 1993a; Campbell and Wood 1988), and mortality levels generally accepted by paleodemographers (e.g., Storey 1992). The model population was designed to grow slowly. These characteristics were built into a Leslie matrix (Leslie 1945), and additional matrices were constructed to simulate years dominated by epidemic events.

The epidemic matrices were built around a series of simple assumptions. The model disease was lethal; 30% of those exposed to the disease for the first time die. Individuals who survive one episode have reduced risk of dying in subsequent epidemics. Specifically, survivors of one epidemic episode have only 10% added risk of death in a second episode; survivors of two episodes have no added risk in subsequent episodes. This reduced risk results either from acquired immunities or the effects of selective mortality. The effects of catastrophic episodes were simulated by projecting the model population and subjecting it to one or more epidemic episodes using the catastrophe model matrices over the course of a 100-year projection. Cumulative deaths were compiled for each projection and analyzed using the same statistical measures as in the child mortality study (for details of the projection procedure see Paine and Boldsen in press; Paine 2000).

Increasing the frequency of epidemic events (up to a point) increases the ratio of older childhood death; more children in the 5–18 year bracket are dying than younger ones. An increase of epidemic events also raises the overall level of age-independent death, yielding age-at-death distributions similar to those found in many archaeological skeletal series. Age-independent mortality affects populations most dramatically at ages for which mortality is usually typically low, especially among older children (beyond infancy), adolescents, and young adults (Figure 9.2).

These results have important implications for life history. Two primary trade-offs are between current and future reproduction, and between

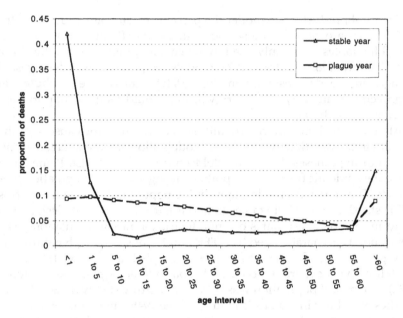

Figure 9.2. Comparison of age-at-death distribution, expressed as proportions, stable year versus plague year. A single plague year produces as many raw deaths as ten stable years.

quantity and quality of offspring. Natural selection favors those organisms that allocate available energy in ways that maximize their reproductive success. Where age-independent (extrinsic) mortality is high and there is uncertainty over reproductive outcomes, natural selection should favor individuals who reproduce early and often. Therefore, the epidemic frequency hypothesis would predict pressure for high fertility in prehistoric populations after the transition to agriculture to offset their high and potentially early mortality.

Differences in male-female survival through the reproductive ages support this contention. Reproduction has, until relatively recently, posed a high risk for female morbidity and mortality. According to the World Health Organization (1991), complications of pregnancy and childbirth cause 1 in 5 deaths to women of reproductive age in the developing world. Changes in the level of fertility would be expected to affect female survival rates through the reproductive years. Again, using the HPHD database, Paine and Boldsen (in press) traced sex differences in survivorship through the female reproductive years from the Mesolithic period through the later Middle Ages. The study included 8,165 adult skeletal records

(3,783 female, 4,382 male) from the same 105 skeletal series used in the childhood mortality study cited earlier (Boldsen and Paine in press). Male-female mortality pattern comparisons are useful in a paleodemographic context because they minimize the influence of growth rate changes on the population at risk, assuming growth rates were the same from both sexes.

Survival analysis indicates male and female adult mortality patterns were similar in the Mesolithic (Figure 9.3). During the Neolithic and all subsequent periods, however, female conditional survivorship through the reproductive years was lower than that of males. Differences between male and female survivorship are significant for all the samples from agricultural periods. Boldsen and Paine (1995; Paine and Boldsen 1997) found no significant differences in male versus female survival beyond the female reproductive years. Higher fertility rates would be expected to lead to a decrease in female survivorship through the reproductive years. The

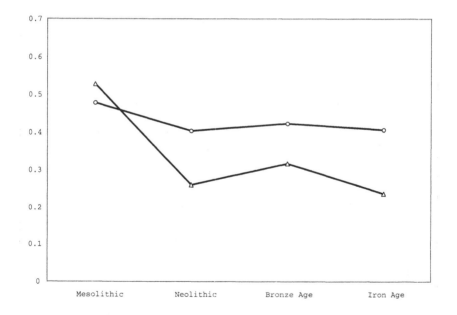

Figure 9.3. Conditional survival through the female reproductive years, approximated in the "adultus" skeletal age category (20–40 years), tracked from the Mesolithic through the Iron Age. Triangles represent male conditional survival. Circles represent female conditional survival. Dotted lines represent bootstrapped upper and lower 95% confidence intervals

differences in male and female survival observed in the HPHD database may therefore be an indication of higher fertility.

Paleodemography cannot, at present, offer definitive conclusions about the effect of agriculture on human fertility. It does raise some interesting questions about selective pressures in the early Holocene. Did changes in the shape of child mortality relieve pressure on fertility or increase it? The two scenarios for child mortality presented here (Paine and Boldsen in press; Pennington 1996) have very different implications for fertility decision-making. Sex differences in survival through the reproductive years after the adoption of agriculture suggest reproduction assumed a greater risk for women after the Mesolithic.

DISCUSSION

Reproductive ecology provides good supporting evidence that increased fertility could be achieved with the advent of agriculture. The availability of weaning foods and their effect on lactational practices is likely to have been a particularly important factor in reducing interbirth intervals. It is more likely that effects of changes in energy expenditure were not visible until much later in the process of agricultural development, and possibly only in Eurasia where the plow was introduced. This technological innovation is associated with a significant change in the division of labor, with men assuming more responsibility for farm labor (Ember 1983; Goody 1976). The plow has also been associated with other agricultural changes, such as the use of draft animals for traction and the use of milk and wool from domesticated animals. This suite of changes has been referred to as the "Secondary Products Revolution" (Sherratt 1981). Nevertheless, the lack of clear fertility differences between contemporary foragers and agriculturalists (Bentley et al. 1993a; Campbell and Wood 1988; Pennington 2001) begs the question, "Is the *potential* for increased fertility with agriculture necessarily *evidence of* increased fertility after the adoption of agriculture?"

Paleodemography provides evidence that the selective environment of early agricultural societies might have favored high fertility. Changes in the shape of child mortality, and apparent increases in the overall level of age-independent mortality, though subject to alternative interpretation, present evidence of a selective environment where early onset of reproduction and short interbirth intervals would have been favored. Paleodemography also offers evidence of fertility increase in the form of reduced female survivorship through the reproductive years.

There has also been a prior tendency in the literature to view demographic changes that took place with advent of agriculture in either/or terms: either fertility increased or mortality decreased. These two positions are far from mutually exclusive. Neither reproductive ecology nor paleodemography, by themselves, provide unambiguous conclusions about the relative roles of fertility and mortality in the increase in population growth that followed the adoption of agriculture. However, taken together they make a stronger case for increased fertility.

We would like to thank Jane Buikstra, Catherine Panter-Brick and Renee Pennington for helpful comments on earlier versions of the paper. This research was supported by the Royal Society, the Danish Center for Demographic Research, the A. P. Sloan Foundation, the Carlsberg Foundation, and the University Research Committee, University of Utah.

NOTES

1.   Although information about whether average TFRs differ between foragers and agriculturalists is contradictory, the upper end of the range among agriculturalists is much higher.

2.   We do not include young children below the age of two. The proportions of infants and young children in archaeologically recovered skeletal series vary widely, seldom approaching demographic expectations. This is most likely an artifact of archaeological preservation and recovery. The skeletons of infants and very young children are small and incompletely calcified. Many paleodemographic studies (e.g., Buikstra et al. 1986) have attempted to deal with this problem by creating statistics that omit very young children.

3.   Paine and Boldsen (in press) employed a statistic referred to as the death rate ratio (drr), which is designed to compare changes in child mortality over time but is relatively insensitive to changes in population growth.

$$drr = d_{5-18}/d_{2-5}$$
$$d_{2-18} = 1 - [S_{18}/S_5]1/13$$
$$d_{2-5} = 1 - [S_5/S_2]1/3$$

where d_{5-18} is the mean death rate from age 5 to 18 years, d_{2-5} is the mean death rate from age 2 to 5 years, and S is survivorship.

Analyses of simulated populations show that drr is insensitive to changes (up to 4%) in the intrinsic growth rate (r), though each of the two components is sensitive to changes in r.

REFERENCES

Acsádi G, Nemeskéri J (1970) *History of Human Lifespan and Mortality* (Budapest, Akademiai Kiado).

Adlercreutz H, Martin F (1980) Biliary excretion and intestinal metabolism of progesterone and estrogen in man. *Journal of Steroid Biochemistry* 13:231–244.

Anderson K, Rosner W, Khan M, New M, Pang S, Wissel P, Kappas A (1987) Diethormone interactions: protein/carbohydrate ratio alters reciprocally the plasma levels of testosterone and cortisol and their respective binding globulins in man. *Life Sciences* 40:1761–1768.

Angel JL (1964) Osteoporosis: Thalassemia? *American Journal of Physical Anthropology* 22:369–374.

Angel JL (1984) Health as a crucial factor in the changes from hunting to developed farming in the eastern Mediterranean. In MN Cohen, GR Armelagos (Eds) *Paleopathology at the Origins of Agriculture* (New York, Academic Press), 51–73.

Bailey R, Jenike M, Ellison P, Bentley G, Harrigan A, Peacock N (1992) The ecology of birth seasonality among agriculturalists in Central Africa. *Journal of Biosocial Science* 24:393–412.

Bailey RC, Peacock NR (1988) Efe pygmies of northeast Zaire: subsistence strategies in the Ituri Forest. In I de Garine, G Harrison (Eds) *Coping with Uncertainty in Food Supply* (Oxford, Clarendon Press), 88–117.

Baker BJ, Armelagos GJ (1988) The origin and antiquity of syphilis. *Current Anthropology* 29:703–737.

Bates GW, Bates SR, Whitworth NS (1982) Reproductive failure in women who practice weight control. *Fertility and Sterility* 37:373–378.

Beitins I, McArthur J, Turnbull B, Skrinar G, Bullen B (1991) Exercise induces two types of human luteal dysfunction: confirmation by urinary free progesterone. *Journal of Clinical Endocrinology and Metabolism* 72:1250–1358.

Bentley GR (1985) Hunter-gatherer energetics and fertility: a reassessment of the !Kung San. *Human Ecology* 13:79–109.

Bentley GR (2000) Environmental pollutants and fertility. In GR Bentley, C Mascie-Taylor (Eds) *Infertility in the Modern World: Present and Future Prospects* (Cambridge, Cambridge University Press), 85–152.

Bentley GR, Goldberg T, Jasienska G (1993a) The fertility of agricultural and non-agricultural traditional societies. *Population Studies* 47:269–281.

Bentley G, Harrigan A, Ellison P (1998a) Dietary composition and ovarian function among Lese horticulturalist women of the Ituri Forest, Democratic Republic of Congo. *European Journal of Clinical Nutrition* 52:261–270.

Bentley GR, Jasienska G, Goldberg T (1993b) Is the fertility of agriculturalists higher than that of non-agriculturalists? *Current Anthropology* 34:778–785.

Bentley GR, Vitzthum VJ, Caceres E, Spielvogel H, Bovenkerk SD, Lu YC, Chatterton RT (2000) Salivary estradiol levels from conception and nonconception cycles in rural Bolivian women. *American Journal of Human Biology* 12:279.

Bentley GR, Vitzthum VJ, Caceres E, Spielvogel H, Crone K, May L, Chatterton R (1998b) Reproduction and ecology in Provincia Aroma, Bolivia: fecundity of women with low levels of salivary progesterone. *American Journal of Physical Anthropology,* Supplement 26:110.

Bocquet-Appel J, Masset C (1982) Farewell to palaeodemography. *Journal of Human Evolution* 11:321–333.

Bocquet-Appel J, Masset C (1996) Paleodemography: expectancy and false hope. *American Journal of Physical Anthropology* 99:571–583.

Boldsen J (1984) Palaeodemography of two southern Scandinavian Medieval communities. *Meddelanden fran Lunds Universitets Historiska Museen* 6:107–115.

Boldsen JE, Paine RR (1995) Defining extreme longevity from the Mesolithic to the Middle Ages: estimates based on skeletal data. In B Jeune, JW Vaupel (Eds)

Exceptional Longevity: From Prehistory to Present, Odense Monographs on Population Aging 2 (Denmark, Odense University Press), 25–36.

Brass W (1971) On the scale of mortality. In W Brass (Ed) *Biological Aspects of Demography* (London, Taylor and Francis), 69–110.

Bridges PS (1985) *Changes in Long Bone Structure with the Transition to Agriculture: Implications for Prehistoric Activities*. PhD dissertation (Ann Arbor, University Microfilms International).

Bridges PS (1992) Prehistoric arthritis in the Americas. *Annual Review of Anthropology* 21:67–91.

Bridges PS, Blitz JH, Solano MC (2000) Changes in long bone diaphyseal strength with horticultural intensification in west-central Illinois. *American Journal of Physical Anthropology* 112:217–238.

Buikstra JE (1997) Paleodemography: context and promise. In RR Paine (Ed) *Integrating Archaeological Demography: Multidisciplinary Approaches to Prehistoric Population*, Center for Archaeological Investigations, Occasional Papers 24 (Carbondale, Southern Illinois University), 367–380.

Buikstra JE, Konigsberg LW (1985) Paleodemography: critiques and controversies. *American Anthropologist* 87:316–333.

Buikstra JE, Konigsberg LW, Bullington J (1986) Fertility and the development of agriculture in the prehistoric Midwest. *American Antiquity* 51:528–546.

Buikstra JE, Williams S (1991) Tuberculosis in the Americas: current perspectives. In DJ Ortner, AC Aufderheide (Eds) *Human Paleopathology: Current Syntheses and Future Options* (Washington D.C., Smithsonian Institution Press), 161–172.

Bullen BA, Skrinar GS, Beitins IZ, von Mering G, Turnbull BA, McArthur JW (1985) Induction of menstrual disorders by strenuous exercise in untrained women. *New England Journal of Medicine* 312:1349–1353.

Caldwell JC, Caldwell P (2000) From STD epidemics to AIDS: a socio-demographic and epidemiologic perspective on sub-Saharan Africa. In GR Bentley, CGN Mascie-Taylor (Eds) *Infertility in the Modern World: Present and Future Prospects* (Cambridge, Cambridge University Press), 153–186.

Campbell KL, Wood JW (1988) Fertility in traditional societies. In P Diggory, S Teper, M Potts (Eds) *Natural Human Fertility: Social and Biological Mechanisms* (London, Macmillan), 39–69.

Coale AJ, Demeny P (1983) *Regional Model Life Tables and Stable Populations*, second ed. (New York, Academic Press).

Cohen MN (1977) *The Food Crisis in Prehistory* (New Haven, Yale University Press).

Cohen MN (1989) *Health and the Rise of Civilization* (New Haven, Yale University Press).

Cohen MN, Armelagos GJ (Eds) (1984) *Paleopathology at the Origins of Agriculture* (New York, Academic Press).

Cook DC (1984) Subsistence and health in the lower Illinois Valley: osteological evidence. In MN Cohen, GR Armelagos (Eds) *Paleopathology at the Origins of Agriculture* (New York, Academic Press), 237–269.

Cowgill GL (1975) Of causes and consequences of ancient and modern population changes. *American Anthropologist* 77:505–525.

Cumming DC, Wheeler GD, Harber VJ (1994) Physical activity, nutrition, and reproduction. In KL Campbell, JW Woods (Eds) *Human Reproductive Ecology: Interactions of Environment, Fertility, and Behavior*, Annals of the New York Academy of Sciences 709:5–76.

De Souza M, Miller B, Loucks A, Luciano A, Pescatello L, Campbell C, Lasley B (1998) High frequency of luteal phase deficiency and anovulation in recreational women runners: blunted elevation in follicle-stimulating hormone observed during luteal-follicular transition. *Journal of Clinical Endocrinology and Metabolism* 83:4220–4232.

Delgado H, Lechtig A, Martorell R, Brineman E, Klein R (1978) Nutrition, lactation and post-partum amenorrhea. *American Journal of Clinical Nutrition* 31:322–327.

Dorgan J, Reichman M, Judd J, Brown C, Longcope C, Schatzkin A, Forman M, Campbell W, Franz C, Kahle L, Taylor P (1996) Relation of energy, fat, and fiber intakes to plasma concentrations of estrogens and androgens in pre-menopausal women. *American Journal of Clinical Nutrition* 64:25– 31.

Dufour DL (1984) The time and energy expenditure of indigenous women horti-culturalists in the northwest Amazon. *American Journal of Physical Anthropol-ogy* 65:37–46.

Ellison PT (1990) Human ovarian function and reproductive ecology: new hypotheses. *American Anthropologist* 92:933–952.

Ellison PT (1991) Reproductive ecology and human fertility. In G Lasker, CGN Mascie-Taylor (Eds) *Biological Anthropology and Human Affairs* (Cambridge, Cambridge University Press), 14–54.

Ellison PT (1994) Salivary steroids and natural variation in human ovarian func-tion. In KL Campbell, JW Woods (Eds) *Human Reproductive Ecology: Interac-tions of Environment, Fertility, and Behavior*, Annals of the New York Academy of Sciences 709:287–298.

Ellison PT (1996) Developmental influences on adult ovarian hormonal function. *American Journal of Human Biology* 8:725–734.

Ellison PT, Lipson SF, O'Rourke MT, Bentley GR, Harrigan AM, Panter-Brick C, Vitzthum VJ (1993) Population variation in ovarian function. *Lancet* (Aug 14):433–434.

Ellison PT, Peacock NR, Lager C (1986) Salivary progesterone and luteal function in two low-fertility populations of northeast Zaire. *Human Biology* 58:473–483.

Ellison PT, Peacock NR, Lager C (1989) Ecology and ovarian function among Lese women of the Ituri Forest, Zaire. *American Journal of Physical Anthropology* 78:519–526.

Ember CR (1983) The relative decline in women's contribution to agriculture with intensification. *American Anthropologist* 85:285–304.

Friedman MJ, Trager W (1981) The biochemistry of resistance to malaria. *Scientific American* 244:154–164.

Frisancho AR (1993) *Human Adaptation and Accommodation* (Ann Arbor, University of Michigan Press).

Froment A (2001) Evolutionary biology and health of hunter-gatherer populations. In C Panter-Brick, RH Layton, PA Rowley-Conwy (Eds) *Hunter-Gatherers: An Interdisciplinary Perspective* (Cambridge, Cambridge University Press), 239–266.

Goldin B, Adlercreutz H, Dwyer J, Swenson L, Warram J, Gorbach S (1981) Effect of diet on excretion of estrogens in pre- and post-menopausal women. *Cancer Research* 41:3771–3773.

Goldin B, Adlercreutz H, Gorbach S, Warram J, Dwyer J, Swenson L, Woods M (1982) Estrogen excretion patterns and plasma levels in vegetarian and omniv-orous women. *New England Journal of Medicine* 307:1542–1547.

Goody J (1976) *Production and Reproduction: A Comparative Study of the Domestic Domain* (Cambridge, Cambridge University Press).

Green B, Weiss N, Daling JR (1988) Risk of ovulatory infertility in relation to body weight. *Fertility and Sterility* 50:721–726.

Green B, Daling JR, Weiss NS, Liff JM, Koepsell T (1986) Exercise as a risk factor for infertility with ovulatory dysfunction. *American Journal of Public Health* 76: 1432–1436.

Haaland R (1995) Sedentism, cultivation, and plant domestication in the Holocene Middle Nile region. *Journal of Field Archaeology* 22:157–174.

Hard R, Merrill W (1992) Mobile agriculturalists and the emergence of sedentism: perspectives from northern Mexico. *American Anthropologist* 94:601–620.

Hassan FA (1981) *Demographic Archaeology* (New York, Academic Press).

Hawkes K, O'Connell J, Blurton-Jones N (1997) Hadza women's time allocation, offspring provisioning, and the evolution of long postmenopausal life spans. *Current Anthropology* 38:551–577.

Herring DA, Saunders SR, Katzenberg MA (1998) Investigating the weaning process in past populations. *American Journal of Physical Anthropology* 105: 425–439.

Hewlett, BS (1991) Demography and childcare in preindustrial societies. *Journal of Anthropological Research* 47:1–39.

Hill K, Hawkes K, Hurtado M, Kaplan H (1984) Seasonal variance in the diet of Ache hunter-gatherers in eastern Paraguay. *Human Ecology* 12:101–135.

Howie P, McNeilly A (1982) Effect of breast feeding patterns on human birth intervals. *Journal of Reproduction and Fertility* 65:545–557.

Huffman SL, Chowdhury A, Allen H, Nahar L (1987a) Suckling patterns and postpartum amenorrhea in Bangladesh. *Journal of Biosocial Science* 19:171–179.

Huffman SL, Ford K, Allen H, Streble P (1987b) Nutrition and fertility in Bangladesh: breastfeeding and post partum amenorrhea. *Population Studies* 41:447–462.

Hurtado AM, Hill KR (1990) Seasonality in a foraging society: variation in diet, work effort, fertility, and sexual division of labor among the Hiwi of Venezuela. *Journal of Anthropological Research* 46:293–346.

Hurtado AM, Hawkes K, Hill K, Kaplan H (1985) Female subsistence strategies among Ache hunter-gatherers of eastern Paraguay. *Human Ecology* 13:1–28.

Huss-Ashmore R, Curry JJ, Hitchcock RK (1989) *Coping with Seasonal Constaints.* MASCA Research Papers in Science and Archaeology 5 (Philadelphia, The University Museum).

Hutchinson D, Larsen C, Schoeninger M, Norr L (1998) Regional variation in the pattern of maize adoption and use in Florida and Georgia. *American Antiquity* 63:397–416.

Jasienska G, Ellison PT (1998) Physical work causes suppression of ovarian function in women. *Proceedings of the Royal Society of London,* B 265:1847–1851.

Jenike MR (1995) Variation in body fat and muscle mass: responses to seasonal hunger among tropical horticulturalists, Zaire. *Ecology of Food and Nutrition* 34:227–249.

Jenike MR (2001) Nutritional ecology: diet, physical activity and body size. In C Panter-Brick, R Layton, P Rowley-Conwy (Eds) Hunter-Gatherers: An Interdisciplinary Perspective (Cambridge, Cambridge University Press), 205–238.

Kaldas RS, Hughes CL (1989) Reproductive and general metabolic effects of phytoestrogens in mammals. *Reproductive Toxicology* 3:81–89.

Katzenberg MA, Herring DA, Saunders SR (1996) Weaning and infant mortality: evaluating the skeletal evidence. *Yearbook of Physical Anthropology* 39:177–199.

Katzenberg MA, Schwarcz HP, Knyf M, Melby FJ (1995) Stable isotope evidence for maize horticulture and paleodiet in southern Ontario, Canada. *American Antiquity* 60:335–350.

Kelly RL (1992) Mobility/sedentism: concepts, archaeological measures, and effects. *Annual Review of Anthropology* 21:43–66.

Kelly RL (1995) *The Foraging Spectrum: Diversity in Hunter-Gatherer Lifeways* (Washington DC, Smithsonian Institution Press).

Kent S (Ed) (1989) *Farmers as Hunters: The Implications of Sedentism* (Cambridge, Cambridge University Press).

Konigsberg LW, Frankenberg S (1992) Estimation of age structure in anthropological demography. *American Journal of Physical Anthropology* 89:235–256.

Konigsberg LW, Frankenberg S (1994) Paleodemography: not quite dead. *Evolutionary Anthropology* 3:92–105.

Konigsberg LW, Frankenberg S, Walker R (1997) Regress what on what? Paleodemographic age estimation as a calibration problem. In RR Paine (Ed) *Integrating Archaeological Demography: Multidisciplinary Approaches to Prehistoric Population*, Center for Archaeological Investigations, Occasional Papers 24 (Carbondale, Southern Illinois University), 64–88.

Kurzer M, Calloway D (1986) Effects of energy deprivation on sex hormone patterns in healthy menstruating women. *American Journal of Physiology* 251:E483–E488.

Larsen CS (1984) Health and disease in prehistoric Georgia: the transition to agriculture. In MN Cohen, GR Armelagos (Eds) *Paleopathology at the Origins of Agriculture* (New York, Academic Press), 367–392.

Larsen CS (1987) Biological interpretations of subsistence economy and behavior from human skeletal remains. In MB Schiffer (Ed) *Advances in Archaeological Method and Theory* 10 (New York, Academic Press), 339–445.

Larsen CS (1995) Biological changes in human populations with agriculture. *Annual Review of Anthropology* 24:185–213.

Layton R, Foley R, Williams E (1991) The transition between hunting and gathering and the specialized husbandry of resources: a socio-ecological approach. *Current Anthropology* 32:255–274.

Lee RB (1979) *The !Kung San: Men, Women, and Work in a Foraging Society* (New York, Cambridge University Press).

Leslie P (1945) On the uses of matrices in certain population mathematics. *Biometrika* 33:186–212.

Lieberman D (1993) The rise and fall of seasonal mobility among hunter-gatherers: the case of the southern Levant. *Current Anthropology* 34:599–631.

Little MA, Leslie PW, Campbell KL (1992) Energy reserves and parity of nomadic and settled Turkana women. *American Journal of Human Biology* 4:729–738.

Longcope C (1990) Relationship of estrogen to breast cancer, of diet to breast cancer, and of diet to estradiol metabolism. *Journal of the National Cancer Institute* 82:896–897.

Lunn PG, Austin S, Prentice AM, Whitehead RG (1984) The effect of improved nutrition on plasma prolactin concentrations and postpartum infertility in lactating Gambian women. *American Journal of Clinical Nutrition* 39:227–235.

Lunn PG, Prentice AM, Austin S, Whitehead RG (1980) Influence of maternal diet on plasma-prolactin levels during lactation. *Lancet* 1:623–625.

McFalls JA, McFalls MH (1984) *Disease and Fertility* (New York, Academic Press).

Meiklejohn C, Schentag C, Venema A, Key P (1984) Socioeconomic change and patterns of pathology and variation in the Mesolithic and Neolithic of western Europe: some suggestions. In MN Cohen, GR Armelagos (Eds) *Paleopathology at the Origins of Agriculture* (New York, Academic Press), 75–100.

Meiklejohn C, Wyman J, Jacobs K, Jackes M (1997) Issues in the archaeological demography of the agricultural transition in western and northern Europe: a view from the Mesolithic. In RR Paine (Ed) *Integrating Archaeological Demogra-*

phy: *Multidisciplinary Approaches to Prehistoric Population*, Center for Archaeological Investigations, Occasional Papers 24 (Carbondale, Southern Illinois University), 311–326.

Meindl R, Lovejoy CO, Mensforth R, Walker R (1985) A revised method of age determination using the *os pubis* with a review of tests of accuracy of other current methods of pubic symphiseal aging. *American Journal of Physical Anthropology* 68:29–45.

Miller J, Rodriguez G, Pebley A (1994) Lactation, seasonality, and mothers' postpartum weight change in Bangladesh: an analysis of maternal depletion. *American Journal of Human Biology* 6:511–524.

Milner GR (1991) Health and cultural change in the late prehistoric American Bottom, Illinois. In ML Powell, PS Bridges, A Mires (Eds) *What Mean These Bones: Issues in Southeastern Bioarchaeology* (Tuscaloosa, University of Alabama Press), 52–69.

Mølleson T (1995) The importance of porridge. In M Otte (Ed) *Nature et culture*, Actes du colloque international de Liège 68:479–486 (Études et Recherches Archéologiques de l'université de Liège).

Pagezy H (1982) Seasonal hunger as experienced by the Oto and the Twa of Ntomba village in the equatorial forest (Lake Tumba, Zaire). *Ecology of Food and Nutrition* 12:139–153.

Paine RR (1997) The need for a multidisciplinary approach to prehistoric demography. In RR Paine (Ed) *Integrating Archaeological Demography: Multidisciplinary Approaches to Prehistoric Population*, Center for Archaeological Investigations, Occasional Papers 24 (Carbondale, Southern Illinois University), 1–18.

Paine RR (2000) If a population crashes in prehistory and there is no paleodemographer there to hear it, does it make a sound? *American Journal of Physical Anthropology*, 112:181–190.

Paine RR, Boldsen JL (1997) Long-term trends in mortality patterns in preindustrial Europe. *American Journal of Physical Anthropology* (Suppl 24):183.

Paine RR, Boldsen JL (in press) Linking mortality and population dynamics. In R Hoppa, J Vaupel (Eds), *Palaeodemography: Age Distributions from Skeletal Samples*, Cambridge Studies in Biological and Evolutionary Anthropology (Cambridge, Cambridge University Press).

Paine R, Harpending HC (1998) The effect of sample bias on paleodemographic fertility estimates. *American Journal of Physical Anthropology* 105:231–240.

Panter-Brick C (1991) Lactation, birth-spacing and maternal work-loads among two castes in rural Nepal. *Journal of Biosocial Science* 23:137–154.

Panter-Brick C, Pollard TM (1999) Work and hormonal variation in subsistence and industrial contexts. In C Panter-Brick, CM Worthman (Eds) *Hormones, Health, and Behavior* (Cambridge, Cambridge University Press), 139–183.

Paul A, Muller E, Whitehead RG (1979) The quantitative effects of maternal dietary intake on pregnancy and lactation in rural Gambian women. *Transactions of the Royal Society of Tropical Medicine and Hygiene* 73:686–692.

Peacock N (1985) *Time Allocation, Work and Fertility among Efe Pygmy Women of Northeast Zaire*, PhD dissertation (Ann Arbor, University Microfilms).

Pennington RL (1996) Causes of early human population growth. *American Journal of Physical Anthropology* 105:231–240.

Pennington R (2001) Hunter-gatherer demography. In C Panter-Brick, RH Layton, PA Rowley-Conwy (Eds) *Hunter-Gatherers: An Interdisciplinary Perspective* (Cambridge, Cambridge University Press), 170–204.

Price TD, Brown J (1985) *Prehistoric Hunter-Gatherers: The Emergence of Cultural Complexity* (New York, Academic Press).

Rafferty J (1985) The archaeological record on sedentariness: recognition, development and implications. *Advances in Archaeological Method and Theory* 8:113–156.

Roberts C, Manchester K (1995) *Archaeology of Disease,* second ed. (Stroud, Gloucestershire, Alan Sutton).

Rocek T (1995) Sedentarization and agricultural dependence: perspectives from the pithouse-to-pueblo transition in the American Southwest. *American Antiquity* 60:218–239.

Rose JC, Burnett B, Blaeuer M, Nassaney M (1984) Paleopathology and the origins of maize agriculture in the lower Mississippi Valley and the Caddoan culture areas. In MN Cohen, GR Armelagos (Eds) *Paleopathology at the Origins of Agriculture* (New York, Academic Press), 51–73.

Rosenberg M (1998) Cheating at musical chairs: territoriality and sedentism in an evolutionary context. *Current Anthropology* 39:653–681.

Sackett RD (1996) *Time, Energy and the Indolent Savage,* PhD dissertation (Ann Arbor, University Microfilms International).

Sattenspiel LR, Harpending HC (1983) Stable populations and skeletal age. *American Antiquity* 48:489–498.

Schurr MR (1997) Stable nitrogen isotopes as evidence for the age of weaning at the Angel site: a comparison of isotopic and demographic measures of weaning age. *Journal of Archaeological Science* 24:919–927.

Sellen DW, Mace R (1997) Fertility and mode of subsistence: a phylogenetic analysis. *Current Anthropology* 38:878–889.

Sellen DW, Mace R (1999) A phylogenetic analysis of the relationship between subadult mortality and mode of subsistence. *Journal of Biosocial Science* 31:1–16.

Sellen DW, Smay DB (2001) Relationship between subsistence and age at weaning in "preindustrial" societies. *Human Nature* 12:47–87.

Sherratt A (1981) Plough and pastoralism: aspects of the Secondary Products Revolution. In I Hodder, G Issac, N Hammond (Eds) *Patterns of the Past: Studies in Honour of David Clarke* (Cambridge, Cambridge University Press), 261–307.

Steinbok RT (1976) *Palaeopathological Diagnosis and Interpretation* (Springfield, CC Thomas).

Storey R (1992) *Life and Death in the Ancient City of Teotihuacan: A Modern Paleodemographic Synthesis* (Tuscaloosa, University of Alabama Press).

Stuart-Macadam P (1995) Breastfeeding in prehistory. In P Stuart-Macadam, KA Dettwyler (Eds) *Breastfeeding: Biocultural Perspectives* (New York, Aldine de Gruyter), 75–99.

Szuter CR, Bayham FE (1989) Sedentism and prehistoric animal procurement among desert horticulturalists of the North American Southwest. In S Kent (Ed) *Farmers as Hunters: The Implications of Sedentism* (Cambridge, Cambridge University Press), 80–95.

Tracer DP (1991) Fertility-related changes in maternal body-composition among the Au of Papua New Guinea. *American Journal of Physical Anthropology* 85:393–405.

Ubelaker DH (1984) Prehistoric human biology of Ecuador: possible temporal trends and cultural correlations. In MN Cohen, GR Armelagos (Eds) *Paleopathology at the Origins of Agriculture* (New York, Academic Press), 491–513.

Ulijaszek SJ, Strickland SS (1993) *Seasonality and Human Ecology* (Cambridge, Cambridge University Press).

Vitzthum VJ (1990) *An Adaptational Model of Ovarian Function.* Research Report of the Population Studies Center (Ann Arbor, University of Michigan).

Vitzthum VJ (1992) The physiological basis of developmental calibration. Paper presented at the Annual Meeting of the American Anthropological Association, San Francisco.

Vitzthum VJ (1994) The comparative study of breastfeeding structure and its relation to human reproductive ecology. *Yearbook of Physical Anthropology* 37: 307–349.

Vitzthum VJ (1997) Flexibility and paradox: the nature of adaptation in human reproduction. In M Morbeck, A Galloway, A Zihlman (Eds) *The Evolving Female: A Life History Perspective* (Princeton, Princeton University Press), 242–258.

Vitzthum VJ, Bentley GR, Spielvogel H, Caceres E, Heidelberg K, Crone K, Chatterton RT (1998) Salivary progesterone levels at conception and during gestation in rural Bolivian women. *FASEB Journal* 12(SS):4211.

Walker P (1995) Problems of preservation and sexism in sexing: some lessons from historical collections for paleodemographers. In S Saunders, A Herring (Eds) *Grave Reflections: Portraying the Past through Cemetery Studies* (Toronto, Canadian Scholars Press), 31–47.

Warren M (1983) Effects of undernutrition on reproductive function in the human. *Endocrine Reviews* 4:363–377.

Wenlock R, Wenlock R (1981) Maternal nutrition, prolonged lactation and birth spacing in Ethiopia. *Journal of Biosocial Science* 13:261–268.

Whitten PL (1999) Diet, hormones, and health: an evolutionary-ecological perspective. In C Panter-Brick, CM Worthman (Eds) *Hormones, Health, and Behavior* (Cambridge, Cambridge University Press), 210–243.

Whittle AW (1996) *Europe in the Neolithic: The Creation of New Worlds* (Cambridge, Cambridge University Press).

Winkvist A, Rasmussen K, Habicht J (1992) A new definition of maternal depletion syndrome. *American Journal of Public Health* 82:691–694.

Wood JW, Milner GR, Harpending HC, Weiss KM (1992) The osteological paradox: problems of inferring prehistoric health from skeletal samples. *Current Anthropology* 33:343–370.

World Health Organization (1991) *Maternal Mortality: A Global Factbook*, compiled by C Abou Zahr and E Royston (Geneva, WHO).

Wright LE, Schwarcz HP (1998) Stable carbon and oxygen isotopes in human tooth enamel: identifying breastfeeding and weaning in prehistory. *American Journal of Physical Anthropology* 106:1–18.

Part III

DEVELOPMENTAL CONTEXT

10

Metabolism, Maturation, and Ovarian Function

SUSAN F. LIPSON

The responsivity of female reproductive function to energetic conditions is now widely recognized. Numerous studies have documented the effects—ranging from suppression of ovarian hormone levels through cessation of menstrual cycling—of energetic "stress" resulting from low energy intake, high energy expenditure, or a combination of the two.

Initially, most of these studies were motivated by the concerns of clinicians. As a result, they tended to focus on extreme forms of energetic stress—for instance, women subjected to starvation and patients with anorexia nervosa, or women who were elite or professional athletes and dancers. Among such individuals, delayed menarche and amenorrhea are frequent results of severely reduced caloric intake and/or rigorous training regimes (Katz and Weiner 1981; Malina et al. 1978; Warren 1980). But subsequently, many studies have shown that much less extreme levels of energetic stress also have significant, though less profound, effects on reproductive function. Thus, for example, moderate weight loss (Lager and Ellison 1990; Pirke et al. 1985; Vigersky et al. 1977), recreational exercise/jogging (Broocks et al. 1990; Ellison and Lager 1986), and even a pattern of "restrained eating" (Schweiger et al. 1992) have been related to disruptions of menstrual function (Feicht et al. 1978), suppressed ovarian hormone levels, sometimes leading to anovulation and/or luteal insufficiency (Bonen 1994; Broocks et al. 1990; Bullen et al. 1985; Ellison and Lager 1986; Lager and Ellison 1990), and infertility (Bates et al. 1982; Green et al. 1986, 1988). These studies have, in addition, shown that such effects, even if severe, are generally reversible by alleviation of the energetic stress—that is, by weight gain (Bates et al. 1982; McArthur et al. 1976) and/or cessation of exercise (Bullen et al. 1985; Prior et al. 1982).

Similar effects have now also been reported among nonwestern populations in response to involuntary, ecologically determined conditions of energetic stress. Particularly among agricultural populations, weight loss resulting from low food availability and/or high workload is often observed because of poor harvests or seasonal food shortages and as a consequence of seasonally variable workloads. Seasonally suppressed hormonal profiles have been demonstrated in conjunction with seasonal weight loss among horticulturalist Lese women in Zaire (now the Democratic Republic of Congo; Ellison et al. 1989), and among agro-pastoralist Tamang women in Nepal (Panter-Brick et al. 1993), and in conjunction with seasonal intensification of work among Polish farm women (Jasienska and Ellison 1998). Variability in fecundity correlated with variations in levels of ovarian function and patterns of weight loss and gain has been documented in the Lese population (Bailey et al. 1992). For more discussion of energy expenditure and ovarian function, see chapter 3, this volume (Jasienska).

Such studies have helped change the interpretation of these phenomena. Given that clinicians are likely to see the most extreme manifestations of reproductive responsivity, and given the "normal vs. abnormal" paradigm that guides clinical practice, it is not surprising that the suppression of ovarian function in response to extreme weight loss or strenuous exercise was initially viewed as dysfunction (Cumming 1989; Rosetta 1993). But with increased awareness that these effects often also occur in the course of "normal" behavior, there has been a growing acceptance of the idea that the responsivity of the female reproductive system is functional (Wasser and Isenberg 1986). According to this view, which has now penetrated even into the clinical literature (e.g., Bonen 1994), the suppression of reproductive function in response to energetic stress enables female reproductive effort to be conserved in the face of unfavorable energetic conditions (Bonen 1994; Wade and Schneider 1992).

CHRONIC EFFECTS

In addition to the short-term, reversible effects of energetic conditions on female reproductive function, it appears that there are also chronic, irreversible effects. That is, as a result of the responsiveness of reproductive function to energetic stress, the conditions that exist during an individual's development may help establish a set point for her reproductive system, thereby affecting all subsequent function.

Several observations, taken together, provide support for this hypothesis. First, there is evidence that energetic stress can affect menarcheal age. Menarche among young female competitive athletes is delayed relative to unathletic girls (Frisch et al. 1981; Malina et al. 1978; Warren 1980). Studies of young female ballet dancers, in particular, have demonstrated a marked delay in menarche among the dancers compared with normal controls (mean 15.4 yr vs. 12.5 yr); in these studies, it appears that the primary energetic stress is very high levels of energy expenditure, as changes in activity level, rather than changes in weight, were correlated with delay or onset of menarche (Warren 1980). Severely restricted energy intake, as seen in starvation or malnutrition, is also associated with delayed menarche (Chowdhury et al. 1977; Frisch and McArthur 1974). Conversely, studies of sexual maturation among American girls indicate that increased lower-thoracic fat thickness (measured on radiographs) or weight-for-height up to 30% greater than normal are correlated with earlier menarche, compared with less fat or normal weight-for-height girls (Garn and Haskell 1959; Zacharias et al. 1970). The effect of weight gain during childhood on menarcheal age is also demonstrated in a study of girls in the U.K., which found that the heaviest girls at age seven subsequently had a significantly earlier age of menarche than the lightest girls (Cooper et al. 1996).

A second line of evidence suggests that differences in menarcheal age are significantly correlated with ovarian hormone levels, even in adulthood. Longitudinal studies of Finnish girls, followed from prepuberty to adulthood, show that girls with early menarche (11–13 yr) had a greater prepubertal (about age 10 yr) increase in serum estradiol concentration and consistently higher estradiol levels thereafter, and had faster pubertal development, including a more rapid onset of ovulatory and luteally sufficient cycles, than girls with later menarche (13–15 yr) (Apter 1996; Apter and Vihko 1985; Vihko and Apter 1984). Follow-up studies reveal that throughout the teenage years and into adulthood (20–30 yr), young women with early menarche had higher serum estradiol concentrations than those with late menarche, and this difference persisted even after the difference in ovulatory frequency had disappeared. A similar result is reported on the basis of a large cross-sectional study of women from 12 different populations, which found that among both young women (15–19 yr) and older women (30–39 yr), age at menarche showed an inverse relationship with (urinary) follicular estrogen levels (MacMahon et al. 1982)

Based on these characteristics, Apter and Vihko suggest that girls with early menarche have "a more profound decrease" in hypothalamic-pituitary sensitivity to negative feedback by circulating steroids than girls with later menarche (Apter and Vihko 1985). This desensitization, which increases the set point for feedback regulation of gonadotropin secretion by ovarian steroids, underlies the progressive rise in gonadatropin and ovarian steroid concentrations during puberty. These researchers suggest that the decrease in sensitivity is slower, as well as less profound, in girls with later menarche; this would account for their more gradual attainment of fully mature ovarian function, as well as their lower estradiol levels in adulthood. Interestingly, there is some evidence that hypothalamic responsiveness may be influenced by energetic conditions affecting prenatal growth (as reflected by birth weight). Studies have shown that intrauterine (and infant) growth rates are correlated with the risk of a number of diseases in later life, including cardiovascular disease, non-insulin-dependent diabetes, and ovarian cancer (Barker et al. 1995; Reynolds and Phillips 1998). These studies raise the possibility that maternal nutrition, directly and through its influence on hormonal levels, may alter the "imprinting" of the fetal hypothalamus, and consequently affect patterns of gonadotropin release during puberty (Barker et al. 1995; Cooper et al. 1996).

Taken together, these lines of evidence—that energetic conditions can affect menarcheal age, and that menarcheal age is correlated with the level of adult ovarian function—predict that differences between populations in energetic conditions would be correlated with differences in levels of adult ovarian function. In particular, we would expect that populations subject to chronic energetic stress would show slower maturation and a lower level of adult function, while populations that enjoy energetic abundance would show faster maturation and a higher level of adult function. Though there are few available data on which to base such interpopulation comparisons, what is known is consistent with these patterns.

Comparison of ovarian function, as reflected in luteal progesterone levels, in regularly cycling adult women from five populations (middle-class women in Boston, rural farmers in southern Poland, Quechua Indians in highland Bolivia, Lese horticulturalists in the Ituri Forest of Zaire, and Tamang agro-pastoralists in central Nepal) living under variable energetic conditions (due to nutritional, workload, and health factors) reveals significant variability (Ellison 1996; Ellison et al. 1993). Reported mean menarcheal age also varies among these populations, and the relationship between mean luteal progesterone level and menarcheal age is, as expected, negative, with the youngest mean menarcheal age and highest luteal progesterone level observed for the Boston women and the oldest mean menarcheal age and lowest progesterone level observed among the Nepali women (Ellison 1996).

MECHANISMS

Both the acute and chronic effects of energetic stress on reproductive function may be achieved through similar mechanisms. There is now considerable evidence that the metabolic hormones, particularly insulin, insulin-like growth factor (IGF)-I, and leptin, have important effects on several aspects of reproductive function (Poretsky et al. 1999). Hence, they may serve as signals to the reproductive system of energetic conditions.

Evidence of the direct effect of metabolic hormones on ovarian function comes, firstly, from experimental studies of hormonal action at the cellular level. Thus, for example, in vitro incubation of granulosa cells with insulin both increases basal production of estradiol and progesterone and enhances luteinizing hormone (LH)–stimulated steroid production (Willis et al. 1996). Similarly, both insulin and IGF-I increase progesterone production by thecal cells (McGee et al. 1996); they also stimulate proliferation of the theca-interstitial cells themselves (Duleba et al. 1998). Insulin (Poretsky et al. 1985; Samoto et al. 1993), IGF-I (Devoto et al. 1995), and leptin (Karlsson et al. 1997) receptors have all been identified on ovarian cells; a study of the expression of the insulin receptor, for instance, indicates that insulin has numerous effects on oocyte maturation, follicular growth, and stromal cell function (Samoto et al. 1993). Experimental studies in animals provide further data on the effects of metabolic hormones on reproductive function. In pharmacologically induced diabetic pigs, a short-term (six-day) withdrawal of insulin significantly increased follicular atresia and reduced follicular growth in preovulatory follicles, demonstrating the necessity of insulin for follicular function and, particularly, for follicular growth (Edwards et al. 1996).

In addition to documenting these ovarian effects, experimental studies indicate that metabolic hormones may also have effects at the hypothalamic level; for instance, IGF-I has been shown to stimulate the release of luteinizing hormone releasing hormone (LH-RH) in cells from the median eminence (of female rats) (Hiney et al. 1991). Such actions may result in acceleration of the process of pubertal development; in adolescent female rhesus monkeys, treatment with IGF-I significantly advanced the maturational decrease in hypothalamic sensitivity to negative feedback by estradiol (Wilson 1995). Similarly, leptin receptors have been demonstrated in the hypothalamus, and leptin has been shown to stimulate gonadotropin releasing hormone (Gn-RH) release in hypothalamic cells (Hileman et al. 2000); also, treatment with leptin induced early onset of reproductive function in female mice (Chehab et al. 1997). Recently, Suter et al. (2000) have demonstrated increased IGF-I and nocturnal leptin secretion in the 30 days preceding nocturnal pulsatile LH secretion in agonadal male monkeys. Such evidence suggests an important role for these metabolic hormones in the onset of puberty (Foster and Nagatani 1999).

Other evidence for a relation between metabolic hormones and ovarian function comes from correlational studies of reproductive function and metabolic hormone levels among women in various energetic conditions. In one such study, sedentary, regularly cycling women were compared with intensively training cycling women and with intensively training amenorrheic women; the amenorrheic athletes were distinguishable not only from the sedentary women but also from the cycling athletes. Thus, among the amenorrheic athletes, disrupted menstrual function was associated with a number of physiological and hormonal indicators of high energy expenditure, including decreased insulin levels, decreased levels of available IGF-I (due to elevated levels of insulin-like growth factor binding protein (IGFBP)-I), and elevated cortisol concentrations (Laughlin and Yen 1996), as well as low concentrations and altered diurnal rhythms of leptin (Laughlin and Yen 1997). Similarly, in another study of elite athletes and dancers, menstrual irregularity was correlated with increased levels of cortisol and IGFBP-I (which modulates IGF-I bioactivity) and decreased levels of insulin (Jenkins et al. 1993). In a study of more subtle manifestations of variability in ovarian function, indices of energy balance (calculated from measures of energy intake and expenditure) were strongly correlated with levels of IGF-I and thyroid hormone, and all three of these were significant predictors of serum estradiol concentration (Zanker and Swaine 1998). In all of these studies, levels of metabolic hormones indicative of an energy deficit were associated with disrupted or reduced ovarian function. Given the evidence that these metabolic hormones can affect reproductive function at both the ovarian and hypothalamic levels, these results suggest that metabolic hormones may provide a signal to the reproductive system indicating current energetic conditions (Jenkins et al. 1993).

In addition to communicating information about current energetic status, metabolic hormones have important roles in determining the onset and course of sexual maturation. While plasma insulin levels increase throughout childhood, there is a particularly pronounced rise in insulin levels during puberty (Hindmarsh et al. 1988). At the same time, insulin resistance increases; increased insulin levels are either a cause or a consequence of reduced insulin sensitivity (Potau et al. 1997; Smith et al. 1989; Stoll et al. 1994). IGF-I and leptin levels also rise markedly just before and during puberty (Apter 1997; Hiney et al. 1991; Smith et al. 1989; Suter et al. 2000). IGF-I and insulin appear to be related not only to normal growth during childhood but also to height velocity, and thus the timing of the growth spurt, and the concurrent increase in steroid levels and onset of pubertal development (Smith et al. 1989; Stoll 1995; Stoll et al. 1994). Since insulin and leptin levels reflect nutritional conditions, at least in part, childhood nutrition may have an important effect on the timing of physical and sexual maturation. It has been shown that menarche occurs earlier in girls who are fatter than average (Garn and Haskell 1959; Maclure et al. 1991), or whose weight is greater (up to 30%) than normal (Zacharias et al. 1970), whereas it is delayed in girls whose weight is below normal (Johnston et al. 1971), and this may be a consequence of increased insulin concentrations in overweight girls and reduced insulin concentrations in underweight girls (Conway and Jacobs 1993; Matkovic et al. 1997).

Since the beginning of the twentieth century, there has been a significant secular trend toward earlier menarche (from a mean of about 16 yr to a mean of about 12.5 yr) among western women (Tanner 1973). At the same time, there has been a secular trend in height, resulting in both earlier achievement of adult height and greater adult height. In contemporary western populations where conditions are consistently adequate, girls with relatively early menarche are taller during childhood, though their eventual adult height is similar to the adult height of women with later menarche. But in populations where conditions (particularly nutritional intake) vary substantially among different segments of the population, early menarche may be linked not only to earlier growth but to greater adult height as well (Stoll et al. 1994); in such populations, an association is also found between height and breast cancer incidence (Vatten et al. 1992). In either case, early menarche is associated with an increased risk of breast cancer (Apter 1996). Childhood nutritional conditions appear to underlie all of these trends and provide links among them. That is, improved nutritional conditions during childhood, by leading to levels of insulin and IGF-I which rise sooner and remain higher, may lead, first, to an earlier growth spurt and earlier menarche, and subsequently, to greater adult height and higher adult ovarian steroid concentrations (with consequently elevated breast cancer risk).

Thus the actions of the metabolic hormones seem to provide possible mechanisms for the observed effects of energetic conditions on reproductive function. Clearly, levels of metabolic hormones are intimately tied to energetic conditions. The suite of responses to energetic stress includes increased insulin sensitivity and increased concentrations of IGFBP-I; consequently, both insulin and IGF-I concentration and bioactivity are reduced. This suite of responses, along with others such as elevated cortisol and reduced thyroid hormone levels, has been observed in conjunction with caloric restriction and physical training (Jenkins et al. 1993; Laughlin and Yen 1996; Zanker and Swaine 1998). Whether in response to low energy intake or high energy expenditure, they constitute adaptive mechanisms that direct energy resources toward attempting to meet immediate requirements.

In addition to their glucoregulatory and growth effects, these metabolic hormones also have effects on the hypothalamic-pituitary-ovarian axis at many levels. Via actions ranging from enhancement of steroid production by granulosa cells in the ovary to stimulation of Gn-RH secretion by cells of the median eminence of the hypothalamus, the metabolic hormones may have effects on the timing and tempo of pubertal development and on the subsequent level of adult function, as well as on short-term fluctuations in ovarian function. Thus, through their multiple effects, the metabolic hormones coordinate the individual's response to energetic conditions by providing a signal that determines how the available energy will be partitioned among the demands of growth, maintenance, and reproduction.

SYNTHESIS

The data presented here can be synthesized into a model for understanding the relationship between energetic conditions and human female reproductive function. Such models have been proposed previously, mainly in response to data demonstrating that energetic conditions have an *acute* effect on adult reproductive function. One of the earliest and most influential of such models proposes that a minimum level of stored body fat is necessary in order to meet the energetic requirements of pregnancy and lactation (Frisch 1987; Frisch and McArthur 1974), and that failure to achieve or maintain this critical level leads to loss of reproductive function. According to this model, mechanisms that linked hypothalamic control of reproduction to fatness would be evolutionarily advantageous because they would delay menarche and/or secondarily suppress cycling if a woman lacked sufficient energy stores to support a successful reproductive effort. In this way, reproductive attempts would be curtailed during periods of energy shortage and (re)established when conditions improved.

Subsequent work has challenged several aspects of this model, particularly the existence of a minimum fat threshold for reproduction (Ellison 1982, 2001; Johnston et al. 1975; Trussell 1978). Studies have shown, rather, that reproductive function is more responsive to energy intake and energy expenditure than to energy reserves (Bronson and Manning 1991), and that there is a continuum of response of reproductive function to energetic stress (Ellison 1990; Prior 1985; Rosetta 1993). Still, the view that the female reproductive system has evolved to make acute adjustments relative to some standard of normal function (be it percent body fat or some other) has become widespread (for example, Conway and Jacobs 1997; Karlsson et al. 1997).

The idea that the suppression of reproductive function in the face of unfavorable energetic conditions might represent an adaptive response, preventing the investment by a female of time and energy in a reproductive attempt that has a low likelihood of success, has been espoused particularly by biological anthropologists (e.g., Ellison 1990; Peacock 1991; Vitzthum 1997). Recognizing that time and energy are limiting constraints on female reproduction, they suggest that physiological mechanisms have evolved to protect a woman from initiating a pregnancy when conditions are unfavorable, instead postponing an attempt until conditions are better. But what if conditions will not improve? In the face of long-term poor conditions, continued postponement may result in significant loss of reproductive chances. Peacock (1991) and Vitzthum (1997) have both argued that mechanisms "should" exist enabling a woman to sustain reproductive function when poor conditions persist. Thus, Vitzthum has proposed that "acclimatization" might occur, allowing ovulation to resume even under unfavorable conditions (Vitzthum 1997), and Peacock has suggested that, under unfavorable conditions, a woman might be able to lessen her investment in each infant (Peacock 1991). For further discussion of Vitzthum's perspective, see chapter 8, this volume.

In contrast to previous arguments which focus on acute effects, I propose a model in which the *chronic* effects of energetic conditions on reproductive function are primary. This model emphasizes the role of energetic conditions during development in determining the *level* of adult reproductive function that will yield the maximum lifetime reproductive output. In this model, factors that affect the survival of the woman are as relevant as those that affect her fecundity.[1]

Under conditions of chronic energetic stress, slow growth, delayed maturation, and low levels of adult ovarian function are physiological adaptations which reduce the costs of maintenance, growth, and, especially, of reproduction in the face of low energy availability. Thus, when energy resources are scarce, it will not only take longer to reach menarche, but adult levels of ovarian production will be lower than if energy were abundant. And, if lower levels of ovarian hormones are associated with a lower *(but not zero)* probability of pregnancy, a woman subjected to chronically low energy availability will tend to have fewer pregnancies over the course of her reproductive lifetime, with longer intervening intervals during which energy can be alloted to her own maintenance needs, improving her chances for survival.

According to this view, the *primary* effect of energetic conditions on reproductive function occurs during development. That is, energy availability during childhood is an important determinant, via the metabolic hormones, of menarcheal age and the pace of subsequent maturation, and, consequently, of the level of adult ovarian function. This establishes a basic pattern and level for energy allocation to reproductive function. But in addition, the ability of metabolic hormones to affect ovarian function means that, even after the basic pattern and level are set, acute adjustments occur throughout the reproductive span, which may temporarily increase or decrease the probability of pregnancy in response to short-term fluctuations in energy availability.

Limited energy availability, and the resulting necessity to make energetic trade-offs among maintenance, growth, and reproduction, has probably been the usual condition for human populations. Thus, while levels of ovarian function among nonwestern and historical populations are often considered "suppressed" relative to levels observed among contemporary western populations, it might be that they are actually relatively "typical." Indeed, the conditions of energetic surplus experienced by at least some of the members of contemporary western populations are probably quite unusual. If so, the patterns and levels of ovarian function observed among such women may, likewise, be rather atypical. In this view, an average menarcheal age of 12.5 yr (for populations in the Americas, Western Europe, and Asia in the 1960s and 1970s; Wood 1994), average interbirth intervals of just over one and a half years (for North American Hutterite women in the 1920s; Wood 1994), and dramatically increased incidences of ovarian and breast cancers (estimated as 10–100 times greater for modern western women compared with preagricultural women; Eaton et al. 1994) may be considered as outcomes arising when the energetic constraints under which the system was designed to operate have largely been removed.

NOTE

1. Several aspects of this model are similar to proposals made previously by Ellison (for example, 1990, 1994, 1996).

REFERENCES

Apter D (1996) Hormonal events during female puberty in relation to breast cancer risk. *European Journal of Cancer Prevention* 5:476–482.

Apter D (1997) Leptin in puberty. *Clinical Endocrinology* 47:175–176.

Apter D, Vihko R (1985) Premenarcheal endocrine changes in relation to age at menarche. *Clinical Endocrinology* 22:753–760.

Bailey RC, Jenike MR, Ellison PT, Bentley GR, Harrigan AM, Peacock NR (1992) The ecology of birth seasonality among agriculturalists in central Africa. *Journal of Biosocial Science* 24:393–412.

Barker DJP, Winter PD, Osmond C, Phillips DIW, Sultan HY (1995) Weight gain in infancy and cancer of the ovary. *Lancet* 345:1087–1088.

Bates GW, Bates SR, Whitworth NS (1982) Reproductive failure in women who practice weight control. *Fertility and Sterility* 37:373–378.

Bonen A (1994) Exercise-induced menstrual cycle changes: a functional, temporary adaptation to metabolic stress. *Sports Medicine* 17:373–392.

Bronson FH, Manning JM (1991) The energetic regulation of ovulation: a realistic role for body fat. *Biology of Reproduction* 44:945–950.

Broocks A, Pirke KM, Schweiger U, Tuschl RJ, Laessle RG, Strowitzki T, Hörl E, Hörl T, Haas W, Jeschke D (1990) Cyclic ovarian function in recreational athletes. *Journal of Applied Physiology* 68:2083–2086.

Bullen BA, Skrinar GS, Beitins IZ, von Mering G, Turnbull BA, McArthur JW (1985) Induction of menstrual disorders by strenuous exercise in untrained women. *New England Journal of Medicine* 312:1349–1353.

Chehab FF, Mounzih K, Lu R, Lim ME (1997) Early onset of reproductive function in normal female mice treated with leptin. *Science* 275:88–90.

Chowdhury AKMA, Huffman SL, Curlin GT (1977) Malnutrition, menarche, and marriage in rural Bangladesh. *Social Biology* 24:316–325.

Conway GS, Jacobs HS (1993) Clinical implications of hyperinsulinaemia in women. *Clinical Endocrinology* 39:623–632.

Conway GS, Jacobs HS (1997) Leptin: a hormone of reproduction. *Human Reproduction* 12:633–635.

Cooper C, Kuh D, Egger P, Wadsworth M, Barker D (1996) Childhood growth and age at menarche. *British Journal of Obstetrics and Gynæcology* 103:814–817.

Cumming DC (1989) Menstrual disturbances caused by exercise. In KM Pirke, W Wuttke, U Schweiger (Eds) *The Menstrual Cycle and Its Disorders* (Berlin, Springer-Verlag), pp. 150–160.

Devoto L, Kohen P, Castro O, Vega M, Troncoso JL, Charreau E (1995) Multihormonal regulation of progesterone synthesis in cultured human midluteal cells. *Journal of Clinical Endocrinology and Metabolism* 80:1566–1570.

Duleba AJ, Spaczynski RZ, Olive DL (1998) Insulin and insulin-like growth factor I stimulate the proliferation of human ovarian theca-interstitial cells. *Fertility and Sterility* 69:335–340.

Eaton SB, Pike MC, Short RV, Lee NC, Trussell J, Hatcher RA, Wood JW, Worthman CM, Blurton Jones NG, Konner MJ, Hill KR, Bailey R, Hurtado AM (1994) Women's reproductive cancers in evolutionary context. *Quarterly Review of Biology* 69:353–367.

Edwards JL, Hughey TC, Moore AB, Cox NM (1996) Depletion of insulin in streptozocin-induced-diabetic pigs alters estradiol, insulin-like growth factor (IGF)-I, and IGF binding proteins in cultured ovarian follicles. *Biology of Reproduction* 55:775–781.

Ellison PT (1982) Skeletal growth, fatness, and menarcheal age: a comparison of two hypotheses. *Human Biology* 54:269–281.

Ellison PT (1990) Human ovarian function and reproductive ecology: new hypotheses. *American Anthropologist* 92:933–952.

Ellison PT (1994) Understanding natural variation in human ovarian function. In RIM Dunbar (Ed) *Human Reproductive Decisions: Biological and Social Perspectives* (London, Macmillan), pp. 22–51.

Ellison PT (1996) Age and developmental effects on human ovarian function. In L Rosetta, CGN Mascie-Taylor (Eds) *Variability in Human Fertility* (Cambridge, Cambridge University Press), pp. 69–90.

Ellison PT (2001) *On Fertile Ground* (Cambridge, Harvard University Press).

Ellison PT, Lager C (1986) Moderate recreational running is associated with lowered salivary progesterone profiles in women. *American Journal of Obstetrics and Gynecology* 154:1000–1003.

Ellison PT, Peacock NR, Lager C (1989) Ecology and ovarian function among Lese women of the Ituri Forest, Zaire. *American Journal of Physical Anthropology* 78:519–526.

Ellison PT, Panter-Brick C, Lipson SF, O'Rourke MT (1993) The ecological context of human ovarian function. *Human Reproduction* 8:2248–2258.

Feicht CB, Johnson TS, Martin BJ, Sparkes KE, Wagner WW Jr (1978) Secondary amenorrhoea in athletes. *Lancet* 2:1145–1146.

Foster DL, Nagatani S (1999) Physiological perspectives on leptin as a regulator of reproduction: role in timing puberty. *Biology of Reproduction* 60:205–215.

Frisch RE (1987) Body fat, menarche, fitness and fertility. *Human Reproduction* 2:521–533.

Frisch RE, McArthur JW (1974) Menstrual cycles: fatness as a determinant of minimum weight for height necessary for their maintenance or onset. *Science* 185:949–951.

Frisch RE, von Gotz-Welbergen A, McArthur JW, Albright T, Witschi J, Bullen B, Birnholz J, Reed RB, Hermann H (1981) Delayed menarche and amenorrhea of college athletes in relation to age of onset of training. *Journal of the American Medical Association* 246:1559–1563.

Garn SM, Haskell JA (1959) Fat and growth during childhood. *Science* 130: 1171–1172.

Green BB, Daling JR, Weiss NS, Liff JM, Koepsell T (1986) Exercise as a risk factor for infertility with ovulatory dysfunction. *American Journal of Public Health* 76:1432–1436.

Green BB, Weiss NS, Daling JR (1988) Risk of ovulatory infertility in relation to body weight. *Fertility and Sterility* 50:721–726.

Hileman SM, Pierroz DD, Flier JS (2000) Leptin, nutrition, and reproduction: timing is everything. *Journal of Clinical Endocrinology and Metabolism* 85:804–807.

Hindmarsh PC, Matthews DR, Di Silvio L, Kurtz AB, Brook CGD (1988) Relation between height velocity and fasting insulin concentrations. *Archives of Diseases in Childhood* 63:665–666.

Hiney JK, Ojeda SR, Dees WL (1991) Insulin-like growth factor I: a possible metabolic signal involved in the regulation of female puberty. *Neuroendocrinology* 54:420–423.

Jasienska G, Ellison PT (1998) Physical work causes suppression of ovarian function in women. *Proceedings of the Royal Society of London* B 265:1847–1851.

Jenkins PJ, Ibanez-Santos X, Holly J, Cotterill A, Perry L, Wolman R, Harries M, Grossman A (1993) IGFBP-1: a metabolic signal associated with exercise-induced amenorrhoea. *Neuroendocrinology* 57:600–604.

Johnston FE, Malina RM, Galbraith MA (1971) Height, weight and age at menarche and the "critical weight" hypothesis. *Science* 174:1148–1149.

Johnston FE, Roche AF, Schell LM, Wettenhall NB (1975) Critical weight at menarche: critique of a hypothesis. *American Journal of Diseases of Childhood* 129:19–23.

Karlsson C, Lindell K, Svensson E, Bergh C, Lind P, Billig H, Carlsson LMS, Carlsson B (1997) Expression of functional leptin receptors in the human ovary. *Journal of Clinical Endocrinology and Metabolism* 82:4144–4148.

Katz JL, Weiner H (1981) The abberant reproductive endocrinology of anorexia nervosa. In H Weiner, MA Hofer, AJ Stunkard (Eds) *Brain, Behavior, and Bodily Disease* (New York, Raven Press), pp. 165–180.

Lager C, Ellison PT (1990) Effect of moderate weight loss on ovarian function assessed by salivary progesterone measurements. *American Journal of Human Biology* 2:303–312.

Laughlin GA, Yen SSC (1996) Nutritional and endocrine-metabolic aberrations in amenorrheic athletes. *Journal of Clinical Endocrinology and Metabolism* 81: 4301–4309.

Laughlin GA, Yen SSC (1997) Hypoleptinemia in women athletes: absence of a diurnal rhythm with amenorrhea. *Journal of Clinical Endocrinology and Metabolism* 82:318–321.

Maclure M, Travis LB, Willett W, MacMahon B (1991) A prospective cohort study of nutrient intake and age at menarche. *American Journal of Clinical Nutrition* 54:649–656.

MacMahon B, Trichopoulos D, Brown J, Andersen AP, Cole P, DeWaard F, Kauraniemi T, Polychronopoulou A, Ravnhar B, Stormby N, Westlund K (1982) Age at menarche, urine estrogens and breast cancer risk. *International Journal of Cancer* 30:427–431.

Malina RM, Spirduso WW, Tate C, Baylor AM (1978) Age at menarche and selected menstrual characteristics in athletes at different competitive levels and in different sports. *Medical Science in Sports and Exercise* 10:218–222.

Matkovic V, Ilich JZ, Skugor M, Badenhop NE, Goel P, Clairmont A, Klisovic D, Nahhas RW, Landoll JD (1997) Leptin is inversely related to age at menarche in human females. *Journal of Clinical Endocrinology and Metabolism* 82:3239–3245.

McArthur JW, O'Loughlin KM, Johnson L, Hourihan J, Alonso C (1976) Endocrine studies during the refeeding of young women with nutritional amenorrhea and infertility. *Mayo Clinic Proceedings* 51:607–616.

McGee EA, Sawetawan C, Bird I, Rainey WE, Carr BR (1996) The effect of insulin and insulin-like growth factors on the expression of steroidogenic enzymes in a human ovarian thecal-like tumor cell model. *Fertility and Sterility* 65:87–93.

Panter-Brick C, Lotstein DS, Ellison PT (1993) Seasonality of reproductive function and weight loss in rural Nepali women. *Human Reproduction* 8:684–690.

Peacock N (1991) An evolutionary perspective on the patterning of maternal investment in pregnancy. *Human Nature* 2:351–385.

Pirke KM, Schweiger U, Lemmel W, Krief JC, Berger M (1985) The influence of dieting on the menstrual cycle of healthy young women. *Journal of Clinical Endocrinology and Metabolism* 60:1174–1179.

Poretsky L, Grigorescu F, Seibel M, Moses AC, Flier JS (1985) Distribution and characterization of insulin and insulin-like growth factor I receptors in normal human ovary. *Journal of Clinical Endocrinology and Metabolism* 61:728–734.

Poretsky L, Cataldo NA, Rosenwaks Z, Giudice LC (1999) The insulin-related ovarian regulatory system in health and disease. *Endocrine Reviews* 20:535–582.

Potau N, Ibañez L, Riqué S, Carrascosa A (1997) Pubertal changes in insulin secretion and peripheral insulin sensitivity. *Hormone Research* 48:219–226.

Prior JC (1985) Luteal phase defects and anovulation: adaptive alterations occurring with conditioning exercise. *Seminars in Reproductive Endocrinology* 3:27–33.

Prior JC, Yuen BH, Clement P, Bowie L, Thomas J (1982) Reversible luteal phase changes and infertility associated with marathon training. *Lancet* 1:269–270.

Reynolds RM, Phillips DIW (1998) Long-term consequences of intrauterine growth retardation. *Hormone Research* 49 (Supplement):28–31.

Rosetta L (1993) Female reproductive dysfunction and intense physical training. *Oxford Reviews of Reproductive Biology* 15:113–141.

Samoto T, Maruo T, Ladines-Llave CA, Matsuo H, Deguchi J, Barnea ER, Mochizuki M (1993) Insulin receptor expression in follicular and stromal compartments of the human ovary over the course of follicular growth, regression and atresia. *Endocrine Journal* 40:715–726.

Schweiger U, Tuschl RJ, Platte P, Broocks A, Laessle RG, Pirke KM (1992) Everyday eating behavior and menstrual function in young women. *Fertility and Sterility* 57:771–775.

Smith CP, Dunger DB, Williams AJK, Taylor AM, Perry LA, Gale EAM, Preece MA, Savage MO (1989) Relationship between insulin, insulin-like growth factor I, and dehydroepiandrosterone sulfate concentrations during childhood, puberty, and adult life. *Journal of Clinical Endocrinology and Metabolism* 68:932–937.

Stoll BA (1995) Timing of weight gain in relation to breast cancer risk. *Annals of Oncology* 6:245–248.

Stoll BA, Vatten LJ, Kvinnsland S (1994) Does early physical maturity influence breast cancer risk? *Acta Oncologica* 33:171–176.

Suter KJ, Pohl CR, Wilson ME (2000) Circulating concentrations of nocturnal leptin, growth hormone, and insulin-like growth factor-I increase before the onset of puberty in agonadal male monkeys: potential signals for the initiation of puberty. *Journal of Clinical Endocrinology and Metabolism* 85:808–814.

Tanner JM (1973) Trend towards earlier menarche in London, Oslo, Copenhagen, the Netherlands and Hungary. *Nature* 243:95–96.

Trussell J (1978) Menarche and fatness: reexamination of the critical body composition hypothesis. *Science* 200:1506–1509.

Vatten LJ, Kvikstad A, Nymoen EH (1992) Incidence and mortality of breast cancer related to body height and living conditions during childhood and adolescence. *European Journal of Cancer* 28:128– 131.

Vigersky RA, Andersen AE, Thompson RH, Loriaux DL (1977) Hypothalamic dysfunction in secondary amenorrhea associated with simple weight loss. *New England Journal of Medicine* 297:1141–1145.

Vihko R, Apter D (1984) Endocrine characteristics of adolescent menstrual cycles: impact of early menarche. *Journal of Steroid Biochemistry* 20:231–236.

Vitzthum VJ (1997) Flexibility and paradox: the nature of adaptation in human reproduction. In ME Morbeck, A Galloway, A Zihlman (Eds) *The Evolving Female: A Life-History Perspective* (Princeton, Princeton University Press), pp. 242–258.

Wade GN, Schneider JE (1992) Metabolic fuels and reproduction in female mammals. *Neuroscience and Biobehavioral Reviews* 16:235–272.

Warren MP (1980) The effects of exercise on pubertal progression and reproductive function in girls. *Journal of Clinical Endocrinology and Metabolism* 51:1150–1157.

Wasser SK, Isenberg DY (1986) Reproductive failure among women: pathology or adaptation? *Journal of Psychosomatic Obstetrics and Gynaecology* 5:153–175.

Willis D, Mason H, Gilling-Smith C, Franks S (1996) Modulation by insulin of follicle-stimulating hormone and luteinizing hormone actions in human granulosa cells of normal and polycystic ovaries. *Journal of Clinical Endocrinology and Metabolism* 81:302–309.

Wilson ME (1995) IGF-I administration advances the decrease in hypersensitivity to oestradiol negative feedback inhibition of serum LH in adolescent female rhesus monkeys. *Journal of Endocrinology* 145:121–130.

Wood JW (1994) *Dynamics of Human Reproduction* (New York, Aldine de Gruyter).

Zacharias L, Wurtman RJ, Schatzoff M (1970) Sexual maturation in contemporary American girls. *American Journal of Obstetrics and Gynecology* 108:833–846.

Zanker CL, Swaine IL (1998) The relationship between serum oestradiol concentration and energy balance in young women distance runners. *International Journal of Sports Medicine* 19:104–108.

11

Child Survival and the Modulation of Parental Investment

Physiological and Hormonal Considerations

HELEN BALL and CATHERINE PANTER-BRICK

POSTNATAL REPRODUCTIVE INVESTMENTS

Human reproduction involves substantial investments of time and effort after parturition to keep children alive and well until maturity or independence. Indeed the ultimate postnatal reproductive "failure"—the death of a child—is an event of great significance, involving the termination of a current child-care effort, possible replacement of the child with a new pregnancy, or increased investment in existing children. This fundamentally alters the landscape of both behavioral and biological reproductive investments.

The extent to which humans modulate parental investment has long been of interest to anthropologists, who correlate child-care behaviors with a large number of socioecological variables, and to evolutionary ecologists, who evaluate reproductive decisions in terms of reproductive fitness over the lifespan. Differential child-care behaviors have thus been examined as a set of strategies for modulating reproductive investments. These behaviors are highly variable, yet finely tuned to social, ecological, and life history constraints (Hrdy 1999). As such, child-care strategies are adaptive responses to selective pressures of varying intensity, particularly with respect to the risks of infant mortality and the opportunity costs for investing in other children. Ethnographic cases of poor maternal bonding, curtailed lactation, benign neglect, or discriminative solicitude are all examples of the plasticity of postnatal reproductive decisions, which have been debated in terms of their possible adaptive outcomes.

In this chapter, we examine how parental reproductive investments have been shaped by evolutionary considerations and, tentatively, ways in which reproductive physiology is implicated in the human ability to vary the amount and timing of postnatal reproductive effort. We contrast humans and other primates with respect to the opportunity to make facultative investments in offspring and we examine several physiological correlates of differential parental investments during the periods of birth, early infancy, and later childhood.

FACULTATIVE RESPONSES IN EVOLUTIONARY CONTEXT

To what extent is parental love for children coded in our genetic blueprint or amenable to individual choice? In modern western societies, the predominant discourse on motherhood (but not fatherhood) promotes the view that maternal attachment to babies arises from the natural expression of "mother love," such that mothers who fail to nurture their children are deviant to the human condition. Nancy Scheper-Hughes (1992) forcefully argues that there is no such "natural" expression. Conversely, Sarah Hrdy (1999) favors biological expression—but argues that human mothers are highly discriminating in the amount of care they lavish on particular children, and in the timing or duration of their child-care investments. Despite a powerful "cocktail of hormones" priming mothers to love their children, maternal attachment is facultative, not obligate or automatic (Hrdy 1999).

On the part of fathers, child-care investments are generally portrayed as optional. Fathers are more likely than mothers to allocate considerable effort to mating costs, and their reproductive strategies towards children are sensitive to such variables as paternity certainty, the ability to command resources, and lost mating opportunities (Borgerhoff Mulder 1992). The evolutionary—and the physiological—ramifications of parental care are very different for men and women. This chapter will focus on women, for whom reproductive costs are more intimately linked to both biology and child- care behavior.

Hrdy argues that there is a striking difference between humans and other primates with respect to their aptitude to terminate reproductive investments postnatally. Simian mothers, she claims, care for each of their offspring regardless of infant attributes (weight, sex, birth order, physical condition, etc.), given the extraordinarily low incidence of failure to bond with a baby. This is a departure from the mammalian pattern where females bear large litters and exercise discrimination regarding their investment in a particular infant: primate mothers, producing a singleton in each gestation, simply do not have the same latitude for choice. Even "defective" infant monkeys are invested in assiduously so long as they can initially cling to their mothers (Hrdy 1999:178). Humans are unable to cling at the moment of birth, a departure from the primate pattern and a consequence of the trade-offs between bipedalism and brain development causing infants to be "secondarily altricial" or less neurologically mature.

Hrdy suggests that being able to cling is the only viability test a nonhuman primate applies to her newborn, a viability test inapplicable to humans.

The fact that human females show a degree of maternal ambivalence, causing them to reject their babies under particular circumstances, is therefore surprising given our primate heritage. Hrdy (1999:182) poses a pertinent question: "What happened in the course of human evolution and history to make mothers in our own species so much more discriminating than other primates?" Or to rephrase this question, what allowed human mothers to be more discriminating? Hrdy also postulates that selective advantage accrued to human mothers who could adjust (modulate) maternal investment from infant to infant, in contrast to nonhuman primate females who appear committed to investing wholesale in each infant produced.

It is true that humans show great flexibility in adjusting their reproductive investments postnatally. This is conventionally related to the evolutionary costs associated with caring for children, which are much greater among humans than in other primates because of an extended period of childhood vulnerability and dependency. Bogin (1998) has argued that the human reproductive strategy, in contrast to that of apes and early hominids, hinges on the insertion of a new life stage (childhood) between the end of infancy and the juvenile period—a stage of development during which an offspring is no longer nursed but still cannot feed independently. This life stage is most prolonged in *Homo sapiens* to allow for brain development and social learning. The links between brain size and parental support required to feed dependent children are further explored in Kaplan et al. (chapter 13, this volume). The development of an expanded neocortex in humans is no doubt linked to their ability, in contrast to other primates, to calculate and foresee the costs and opportunities entailed by reproductive investments in children.

Thus the ability to make facultative reproductive investments after the birth of an offspring has flourished in humans. Moreover, the opportunity for differential allocation of parental effort varies as the life cycle of the child unfolds, as we shall see by contrasting the first few days postpartum, early infancy, and the period of childhood. We know from past research that human reproductive investments are behaviors shaped by evolutionary considerations. We consider in this chapter how they may also intersect with maternal reproductive physiology.

BONDING OR INFANT REJECTION

While the debate regarding the obligate or facultative nature of human mother-infant bonding is confounded by sociopolitical sensibilities, the role of physiological mechanisms underpinning mother-infant bonding is well accepted by biologists. The infant, in the act of suckling, triggers the hormonal reflexes that elicit those particular maternal care-giving behaviors characterized as "bonding." Suckling stimulates the nerve endings in the areola and the nipple and, by reflex, causes the pituitary gland to release prolactin and oxytocin. Prolactin has been called the "mothering hormone," having a relaxing effect on the mother and enhancing her desire for proximity with the infant, as well as being responsible for lactational amenorrhea (Stuart-Macadam 1995:8). Oxytocin has been called the "hormone of love" because it is involved in orgasm, birth, breastfeeding, and bonding (Stuart-Macadam, citing Newton 1978). Prolactin is also associated with the production of β-endorphins which suppress the nervous system's hormonal response to stress (Franceschini et al. 1989; Kitzinger 1987).

Current research is exploring the exact hormonal pathways involved in bonding across different species. Animal studies have shown that prolactin and oxytocin enhance nurturing behavior such as retrieval, nest-building, licking, and proximity to pups in rats, and researchers have postulated in mice a possible role for norepinephrine in conjunction with oxytocin (Insel 1990). In humans, Dettwyler (1995:171) comments that oxytocin and prolactin affect maternal feelings and behavior, "leading to more appropriate child promoting behaviors on the part of the mother, and strong feelings of acceptance and nurturance in the child." By contrast, Stuart-Macadam (1995:10) asserts that it is unlikely that any maternal behavior in humans is entirely hormonally regulated, although vestiges of such behavior exist and hormones such as oxytocin play a part in the preparation of the female for maternity. In brief, maternal physiology ensures maternal bonding and promotes reproductive investment, suggesting that such hormonally mediated maternal investment is a (mammalian) evolutionary trait. However, natural selection may have favored parental behavioral strategies which could disrupt or alter this evolved physiological mechanism under certain circumstances. Indeed bonding responses to infants can be circumvented in humans, providing the opportunity for mothers to reject their infants, even to the point of infanticide.

In humans, a "hormonal storm" will promote "mother love" within minutes of birth, but only if the mother plays her part in the scenario. When a mother puts a neonate to nurse at the breast, release of oxytocin stimulates the contraction of the uterus, the constriction of uterine blood vessels, and (in some way) the onset of mother-infant bonding. If the initiation of body or nipple contact is delayed, however, bonding is not obligate: there is a window of opportunity during which the mother may reject the infant. Hrdy (1999) argues that this "window of opportunity" is a consequence of the human neonate's inability to cling to its mother, allowing her to reject it before "bonding" has been established. Monkey infants, who have a well-developed clinging reflex immediately following birth, are able to crawl up their mothers' bodies and find a nipple independent of maternal assistance (Jolly 1985). Ape and human infants are less adept at clinging in the immediate postnatal period: gorilla and chimpanzee neonates are dependent on their mothers for physical support for the first 2 or 3 months of life, human neonates for even longer. At least in humans, this means that important physiological mechanisms promoting bonding will only be activated if maternal behavior actually facilitates physical contact and breastfeeding. While data on the propensity of gorilla and chimpanzee mothers to reject their neonates and thereby modulate reproductive investment are lacking, the evidence for humans indicates that the majority of maternal rejections occur in the first few hours and days following birth (Bugos and McCarthy 1984; Minturn and Stashak 1982; Schiefenhövel 1989)—before the establishment of lactation and hormonal changes inducing bonding (Hrdy 1999). Once bonding mechanisms are initiated, maternal nurturing behavior is promoted hormonally, particularly through breastfeeding—mothers who begin to invest in their infants generally do not withdraw that investment in early infancy except under extreme or unusual circumstances.

Some extreme cases of failed maternal bonding have been related in the literature to postpartum depression and infanticide. The western biomedical perspective on postnatal depression is one of a situation of bonding failure in which mothers exhibit little care-giving behaviors and a lack of interest in infants. In its most extreme form (called "postnatal psychosis"), women who attempt infanticide several weeks or months after birth are characterized as lacking maternal instinct, although mothers themselves rationalize their behavior as being in the actual interests of the child (Jan Cubison, Research Health Visitor, University of Sheffield, personal communication 1999). Research on the hormonal basis for this "syndrome" has postulated associations between early postnatal depression (6–10 weeks after delivery) and changing concentrations of steroid hormones and prolactin, noting the dramatic fall of cortisol, plasma progesterone (a hundredfold fall), and estradiol (a tenfold fall) in the first few days after delivery, and the rise in prolactin levels which is sustained with established breastfeeding (Harris et al. 1989). Indeed Harris and colleagues (1989) found that depressed women who were breast-feeding had "inappropriately low" plasma prolactin levels and some deficits in progesterone, but also that associations with progesterone were different in the case of breast and bottle feeders. In turn, Abou-Saleh et al. (1998) found lower prolactin and higher progesterone levels in depressed mothers relative to controls, noting that breastfeeders showed comparatively lower depression scores and higher prolactin levels. This work raises the possibility that breastfeeding and its associated hormones might mediate both the biological aspects of maternal investment and the intensity of emotional attachment, with consequences for the modulation of infant care (or rejection and infanticide). But while it might be tempting to link "defective" maternal behavior to failed maternal "instinct" and "abnormal" maternal physiology, the complexities of hormonal functioning (and interactions with nursing behavior and prolactin) are barely uncovered.

Hagen (1999), for instance, warns that postpartum depression cannot be a simple by-product of hormonal changes—intriguingly, fathers experience postpartum depression at rates half or more as high as those of mothers. He argues that clinical depression may be an evolutionarily adaptive strategy to negotiate postnatal parental investments in offspring, a "defection" strategy on the part of a mother to enlist greater investment from the father or kin in circumstances where she perceives a lack of support or problems with pregnancy and infant viability.

In the case of infanticide, as described in "classic" ethnographic examples, infant rejection is hardly related to bonding physiology between particular mother-infant pairs. It is governed by reproductive decisions related to cultural factors (Hill and Ball 1996). The reasons for killing babies right after birth—in the first few hours or days—are related to cultural rules and personal decisions established *prior* to the birth of a particular infant. For example, multiple births, deformities, or babies born breech or with teeth or red hair must be killed even though mothers themselves may attempt to prevent it (Hill and Ball 1996). The traditional practice among Netsilik Eskimo, who eliminated a baby girl born into a family lacking a male cross-cousin for marriage, is a good example of an a priori cultural norm, while the case of Ayoreo women in Paraguay and Bolivia who articulate their infanticide decisions based on current family size and composition illustrates ad hoc personal decisions (Bugos and McCarthy 1984). Interestingly, the cultural prescription among the !Kung San enjoining mothers to kill neonates if still nursing an older child is one case where infanticide relates explicitly to maternal physiology, but in no way does it relate to "defective" bonding or physiology (and the cultural practice can be overridden by personal decisions, as depicted by Nisa in Shostak 1981). Human infanticide has been described as an optimization of reproductive effort in response to infant characteristics, maternal condition, and socioecological and life history parameters, which include the perception of a given infant's survival chances weighed against previous and future reproductive investments (Hrdy 1992). Certainly infanticide in humans differs from that in simians, for whom there are no known cases in the wild of parents killing their own progeny (Hrdy and Hausfater 1984).

The practices of infant "exposure" and "abandonment" in historical western societies, practices which effectively side-stepped overt infanticide and held an infant's fate to the "kindness of strangers" (Boswell 1988), were also related to dire individual circumstances such as poverty and to a cultural distaste for illegitimacy, rather than to abnormal mothering. Even wet-nursing, associated with appalling infant mortality, has been related to perceptions that infants may have a better chance of survival if raised elsewhere than with biological parents. Such decisions to "retrench" direct parental investment and to "dilute" the costs of reproductive effort may even ultimately promote reproductive fitness (Hrdy 1992).

Perhaps it is the "window of opportunity" for rejection of an infant immediately after parturition among humans that has facilitated the proliferation of cultural rules and the latitude for personal decisions regarding the termination of parental investment. Humans, in contrast to other animals, are exploiting the fact that maternal bonding is for them neither necessarily obligate nor immediate. Cases of bonding failure such as those found in relation to postnatal depression seem to some degree of hormonal basis, but they are also mediated by individual circumstances and behaviors such as breastfeeding practices. Infanticide in the first 72 hours after birth is best characterized as bonding interference rather than bonding failure, since purposeful decisions are made not to invest in a given child before biological bonding takes place. Other cases of "retrenchment" of direct parental investment are further examples of the highly facultative human responses to a dependent infant. Despite hormonal priming for attachment, human maternal behavior is effectively contingent upon parental investment decisions and early opportunities to evaluate given reproductive investments.

BREAST MILK SUPPLY AND INFANT DEMAND

An infant who survives the immediate postpartum period is still completely dependent upon adults for survival, requiring continuing investment. The primary investments (for human caretakers as well as for nonhuman primates) involve carrying and feeding the baby. Both these behaviors place energetic demands on a mother, but the most critical for infant survival is adequate lactation. Indeed the infant is so vulnerable during this period that its growth is ensured in the face of its mother's inadequate nutritional status. Even in the Dutch famine of 1944–1945 (Stein and Susser 1975), women were able to sustain pregnancies and successfully breast-feed their infants though their dietary intakes fell to starvation levels. Marginally nourished women in Bangladesh, Guatemala, and The Gambia can still produce breast-milk volumes and compositions within the range expected for well-nourished mothers. From an evolutionary perspective, natural selection has favored an interaction between mother and child that is heavily tipped towards the baby at this early juncture. Even so, how could this interaction be modulated under conditions of poor maternal fitness, and how do maternal trade-offs during fetal growth, and during early and established lactation, affect the offspring's survival prospects?

Maternal undernutrition does have some impact on fetal growth, birth weight, neonatal morbidity, and subsequent offspring mortality. Notwithstanding existing controversy in the literature, direct trials show that the effects of maternal dietary supplementation on fetal growth are relatively modest. Kramer's (1993) meta-analysis of the literature found but small increases in maternal weight gain and fetal growth with maternal supplementation, while Prentice and Whitehead (1987) reported that birth weight is never enhanced by more than 10%. However, a recent randomized trial in The Gambia showed that supplementation of third-trimester pregnant women not only increased birth weight (by 200 g) in the hungry season but also reduced both the prevalence of stillbirths and early neonatal mortality (Ceesay et al. 1997). Even though Gambian women prioritize fetal growth at the expense of maternal condition (their ratio of fetal weight to pregnancy weight gain is 40% compared with 25% in well-nourished U.K. women), the poor maternal environment fails to protect fetal growth fully. Moreover, there is intriguing new evidence in The Gambia that early fetal retardation strongly influences vulnerability to infections and survival prospects during adulthood, possibly through impairment of immune competence (Moore et al. 1997) and/or fetal exposure to hypercortisolaemia resulting from maternal infections in the hungry season (Moore et al. 1999; Prentice et al. 1999).

The impact of poor maternal condition on lactational performance is also extensively debated since the relationship is confounded by infant demand, particularly infant weight and nursing time. Perhaps not surprisingly, maternal physiology does appear to influence early lactation. Breast milk output one week into the neonatal period has been positively related to antenatal progesterone and prolactin levels of the mother, controlling for strong associations with parity and time spent nursing, while at 4 weeks, maternal hormonal factors (progesterone and estradiol) matter less to milk output than the infant's current weight (Ingram et al. 1999). Once nursing is initiated, however, it seems that lactational performance is driven by infant demand rather than by maternal factors. For western mothers, Daly and Hartmann (1995:21) maintain that with demand feeding "a mother's milk production is likely to be a reflection of her infant's appetite, rather than her ability to produce milk" and, specifically, the degree to which an infant empties the breast at each breast-feed. Women who express for a milk bank, nurse twins or triplets, or breast-feed an infant and sibling in tandem produce considerably more (e.g., >2,000 g/day) than the "average" production of 700 to 800 g/day for exclusively breast-fed infants in the first 5 months postpartum. Dewey et al. (1991) also concluded for a U.S. population that infants self-regulate their intakes while nursing on demand, and that even infants with poor intakes (650 g/day) left as much milk unconsumed (residual in the breast) as did infants with intakes in the "normal" range. Among both affluent and marginally nourished mothers, lactational performance is not only generally excellent but also highly variable, demonstrating physiological "plasticity." Yet milk volumes are largely unaffected by maternal dietary intakes, body weight, or socioeconomic status (Prentice and Prentice 1995; Villalpando et al. 1991). In The Gambia, where one of the more detailed studies of a marginally nourished population has been undertaken to date, significant changes in milk output were noted in the hungry season (although milk consumption dropped by less than 10%). Initially correlated with maternal nutritional stress, the drop in milk output was related to changes in infant demand: infants who were left at home when their mothers went to work in the fields suffered the anorexic effects of prevalent infections during the rainy season and suckled less vigorously (Prentice and Prentice 1995). Even the effect of parity on milk volume (observed only for Gambian women with very high parity—namely, more than 10 children) have been related to gland secretion capacity rather than to maternal nutritional depletion (see Dewey et al. 1991).

Is breast-milk quality, rather than quantity, affected, and how might this relate to infant suckling? There is some evidence that milk fat and milk vitamins may be affected by poor maternal nutritional status, even if milk volume and milk protein are not (Lönnerdal 1986; Prentice and Prentice 1995). In The Gambia, breast-milk fat concentration showed marked seasonal variations as well as associations with parity (Prentice et al. 1981), although after dietary supplementation, increases in milk fat concentration were offset by decreases in lactose, leaving milk energy content unchanged (Prentice et al. 1983a), possibly because mothers relaxed from a state of high metabolic efficiency (Prentice et al. 1983b). It is important to note, however, that feed frequency will significantly influence milk fat concentrations—the longer the feed interval, the lower the fat content—and that fat (rather than calories per se) may be the key trigger to infant satiety, which itself regulates infant demand (Woolridge 1995). Woolridge surmises that maternal practices that promote frequent feeding would lead to more settled behavior on the part of infants, whereas mothers' attempts to curtail nighttime feeding may induce the high incidence of sleep pathologies found in western countries. He also notes that the lower fat concentration in breast milk alters infant suckling behavior—infants are less easily satiated in any one feed—and this alone can lead to maternal perceptions of lactational insufficiency. Insufficient milk supply is the major reason reported by mothers worldwide for early termination of breastfeeding (Hill 1992), and early weaning itself will induce significant changes in milk volume and composition (Dewey et al. 1984). Thus perhaps the quality of breast milk (rather than mere volume) together with infant demand can influence the timing of food supplementation. If so, it would affect a crucial aspect of parental child-care practices and also infant survival. Hence while maternal physiology for the most part operates to protect infant growth from the vagaries of the maternal nutritional environment, a mother's breastfeeding behavior can easily disrupt this interaction.

The complex trade-offs between infant needs and maternal constraints (including the demands of time and energy involved in breastfeeding, and attempts to maintain maternal condition while promoting infant growth and survival) have been well elaborated by McDade and Worthman (1998). They highlight the variables affecting maternal decisions regarding early or late food supplementation under varying circumstances in terms of nutrition and pathogen exposure, aiming for a framework to formulate testable hypotheses. Maternal decisions to over- or under-invest in infants are context-specific. In Brazilian slums, as described by Scheper-Hughes (1992), dire circumstances led mothers to selectively invest in "feisty" infants and neglect those who appeared in poor health. In the West, it is easily assumed that exhausted mothers would reject "colicky" infants, and indeed poor infant temperament has been associated with maternal postpartum depression (Beck 1996). Among the Masai, however, in conditions of drought and marginal nutrition, De Vries (1987) reported that infants with a fussy or difficult temperament showed better chances of survival than "easy" infants who demanded less maternal attention and suckling time. Among British mothers, a "good" baby is perceived as one who sleeps heavily, cries little, and generally requires minimal maternal investment, while a "cranky" baby is entertained, cuddled, and nursed repeatedly both day and night (Ball et al. 1999). Little do these mothers realize that good babies left alone in their rooms requiring so little attention are more at risk of SIDS (cot death) than are infants who constantly demand to be in their mothers' presence (Blair et al. 1999). Such child-care decisions play themselves out for infant survival and maternal biology and reproductive success.

Infant care strategies crucially affect the amount of contact a mother will have with her baby, and thus how frequently it can access the breast. In contrast to ape and monkey infants, who ensure their own proximity both day and night, human babies are helpless at the hands of mothers who sleep apart from them at night, and who choose not to carry them continuously during the day. In our evolutionary past, continuous and close proximity of the infant to a mother would have been a dire necessity for infant survival (Eaton et al. 1988; Lancaster and Lancaster 1987; McKenna and Bernshaw 1995). Presently, however, the cultural variation in the ways in which maternal biological investments are modulated through patterns of infant care is enormous. In western, industrialized society, infant care strategies primarily function to facilitate the social best interests of the parents as opposed to the biological best interests of the infant (Trevathan and McKenna 1994). The contemporary western goals of promoting early infant independence via separate sleeping arrangements, intermittent and prolonged day-time separation of mother and child, and regimented breast- or bottle feeding have been described as a set of particular cultural practices that are both historically and culturally unusual (Stuart-Macadam and Dettwyler 1995; Trevathan and McKenna 1994). These practices can be contrasted to wet-nursing and the movement of children out of the home in historical Europe, which have been held as prominent examples of "delegated motherhood" (Hrdy 1992; Panter-Brick 2000). Not only is there massive cross-cultural variation in child-rearing practices, tied to the goals of parents (LeVine 1998), there is also extreme cultural relativism in what can be interpreted as "proper" maternal attention or "neglect" (Morelli et al. 1992). In essence, these cultural norms are setting the parameters under which child-care investment decisions are made.

These differential investment strategies in the two primary facets of child-care, proximity and breastfeeding, have fundamental consequences for the biological nature of mother-infant relationships. For instance, co-sleeping has been shown to promote breastfeeding in terms of duration and suckling frequency, which has consequences for both maternal reproductive physiology and aspects of child health ranging from growth to the risk of cot death (McKenna and Bernshaw 1995). The daytime proximity of mothers and babies has been implicated not only in patterns of secure attachment and infant intellectual development (Trevathan and McKenna 1994) but in the intensity of nursing patterns and hormonal mechanisms underlying postpartum amenorrhea (see Valeggia and Ellison, chapter 4, this volume). The immense literature on breastfeeding patterns has highlighted dramatic consequences on birth spacing, maternal nutrition, and reproductive health, as well as child survival and morbidity.

PROVISIONING AND CARRYING

The next few years of a child's life provide human parents with an even greater opportunity to modulate reproductive effort. There are both biological and cultural parameters to the palette of reproductive decisions. One of the main biological considerations is the energetic correlates of child care and the point at which a mother ceases to invest her resources in the current infant and diverts time and energy to her own replenishment and/or future reproductive effort. This trade-off is very delicate because short reproductive intervals can lead to maternal depletion and can compromise child survival. Patterns of parental investment are also demonstrably linked to human reproductive biology and are ultimately shaped by our evolutionary history to constitute "the hominid adaptation" (Lancaster and Lancaster 1983).

The energetic demands placed on the mother are tied to both child care and her subsistence behavior. Whereas in infancy the primary cost of child care to the mother was lactation, in early childhood the cost of carrying that child assumes greater significance, with or without prolonged lactation. For example, it has been estimated that !Kung San women of Botswana walk 2,400 km annually (6.6 km/day) while carrying equipment, food, and a child—a child, weighing 3 kg at birth and 11–15 kg at age 4 is carried some 7,800 km during its first 4 years of life (Bentley 1985; Eaton and Eaton 1999; Lee 1979:312). Evolutionary considerations have been explicitly modeled in the energetic trade-offs between maternal investments in reproduction and production (for instance, the backload model tests the adaptiveness of given birth spacing intervals with data on offspring survivorship: Blurton Jones 1986; Blurton Jones and Sibly 1978; see also Pennington and Harpending 1988; Jasienska, this volume). Studies of the San have thus illustrated the cost of child transport during maternal subsistence work, and the role of energetic factors rather than intense lactation in maintaining long birth intervals (Bentley 1985). In other societies, working mothers may elect to leave their dependent children behind (Harpending et al. 1990; McDade and Worthman 1998; Tronick et al. 1985), thus affecting the opportunities for "contact" between mother and child and potentially both the reproductive physiology of the mother and the health or survival of the child. For instance, work away from home is one of the most significant variables influencing the timing of supplementation (van Esterik and Greiner 1981; McDade and Worthman 1998), and weaning itself is perhaps the most dangerous time of life for a child; both have consequences for a mother's return to fecundity.

Arguably the most effective mechanism for modulating female parental investment is to manipulate birth spacing through lactational amenorrhea. As Ellison (1995:338) comments, postpartum amennorhea "helps to modulate natural reproductive effort over the life span" of the mother, and two important variables, maternal nutritional condition and maternal age, influence this. Where a mother is energetically stressed, the sensitivity of neuroendocrine responses to suckling is heightened, prolonging amenorrhea. In The Gambia, for example, dietary supplementation of hardworking, undernourished women had little impact on their body weight or lactational performance, but it did lower their prolactin levels and shorten postpartum amenorrhea, thereby increasing fecundity (Lunn 1996). In brief, lactational amenorrhea is modulated by maternal biology as well as infant nursing demand (Valeggia and Ellison, chapter 4, this volume).

The primary strategy of the mother is to lengthen birth intervals until she can invest wholesale in a new conception. As with early lactation, there is a complex physiological and behavioral relationship affecting the feedback mechanism of postpartum infecundability. But in contrast to early lactation, the balance in terms of physiology seems tipped towards the mother. Temporary infecundability provides the opportunity for maternal repletion prior to undertaking another pregnancy—frequent reproductive cycling has been linked to maternal nutritional depletion (Merchant and Martorell 1988; Winkvist et al. 1992). The "window of depletion" is particularly wide for the Gainj women of highland Papua New Guinea, for example, because of their heavy workloads in addition to prolonged breastfeeding (McDade and Worthman 1998). For more on these issues see Valeggia and Ellison, this volume.

Of course, a woman may regulate birth intervals through a variety of behaviors, such as lactation practices, abortion and infanticide, postpartum sex taboos, and contraception. Another means of modulating investment is through child neglect or retrenchment of parental solicitude (Hrdy 1992), which can lead to child mortality and child replacement (Scheper-Hughes 1992). These types of investment modulations are influenced by demographic and socioecological contexts shaping the adaptive role of mother-infant attachments (Wiley and Carlin 1999). For instance, where chances of child survival are improved by parental care, intensive parental investments are expected (Harpending et al. 1990), and where fertility increases, decreased parental care is likely (Wiley and Carlin 1999). This perspective looks at different types of attachment as adaptive in different local environments. For example, only in an environment of low mortality and low fertility is exclusivity in maternal attachment promoted.

Harpending, Draper, and Pennington (1990) have characterized the variation in human parental effort in terms of a contrast between peer-raising and parent-raising societies (illustrated with the Polynesians, Kpelle, and nomadic !Kung, as well as societies in transition) and further discriminate within the parent-raising societies between those conforming to western cultural assumptions in the practice of "intense saturating infant care" and those practicing "measured investment" infant care strategies. They posit that natural selection would act on human "learning propensities" to allocate effort among competing demands, including those of parental care, arguing that "from an evolutionary scenario, a measured allocation of parental resources would have been favored by selection in competition with intense saturating infant care" (1990:252). Their model explicitly tried to incorporate the human cultural milieu shaping child-care patterns and to generate testable hypotheses using data on life history survivorship and the energetic demands of lactation. However, the ramifications for maternal reproductive physiology are not explored by these authors. We expect that different maternal investment and attachment strategies have an impact on maternal reproductive biology via the production of different hormonal profiles, and that these, as discussed above, have concomitant links with bonding, depression, breast milk sufficiency, maternal condition, and amenorrhea.

CONCLUSION: PHYSIOLOGY AND THE BIOCULTURAL MILIEU OF PARENTAL INVESTMENT

Parental child-care investments can be usefully examined as strategies effectively modulating reproductive behavior. In contrast to nonhuman primates, humans have evolved a highly flexible set of behaviors governing parent-child interactions. We have stressed that human parental investments are facultative for many births, highly variable in the amount of care lavished onto children, and responsive to culturally defined parental goals, to extrinsic environmental conditions, and to intrinsic attributes of mothers and their children.

As humans invest an enormous amount in a few births, their reproductive success depends on raising infants through a long period of dependency until maturity. How maternal physiology factors into parental investment decisions is considerably under-researched. A decade ago, Harpending, Draper, and Pennington (1990:255) remarked: "Anthropology, with the most interesting species and the richest set of models, is cursed with the worst data of any biological science. Here we can only muster a motley collection of anecdotes, poor data, and corrupt information." We suggest that further investigation of hormonal characteristics would provide new ways of linking reproductive physiology with parental investment decisions. We argue that the physiological consequences of reproductive decisions and indeed the role of physiology in underpinning and catalyzing reproductive decisions are arenas worthy of further exploration.

REFERENCES

Abou-Saleh MT, Ghubash R, Karim L, Krymski M, Bhai I (1998) Hormonal aspects of postpartum depression. *Psychoneuroendocrinology* 23:465–475.
Ball HL, Hooker E, Kelly PJ (1999) Where will the baby sleep? attitudes and practices of new and experienced parents regarding cosleeping with their newborn infants. *American Anthropologist* 10:143–151.

Beck CT (1996) A meta-analysis of the relationship between postpartum depression and infant temperament. *Nursing Research* 45:225–230.

Bentley GR (1985) Hunter-gatherer energetics and fertility: a reassessment of the !Kung San. *Human Ecology* 13:79–109.

Blair PS, Fleming PJ, Smith IJ, Platt MW, Young J, Nadin P, Berry PJ, Golding J (1999) Babies sleeping with parents: case-control study of factors influencing the risk of the sudden infant death syndrome. *British Medical Journal* 319: 1457–1461.

Blurton Jones N (1986) Bushman birth spacing: a test for optimal interbirth interval. *Ethology and Sociobiology* 7(2):91–105.

Blurton Jones N, Sibly R (1978) Testing adaptiveness of culturally determined behavior: do Bushman women maximise their reproductive success by spacing births widely and foraging seldom? In N Blurton Jones, V Reynolds (Eds) *Human Adaptation and Behaviour* (London, Taylor & Francis), 135–158.

Bogin B (1998) Evolutionary and biological aspects of childhood. In C Panter-Brick (Ed) *Biosocial Perspectives on Children* (Cambridge, Cambridge University Press), 10–44.

Borgerhoff Mulder M (1992) Reproductive decisions. In EA Smith, B Winterhalder (Eds) *Evolutionary Ecology and Human Behavior* (New York, Aldine de Gruyter), 339–374.

Boswell J (1988) *The Kindness of Strangers: The Abandonment of Children in Western Europe from Late Antiquity to the Renaissance* (New York, Pantheon Books).

Bugos P, McCarthy L (1984). Ayoreo infanticide: a case study. In G Hausfater, SB Hrdy (Eds) *Infanticide: Comparative and Evolutionary Perspectives* (Hawthorne, New York, Aldine de Gryuter), 503–520.

Ceesay SM, Prentice AM, Cole TJ et al. (1997) Effects on birth weight and perinatal mortality of maternal dietary supplements in rural Gambia: 5 year randomised controlled trial. *British Medical Journal* 315:786–790.

Daly SEJ, Hartmann PE (1995) Infant demand and milk supply, 1: infant demand and milk production in lactating women. *Journal of Human Lactation* 11:21–26.

Dettwyler KA (1995) Beauty and the breast: the cultural context of breastfeeding in the United States. In P Stuart Macadam, KA Dettwyler (Eds) *Breastfeeding: Biocultural Perspectives* (New York, Aldine de Gruyter),167–216.

De Vries MW (1987) Cry babies, culture, and catastrophe: infant temperament among the Masai. In N Scheper-Hughes (Ed) *Child Survival: Anthropological Perspectives on the Treatment and Maltreatment of Children* (Dordrecht, D. Reidel), 165–185.

Dewey KG, Finley DA, Lönnerdal B (1984) Breast milk volume and composition during late lactation (7–20 months). *Journal of Pediatric Gastroenterolgy and Nutrition* 3:713–720.

Dewey KG, Heining MJ, Nommsen LA, Lönnerdal B (1991) Maternal versus infant factors related to breast milk intake and residual milk volume: the DARLING Study. *Pediatrics* 87:829–837.

Eaton SB, Shostak M, Konner M (1988) *The Paleolithic Prescription* (New York, Harper & Row).

Eaton SB, Eaton SB III (1999) Hunter-gatherers and human health. In RB Lee, R Daly (Eds) *The Cambridge Encyclopedia of Hunters and Gatherers* (Cambridge, Cambridge University Press), 449–456.

Ellison PT (1995) Breastfeeding, fertility, and maternal condition. In P Stuart-Macadam, KA Dettwyler (Eds) *Breastfeeding: Biocultural Perspectives* (New York, Aldine de Gruyter), 305–345.

Franceschini R, Venturini PL, Cataldi A, Barreca T, Ragni N, Rolandi E (1989) Plasma beta-endorphin concentrations during suckling in lactating women. *British Journal of Obstetrics and Gynæcology* 96:711–713.

Hagen EH (1999) The functions of postpartum depression. *Evolution and Human Behavior* 20:325–359.

Harris B, Johns S, Fung H, Thomas R, Walker R, Read G, Riad-Fahmy D 989) The hormonal environment of post-natal depression. *British Journal of Psychiatry* 154:660–667.

Harpending HC, Draper P, Pennington R (1990) Cultural evolution, parental care, and mortality. In AC Swedlund, GJ Armelagos (Eds) *Disease in Populations in Transition: Anthropological and Epidemiological Perspectives* (New York, Bergin and Garvey), 252–265.

Hill CM, Ball HL (1996) Abnormal births and other "ill omens": the adaptive case for infanticide. *Human Nature* 7:381–402.

Hill PD (1992) Insufficient milk supply syndrome. *Clinical Issues* 3:605–612. NAACOG.

Hrdy SB (1992) Fitness tradeoffs in the history and evolution of delegated mothering with special reference to wet-nursing, abandonment, and infanticide. *Ethology and Sociobiology* 13:409–442.

Hrdy SB (1999) *Mother Nature: A History of Mothers, Infants, and Natural Selection* (New York, Pantheon Books).

Hrdy SB, Hausfater G (Eds) (1984) *Infanticide: Comparative and Evolutionary Perspectives* (New York, Aldine).

Ingram JC, Woolridge MW, Greenwood RJ, McGrath L (1999) Maternal predictors of early breast milk output. *Acta Paediatrica* 88:493–499.

Insel TR (1990) Oxytocin and maternal behavior. In NA Krasnegor, RS Bridges (Eds) *Mammalian Parenting* (New York, Oxford University Press), 260–280.

Jolly A (1985) *The Evolution of Primate Behavior* (New York, Macmillan).

Kitzinger SA (1987) *The Experience of Breastfeeding* (London, Penguin).

Kramer MS (1993) Effects of energy and protein intakes on pregnancy outcome: an overview of the research evidence from controlled clinical trails. *American Journal of Clinical Nutrition* 58:627–635.

Lancaster JB, Lancaster CS (1983) Parental investment: the hominid adaptation. In DJ Ortner (Ed) *How Humans Adapt: A Biocultural Odyssey* (Washington DC, Smithsonian Institution Press), 33–56.

Lancaster JB, Lancaster CS (1987) The watershed: change in parental investment and family formation strategies in the course of human evolution. In J Lancaster, J Altmann, A Rossi, L Sherrod (Eds) *Parenting across the Life Span: Biosocial Dimensions* (New York, Aldine de Gruyter), 187–205.

Lee RB (1979) *The !Kung San: Men, Women and Work in a Foraging Society* (Cambridge, Cambridge University Press).

LeVine RA (1998) Child psychology and anthropology: an environmental view. In C Panter-Brick (Ed) *Biosocial Perspectives on Children* (Cambridge, Cambridge University Press), 102–130.

Lönnerdal B (1986) Effects of maternal dietary intake on human milk composition. *Journal of Nutrition* 116:499–513.

Lunn PG (1996) Breast-feeding practices and other metabolic loads affecting human reproduction. In L Rosetta, CGN Mascie-Taylor (Eds) *Variability in Human Fertility* (Cambridge, Cambridge University Press), 195–216.

McDade TW, Worthman CN (1998) The weanling's dilemma reconsidered: a biocultural analysis of breastfeeding ecology. *Journal of Developmental and Behavioral Pediatrics* 19:286–299.

McKenna JJ, Bernshaw NJ (1995) Breastfeeding and infant-parent co-sleeping as adaptive strategies: are they protective against SIDS? In P Stuart-Macadam, KA Dettwyler (Eds) *Breastfeeding: Biocultural Perspectives* (New York, Aldine de Gruyter), 265–303.

Merchant K, Martorell R (1988) Frequent reproductive cycling: does it lead to nutritional depletion of mothers? *Progress in Food and Nutrition Science* 12: 339–369.

Minturn L, Stashak J (1982) Infanticide as a terminal abortion procedure. *Behavior Science Research* 17:70–90.

Moore SE, Cole TJ, Poskitt EME et al. (1997) Season of birth predicts mortality in rural Gambia. *Nature* 338:434.

Moore SE, Cole TJ, Collinson AC, Poskitt EME, McGregor IA, Prentice AM (1999) Prenatal or early postnatal events predict infectious deaths in young adulthood in rural Africa. *International Journal of Epidemiology* 28:1088–1095.

Morelli GA, Rogoff B, Oppenheim D, Goldsmith D (1992) Cultural variations in infants' sleeping arrangements: questions of independence. *Developmental Psychology* 28:604–613.

Newton N (1978) The role of oxytocin reflexes in three interpersonal reproductive acts: coitus, birth and breastfeeding. In L Carenza, P Pancheri, L Zichella (Eds) *Clinical Psychoneuroendocrinology in Reproduction: Proceedings of the Serono Symposia* 22 (New York, Academic Press), 411–418.

Panter-Brick C (2000) Nobody's children? A reconsideration of child abandonment. In C Panter-Brick, MT Smith (Eds) *Abandoned Children* (Cambridge, Cambridge University Press), 1–26.

Pennington R, Harpending H (1988) Fitness and fertility among Kalahari !Kung. *American Journal of Physical Anthropology* 77:303–319.

Prentice A, Prentice AM, Whitehead RG (1981) Breast-milk fat concentrations of rural African women, 2. Long-term variations within a community. *British Journal of Nutrition* 45:495–503.

Prentice AM, Roberts SB, Prentice A, Paul AA, Watkinson M, Watkinson AA, Whitehead RG (1983a) Dietary supplementation of lactating Gambian women, I. Effect on breast-milk volume and quality. *Human Nutrition: Clinical Nutrition* 37C:53–64.

Prentice AM, Lunn PG, Watkinson M, Whitehead RG (1983b) Dietary supplementation of lactating Gambian women, II. Effect on maternal health, nutritional satus and biochemistry. *Human Nutrition: Clinical Nutrition* 37C:65–74.

Prentice AM, Whitehead RG (1987) The energetics of human reproduction. *Symposia of the Zoological Society of London* 57:275–304.

Prentice AM, Prentice A (1995) Evolutionary and environmental influences of human lactation. *Proceedings of the Nutrition Society* 54:391–400.

Prentice AM, Cole TJ, Moore SE, Collinson AC (1999) Programming the adult immune system. In PMS O'Brien, T Wheeler, DJP Baker (Eds) *Fetal Programming: Influences on Development and Disease in Later Life* (London, Royal College of Obstetricians and Gynaecologists Press), 399–413.

Scheper-Hughes N (1992) *Death without Weeping: The Violence of Everyday Life in Brazil* (Berkeley, University of California Press).

Schiefenhövel W (1989) Reproduction and sex-ratio manipulation through preferential female infanticide among the Eipo, in the highlands of West New Guinea. In AE Rasa, C Vogel, E Voland (Eds) *The Sociobiology of Sexual and Reproductive Strategies* (London, Chapman & Hall), 170–193.

Shostak M (1981) *Nisa: The Life and Words of a !Kung Woman* (Cambridge, Harvard University Press).

Stein Z, Susser M (1975) The Dutch famine, 1944–1945, and the reproductive process, I. Effects on six indices at birth. *Pediatric Research* 9:70–76.

Stuart-Macadam P (1995) Biocultural perspectives on breastfeeding. In P Stuart-Macadam, KA Dettwyler (Eds) *Breastfeeding: Biocultural Perspectives* (New York, Aldine de Gruyter), 1–38.

Stuart-Macadam P, Dettwyler KA (Eds) *Breastfeeding: Biocultural Perspectives* (New York, Aldine de Gruyter).

Trevathan WR, McKenna JJ (1994) Evolutionary environments of human birth and infancy: insights to apply to contemporary life. *Children's Environments* 11: 88–104.

Tronick EZ, Winn S, Morlli GA (1985) Multiple caretaking in the context of human evolution: why don't the Efé know the Western prescription for child care? In M Reite, T Field (Eds) *The Psychobiology of Attachment and Separation* (London, Academic Press), 293–322.

van Esterik P, Greiner T (1981) Breastfeeding and women's work: constraints and opportunities. *Studies in Family Planning* 12:184–197.

Villalpando S, de Santiago S, Flores-Huerta S (1991) Maternal nutritional status and milk volume: is there a cause-effect relationship? *Archivos Latin Americanos de Nutrición* 41:293–303.

Wiley AS, Carlin LE (1999) Demographic contexts and the adaptive role of mother-infant attachment: a hypothesis. *Human Nature* 10:135–161.

Winkvist A, Rasmussen KM, Habicht J (1992) A new definition of maternal depletion syndrome. *American Journal of Public Health* 82:691–694.

Woolridge MW (1995) Baby-controlled breastfeeding: biocultural implications. In P Stuart-Macadam, KA Dettwyler (Eds) *Breastfeeding: Biocultural Perspectives* (New York, Aldine de Gruyter), 217–242.

12

Aging and Reproductive Senescence

LYNNETTE LEIDY SIEVERT

Aging, as differentiated from disease, is progressive, irreversible, and universal (Kohn 1971). Senescence, a more restrictive term, refers to "a decrease in the efficient functioning of an organism with increasing age" (Spence 1989:8). Reproductive senescence is part of the aging process in the sense that it is progressive—the ability to conceive and bear offspring declines with age (Finch 1990; Wood 1994). Reproductive senescence is not, however, a species universal or necessarily irreversible; it is better characterized as sex- and culture-specific.

Reproductive senescence is *sex-specific* in that human females experience a universal menopause if they live to the age of 60 (Diczfalusy 1986); human males share no similar, universal endpoint to their ability to reproduce (Merry and Holehan 1994b; Wood 1994). In terms of the general theories of aging (Spence 1989), changes in female fecundity with age appear to be genetically programmed, while changes in male fecundity are the consequence of wear and tear.[1] In all women, the ability to become pregnant declines with the loss of oocytes (undeveloped eggs) from the ovary. In individual men, the ability to impregnate declines with cellular atrophy and loss of tissue elasticity in reproductive organs. In both females and males, aging processes are regulated by the neuroendocrine system, which controls or influences the function of every organ and tissue in the body (Meites and Lu 1994). Therefore, many aspects of aging appear to be sex-specific because most sex differences in disease risk with age (e.g., the protective effect of ovarian estrogen on skeletal health in premenopausal women) can be traced to differential senescence in the female/male hypothalamic-pituitary-gonadal axis.

Reproductive senescence is *culture-specific* in that gender roles determine occupational hazards that affect the ability to conceive and bear healthy offspring at advanced ages (Manderson 1999). For example, a history of military service in Vietnam is associated with lower sperm concentrations and fewer morphologically normal sperm cells (DeStefano et al.

1989), and male workers exposed to dibromocholoropropane (DBCP) demonstrate cumulative effects that result in subfertility or infertility (Schrader 1993; Whorton 1984). For women, more subtle cultural norms, (e.g., those affecting marital practices and whether or not it is acceptable to smoke) can affect age at menopause (Kaufman et al. 1980; Leidy Sievert et al. 2001; Willet et al. 1983). Finally, reproductive senescence is culture-specific in that certain societies are able to prolong female reproduction beyond the biological parameter of menopause through egg donation and exogenous hormonal support (Lutjen et al. 1984; Paulson and Sauer 1994).

Across industrialized (and some nonindustrialized) countries, delayed childbearing is becoming more acceptable; however, the biological parameter of menopause is not likely to demonstrate change (Flint 1997). Instead, as reproduction is delayed to later ages, reproductive technologies (e.g., postmenopausal, medically assisted pregnancies) provide the possibility of a "cultural menopause" (Cavalli-Sforza 1983) well after the biological event. However, in the much publicized postmenopausal pregnancy, genetic success is enjoyed by the spouse and the egg donor, not the pregnant woman herself (Smith 1993). The story is far from finished, however, as medicine and pharmaceuticals continue to expand the reproductive options for future generations, including the technological capacity for women to freeze ovarian tissue for later use (Highfield 1999).

Reproductive senescence is organ-specific, and this observation is particularly prominent in comparisons between rodents and primates (Meites and Lu 1994). This chapter begins with a brief review of the biology of the hypothalamic-pituitary-gonadal axis in both females and males. Then, senescent changes specific to this axis are examined. Cross-species comparisons demonstrate that human females are unusual in their experience of menopause at the midpoint of the species' maximum lifespan potential (Leidy 1999; Pavelka and Fedigan 1991). Finally, the relationship between culture (e.g., medicine) and biology is explored specific to human reproductive senescence, along with the evolutionary implications of postmenopausal pregnancies and the treatment of age-related sexual dysfunction in men.

THE NEUROENDOCRINE SYSTEM

The discussion begins with the brain, an arbitrary starting point. In both males and females the hypothalamus transmits a polypeptide gonadotropin releasing hormone (GnRH) in episodic pulses directly to the anterior pituitary. In the anterior pituitary, plasma membrane receptors sense the pulse frequency and amplitude of GnRH and direct the production of two gonadotropins, follicle-stimulating hormone (FSH) and luteinizing hormone (LH). FSH and LH are also characterized by episodic secretion (Leidy 1994; Meites and Lu 1994; Merry and Holehan 1994a).

Catecholamines (dopamine and norepinephrine), serotonin, endogenous opioid peptides (enkephalins and B-endorphin), and hypothalamic peptides (such as vasoactive intestinal peptide) influence the secretion of GnRH (Ferin et al. 1984; Kaiser et al. 1993; Meites et al. 1982). The daily rhythmicity in the activity of neurotransmitters, "the density of their receptors, and/or the level of gene expression is greatly dampened or altered with age" (Wise et al. 1997:288). Environmental stimuli carried by the central nervous system can also affect the secretion of GnRH (Meites and Lu 1994). Although FSH and LH are both stimulated by GnRH, they are under separate regulatory control. In women this is evidenced by higher levels of FSH during the follicular phase of menstrual cycles, an earlier rise in FSH levels prior to menopause, and an age-related loss of concordance between LH and FSH pulses (Backstrom et al. 1982; Channing et al. 1985; Genazzani et al. 1997; Rannevik et al. 1995). In men, there is also a greater rise with age in FSH than in LH (Meites and Lu 1994).

Within the ovaries, FSH and LH stimulate oogenesis, follicular growth, and the production of estrogens (in order of potency: estradiol, estrone, estriol), progesterone, inhibin, and small amounts of androgens, e.g., testosterone and dehydroepiandrosterone (DHEA). Estrogen, progesterone, and inhibin send feedback signals to the brain, regulating the secretion of FSH and LH, as shown in Figure 12.1 (Channing et al. 1985; Guraya 1985; Merry and Holehan 1994a; Wood 1994). The sex steroids (e.g., estradiol) are transported via sex hormone binding globulin (SHBG), which is the main factor influencing their biological activity (Rannevik et al. 1995). Secondary sex characteristics affected by ovarian hormones include stature and adipose tissue distribution. In addition, estrogen receptors are found in the vulva, vagina, cervix, uterus, ovary, skin, breast, bladder, and urethra and are associated with cardiovascular and skeletal tissues (Merry and Holehan 1994a; Whitehead et al. 1993).

Within the testes, FSH stimulates Sertoli cells in the seminiferous tubules to produce inhibin, which in turn acts to inhibit FSH secretion. FSH also acts on Sertoli cells to stimulate the differentiation and division of germ cells. LH stimulates Leydig cells to produce testosterone, which stimulates growth, mediates the expression of sexual characteristics, and provides the feedback regulation of LH (Figure 12.1). Testosterone circulates in the blood plasma bound to SHBG and albumin, with only about 2% of testosterone free to circulate in its biologically active form. Testosterone may be actively metabolized to estradiol by aromatization and, within the testes and other tissues, to dihydrotestosterone (DHT) by 5 alpha reduction. The testes also secrete extremely small amounts of estradiol (Matsumoto 1993; Merry and Holehan 1994b). Target organs for

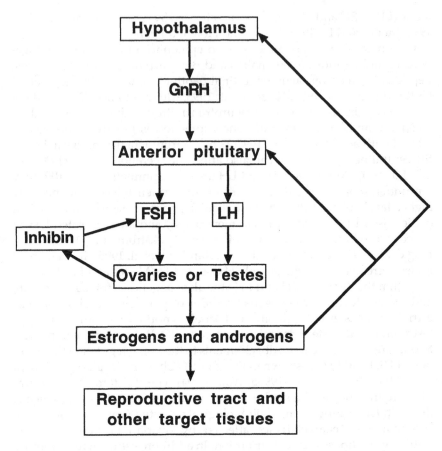

Figure 12.1 Hypothalamic-pituitary-gonadal axis.

testosterone include the penis, prostate, muscle, and skin (body hair). Testosterone is also associated with hematopoiesis as well as with cardio-vascular and skeletal tissues (Tenover 1993).

NEUROENDOCRINE AND TARGET TISSUE CHANGES WITH ADVANCED AGE

Females

The trigger of reproductive decline differs substantially between rodents and primates. In the former a "neural clock" is more critical, in the latter a "pelvic clock" appears to be the locus of control (Bennett and Whitehead 1983). In old female rats, the hypothalamus is the core of reproductive function and decline. The pituitary and ovaries remain functional, as demonstrated by the transplantation of these organs from old rats into young rats, and by the administration of Gn-RH which can elicit an LH response and ovulation in aged rats. The declines in two catecholamines, dopamine and noradrenaline, appear to be mainly responsible for the loss of estrous cycles in aging female rats (see review in Meites and Lu 1994). Among female rats there is an uneven decline in regular cycles and fertile gestations. At four months, 93% demonstrate fertile gestations; at 10 months, 62% have regular cycles but only 38% have fertile gestations; at 12 months, there is a decline to 40% with regular cycles and 23% with fertile gestations. Litter size also decreases with age (Matt et al. 1986).

Specific to women, the sequence of hormonal feedback remains the same, but hormonal levels are modified with age. Estrogen levels increase with age during the late follicular phase, and both estrogen and progesterone levels decline with age during the luteal phase (Korenman et al. 1978). In women over the age of 45, the length of the follicular but not the luteal phase is decreased and FSH levels increase, particularly during the early follicular phase (Sherman 1987). The age-related increase in FSH occurs before the age-related increase of LH and is thought to be the result of lower inhibin secretion by the ovaries (Baird and Smith 1993). Significant increases in serum FSH and LH begin 4.75 years prior to menopause (Rannevik et al. 1995), although hormonal changes are transient and vary greatly with age (Metcalf et al. 1981; Reame et al. 1996).

There is no definitive hormonal marker of the inception of "perimenopause" (Rannevik et al. 1995; Santoro 1996); however, as the ovarian follicular supply is exhausted, there is a marked decrease in estradiol and estrone, along with a significant decline in testosterone, androstenedione, and SHBG (Rannevik et al. 1995). FSH and LH remain elevated (Longcope et al. 1986). Figure 12.2 summarizes the hormonal changes of 160 women who were observed for 7–12 years around menopause. Mean age at menopause was 52.1 years, ranging from 48.3 to 57.4 years (Rannevik et al. 1995:107).

Prior to menopause, menstrual cycles become increasingly irregular (Treloar 1981) and there is an increase in anovulatory cycles (O'Connor et al. 1998). Fertility declines with age in women aged 25 and older who receive sperm donation (Federation CECOS et al. 1982) and oocyte donation (Abdalla et al. 1990), and both historical and cross-cultural evidence demonstrate an end to female fecundity 5 to 10 years prior to the end of menstruation (Gage et al. 1989; Wood 1994). This pattern of "senescent subfertility" prior to menopause is characterized as "long and variable cycles, a higher fraction of anovulatory cycles, and an elevated risk of fetal

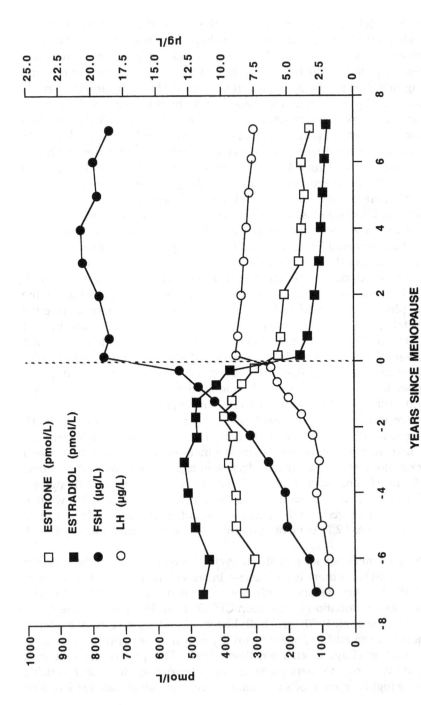

Figure 12.2. Mean serum levels of FSH, LH, estradiol and estrone during the perimenopausal transition (from Rannevik et al. 1995:107; reprinted with permission from Elsevier Science)

loss" (Wood 1994:465). Primordial follicles continue to exist in the ovaries of women over the age of 50 years (Costoff and Mahesh 1975; Novak 1970); however, there appears to be a threshold number of follicles below which menstrual cyclicity and fecundity are lost (Nelson and Felicio 1985). For further discussion, see Holman and Wood in this volume.

It used to be thought that an aging uterus made pregnancy unlikely or impossible beyond the age of 50 years, but this view has since been challenged by successful postmenopausal pregnancies using donor eggs (Antinori et al. 1993; Sauer et al. 1992). It is now generally agreed that, given appropriate exogenous hormonal support (Meldrum 1993), the uterus is capable of supporting a pregnancy well beyond the ticking of the ovarian "biological clock" (Levran et al. 1991; Navot et al. 1991).

After menopause, serum levels of LH and FSH decline but remain higher than premenopausal levels (Genazzani et al. 1997). From 12 months to 10 years after menopause, estrone levels appear to be relatively stable, while levels of estradiol, the most physiologically active estrogen, continue to decline (Jiroutek et al. 1998). Estrone continues to be produced through the peripheral conversion (aromatization) of adrenal and ovarian androstenedione in muscle, fat, and other tissues. The production of progesterone decreases markedly, although the postmenopausal ovary continues to secrete testosterone and androstenedione (Casey and MacDonald 1983; Judd et al. 1974; Korenman et al. 1978; Metcalf et al. 1981). There is a rise, then fall, of SHBG (Jiroutek et al. 1998).

The decline in estradiol levels associated with menopause is related to the specific symptoms of hot flashes, sweating, and vaginal dryness (Whitehead et al. 1993). Although these symptoms decrease with estrogen therapy (Kronenberg 1994), implying a common biological basis, they are not universal across populations (Avis et al. 1993; Beyene 1989; Lock 1993, 1998; Obermeyer 2000). How the experience of menopause varies across cultures is illustrated by Table 12.1 which lists symptom frequencies gathered via very similar survey instruments in different populations.

The biology of hot flashes, a frequent marker of menopause in the United States, is still not completely understood (Freedman 2000). Hot flashes involve an increase in peripheral blood flow and an elevation in peripheral temperature which coincides with a fall in core body temperature (Freedman 1989; Freedman et al. 1995). Hot flashes are associated with low estrogen levels, pulses of pituitary LH (although these are not causal), and increased levels of brain norepinephrine (Freedman 1998, 2000; Kronenberg 1994). Although associated with the menopause transition, episodes of chills and sweats are also reported by women in their reproductive years who have regular menstrual cycles and experience premenstrual syndrome (Hahn et al. 1998), possibly due to an estrogen deficiency during the

Table 12.1. Percent of Women Reporting Symptoms during Two Weeks Prior to Interview

Symptom	Japan[1] N = 1225	Canada[2] N = 1307	U.S.[3] N = 7802	Australia[4] N = 549	Mexico[5] N = 755
Vasomotor					
Hot flash	12	31	35	32	50
Sweats	4	20	11	10	31
Neurological					
Headache	28	34	37	36	53
Dizziness	7	12	11	10	36
Trouble sleeping	12	30	31	35	52
Lack of energy	6	40	38	46	70
Mood					
Irritability	12	17	30	—	—
Nervousness	—	—	—	41	66
Feeling blue/depressed	10	23	36	33	52
Musculoskeletal					
Back pain	24	27	30	38	56
Joint aches/stiffness	15	31	39	52	56

[1] Japanese women age 45–55 from southern Nagano, Kyoto, and Kobe (Lock 1998)
[2] Canadian women age 45–55 from Manitoba (Lock 1998)
[3] Massachusetts women age 45–55 (Lock 1998)
[4] Perimenopausal Australian women age 45 to 55. "Perimenopause" defined as changes in menstrual frequency or flow in the previous 12 months (Dennerstein et al. 1993).
[5] Mexican women age 40–60 living in Puebla, Mexico (Leidy Sievert, unpublished data)

luteal phase. The Melbourne Women's Midlife Health Project found that 13% of premenopausal, 37% of perimenopausal, 62% of postmenopausal women, and 15% of women on hormone therapy reported at least one hot flash in the two weeks prior to interview (Guthrie et al. 1996).

Psychiatric symptoms do not significantly increase in frequency during the change from premenopause to the first six-month-postmenopausal period, as opposed to vasomotor symptoms, such as hot flashes, which do increase significantly during this same period (Obermeyer 2000; Rannevik et al. 1995). Mood disorders attributed to hypoestrogenic states (e.g., post-partum blues, PMS, and depression associated with menopause) may be more directly related to changes in a variety of neurotransmitters (Hahn et al. 1998). The serotoninergic system has received the most attention, in part due to the availability of selective serotonin re-uptake inhibitors (e.g., Prozac) which allow for clinical trials.

Following menopause there is an increased risk in cardiovascular disease and loss in bone density. Although estrogen replacement effectively halts bone loss (Whitehead et al. 1993), cross-cultural studies suggest that menopause is not the most important risk factor for osteoporotic fractures

(Beall 1987; Martin et al. 1993) or heart disease (Crews and Gerber 1994; Gerber and Crews 1999).

In summary, female reproductive senescence in humans appears to be genetically programmed. The species universal loss of ovarian follicles across time is ultimately related to a rise in pituitary hormones and a decline in ovarian hormones which, along with age-related changes in neurotransmitters (e.g., norepinephrine), induces negative effects in various target tissues. There is an accompanying decline in fertility with age, and menopause results when the number of oocytes remaining in the ovaries drops below a threshold value (discussed below). At present there is no way to assess "ovarian age," although ovarian volume measured by transvaginal ultrasound technology may allow for an indirect estimation of follicular numbers (Flaws et al. 2000).

Males

In the aging male rat, FSH and LH secretion decrease, leading to a decline in the secretion of testosterone. As summarized by Meites and Lu (1994), the reduced FSH and LH secretion is due to the diminished release of GnRH associated with a reduction in hypothalamic catecholamines, dopamine and norepinephrine (Simpkins et al. 1977), as well as the reduced responsiveness of the pituitary to Gn-RH. In old rats, Leydig cell numbers increase, but there is a decreased responsiveness to gonadotropins and a decline in sperm production as well as an increase in sperm abnormalities. There is no significant loss in Sertoli cells (Meites and Lu 1994; Merry and Holehan 1994b).

Unlike rats, mice and golden hamsters do not show an age-related decline in testosterone (reviewed in Merry and Holehan 1994b); there is evidence, however, of a decline in fertility. For example, the spermatozoa from mice 7 months old fertilized 80–86% of oocytes in vitro, while the spermatozoa from aged males fertilized only 11–19% of oocytes. Sperm motility was reduced in aged mice compared to younger mice, and superovulated females artificially inseminated with spermatazoa from 25-month-old males did not become pregnant (Parkening 1989).

Specific to men, there are conflicting reports with regard to changes in serum levels of FSH and LH (Merry and Holehan 1994b). A reduced response to GnRH by pituitary gonadotropins with age (Kaiser et al. 1993) begins at about 45–50 years of age along with a decrease in inhibin secretion. There is, however, considerable individual variation. Changes in the nature of GnRH release are suggested by the absence of a pulsatile pattern of LH secretion in older men and a reduction of noradrenaline and dopamine in the hypothalamus (reviewed by Meites and Lu 1994).

Most studies report a progressive decline in testosterone production and secretion beginning at about 40–50 years of age; however, there are considerable individual differences (Wood 1994). Korenman et al. (1990) report an age-related drop in bioavailable testosterone owing to an increased binding with SHBG. Testosterone was found to decrease with age in monks 26 to 90 years of age (Deslypere and Vermeulen 1984). In contrast, others have shown no decline in testosterone with age (Nieschlag et al. 1982). In the Baltimore Longitudinal Study on Aging, there was no decline in serum testosterone, DHT, or estrogens between ages 25 and 89 years (Harman and Tsitouras 1980).

There is general agreement regarding a loss of circadian rhythm in testosterone, a blunting of the morning peak in testosterone secretion, and reduced inhibin secretion (Matsumoto 1993; Meites and Lu 1994). As with women, plasma levels of estrogens increase in older men because of the increased peripheral conversion of androgens to estrone (Merry and Holehan 1994b).

With age, there are structural alterations in the testis, accessory sexual glands, and penis (Matsumoto 1993). In the penis, smooth muscle cells decrease, collagen fibers increase, and there is a loss of sinusoidal endothelium. Nerve fiber changes also occur (Donatucci and Lue 1993). Testis weight does not change with age in men over 40 years of age (Merry and Holehan 1994b). There is, however, some atrophy of the seminiferous tubules, a loss of Sertoli cells (Johnson et al. 1984), and a loss of Leydig cells (Neaves et al. 1984). Other degenerative changes include peritubular fibrosis and failure of spermatogenic maturation owing to sclerosis and closing of the tubular lumen (Nieschlag et al. 1982; Nieschlag and Michel 1986).

Impotence (the inability to sustain an erection sufficient for coitus) occurs with increasing frequency with advancing age so that by 50 years of age 6.7% of men are impotent, 25% by 65 years, and 55% by 75 years (Kinsey et al. 1948). More recent research in the United States, using the National Health and Social Life Survey, found men aged 50–59 were three times as likely to experience erection problems and low sexual desire as were men aged 18–29 (Laumann et al. 1999).

The most important physiologic event in an erection is the relaxation of the smooth muscle lining the sinusoids—an endothelial-lined network of spaces that function as a "scaffold" for the erectile tissue (Donatucci and Lue 1993:56). What appears to be an age-related dysfunction of the penile scaffolding is more often related to illness (e.g., hypertension, diabetes mellitus, incontinence), medications (e.g., antidepressants), recreational drugs (e.g., alcohol), hormonal dysfunctions, and subjective poor health than to advanced age (Mulligan et al.1988). Declining free testosterone levels and sexual thoughts or sexual activity demonstrate very low coefficients of correlation (Davidson et al. 1983). Korenman et al. (1990) found that impotent older men, mostly with medical conditions, had testosterone, bioavailable testosterone, and LH concentrations at least as high as those in age-matched controls. Nevertheless, although testosterone levels and impotence are independent, decreased levels of testosterone will exacerbate erectile dysfunction (Donatucci and Lue 1993).

In the prostate, between the ages of 40 and 60 years there is a loss of smooth muscle and a proliferation of fibrous tissue (Timiras 1994), and as demonstrated in the longitudinal Veterans Administration Normative Aging Study of healthy volunteers in Boston, there is an increased incidence of benign prostatic hyperplasia (BPH) with age (Glynn et al. 1985). This nodular enlargement of the prostate gland, experienced by one third or more of males older than 60 years, can lead to obstruction of the urethra and urine outflow which can cause changes in the bladder, ureters, and kidney (Timiras 1994). There is also, with age, an increased incidence of prostate cancer, the most frequently diagnosed cancer in men in most western countries (Hsing et al. 2000). Both BPH and prostate cancer are androgen dependent (Timiras 1994). With regard to testosterone's other target organs, there are conflicting opinions on the importance of declining testosterone levels on bone, blood, and cardiovascular health (Tenover 1993).

There is an increased frequency of structural chromosomal abnormalities in sperm with paternal age (Martin and Rademaker 1987). However, and in summary, the single biggest difference between women and men in fecundity and reproductive senescence is that women are born with all of the oocytes they will ever have, while men retain the ability to make sperm, potentially, for all their lives.[2] Unlike in human females, in males senescence is not a programmed universal. Gametic production continues so that sperm is found in the ejaculate of 48% of men aged 80–90 (Merry and Holehan 1994b). Nieschlag et al. (1982) found no difference in ejaculate volume, sperm morphology, or fertilizing capacity between unrelated fathers (aged 24–37 years) and grandfathers (aged 60–88), although sperm motility did decline with age. As with women, men demonstrate changes in the hypothalamic-pituitary-gonadal axis with age. However, these changes are highly individualized, as are age-related alterations in the reproductive support structures. Many of these changes are, in fact, amenable to medical treatment (discussed below).

THE BIOLOGY AND EPIDEMIOLOGY OF MENOPAUSE

Menopause, defined as the last menstrual period, is identified in retrospect after 12 months of amenorrhea (WHO 1981). Age at menopause is determined by three factors: the number of oocytes formed in the female ovary through mitotic division by the fifth month of fetal development, the rate of oocyte loss across the lifespan through the processes of ovulation and degenerative atresia, and the threshold number of ovarian follicles required to support menstruation (Gosden 1985a; Gougeon 1996; Leidy 1994; Richardson et al. 1987; Wood 1994). Although Wise et al. (1997:280) contend that "the brain is a critical pacemaker in the sequence of events leading to reproductive senescence," most investigators view human menopause as driven by the process of follicular decline.

Fish, amphibians, and reptiles continue oogenesis—germ cell mitosis—throughout adult life (Sadleir 1973). Birds and mammals, however, cease oogenesis prior to or just after birth (Guraya 1985; Peters and McNatty 1980). In the human ovary, approximately 7 million oogonia proliferate by the fifth month of fetal development. This number declines to 2 million oocytes in the human ovaries at birth (Baker 1986) and 400,000 oocytes by the onset of puberty (Byskov 1978). Following puberty, monthly ovulation accounts for the disappearance of a maximum of 400 or so oocytes. Thousands more simply degenerate until comparatively few remain at the time of menopause (Nelson and Felicio 1985; Novak 1970; Richardson et al. 1987; Thomford et al. 1987). The degeneration of oocytes occurs through follicular atresia, a process that involves the shrinking of either the oocyte itself or its surrounding follicle (Byskov 1978; Crisp 1992; Gougeon 1996; Guraya 1985).

Until recently, it was believed that oocyte depletion accelerated near the onset of menopause, beginning at around age 38 or 40 years, as shown by log-linear plots of follicle number vs. age (Faddy et al. 1992; Gougeon et al. 1994; Richardson et al. 1987; Wood et al. 1994; WHO 1996). Reanalyses of these plots demonstrate the opposite trend, that the absolute number of follicles lost per unit time is lowest during the years prior to menopause (Leidy et al. 1998; McDonough 1999).

Cross-sectional, retrospective, and longitudinal studies place the median age of menopause at 50–51 years in well-nourished, industrialized societies. In less nourished populations mean and median ages at menopause are 43 to 47 years (Gosden 1985a; Gray 1976; Wood 1994). Variables associated with age at menopause include smoking, body size, marital status, parity, age at first pregnancy, education, socioeconomic status, and regularity of menstrual cycles (Leidy 1994, 1996; Leidy Sievert et al. 2001; Luoto et al. 1994; Parazzini et al. 1992; Stanford et al. 1987; Whelan et al. 1990).

EVOLUTION OF FEMALE MENOPAUSE

While other mammals experience reproductive senescence (Comfort 1979; Finch 1990) and individual primates have demonstrated changes similar to the human menopause (Caro et al. 1995; Gould et al. 1981; Hodgen et al. 1977; Lapin et al. 1979; Pavelka and Fedigan 1999; Walker 1995), no other species of primates have demonstrated a universally experienced, permanent cessation of reproductive cyclicity followed by a prolonged period of postreproductive life (Lancaster and Lancaster 1983; Pavelka and Fedigan 1991).

It has been suggested that female menopause is an adaptation related to differential parental investment (Gaulin 1980), that females make a greater investment in offspring (e.g., lactation and protection of altricial young) compared with males. Menopause coupled with a long postreproductive life ensures that mothers must be young enough to survive pregnancy, parturition, and the infancy of their offspring (Lancaster and Lancaster 1983; Peacock 1991; Pollard 1994). This argument has recently resurfaced in debates regarding postmenopausal pregnancy (see below). There is, however, a lack of support for this position in quantitative tests of the deleterious effects of maternal mortality on offspring survival (Hill and Hurtado 1991).

From an evolutionary perspective, menopause can be viewed as adaptative or neutral (for a longer review see Leidy 1999). For example, menopause curtails the ovulation of old, possibly abnormal, oocytes (O'Rourke and Ellison 1993; Pollard 1994). Advocates of the popular "grandmother hypothesis" (Donaldson 1994; Gaulin 1980; Hawkes et al. 1997; Turke 1988) speculate that "females can make a greater contribution to the population gene pool by investing in kin (particularly grandchildren) than they could by producing their own offspring" (summarized by Hill and Hurtado 1991:321). Alternatively, menopause can be considered to be adaptive within contemporary, industrialized society in which constant ovulatory cycles, without breaks for multiple pregnancies and lactation, is a recent human condition (Eaton et al. 1994; Harrell 1977). Menopause marks the end of exposure of breast tissue (and other estrogenically sensitive tissue) to high, cyclic levels of estrogen and, therefore, lowers the risk of reproductive cancers. Some adaptive scenarios postulate that the cessation of menses originally occurred at an earlier age (premature ovarian failure) and gradually shifted to a later age (menopause) as the maximum lifespan lengthened (Peccei 1995; Donaldson 1994).

From a more neutral perspective, it is likely that female hominids were originally fertile to the end of the lifespan, similar to present-day chimpanzees, but then the human maximum lifespan potential (MLP) extended—perhaps through the progressive prolongation of life stages and in relation to enlarged brain size (Bogin and Smith 1996; Cutler 1976; Sacher 1978; Watts 1986). The lifespan more than doubled, from the 50-year MLP for chimpanzees to >110 years MLP for humans; however, ovarian characteristics such as oocyte number and rate of atresia did not change to the same extent. Menopause, the cessation of menses, was "uncovered" by the extension of the human lifespan. In this scenario the appearance of menopause is neutral or architectural (Gould and Lewontin 1979). In any case, the loss of follicles leads to the exhaustion of oocyte reserves and menopause is the result.

THE CHANGING "NATURE" OF
REPRODUCTIVE SENESCENCE

Durham (1991) has argued that it is the phenotype which connects evolutionary changes in genotypic and cultural systems across time. Can the genetic limits of reproductive senescence be changed by culturally modifying the expression of reproduction?

Specific to males, as discussed above, changes associated with aging are individualistic, characteristic of disease processes rather than the universal changes of aging. The same arguments applied to the delay of chronic diseases until after *most* childbearing is complete can be applied to the appearance of age-related changes in hormonal profiles, testes, penis, and accessory structures that afflict individual men. Namely, there is reduced selection against disease processes that are expressed late in life. But could microevolutionary consequences occur through changes in the phenotype—in other words, does the ability to have an erection translate directly into increased fertility?

Even with cultural (medical) innovations making erections possible, e.g., penile implants, local papaverine injection and other smooth muscle relaxants, vacuum erection devices, microsurgery (Renshaw 1993), and now sildenafil citrate (Viagra) (Ballard et al. 1998), there is unlikely to be a substantial change in the fitness of individuals. Genes have already, most likely, been passed on by the time impotence becomes a health concern,[3] and despite the extensive media coverage, it is difficult to find literature substantiating pregnancies produced as a result of Viagra, although its use in assisted reproductive technologies is likely to increase (Tur-Kaspa et al. 1999). In contrast, there is some evidence that Viagra decreases fitnesses through untimely death: officials in the German Embassy blame Viagra and subsequent overexertion for the death of more than one hundred German tourists in Bangkok in 1999, a 20% increase from 1998 (O'Donnell et al. 1999).

Specific to women, in western society delayed childbirth is related to changing social norms, the postponement of marriage, expanded educational and career opportunities, increased rates of divorce and remarriage, as well as the availability of birth control (Benshushan and Schenker 1993; Stein 1985). Difficulties associated with late childbearing include endometriosis, anovulation, tubal obstruction subsequent to pelvic inflammatory disease, sperm antibodies, contraceptive sequelae, gonadal dysgenesis, premature ovarian failure (POF), and even natural menopause itself—all of which can be assisted or amended through infertility treatment (Benshushan and Schenker 1993; Bustillo et al. 1984).

It is estimated that 100 women over age 50 have had babies through medical intervention (Belkin 1997). According to Sauer et al. (1992:1276), women over 50 seek egg donation for many reasons, including ovarian failure (31%), failure of traditional infertility therapies (62%), and concerns about age-related pregnancy miscarriage rates and genetic anomalies (7%). In Sauer et al.'s (1993) report, ages of women ranged from 50 to 59 (mean 52.2 years), ages of husbands ranged from 27 to 70 (mean 47.8 years), and ages of donors ranged from 24 to 32 (mean 28.1 years). Of 14 couples assisted, eight women had never had a child, three were grandparents, and nine of the couples were married for the second time. In another report, a 63-year-old California woman had never had any children and had been married for 13 years. Her 57-year-old husband's sperm was used to fertilize the donated eggs and a healthy female infant was delivered by cesarean section at 38 weeks, weighed 2,844 g, and was breast-fed (Paulson et al. 1997).

While in vitro fertilization (IVF) success rates are very low for women older than 40 using their own eggs (Chetkowski et al. 1991; Meldrum 1993; Navot et al. 1991), success rates are equal to those of younger women when women use eggs from a younger donor. In one of the first clinical trials, the ratio of ongoing pregnancies or deliveries per embryo transfer was 8.6% for women 40 years or older using their own oocytes and standard IVF, 30.2% for women younger than 40 with donor IVF, and 33.7% for women 40 and older using donor IVF (Sauer et al. 1992).

Oocyte donation has become a successful "treatment" for menopause in women older than 50 (Antinori et al. 1993; Sauer et al. 1993), including the much publicized success of two women older than 60 years of age (Antinori et al. 1995; Kolata 1997; Paulson et al. 1997). Physicians tout that "the age-related decline in female fertility may be *reversed"*; that woman will *"conceive*, carry and give birth" to an infant with an oocyte donated from a younger woman (Sauer et al. 1992:1275, emphasis added). The word "conceive" is used loosely, since the egg is fertilized outside the body and recipients are prepared for the pregnancy with exogenous estradiol for 3 days and then progesterone replacement. Once pregnant, they continue to receive estradiol orally and progesterone intramuscularly for an additional 100 days (Sauer et al. 1992).

Ethical concerns specific to postmenopausal pregnancy revolve around the health of the woman involved and the future of the children. With age, there is an increased risk of obstetric complication (Cnattingius et al. 1992; Kirz et al. 1985), maternal mortality (Buehler et al. 1986; *Lancet* 1993), an increased rate of chromosomal abnormalities in the oocytes (Gosden

1985b; Wood 1994), and an increased risk of fetal loss (Fretts et al. 1995; Meldrum 1993; O'Connor et al. 1998; Stein 1985). In one hospital population, Berkowitz et al. (1990) noted an increase in pregnancy-induced hypertension, gestational diabetes, low birth weight babies, abruptio placentae, and placenta previa in women over the age of 35 (see also Kirz et al. 1985). However, Edwards (1993:1543) observed that more than 50 women older than 50 years of age have carried pregnancies to term and "there have been no signs of sharp increases in the frequency of mid-gestational fetal deaths, hydramnios or other disorders. . . . Nor have fears of hypertension, pre-eclampsia, diabetes and vascular complications been realized in mothers up to 65 years." More recently, Schmidt-Sarosi (1998) reviewed the complications of pregnancies in women older than 50 years following oocyte donation and concluded that a considerable maternal morbidity exists. In 17 viable pregnancies detailed by Sauer et al. (1995), nine were multiple gestations (6 twins, 1 triplet, and 2 quadruplets selectively terminated to twins) and complications were described in eight patients (including gestational hypertension, gestational diabetes, and preeclampsia.)

Regarding the health of the children, worries expressed include whether or not aging mothers can deal with the physical demands of childrearing (Belkin 1997), but children have often been raised by grandparents (Paulson and Sauer 1994; Sauer et al. 1993). Others worry that older mothers will leave orphans (Benshushan and Schenker 1993). In answer, it is pointed out that the expected lifespan has never been longer (Mori 1994) and "there was no talk of orphans when only men could conceive into their 70s or older" (Edwards 1993:1543). In addition, advocates of postmenopausal pregnancy ask whether or not women with systemic lupus erythematosus, diabetes mellitus, or chronic renal failure should also be prohibited from reproducing, and point out that men known to be dying occasionally wish to reproduce prior to or, with banked spermatozoa, even after death (Paulson and Sauer 1994).

In terms of genetic success, egg donation to postmenopausal women increases the reproductive fitness of the spouse (assuming it is his sperm) and of the donor, but not of the woman—the recipient—herself (Smith 1993). For the woman herself, the use of another's egg(s) is akin to adoption—albeit a very intensive, costly form of adoption. She has not had her *own* baby, although genetic relatedness is possible when an egg donated by the woman's sister makes her an aunt, or an egg from her daughter makes her a grandmother to the infant she bears (Belkin 1997; *Lancet* 1993). Thinking beyond the individual, Takahide Mori (1994:187) of Japan suggests that the new opportunities for postmenopausal pregnancies "may contribute considerably to normalize age distribution of developed countries which are suffering from a continuous decrease in birth rates." In contrast, Sauer et al. (1993:323) postulate that few individuals will choose to become parents late in life; therefore, "it is unlikely that this new technology will have a serious influence on the fabric of society."

The influence of medically assisted postmenopausal pregnancy will be that women may someday be released from the tyranny of aging eggs. Although the ethics committee for the American Society for Reproductive Medicine stated in 1996 that "Just as fertility is the norm during the reproductive years . . . infertility should remain the natural characteristic of menopause," an expert in reproductive law responded "Why is [postmenopausal pregnancy] any more unnatural than coronary-bypass surgery?" (in Belkin 1997:49, 67). Roger Gosden speculates that within a few years a test will be developed to allow a woman to assess her "ovarian age," or how close she is to running out of eggs (Highfield 1999). Perhaps ovarian volume will be refined to offer that information (Flaws et al. 2000). Following the success of ovarian grafting (Grady 1999), women will be able to freeze their eggs when they are young to protect them "from the ravages of time" (Highfield 1999) for use later, when they are older and their eggs are of poorer quality (Belkin 1997).

SUMMARY

Reproductive senescence is sex- and culture-specific. Changes in female fecundity with age appear to be a species universal, whereas changes in male fecundity are the consequence of cellular atrophy, loss of tissue elasticity, and other idiosyncratic changes. One way in which reproductive senescence is culture-specific is that certain societies are able to prolong female reproduction beyond menopause through egg donation and exogenous hormonal support. This ability to "treat" or "cure" post-menopausal women of infertility makes menopause a disease (Kluge 1994) and therefore idiosyncratic in the way that reproductive senescence in males is idiosyncratic. As medicine continues to expand reproductive options—e.g., the treatment of male impotence, the freezing of a woman's ovarian tissue for later use—the experience of reproductive senescence will be altered for some. However, there will be few, if any, evolutionary consequences.

I am indebted to Claire Wendland for her assistance in finding some particularly helpful references.

NOTES

1. The use of *fecundity* to apply to males is stretched from the demographic use of *fecundability* to mean "the probability that a fecund couple will conceive during a month of exposure to unprotected intercourse" (Wood 1994:72). Fecundability is determined by both behavioral and physiological factors.

2.   Author Saul Bellow, age 84, just fathered his fourth child (*Newsweek*, Feb. 7, 2000:68).
3.   Saul Bellow being an exception.

REFERENCES

Abdalla HI, Baber R, Kirkland A, Leonard T, Power M, Studd JWW (1990) A report on 100 cycles of oocyte donation: factors affecting the outcome. *Human Reproduction* 5:1018–1022.

Antinori S, Versaci C, Gholami GH, Panci C, Caffa B (1993) Oocyte donation in menopausal women. *Human Reproduction* 8:1487–1490.

Antinori S, Versaci C, Panci C, Caffa B, Gholami GH (1995) Fetal and maternal morbidity and mortality in menopausal women aged 45–63 years. *Human Reproduction* 10:464–469.

Avis NE, Kaufert PA, Lock M, McKinlay SM, Vass K (1993) The evolution of menopausal symptoms. *Bailliere's Clinical Endocrinology and Metabolism* 7:17–32.

Backstrom CT, McNeilly A, Leask RM, Bird DT (1982) Pulsatile secretion of LH, FSH, prolactin, estradiol, and progesterone during the human menstrual cycle. *Clinical Endocrinology* 17:29–42.

Baker TG (1986) Gametogenesis. In WR Dukelow, J Erwin (Eds) *Comparative Primate Biology*, 3: Reproduction and Development (New York, Alan R. Liss), 195–213.

Baird DT, Smith KB (1993) Inhibin and related peptides in the regulation of reproduction. *Oxford Reviews of Reproductive Biology* 15:191–232.

Ballard SA, Gingell CJ, Tang K, Turner LA, Price ME, Naylor AM (1998) Effects of Sildenafil on the relaxation of human corpus cavernosum tissue in vitro and on the activities of cyclic nucleotide phosphodiesterase isozymes. *Journal of Urology* 159:2164–2171.

Beall CM (1987) Nutrition and variation in biological anthropology. In FE Johnson (Ed) *Nutritional Anthropology* (New York, Alan R. Liss), 197–221.

Belkin L (1997) How old is too old? *New York Times Magazine* (October 26):35–39, 48–49, 67–68.

Bennett GW, Whitehead SA (1983) *Mammalian Neuroendocrinology* (New York, Oxford University Press).

Benshushan A, Schenker JG (1993) Age limitation in human reproduction: is it justified? *Journal of Assisted Reproduction and Genetics* 10:321–331.

Berkowitz GS, Skovron ML, Lapinski RH, Berkowitz RL (1990) Delayed childbearing and the outcome of pregnancy. *New England Journal of Medicine* 322:659–664.

Beyene Y (1989) *From Menarche to Menopause: Reproductive Lives of Peasant Women in Two Cultures* (Albany, State University of New York Press).

Bogin B, Smith BH (1996) Evolution of the human life cycle. *American Journal of Human Biology* 8:703–716.

Buehler JW, Kaunitz AM, Hogue CJR, Hughes JM, Smith JC, Rochat RW (1986) Maternal mortality in women aged 35 years and older: United States. *Journal of the American Medical Association* 255:53–57.

Bustillo M, Buster JE, Cohen SW, Thorneycroft IH, Simon JA, Boyers SP, Marshall JR, Seed RW, Louw JA, Seed RG (1984) Non-surgical ovum transfer as a treatment in infertile women: a preliminary report. *Journal of the American Medical Association* 251:1171–1173.

Byskov AG (1978) Follicular atresia. In RE Jones (Ed) *The Vertebrate Ovary* (New York, Plenum), 533–562.

Caro TM, Sellen DW, Parish A, Frank R, Brown DM, Voland E, Borgerhoff Mulder M (1995) Termination of reproduction in nonhuman and human female primates. *International Journal of Primatology* 16:205–220.

Casey ML, MacDonald PC (1983) Origin of estrogen and regulation of its formation in postmenopausal women. In HJ Buchsbaum (Ed) *The Menopause* (New York, Springer-Verlag), 1–12.

Cavalli-Sforza LL (1983) The transition to agriculture and some of its consequences. In DJ Ortner (Ed) *How Humans Adapt: A Biocultural Odyssey* (Washington DC, Smithsonian Institution Press), 103–126.

Channing CP, Gordon WL, Liu WK, Ward DN (1985) Physiology and biochemistry of ovarian inhibin. *Proceedings of the Society for Experimental Biology and Medicine* 178:339–361.

Chetkowski RJ, Rode RA, Burruel V, Nass TE (1991) The effect of pituitary suppression and the women's age on embryo viability and uterine receptivity. *Fertility and Sterility* 56:1095–1103.

Cnattingius S, Forman MR, Berenedes HW, Isotalo L (1992) Delayed childbearing and risk of adverse perinatal outcome: a population-based study. *Journal of the American Medical Association* 268:886–890.

Comfort A (1979) *The Biology of Senescence* (New York, Elsevier).

Costoff A, Mahesh VB (1975) Primordial follicles with normal oocytes in the ovaries of postmenopausal women. *Journal of the American Geriatric Society* 23:193–196.

Crews DE, Gerber LM (1994) Chronic degenerative diseases and aging. In DE Crews, RM Garruto (Eds) *Biological Anthropology and Aging: Perspectives on Human Variation over the Life Span* (New York, Oxford University Press), 154–181.

Crisp TM (1992) Organization of the ovarian follicle and events in its biology: oogenesis, ovulation or atresia. *Mutation Research* 296:89–106.

Cutler RG (1976) Evolution of longevity in primates. *Journal of Human Evolution* 5:169–202.

Davidson JM, Chen JJ, Crapo L, Gray GD, Greenleaf WJ, Catania JA (1983) Hormonal changes and sexual function in aging men. *Journal of Clinical Endocrinology and Metabolism* 57:71–77.

Dennerstein L, Smith AMA, Morse C, Burger H, Green A, Hopper J, Ryan M (1993) Menopausal symptoms in Australian women. *Medical Journal of Australia* 159:232–236.

Deslypere JP, Vermeulen A (1984) Leydig cell function in normal men: effect of age, life style, residence, diet, and activity. *Journal of Clinical Endocrinology and Metabolism* 59:955–962.

DeStefano F, Annest JL, Kresnow MJ, Schrader SM, Katz DF (1989) Semen characteristics of Vietnam veterans. *Reproductive Toxicology* 3:165–173.

Diczfalusy E (1986) Menopause, developing countries and the 21st century. *Acta Obstetricia et Gynecologica Scandinavica* 134:45–57.

Donatucci CF, Lue TF (1993) Fibromuscular changes and the aging penis. In F Haseltine, CA Paulsen, C Wang (Eds) *Reproductive Issues and the Aging Male* (Washington DC, AAAS Publication 93-22S), 55–64.

Donaldson, JF (1994) How did the human menopause arise? *Menopause* 1:211–221.

Durham WH (1991) *Coevolution: Genes, Culture, and Human Diversity* (Stanford, Stanford University Press).

Eaton SB, Pike MC, Short RV, Lee NC, Trussell J, Hatcher RA, Wood JW, Worthman CM, Blurton Jones NG, Konner MJ, Hill KR, Bailey R, Hurtado AM (1994) Women's reproductive cancers in evolutionary context. *Quarterly Review of Biology* 69:353–366.

Edwards RG (1993) Pregnancies are acceptable in post-menopausal women. *Human Reproduction* 8:1542–1544.

Faddy MJ, Gosden RG, Gougeon A, Richardson SJ, Nelson JF (1992) Accelerated disappearance of ovarian follicles in mid-life: implications for forecasting menopause. *Human Reproduction* 7:1342–1346.

Federation CECOS, Schwartz D, Mayaux MJ (1982) Female fecundity as a function of age: results of artificial insemination in 2193 nulliparous women with azoospermic husbands. *New England Journal of Medicine* 306:404–406.

Ferin M, Van Vugt D, Wardlaw S (1984) The hypothalamic control of the menstrual cycle and the role of the endogenous opioid peptides. *Recent Progress in Hormone Research* 40:441–485.

Finch, CE (1990) *Longevity, Senescence, and the Genome* (Chicago, University of Chicago Press).

Flaws JA, Rhodes JC, Langenberg P, Hirshfield AN, Kjerulff K, Sharara FI (2000) Ovarian volume and menopausal status. *Menopause* 7:53–61.

Flint MP (1997) Secular trends in menopause age. *Journal of Psychosomatic Obstetrics and Gynaecology* 18:65–72.

Freedman RR (1989) Laboratory and ambulatory monitoring of menopausal hot flashes. *Psychophysiology* 26:573–579.

Freedman RR (1998) Biochemical, metabolic, and vascular mechanisms in menopausal hot flashes. *Fertility and Sterility* 70:332–337.

Freedman RR (2000) Hot flashes revisited (Editorial). *Menopause* 7:3–4.

Freedman RR, Norton D, Woodward S, Cornelissen G (1995) Core body temperature and circadian rhythm of hot flashes in menopausal women. *Journal of Clinical Endocrinology and Metabolism* 80:2354–2358.

Fretts RC, Schmittdiel J, McLean FH, Usher RH, Goldman MB (1995) Increased maternal age and the risk of fetal death. *New England Journal of Medicine* 333:953–957.

Gage TB, McCullough JM, Weitz CA, Dutt JS, Abelson A (1989) Demographic studies and human population biology. In MA Little, JD Haas (Eds) *Human Population Biology: A Transdisciplinary Science* (New York, Oxford University Press), 45–65.

Gaulin SJC (1980) Sexual dimorphism in the human post-reproductive life-span: possible causes. *Journal of Human Evolution* 9:227–232.

Genazzani AD, Petraglia F, Sgarbi L, Montanini V, Hartmann B, Surico N, Biolcati A, Volpe A, Genazzani AR (1997) Difference of LH and FSH secretory characteristics and degree of concordance between postmenopausal and aging women. *Maturitas* 26:133–138.

Gerber LM, Crews DE (1999) Evolutionary perspectives on chronic degenerative diseases. In WR Trevathan, EO Smith, JJ McKenna (Eds) *Evolutionary Medicine* (Oxford, Oxford University Press), 443–469.

Glynn RJ, Campion EW, Bouchard GR, Silbert JE (1985) The development of benign prostatic hyperplasia among volunteers in the normative aging study. *American Journal of Epidemiology* 121:78–90.

Gosden RG (1985a) *Biology of Menopause: The Causes and Consequences of Ovarian Ageing* (New York, Academic Press).

Gosden RG (1985b) Maternal age: a major factor affecting the prospects and outcome of pregnancy. *Annals of the New York Academy of Science* 442:45–57.

Gougeon A (1996) Regulation of ovarian follicular development in primates: facts and hypotheses. *Endocrine Reviews* 17:121–155.

Gougeon A, Ecochard R, Thalabard JC (1994) Age-related changes of the population of human ovarian follicles: increase in the disappearance rate of nongrowing and early-growing follicles in aging women. *Biology of Reproduction* 50:653–663.

Gould K, Flint M, Graham C (1981) Chimpanzee reproductive senescence: a possible model for evolution of the menopause. *Maturitas* 3:157–166.

Gould SJ, Lewontin RC (1979) The spandrels of San Marco and the Panglossian paradigm: a critique of the adaptationist programme. *Proceedings of the Royal Society of London, B* 205:581–598.

Grady D (1999) Experiment seeks to protect ovaries from cancer treatment. *The New York Times* (October 26):D7.

Gray RH (1976) The menopause—epidemiological and demographic considerations. In RJ Beard (Ed) *The Menopause* (Baltimore, University Park Press), 25–40.

Guraya SS (1985) *Biology of Ovarian Follicles in Mammals* (New York, Springer-Verlag).

Guthrie JR, Dennerstein L, Hopper JL, Burger HG (1996) Hot flushes, menstrual status, and hormone levels in a population-based sample of midlife women. *Obstetrics and Gynecology* 88:437–442.

Hahn PM, Wong J, Reid RL (1998) Menopausal-like hot flashes reported in women of reproductive age. *Fertility and Sterility* 70:913–918.

Harman SM, Tsitouras PD (1980) Reproductive hormones in aging men, I. Measurement of sex steroids, basal luteinizing hormone, and Leydig cell response to human chorionic gonadotropin. *Journal of Clinical Endocrinology and Metabolism* 51:35–40.

Harrell, BB (1977) Lactation and menstruation in cultural perspective. *American Anthropologist* 83:796–823.

Hawkes K, O'Connell JF, Blurton-Jones NG (1997) Hadza women's time allocation, offspring provisioning, and the evolution of long post-menopausal life spans. *Current Anthropology* 38:551–557.

Highfield R (1999) Menopause reversed: how to beat the biological clock. *The Daily Telegraph* (London) (September 23):2.

Hill K, Hurtado AM (1991) The evolution of premature reproductive sensecence and menopause in human females: an evaluation of the "grandmother hypothesis." *Human Nature* 2:313–350.

Hodgen G, Goodman A, O'Connor A, Johnson D (1977) Menopause in rhesus monkeys: model for study of disorders in the human climacteric. *American Journal of Obstetrics and Gynecology* 127:581–584.

Hsing AW, Tsao L, Devesa SS (2000) International trends and patterns of prostate cancer incidence and mortality. *International Journal of Cancer* 85:60–67.

Jiroutek MR, Chen M-H, Johnston CC, Longcope C (1998) Changes in reproductive hormones and sex hormone-binding globulin in a group of postmenopausal women measured over 10 years. *Menopause* 5(2):90–94.

Johnson L, Zane RS, Petty CS, Neaves WB (1984) Quantification of the human Sertoli cell population: its distribution, relation to germ cell numbers, and age-related decline. *Biology of Reproduction* 31:785–795.

Judd HL, Judd GE, Lucas WE, Yen SSC (1974) Endocrine function of the postmenopausal ovary: concentration of androgens and estrogens in ovarian and peripheral vein blood. *Journal of Clinical Endocrinology and Metabolism* 39: 1020–1024.

Kaiser FE, Morley JE, Korenman SG (1993) Hypothalamic function and its relationship to impotence. In F Haseltine, CA Paulsen, C Wang (Eds) *Reproductive Issues and the Aging Male* (Washington DC, AAAS Publication 93-22S), 77–87.

Kaufman DW, Slone D, Rosenberg L, Miettinen OS, Shapiro S (1980) Cigarette smoking and age at natural menopause. *American Journal of Public Health* 70:420–422.

Kinsey AC, Popmeroy WB, Martin CE (1948) *Sexual Behavior in the Human Male* (Philadelphia, WB Saunders).

Kirz DS, Dorchester W, Freeman RK (1985) Advanced maternal age: the mature gravida. *American Journal of Obstetrics and Gynecology* 152:7–12.

Kluge E-H (1994) Reproductive technology and postmenopausal motherhood. *Canadian Medical Association Journal* 151:353–354.

Kohn, RR (1971) *Principles of Mammalian Aging* (Englewood Cliffs, NJ, Prentice-Hall).

Kolata G (1997) A record and big questions as woman gives birth at 63. *New York Times* (April 24):A1, A25.

Korenman SG, Sherman BM, Korenman JC (1978) Reproductive hormone function: the perimenopausal period and beyond. *Clinics in Endocrinology and Metabolism* 7:625–643.

Korenman SG, Morley JE, Morradian AD, Davis SS, Kaiser FE, Silver AJ, Viosca SP, Garza D (1990) Secondary hypogonadism in older men: its relation to impotence. *Journal of Clinical Endocrinology and Metabolism* 71:963–969.

Kronenberg F (1994) Hot flashes: phenomenology, quality of life, and search for treatment options. *Experimental Gerontology* 29:319–336.

Lancaster, JB, Lancaster CS (1983) Parental investment: the hominid adaptation. In DJ Ortner (Ed) *How Humans Adapt: A Biocultural Odyssey* (Washington DC, Smithsonian Institute Press), 33–65.

Lancet (1993) Editorial: Too old to have a baby? *Lancet* 341:344–345.

Lapin BA, Krilova RI, Cherkovich G, Asanov S (1979) Observations from Sukhumi. In D Bowden (Ed) *Aging in Nonhuman Primates* (New York, Van Nostrand Reinhold), 183–202.

Laumann EO, Paik A, Rosen RC (1999) Sexual dysfunction in the United States: prevalence and predictors. *Journal of the American Medical Association* 281: 537–544.

Leidy LE (1994) Biological aspects of menopause: across the lifespan. *Annual Review of Anthropology* 23:231–253.

Leidy LE (1996) The timing of menopause in relation to body size and weight change. *Human Biology* 68:997–1012.

Leidy LE (1999) Menopause in evolutionary perspective. In WR Trevethan, EO Smith, JJ McKenna (Eds) *Evolutionary Medicine* (Oxford, Oxford University Press), 407–427.

Leidy LE, Godfrey LR, Sutherland MR (1998) Is follicular atresia biphasic? *Fertility and Sterility* 70:851–859.

Leidy Sievert L, Waddle D, Canali K (2001) Marital status and age at menopause: considering pheromonal influence. *American Journal of Human Biology* 13, in press.

Levran D, Ben-Shlomo I, Dor J, Ben-Rafael Z, Nebel L, Mashiach S (1991) Aging of endometrium and oocytes: observations on conception and abortion rates in an egg donation model. *Fertility and Sterility* 56:1091–1094.

Lock M (1993) *Encounters with Aging: Mythologies of Menopause in Japan and North America* (Berkeley, University of California Press).

Lock M (1998) Menopause: lessons from anthropology. *Psychosomatic Medicine* 60:410–419.

Longcope C, Franz C, Morello C, Baker R, Johnston CC (1986) Steroid and gonadotropin levels in women during the perimenopausal years. *Maturitas* 8:189–196.

Luoto R, Kaprio J, Uutela A (1994) Age at natural menopause and sociodemographic status in Finland. *American Journal of Epidemiology* 139:64–76.

Lutjen P, Trounson A, Leeton J, Findlay J, Wood C, Renou P (1984) The establishment and maintenance of pregnancy using in vitro fertilization and embryo donation in a patient with primary ovarian failure. *Nature* 307:174–175.

Manderson L (1999) Social meanings and sexual bodies: gender, sexuality and barriers to women's health care. In TM Pollard, SB Hyatt (Eds) *Sex, Gender and Health* (Cambridge, Cambridge University Press), 75–93.

Martin MC, Block JE, Sanchez SD, Arnaud CD, Beyene Y (1993) Menopause without symptoms: the endocrinology of menopause among rural Mayan Indians. *American Journal of Obstetrics and Gynecology* 168:1839–1845.

Martin RH, Rademaker AW (1987) The effect of age on the frequency of sperm chromosomal abnormalities in normal men. *American Journal of Human Genetics* 41:484–492.

Matsumoto AM (1993) Aging and human male reproductive function. In F Haseltine, CA Paulsen, C Wang (Eds) *Reproductive Issues and the Aging Male* (Washington DC, AAAS Publication 93-22S), 1–14.

Matt DW, Lee J, Sarver PL, Judd HL, Lu JKH (1986) Chronological changes in fertility, fecundity and steroid hormone secretion during consecutive pregnancies in aging rats. *Biology of Reproduction* 34:478–487.

McDonough PG (1999) Factoring in complexity and oocyte memory—Can transformations and cyperpathology distort reality? (Editorial Comment) *Fertility and Sterility* 71:1172–1174.

Meites J, Huang H, Simpkins J, Steger R (1982) Central nervous system neurotransmitters during the decline of reproductive activity. In P Fiorette, L Martini, G Melis, S Yen (Eds) *The Menopause: Clinical, Endocrinological and Pathophysiological Aspects* (New York, Academic Press), 3–13.

Meites J, Lu JKH (1994) Reproductive ageing and neuroendocrine function. *Oxford Reviews of Reproductive Biology* 16:215–247.

Meldrum DR (1993) Female reproductive ageing—ovarian and uterine factors. *Fertility and Sterility* 59:1–5.

Merry BJ, Holehan AM (1994a) Aging of the female reproductive system: the menopause. In PS Timiras (Ed) *Physiological Basis of Aging and Geriatrics*, second ed. (Ann Arbor, CRC Press), 147–170.

Merry BJ, Holehan AM (1994b) Aging of the male reproductive system. In PS Timiras (Ed) *Physiological Basis of Aging and Geriatrics*, second ed. (Ann Arbor, CRC Press), 171–178.

Metcalf MG, Donald RA, Livesey JH (1981) Pituitary-ovarian function in normal women during the menopausal transition. *Clinical Endocrinology* 14:245–255.

Mori T (1994) Post-menopausal pregnancy is permissible for women below 60 years of age. *Human Reproduction* 9:187.

Mulligan T, Retchin SM, Chinchilli VM, Bettinger CB (1988) The role of aging and chronic disease in sexual dysfunction. *Journal of the American Geriatric Society* 36:520–524.

Navot D, Bergh PA, Williams MA, Garrisa GJ, Guzman I, Sandler B, Grunfeld L (1991) Poor oocyte quality rather than implantation failure as a cause of age-related decline in female fertility. *Lancet* 337:1375–1377.

Neaves WB, Johnson L, Porter JC, Parker CR, Petty CS (1984) Leydig cell numbers, daily sperm production, and serum gonadotropin levels in aging men. *Journal of Clinical Endocrinology and Metabolism* 55:756–763.

Nelson JF, Felicio LS (1985) Reproductive aging in the female: an etiological perspective. *Review of Biological Research in Aging* 2:251–314.

Nieschlag E, Michel E (1986) Reproductive functions in grandfathers. In L Mastroianni, CA Paulsen (Eds) *Aging, Reproduction and the Climacteric* (New York, Plenum Press), 59–71.

Nieschlag E, Lammers U, Freischem CW, Langer K, Wickings EJ (1982) Reproductive function in young fathers and grandfathers. *Journal of Clinical Endocrinology and Metabolism* 55:676–681.

Novak ER (1970) Ovulation after fifty. *Obstetrics and Gynecology* 36:903–910.

Obermeyer CM (2000) Menopause across cultures: a review of the evidence. *Menopause* 7:184–192.

O'Connor KA, Holman DJ, Wood JW (1998) Declining fecundity and ovarian aging in natural fertility populations. *Maturitas* 30:127–136.

O'Donnell P, Stevenson S, Stefanakos VS (1999) No Apollos. *Newsweek* (November 29):8.

O'Rourke MT, Ellison PT (1993) Menopause and ovarian senescence in human females. *American Journal of Physical Anthropology* (Suppl.16):154.

Parazzini F, Negri E, La Vecchia C (1992) Reproductive and general lifestyle determinants of age at menopause. *Maturitas* 15:141–149.

Parkening TA (1989) Fertilizing ability of spermatozoa from aged C57BL/6NNia mice. *Journal of Reproduction and Fertility* 87:727–733.

Paulson RJ, Sauer MV (1994) Oocyte donation to women of advanced reproductive age: how old is too old? *Human Reproduction* 9:571–572.

Paulson RJ, Thornton MH, Francis MM, Salvador HS (1997) Successful pregnancy in a 63-year-old woman. *Fertility and Sterility* 67:949–951.

Pavelka MS, Fedigan LM (1991) Menopause: a comparative life history perspective. *Yearbook of Physical Anthropology* 34:13–38.

Pavelka MSM, Fedigan LM (1999) Reproductive termination in female Japanese monkeys: a comparative life history perspective. *American Journal of Physical Anthropology* 109:455–464.

Peacock N (1991) An evolutionary perspective on the patterning of maternal investment in pregnancy. *Human Nature* 2:351–385.

Peccei JS (1995) A hypothesis for the origin and evolution of menopause. *Maturitas* 21:83–89.

Peters H, McNatty KP (1980) *The Ovary* (New York, Granada).

Pollard I (1994) *A Guide to Reproduction: Social Issues and Human Concerns* (Cambridge, Cambridge Univeristy Press).

Rannevik G, Jeppsson S, Johnell O, Bjerre B, Laurell-Borulf Y, Svanberg L (1995) A longitudinal study of the perimenopausal transition: altered profiles of steroid and pituitary hormones, SHBG and bone mineral density. *Maturitas* 21:103–113.

Reame NE, Kelche RP, Beitins IZ, Yu MY, Zawacki CM, Padmanabhan V (1996) Age effects of FSH and pulsatile LH secretion across the menstrual cycle of premenopausal women. *Journal of Clinical Endocrinology and Metabolism* 81:1512–1518.

Renshaw DC (1993) Libido and aging: didactic issues. In F Haseltine, CA Paulsen,

C Wang (Eds) *Reproductive Issues and the Aging Male* (Washington DC, AAAS Publication 93-22S), 49–54.

Richardson SJ, Senika V, Nelson J (1987) Follicular depletion during the menopausal transition: evidence for accelerated loss and ultimate exhaustion. *Journal of Clinical Endocrinology and Metabolism* 65:1231–1237.

Sacher GA (1978) Evolution of longevity and survival characteristics in mammals. In EL Schneider (Ed) *The Genetics of Aging* (New York, Plenum Press), 151–168.

Sadleir RM (1973) *The Reproduction of Vertebrates* (New York, Academic Press).

Santoro N (1996) Hormonal changes in the perimenopause. *Clinical Consultations in Obstetrics and Gynecology* 8:2–8.

Sauer MV, Paulson RJ, Lobo RA (1992) Reversing the natural decline in human fertility: an extended clinical trial of oocyte donation to women of advanced reproductive age. *Journal of the American Medical Association* 268:1275–1279.

Sauer MV, Paulson RJ, Lobo RA (1993) Pregnancy after age 50: application of oocyte donation to women after natural menopause. *Lancet* 341:321–323.

Sauer MV, Paulson RJ, Lobo RA (1995) Pregnancy in women 50 or more years of age: outcomes of 22 consecutively established pregnancies from oocyte donation. *Fertility and Sterility* 64:111–115.

Schmidt-Sarosi C (1998) Infertility in the older woman. *Clinical Obstetrics and Gynecology* 41:940–950.

Schrader SM (1993) Environmental toxicants: identification and impact. In F Haseltine, CA Paulsen, C Wang (Eds) *Reproductive Issues and the Aging Male* (Washington DC, AAAS Publication 93- 22S), 123–129.

Sherman BM (1987) Endocrinologic and menstrual alterations. In DR Mishell (Ed) *Menopause: Physiology and Pharmacology* (Chicago, Year Book Medical), 41–51.

Simpkins JW, Mueller GP, Huang HH, Meites J (1977) Evidence for depressed catecholamine and enhanced serotonin metabolism in aging male rats: possible relation to gonadotropin secretion. *Endocrinology* 100:1672–1678.

Smith P (1993) Selfish genes and maternal myths: a look at postmenopausal pregnancy. In JC Callahan (Ed) *Menopause: A Midlife Passage* (Bloomington, Indiana University Press), 92–119.

Spence AP (1989) *Biology of Human Aging* (Englewood Cliffs, NJ, Prentice Hill)

Stanford JL, Hartge P, Brinton LA, Hoover RN, Brookmeyer R (1987) Factors influencing the age at natural menopause. *Journal of Chronic Disease* 40:955–1002.

Stein ZA (1985) A woman's age: childbearing and child rearing *American Journal of Epidemiology* 121:327–342.

Tenover JS (1993) Systemic effects of testosterone replacement in older men. In F Haseltine, CA Paulsen, C Wang (Eds) *Reproductive Issues and the Aging Male* (Washington DC, AAAS Publication 93-22S), 109–121.

Thomford, PJ, Jelovsek FR, Mattison DR (1987) Effect of oocyte number and rate of atresia on the age of menopause. *Reproductive Toxicology* 1:41–51.

Timiras ML (1994) The kidney, the lower urinary tract, the prostate, and body fluids. In PS Timiras (Ed) *Physiological Basis of Aging and Geriatrics*, second ed. (Ann Arbor, CRC Press), 235–246.

Treloar AE (1981) Menstrual cyclicity and the pre-menopause. *Maturitas* 3:249–264.

Tur-Kaspa I, Segal S, Moffa F, Massobrio M, Meltzer S (1999) Viagra for temporary erectile dysfunction during treatments with assisted reproductive technologies. *Human Reproduction* 14:1783–1784.

Turke PW (1988) Helpers at the nest: childcare networks on Ifaluk. In L Betzig, M Borgerhoff Mulder, P Turke (Eds) *Human Reproductive Behavior: A Darwinian Perspective* (New York, Cambridge University Press), 173–188.

Walker ML (1995) Menopause in female rhesus monkeys. *American Journal of Primatology* 35:59–71.

Watts ES (1986) Evolution of the human growth curve. In F Falkner, JM Tanner (Eds) *Human Growth: A Comprehensive Treatise*, 1 (New York, Plenum Press), 153–166.

Whelan E, Sandler D, McConnaughey D, Weinberg C (1990) Menstrual and reproductive characteristics and age at natural menopause. *American Journal of Epidemiology* 13:625–632.

Whitehead, MI, Whitcroft SIJ, Hillard TC (1993) *An Atlas of the Menopause* (New York, Parthenon).

Whorton MD (1984) Environmental and occupational reproductive hazards. In JM Swanson and KA Forrest (Eds) *Men's Reproductive Health* (New York, Springer), 193–203.

Willet W, Stampfer MJ, Bain C, Lipnick R, Speizer FE, Rosner B, Cramer D, Hennekens CH (1983) Cigarette smoking, relative weight and menopause. *American Journal of Epidemiology* 117:651–658.

Wise PM, Kashon ML, Krajnak KM, Rosewell KL, Cai A, Scarbrough K, Harney JP, McShane T, Lloyd JM, Weiland NG (1997) Aging of the female reproductive system: a window into brain aging. *Recent Progress in Hormone Research* 52:279–305.

Wood JW (1994) *Dynamics of Human Reproduction: Biology, Biometry, Demography* (New York, Aldine de Gruyter).

Wood JW, Weeks SC, Bentley, Weiss KM (1994) Human population biology and the evolution of aging. In DE Crews and RM Garruto (Eds) *Biological Anthropology and Aging: Perspectives on Human Variation over the Life Span* (New York, Oxford University Press), 19–75.

World Health Organization (1981) *Research on Menopause.* Technical Report Series 670 (Geneva, WHO).

World Health Organization (1996) *Summary of Research on Menopause in the 1990s.* Technical Report Series 866 (Geneva, WHO).

13

The Embodied Capital Theory of Human Evolution

HILLARD KAPLAN, KIM HILL, A. MAGDALENA
HURTADO, and JANE LANCASTER

This paper presents a theoretical approach to life history evolution with the goal of shedding new light on important problems in human evolution and the evolution of primates, in general. Life history theory (LHT) in biology organizes research into the evolutionary forces shaping the timing of life events, with a particular focus on age-schedules of fertility and mortality (Cole 1954; Gadgil and Bossert 1970; Partridge and Harvey 1985). We integrate standard approaches to life history evolution with an economic analysis of capital investments and energy production to generate new theoretical models capable of addressing many of the fundamental problems in the evolution of our species. We refer to this approach as *the embodied capital theory of life history evolution*.

After presenting a brief introduction to this theoretical perspective we apply the theory to understanding major trends in primate evolution and the specific characteristics of humans. We first address the evolution of brain size, intelligence, and life histories in the primate order. We then consider the evolution of the human life course, including mortality and longevity, reproduction, learning and development, the timing of energy production, the sexual division of labor, and pair bonding. Together, these analyses illustrate both continuities and discontinuities between humans and other primates.

THE EMBODIED CAPITAL THEORY OF
LIFE HISTORY EVOLUTION

According to the theory of evolution by natural selection, the evolution of life is the result of a process in which variant forms compete to harvest

293

energy from the environment and convert that energy into replicates of those forms. Those forms that can capture more energy than others and can convert the energy they acquire into replicates more efficiently than others become more prevalent through time. This simple issue of harvesting energy and converting energy into offspring generates many complex problems that are time-dependent.

Two fundamental trade-offs determine the action of natural selection on reproductive schedules and mortality rates. The first trade-off is between current and future reproduction. By growing, an organism can increase its future energy capture rates and thus its future fertility. For this reason, organisms typically have a juvenile phase in which fertility is zero until they reach a size at which some allocation to reproduction increases fitness more than allocation to growth would. Similarly, among organisms that engage in repeated bouts of reproduction (humans included), some energy during the reproductive phase is diverted away from reproduction and allocated to maintenance so that it can live to reproduce again. Natural selection is expected to optimize the allocation of energy to current reproduction and to future reproduction (via investments in growth and maintenance) at each point in the life course so that genetic descendents are maximized (Gadgil and Bossert 1970). Variation in optimal energy allocations across taxa and across conditions is shaped by such ecological factors as food supply, disease, and predation rates.

A second fundamental life history trade-off is between offspring number (quantity) and offspring fitness (quality). This trade-off occurs because parents have limited resources in which to invest in offspring and each additional offspring produced necessarily reduces average investment per offspring. Most biological models (Lack 1954; Lloyd 1987; Smith and Fretwell 1974) operationalize this trade-off as number versus survival of offspring. However, parental investment may affect not only survival to adulthood but also the adult productivity and fertility of offspring. This is especially true of humans. Thus, natural selection is expected to shape investment per offspring and offspring number so as to maximize offspring number times their average lifetime fitness.

The embodied capital theory generalizes existing life history theory by treating the processes of growth, development, and maintenance as investments in stocks of somatic or embodied capital. In a physical sense, embodied capital is organized somatic tissue—muscles, digestive organs, brains, and so forth. In a functional sense, embodied capital includes strength, speed, immune function, skill, knowledge, and other abilities. Since such stocks tend to depreciate with time, allocations to maintenance can also be seen as investments in embodied capital. Thus, the present-future reproductive trade-off can be understood in terms of optimal investments in own embodied capital versus reproduction, and the quantity-quality trade-off can be understood in terms of investments in the embodied capital of off-spring versus their number.

The embodied capital theory allows us to address problems that have not been addressed with standard life history models. An exclusive focus on physical growth per se is an impoverished way of understanding development. The large human brain, for example, is a stock of embodied capital that supports a great deal of learning and knowledge acquisition during both the juvenile and adult periods. The growth in knowledge may be as important as growth in body size with respect to providing benefits through time.

Models of investment in embodied capital have produced some fundamental results. Of central interest here, the models show that investments in embodied capital affecting adult income or energy capture coevolve with investments affecting mortality and longevity (Kaplan and Robson 2000b; Kaplan et al. 2000b). The longer the time spent growing and learning prior to reproducing, the more natural selection favors investments in staying alive to reap the benefits of those investments. Similarly, any investments that increase energy capture rates later in life select for additional investments to reach those older ages. The converse is also true. Ecological features or investments that increase the probability of survival to older ages also produce selection for greater investments in income-related embodied capital. A central thesis of this paper is that these co-evolutionary effects have been particularly important in primate and hominid evolution.

EMBODIED-CAPITAL EVOLUTION AMONG PRIMATES

Relative to other mammalian orders, the primate order can be characterized as slow-growing, slow-reproducing, long-lived, and large-brained. Although there is a great deal of variation within the order in terms of life history characteristics and brain size, the radiation of the order over time has involved a series of four directional grade shifts towards slowed life histories and increased encephalization (i.e., brain size relative to body size).[1]

The first grade shift, beginning about 60 mya with the evolution of prosimians, is towards a longer lifespan (Kaplan and Robson 2000a), probably owing to the safety of the arboreal habitat (Austad and Fischer 1991, 1992). The second major grade shift began about 35 mya with the evolution of the anthropoid lineage and involves a large increase in both brain size and lifespan, relative to prosimians. This shift is evident among extant monkeys. The major defining characteristic of the anthropoids is the reorganization of the sensory system from one in which olfaction and hearing are relatively dominant to one dominated by binocular, color vision and by a switch in feeding behavior from insects to plant foods using a manipulating hand and hand-eye coordination (Fleagle 1999). Apes represent the third major grade shift in primates. Controlling for the allometric relations between brain size and body size, the great apes have the largest brains among nonhominid primates and also live more than twice as long as most monkeys. This shift is most likely due to increased emphasis on complex, extractive foraging techniques (Byrne 1997b; Parker and Gibson 1979). Comparison of intercepts among prosimians, monkeys, and apes in regression analyses of brain size on body size confirm the existence of these grade shifts (Allman, McLaughlin, and Hakeem 1993; Barton 1999). The fourth major grade shift occurs with the divergence of the hominid line, particularly the evolution of genus *Homo*. Controlling for body size, *Homo sapiens* has a brain about three times as large and a lifespan about twice as long as chimpanzees and gorillas, our closet living relatives.

The brain is a special form of embodied capital. On the one hand, neural tissue is involved in monitoring the organism's internal and external environment, and organizing physiological and behavioral adjustments to those stimuli. On the other, portions of the brain are involved in transforming present experiences into future performance. This is particularly true of the cerebral cortex, which is specialized towards the storage, retrieval, and processing of experiences. The expansion of the cerebral cortex among higher primates, along with their enhanced learning abilities (Armstrong and Falk 1982; Fleagle 1999), is indicative of increased investment in transforming present experience into future performance.

The action of natural selection on neural tissue involved in learning, memory, and the processing of stored information depends on costs and benefits realized over the organism's lifetime. First are the initial energetic costs of growing the brain. Among mammals, those costs are largely borne by the mother. Second are the energetic costs of maintaining neural tissue. In fact, as much as 65% of all resting energetic expenditure is used to support the maintenance and growth of the brain during the first year of a human's life (Holliday 1978). A third potential cost of the brain is decreased performance early in life. The ability to learn and increased behavioral flexibility may entail reductions in "pre-programmed" behavioral routines, which would enhance early performance. The incompetence of human infants, and even children, in many motor tasks is an example.

The benefits of the brain tissue involved in learning are realized as the organism ages. Those benefits are likely to depend, at least in part, on the impact of learning on food acquisition. Some features of the feeding niche are likely to affect the payoffs to information storage and processing and, hence, brain size. Spatial patchiness of resources tends to be associated with larger home ranges and potentially greater demands on spatial memory. The number of different species consumed potentially adds to demands for

spatial memory, learned motor patterns, processing of resource characteristics, and temporal associations. Large, nutrient-dense packages (such as
big, ripe fruits) tend to be patchily distributed in space and often have very
short windows of availability. There is also significant year-to-year variability in abundance and location of these high-quality packages, increasing the demands for monitoring the environment and predicting the best
time to harvest them. Diets with an emphasis on large, high-quality packages are probably associated with increased brain size through several
routes: by increasing the total number of species exploited, the size of the
home range, and the importance of predicting the timing and location of
availability. In addition, such high-quality foods as nuts, insects, and honey
need to be extracted from protective casings, and their exploitation requires
learned strategies and often tools.

Feeding niches with high demands for learning and information processing should select not only for increased brain size but also for
increased effort at reducing mortality. This is because the brain has high
costs early in life and provides benefits later in life. Thus, living longer is
more beneficial. At the same time, there is ecological variability in mortality risks. Life in or near trees probably increases injury risk but decreases
predation risk to lower mortality risks overall. Other factors such as body
size, daily activity patterns, predator density, and disease risk are also
likely to affect mortality rates. The results from modeling embodied capital investments discussed above suggest that those risks also affect selection on brain size, since higher risks of dying reduce the expected time
over which the brain will confer benefits.

Following others (e.g., Dunbar 1998; Jerison 1976; Milton 1993) we
hypothesize that much of the increase in primate brain size, relative to
other mammals, is due to increases in the ability to store and process
learned information. We hypothesize further that the protection conferred
by the arboreal environment in terms of the ability to escape predation and
the types of foods available in trees favored entry into a learning-intensive
feeding niche and the evolution of large brains.

These hypotheses, together with the analytical results discussed above,
generate three predictions about variation among extant nonhuman primates. The first is that features of the ecology that increase the productivity of a large brain, such as a large home range and a diet emphasizing ripe
fruits (Clutton-Brock and Harvey 1980), would be associated with both
increased brain size and a longer lifespan. Second, a longer lifespan would
be associated with an increased brain size, even after controlling for the
feeding niche. Third, larger-brained species would allocate more effort to
survival, which would be reflected in slower grow rates and later first
reproduction. Results of a path analysis of 101 primate species are fully
consistent with those predictions (Kaplan et al. 2000a). Home range size

and percent of fruit in the diet are strongly associated with both maximum lifespan and brain size. Controlling for feeding niche and body size, maximum lifespan is also positively associated with brain size. Finally, controlling for body size, longer-lived and larger-brained species reach their adult body weight at a later age than shorter-lived, smaller-brained species, indicating slower growth and greater effort towards survival.

THE EVOLUTION OF *HOMO:* CHIMPANZEES AND MODERN HUMANS COMPARED

Can the same principles explain the very long lives and the very large brains characteristic of the genus *Homo* and particularly of modern *Homo sapiens?* Our theory is that these extreme values with respect to brain size and longevity are coevolved responses to an equally extreme commitment to learning-intensive foraging strategies and a dietary shift towards high-quality, nutrient-dense, and difficult-to-acquire food resources. The following logic underlies our proposal. First, high levels of knowledge, skill, coordination, and strength are required to exploit the suite of high-quality, difficult-to-acquire resources humans consume. The attainment of those abilities requires time and a significant commitment to development. Higher productivity during the adult period compensates for this extended learning phase during which productivity is low, with an intergenerational flow of food from old to young. Since productivity increases with age, the time investment in skill acquisition and knowledge leads to selection for lowered mortality rates and greater longevity because the returns on the investments in development occur at older ages.

Second, we believe that the feeding niche specializing on large, valuable food packages, and particularly hunting, promotes cooperation between men and women and high levels of male parental investment because it favors sex-specific specialization in embodied capital investments and generates a complementarity between male and female inputs. The economic and reproductive cooperation between men and women facilitates provisioning of juveniles, which both bankrolls their embodied capital investments and acts to lower mortality during the juvenile and early adult periods. Cooperation between males and females also allows women to allocate more time to child care and increases nutritional status, increasing both survival and reproductive rates. Finally, large packages also appear to promote interfamilial food sharing. Food sharing assists recovery in times of illness and reduces risk of food shortfalls owing both to the vagaries of foraging luck and to variance in family size resulting from stochastic mortality and fertility. These buffers against mortality also favor a longer juvenile period and higher investment in other mechanisms to increase lifespan.

Thus, we propose that the long human lifespan coevolved with the lengthening of the juvenile period, increased brain capacities for information processing and storage, and intergenerational resource flows—all as a result of an important dietary shift. Humans are specialists in that they only consume the highest-quality plant and animal resources in their local ecology and rely on creative, skill-intensive techniques to exploit them. Yet, the capacity to develop new techniques for extractive foraging and hunting allows them to exploit a wide variety of different foods and to colonize all of the Earth's terrestrial and coastal ecosystems.

This theory generates a series of test implications. We must show that (1) humans do, in fact, exhibit lower mortality rates, especially in adulthood, than apes; (2) the human diet differs from the ape diet in the proportional contribution of difficult-to-acquire, high-quality foods; (3) difficulty of acquisition is positively associated with age-effects on return rate for both apes and humans; (4) the greater proportion of high-quality foods in human diets causes a shift in energy production towards older ages, favoring a longer adult lifespan; (5) hunting and the acquisition of large packages of food favor sex-specific investments in embodied capital and male-female cooperation; and (6) large packages also promote interfamilial food sharing and cooperation, and those adaptations lower mortality. In this paper, we consider the first five test implications. We only briefly consider interfamilial sharing and cooperation in the discussion since the sixth prediction has been confirmed elsewhere (Gurven, Hill et al. 2000; Kaplan and Hill 1985; Winterhalder 1996).

Mortality and Survival

About 60% of hunter-gatherer children survive to age 15, compared with 35% of chimpanzees (Table 13.1, Figure 13.1).[2] Chimpanzees spend less time as juveniles than humans, with age at first birth for chimpanzee females about 5 years earlier than among hunter-gatherer women. In natural habitats chimpanzees have a much shorter adult lifespan than humans. At age 15 chimpanzee life expectancy is an additional 15 years, compared with 39 more years among human foragers. Importantly, women spend more than a third of their adult life in a postreproductive phase, whereas very few chimpanzee females survive to reach the postreproductive phase. Less than 10% of chimpanzees ever born survive to age 40, but more than 15% of hunter-gatherers survive to age 70!

Composition of the Diet

There are ten foraging societies and five chimpanzee communities for which caloric production or time spent feeding were monitored systematically (Kaplan et al. 2000a: Table 4). Modern foragers' diets all differ

Table 13.1.   Life History Characteristics and Diet of Human Foragers and Chimpanzees

	Human Foragers	Chimpanzees
LIFE HISTORY CHARACTERISTICS		
Maximum lifespan	~120	~60
Probability of survival to age 15	0.6	0.35
Expected age of death at 15 (years)	54.3	29.7
Mean age first reproduction (years)	19.7	14.3
Mean age last reproduction (years)	39	27.7**
Interbirth interval* (months)	41.3	66.7
Mean weight at age 5 (kg)	15.7	10
Mean weight at age 10 (kg)	24.9	22.5
COMPOSITION OF DIET (%)		
Collected	9	94
Extracted	31	4
Hunted	60	2

CONTRIBUTIONS BY SEX (%)	Men	Women	
Adult calories	68	32	Sexes
Adult protein	88	12	Independent
Caloric support for offspring	97	3	
Protein support for offspring	100	0	

*Mean interbirth interval following a surviving infant.
**Age of last reproduction for chimpanzee females was estimated as two years
    prior to the mean adult life expectancy.

considerably from that of chimpanzees. Measured in calories, the major component of forager diets is vertebrate meat. This ranges from about 30% to around 80% of the diet in the sampled societies with most diets consisting of more than 50% vertebrate meat (equally weighted mean = 60%, Table 13.1), whereas chimpanzees obtain about 2% of their food energy from hunted foods.

The next most important food category in the forager sample is extracted resources, such as roots, nuts, seeds, most invertebrate products, and difficult-to-extract plant parts such as palm fiber or growing shoots. They may be defined as non-mobile resources that are embedded in a protective context such as underground, in hard shells, or bearing toxins that must be removed before they can be consumed. In the sample of ten forager groups, extracted foods account for about 32% of the diet as opposed to 3% among chimpanzees.

In contrast to hunted and extracted resources, which are difficult to acquire, collected resources form the bulk of the chimpanzee diet. Collected resources such as fruits, leaves, flowers, and other easily accessible

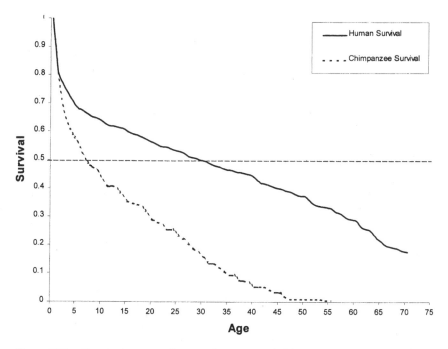

Figure 13.1. Survival curves: Human foragers and chimpanzees

plant parts are simply gathered and consumed. They account for 95% of the chimpanzee diet, on average, and only 8% of the forager diet.

The data suggest that humans specialize in rare but nutrient-dense resource packages or patches (meat, roots, nuts) whereas chimpanzees specialize in ripe fruit and low-nutrient-density plant parts. These differences in nutrient density are also reflected in human and chimpanzee gut morphology and food passage time, with chimpanzees specialized for rapid processing of large quantities and low-nutrient, bulky, fibrous meals (Milton 1999).

The Age Profile of Acquisition for Collected, Extracted, and Hunted Resources

In most environments, fruits are the easiest resources that people acquire. Daily production data among Ache foragers show that both males and females reach their peak daily fruit production by their mid to late teens. Some fruits that are simply picked from the ground are collected by two- to three-year-olds at 30% of the adult maximum rate. Ache children acquire five times as many calories per day during the fruit season as during other seasons of the year (Kaplan 1997). Similarly, among the Hadza, teen girls acquired 1,650 calories per day during the wet season when fruits were available and only 610 calories per day during the dry season when fruits were not. If we weight the wet- and dry-season data equally, Hadza teen girls acquire 53% of their calories from fruits compared with 37% and 19% for reproductive-age and postreproductive women, respectively (all calculated from Hawkes, O'Connell, and Blurton Jones 1989).

The acquisition rate of extracted resources, in contrast to that of fruits, often increases through early adulthood as foragers acquire necessary skills. Data on Hiwi women show that root acquisition rates do not reach an asymptote until about age 35–45 (Kaplan et al. 2000a: Figure 8 for details) and the rate of 10-year-old girls is only 15% of the adult maximum. Hadza women appear to attain maximum root digging rates by early adulthood (Hawkes, O'Connell, and Blurton Jones 1989). Hiwi honey extraction rates by males peak at about age 25. Again the extraction rate of 10-year-olds is less than 10% of the adult maximum. Experiments done with Ache women and girls clearly show that young adult girls are not capable of extracting palm products at the rate attained by older Ache women (see Kaplan et al. 2000a: Figure 9 for details). Ache women do not reach peak return rates until their early twenties. !Kung (Ju/'hoansi) children crack mongongo nuts at a much slower rate than adults (Blurton Jones, Hawkes, and Draper 1994), and Bock (1995) has shown that nut cracking rates among the neighboring Hambukushu do not peak until about age 35. Finally, chimpanzee juveniles also focus on more easily acquired resources than adult chimpanzees. Difficult extraction activities such as termite and ant fishing or nut cracking are practiced less by chimpanzee juveniles than by adults (Boesch and Boesch 1999; Hiraiwa-Hasegawa 1990; Silk 1978).

Human hunting differs qualitatively from hunting by other animals and is the most skill-intensive foraging activity. Unlike most animals that either sit and wait to ambush prey or use stealth and pursuit techniques, human hunters use a wealth of information to make context-specific decisions, both during the search phase of hunting and then after prey are encountered. Specifically, information on ecology, seasonality, current weather, expected animal behavior, and fresh animal signs are all integrated to form multivariate mental models of encounter probabilities that guide the search and are continually updated as conditions change. Various alternative courses of action are constantly compared and referenced to spatial and temporal mental maps of resource availability (Leibenberg 1990). This information is collected, memorized, and processed over much larger spatial areas than chimpanzees ever cover. For example, interviews with Ache men show that fully adult men (aged 35+) had hunted in an area of nearly 12,000 km² of tropical forest in their lifetimes. Almost all foragers surveyed use more than 200 km² in a single year, and many cover more than 1,000 km² in a year (Kelly 1995: Table 4.1). Male chimpanzees, on the other hand, cover only about 10 km² in a lifetime (Wrangham 1975, 1980).

In addition, humans employ a wide variety of techniques to capture and kill prey, using astounding creativity (Kaplan et al. 2000b). Those kill techniques are tailored to many different prey under a wide variety of conditions. For example, from 1980 to 1996 our sample of weighed prey among the Ache includes a minimum of 78 different mammal species, at least 21 species of reptiles and amphibians, probably more than 150 species of birds (more than we have been able to identify), and more than 14 species of fish. Finally, human hunters tend to select prey that is in prime condition from the perspective of human nutritional needs rather than prey made vulnerable by youth, old age, or disease as do so many carnivorous animals (Alvard 1995; Stiner 1991).

The skill-intensive nature of human hunting and the long learning process involved are demonstrated dramatically by data on hunting return rates by age. Hunting return rates among the Hiwi do not peak until age 30–35, with the acquisition rates of 10- and 20-year-old boys reaching only 16% and 50% of the adult maximum, respectively. The hourly return rate for Ache men peaks in their mid thirties. The return rate of 10-year-old boys is about 1% of the adult maximum, and the return rate of 20-year-old juvenile males is still only 25% of the adult maximum. Frank Marlowe (Harvard University, unpublished data) obtains similar results for the Hadza. Also, boys switch from easier tasks, such as fruit collection, shallow tuber extraction, and baobab processing, to honey extraction, and hunting in their mid to late teens among the Hadza, Ache, and Hiwi (Blurton Jones, Hawkes, and O'Connell 1989, 1997; Kaplan et al. 2000b). Even among chimpanzees, hunting is strictly an adult or subadult activity (Boesch and Boesch 1999; Stanford 1998; Teleki 1973).

Net Food Production and Longevity

Figure 13.2 compares humans and chimpanzees in terms of age-profiles of production. The chimpanzee net production curve shows three distinct phases. The first phase, lasting to about age 5, is the period of complete and then partial dependence upon mother's milk. Net production during this phase is negative. The second phase during which net production is zero is independent juvenile growth, lasting until adulthood, about age 13 for females. The third phase is reproductive, during which females, but not males, produce a surplus of calories that they allocate to nursing.

Humans, in contrast, produce less than they consume for close to twenty years! Net production becomes increasingly negative until about

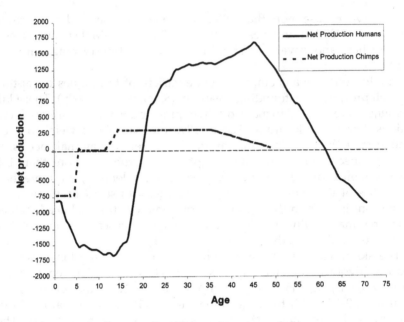

Figure 13.2.   Net food production: Human foragers and chimpanzees

age 14 (with growth in consumption owing to increased body size out-
stripping growth in production) and then begins to climb. Net production
in adulthood among humans is much higher than among chimpanzees
and peaks at a much older age. Peak net production among humans
reflects the payoffs to the long dependency period. It is about 1,750 calories per day, but it is not reached until about age 45. Among chimpanzee
females, peak net production is only about 250 calories per day (Kaplan et
al. 2000b) and since fertility decreases with age, net productivity probably
decreases during the adult period.

The survival curves in Figure 13.1 also reveal why the human age-pro-
file of productivity requires a long adult lifespan. Only about 30% of chimpanzees ever born reach 20, the age when humans produce as much as
they consume, and less than 5% ever born reach 45, when human net production peaks. The relationship between survival rates and age-profiles of
production is made even clearer in Figure 13.3. This panel plots net
expected *cumulative* productivity by age, multiplying the probability of
being alive at each age times the net productivity at that age and then
cumulating over all ages up to the present age. The thin and bold lines
show *cumulative* productivity by age for chimpanzees and humans,
respectively. The long human training period is evident when the troughs

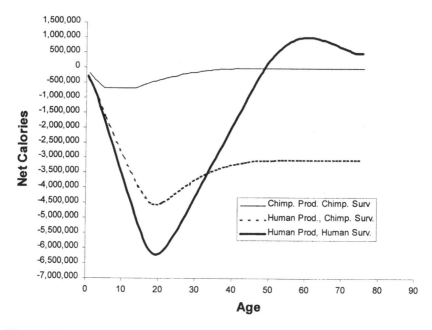

Figure 13.3. Cumulative expected net caloric production by age: Humans and chimpanzees (adapted from Kaplan and Robson 2000a)

in the human and chimpanzee curves are compared. The dashed line is a hypothetical cross of human production profiles with chimpanzee survival rates. It shows that the human production profile would not be viable with chimpanzee survival rates because expected lifetime net production would be negative.

Sex-Specific Embodied Capital Investment and Cooperation between the Sexes

The evidence discussed above suggests that the same principles explaining the covariance among life history traits and brain size among nonhuman primates explains the extreme values exhibited by humans with respect to difficulty of the foraging niche, mortality rates, delay to peak productivity, and investments in intelligence and learning. There is, however, a major discontinuity between humans and other primates. Among humans, men and women specialize in different forms of embodied capital with correspondingly different foraging niches and activity budgets, and then share the fruits of their labor. The reproductive and economic cooperation between men and women is unparalleled in other primates. In this section we present theory to help explain this discontinuity and some of the evidence upon which the theory is based.

Why women gather and men hunt. The analyses in the previous section show that the principal foraging activities of humans are learning-intensive, and as a result, productivity increases with age. Therefore the lifetime payoffs associated with alternative activities depend on the time allocated to those activities. Hunting, as practiced by humans, is largely incompatible with the evolved commitment among primate females towards intensive mothering, carrying of infants, and lactation-on-demand in service of high infant survival rates. First, it often involves rapid travel and encounters with dangerous prey. Second, it is often most efficiently practiced over relatively long periods of time rather than in short stretches, owing to search and travel costs. Third, it is extremely skill-intensive, with improvements in return rate occurring over two decades of daily hunting. Fourth, it provides large (shareable) packages of food that are high in fat and protein.

The first two qualities make hunting a high-cost activity for pregnant and lactating females. The third quality, in interaction with the first and second, generates life course effects such that gathering is a better option for females, *even when they are not lactating*, and hunting is a better option for males.

Figure 13.4, which plots expected *cumulative net lifetime production* by age, disaggregated by sex, shows why this is true for Ache foragers. There is very little variation in men's time allocation to hunting, which averages about seven hours a day. For men, the effects of learning and skill acquisition are clearly visible in the steep increase in productivity until about 35. With their time allocation pattern, hunting provides higher lifetime returns than gathering. Women gather less than two hours a day (about 26% as much as males hunt), and as a result, they remain net consumers throughout their lives. The line with the open squares represents the hypothetical cumulative net production women would achieve if they hunted 26% of the time and learned at the same rate as men. Since women spend about 75% of their time either nursing or more than three months pregnant, a more illuminating way of thinking of this hypothetical line is that it plots the returns they would have if they hunted as much as men when they were unencumbered by pregnancy and lactation. For most of a woman's life, it would not pay to hunt, and she never would get enough practice to make it worthwhile, even when she is postreproductive.

Economic and reproductive cooperation among husbands and wives. We propose that this sex-based specialization in embodied capital investments over the life course, together with the long period of parental invest-

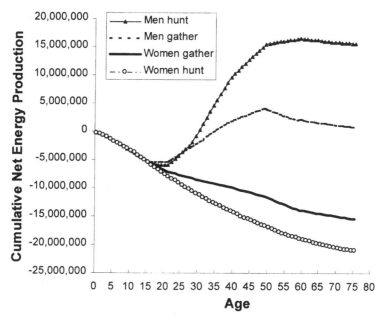

Figure 13.4. Cumulative net energy production by Ache

ment leading to multiple child dependents, is directly responsible for high male parental investment, the universality of the marriage institution, and the extensive economic and reproductive cooperation among husbands and wives. The specialization in different skills and in the procurement of different resources generates a complementarity between human men and women that is rare among mammals. Stated simply, complementarity occurs when the value of male investment in offspring depends *positively* on the amount given by females and vice versa (with fitness held constant).[3] In contrast, male and female inputs are substitutes when the relative values of the two inputs are independent of the amount provided by the other sex (again holding fitness constant).

The specialization generates two forms of complementarity. Hunted foods complement gathered foods because protein, fat, and carbohydrates complement one another with respect to their nutritional functions (see Hill 1988 for a review) and because most gathered foods, such as roots, palm fiber, and fruits, are low in fat and protein (nuts are an exception). The fact that male specialization in hunting produces high delivery rates of large, shareable packages of food leads to another form of complementarity. The meat inputs of men shift the optimal mix of activities for women, increasing time spent in child care and decreasing time spent in food acquisition. They also shift their time to foraging and productive activities that are compatible with child care and away from activities that are dangerous to them and their children.

On average among adults in the ten-group sample, men acquired 68% of the calories and almost 88% of the protein; women acquired the remaining 32% of calories and 12% of protein (Table 13.1). Given that on average these calories are distributed to support adult female consumption (31%), adult male consumption (39%), and offspring (31%), respectively, women supply 3% of the calories to offspring and men provide the remaining 97%! Men not only supply all of the protein to offspring but also the bulk of the protein consumed by women. This contrasts sharply with most mammalian species (>97%), where the female supports all of the energetic needs of the offspring until it begins eating solid foods (Clutton-Brock 1991) and males provide little or no investment.

Complementarity of investments is also evident in the behavior of married couples. For example, as the amount of food that men acquire increases, their spouses forage less and allocate more time to other activities, such as child care. For every 1,000 additional calories that husbands acquire, Hiwi and Ache women decrease time spent foraging by 0.8 and 0.5 hours, respectively (Hurtado et al. 1992). Couples also have a number of behaviors that help each other increase foraging return rates. For example, among the Ache, men cut most of the palms from which their wives extract palm fiber, the main carbohydrate staple. Women often help their husbands spot game. In fact, women spend about 11% of their out-of-camp time helping others acquire food, 55% of which is spent helping their husbands. Among both the Ache and Hiwi (and most other foragers, for that matter), women cook and process most of the food that their husbands acquire and consume (Hurtado et al. 2000). Among the Hiwi, spouses adjust their activities and time use according to what the other spouse is doing and the weaning status of their youngest child. The husbands of nursing women increase time spent in activities in camp that are compatible with child care as their infants get older. This suggests that as breastfeeding duration and frequency decrease, men do more child care. Moreover, reproductive age women are more likely to be out foraging when their husbands are in camp than when their husbands are out of camp. Thus spouses take turns staying in camp with some of their shared offspring while the other goes out to forage, sometimes accompanied by one child (Hurtado et al. 2000).

In this sense, humans are more like birds than mammals. Most bird species produce altricial chicks that cannot fly or defend themselves effectively, and as a result, they are especially vulnerable to predation when they are unprotected. However, finding food for both the parents and the young requires time away from the nest. Male and female investments are complements since the value of the food brought by one sex is greater if the other sex protects the chicks (either through specialization in care and feeding or turn-taking at the nest). Male parental investment and monogamy are extremely common among bird species with altricial young and rare among species with precocial young who feed themselves.

Male and female investments are much less complementary among mammals because mothers and infants tend to stay together to facilitate nursing. Most mammalian young follow their mothers during feeding (or are cached in hidden places) so that care and feeding can be done simultaneously (or do not trade off against one another as sharply). In principle, mammalian males could have evolved to lactate as well. Mother's milk and father's milk would be perfect substitutes because milk is milk, regardless of who provides it.

The extensive cooperation among human men and women would only make sense if the reproductive performance of spouses were linked. Ache juvenile mortality increases when fathers are poor hunters or are deceased (Hurtado and Hill 1992). Thus, for females in a stable pair bond, whatever they can do to increase their husbands' strength and survivorship will be mutually beneficial. Behavioral cooperation between the sexes would also make sense if the probability of defection was relatively low.

The fact that humans are unique in raising multiple dependent offspring of different ages reduces the payoffs to defection and increases the benefits for men and women to link their economic and reproductive lives over the long run. Men and women who divorce and remarry during the time they are raising offspring will face conflicts of interest with new spouses over the division of resources. If they marry someone with children from previous marriages they may disagree with their spouses over the allocation of food and care to their joint children relative to children from the previous marriage. Those conflicts increase the benefits of spouses staying together and having all or most of their children together.

Data on divorce and reproduction show that people are responsive to those costs and benefits. Among the Ache, who marry and divorce frequently when they are young, reproduction solidifies marital bonds. A good measure of pair bond stability is the extent to which there is overlap in the timing of last births between spouses. Among the Ache, most men are five to six years older than their spouses (Hill and Hurtado 1996). When women reach menopause in their late forties, men have the option to continue reproducing with younger women but they do not generally do so. Overall, 83% of all last births for women also represent a last birth for the fathers of these children. In addition, the last child of 90% of Ache men who had fathered at least two children with the same spouse was also the last child of the wife. Last, as the number of shared offspring increases, the difference in spouses' ages at the time of the birth of their last child decreases (Hurtado et al. 2000). For the minority of couples whose year of last birth differed greatly and men established new families with younger women, spouses usually had only one shared offspring.

Finally, human females evidence physiological and behavioral adaptations that are consistent with an evolutionary history involving extensive male parental investment. Human females decrease metabolic rates during pregnancy (suggesting that they lower work effort) and store fat (suggesting that they are being provisioned) (Lawrence and Whitehead 1988; Pike 1999; Poppitt et al. 1993), whereas nonhuman primates do not (Lancaster et al. 2000). In addition, nonhuman primate females increase work effort during lactation and, as a result, have increased risk of mortality. Human female foragers, in contrast, tend to decrease work effort during lactation and focus on high-quality care (Hurtado et al. 1985; Lancaster et al. 2000). These phenotypes could not have evolved if women did not depend on men for most of their food provisioning throughout human history.

Specialization in nutrient extraction and multiple dependency of young may be the critical factors favoring the greater relative importance of selection for cooperative rather than competitive arrangements between human mates. The investments by men may also explain why humans manage to have both shorter interbirth intervals and higher rates of juvenile and adult survival than chimpanzees (see Table 13.1).

DISCUSSION AND CONCLUSIONS

The analyses in this paper have applied embodied capital theory to understanding primate radiations in brain size and longevity, the evolution of the human life course, and sex-specific specialization in embodied capital investments. In each case, the theory has led to new insights and empirical results, some of which contravene alternative theories that have heretofore been widely accepted.

Embodied capital theory organizes the relationships of ecology, brain size, and longevity among primates, which existing debates about primate brain size evolution have failed to do. One debate pits ecological and social intelligence hypotheses against each other. According to "the ecological hypothesis," increases in brain size are largely driven by the complexities of the diet. Jerison (1973, 1976) hypothesized that the need to process information in a complex three-dimensional environment was the cause of the large brain size of primates relative to other mammals. He therefore predicted that differences in brain size, after controlling for body mass, would be associated with an animal's ecological niche and its demands for information processing. Milton (1981, 1993; Milton and Demment 1988) extended this approach by focusing on gut specialization and brain size as two alternative routes to energetic efficiency. Leaves, while abundant, tend to contain high amounts of fiber and often toxins as well. The ability to extract nutrients from leaves depends on the size of the gut and other specializations designed to facilitate fermentation for nutrient extraction. Fruits, on the other hand, are ephemeral resources that are patchily distributed but offer a higher density of easily processed energy.

According to "the social brain" or "Machiavellian intelligence" hypothesis (Barton and Dunbar 1997; Byrne 1995, 1996; Dunbar 1992, 1998; Milton 1981, 1993; Milton and Demment 1988), the expansion of the brain is driven primarily by the complexities of social life in primate groups. Many species of primates exhibit complex dominance hierarchies that are mediated by political alliances and relations among relatives in genetic lineages (Harcourt 1988a, 1988b; Walters and Seyfarth 1987). Discussions of life history associations with brain size have focused primarily on the metabolic costs of growing large brains (Foley and Lee 1991; Martin 1996), or on whether the relationship between brain size and longevity is real or a statistical artifact (Allman et al. 1993; Barton 1999; Economos 1980; Foley and Lee 1991; Martin 1996). There has been virtually no discussion on how selection might work on both longevity and brain size.

The embodied capital theory and our empirical results show how features of ecology, including both mortality risks and information processing demands, interact in determining optimal allocations to the brain and survival. They also suggest an alternative interpretation of primate social intelligence. Coevolutionary selection on brains and longevity owing to the complexity and the navigational demands of the primate diet may have produced preadaptations for the evolution of social intelligence. Given that primates have long lives with enduring social relationships, and given that many species of primates eat foods whose distribution generates within-group competition, there would be selection for the application of existing enhancements in memory and information processing abilities to the management of social interaction. Many animals live in social groups, but primates are notable in terms of the complexity of their social arrangements. Perhaps social pressures alone are not sufficient to select for markedly increased brain size, but they might select for the extension of existing abilities to social problems. This may be why apes display remarkable social intelligence even though group size is not particularly large (Byrne 1995, 1997a). Orangutans, for example, are mostly solitary, but it takes about seven years for a young orangutan to become independent of its mother (presumably because of the learning-intensive nature of the diet). If this view is correct, it also suggests that the assumption of extreme domain-specificity in intelligence may be unwarranted.

There is growing interest in the evolution of human life histories, especially longevity. One model, recently proposed by Hawkes and colleagues (1998) and often referred to as the "Grandmother Hypothesis," proposes that humans have a long lifespan because of the assistance that older postreproductive women contribute to descendant kin through the provisioning of difficult-to-acquire plant foods. Women, therefore, are selected to invest in maintaining their bodies longer than chimpanzee females do. This model offers no explanation for why men live so long. In contrast to this female-centered view, Marlowe (2000) proposes that reproduction by males late in life selects for the lengthening of the human life course, with effects on females being incidental. The data we presented regarding the interdependence of men's and women's economic and reproductive lives cast doubt on both those theories and on the view that the sexual division of labor is primarily caused by conflicts of interest between mates (Bird 1999). Cooperative arrangements between men and women help bolster their individual chances for survival and the number of surviving children they produce.

The embodied capital theory explains why both men and women have long lives. Both men and women exploit high-quality, difficult-to-acquire foods (females extracting plant foods and males hunting animal foods), sacrificing early productivity for later productivity; both have a life history characterized by an extended juvenile period where growth is slow and much is learned; and both make a high investment in mortality reduction to reap the rewards of those investments. It also explains many other facts, such as the expansion of the costly human brain, the sex-specific investments in embodied capital, and the economic and reproductive cooperation among men and women.

The complementarity in embodied capital investments between men and women is a distinctive feature of the human adaptation that is qualitatively different from other primates. It is not just men and women that cooperate in nuclear families, however. Food sharing among families is pervasive in human groups. This is true of both hunted and extracted resources and of the foods acquired by women and men (Gurven, Allen et al. 2000; Gurven, Hill et al. 2000; Kaplan and Hill 1985). Food sharing not only buffers the risk of day-to-day variation in food supply owing to foraging luck, it also allows people to recover from illness and injury (Gurven, Hill, and Hurtado 2000). Food sharing may be one reason why humans have such low mortality rates and can afford to invest in learning-intensive foraging strategies (see Kaplan et al. 2000a for a fuller treatment). Moreover, food sharing buffers variance in family size resulting from unpredictable mortality. Larger families are reported to receive larger shares of food in most societies for which data are available (Gurven, Hill et al. 2000). Interfamilial food sharing may also be a necessary support for long-term child dependence since families with multiple, surviving young could not support themselves without the assistance of families with low dependency ratios.

The human adaptation is broad and flexible in one sense, and very narrow and specialized in another sense. It is broad in the sense that as hunter-gatherers, humans have existed successfully in virtually all of the world's major habitats. This has entailed eating a very wide variety of foods, both plant and animal, and a great deal of flexibility in the contributions of different age and sex classes of individuals. The human adaptation is narrow and specialized in that it is based on extremely high investments in brain tissue and learning. In every environment, human foragers consume the largest, highest-quality, and most difficult-to-acquire foods using techniques that often take years to learn. In terms of embodied capital, males specialize in acquiring hunting skills at the expense of very low productivity during the adolescent and early adult years, and females specialize in extractive activities that are compatible with child care and in the care and training of offspring. The human feeding niche and parental investment system is also specialized in that it depends upon cooperation between men and women and food sharing among families. It is this legacy that modern humans bring to the complex economies existing today, where education-based embodied capital determines income and the economy is a complex web of specialization and cooperation between spouses, families, and larger social units. We are only beginning to explore the implications of this legacy for understanding modern behavior.

NOTES

1. See Kaplan et al. 2000b for details on this section.
2. The hunter-gatherer data come from studies on populations during periods when they were almost completely dependent on wild foods, with little modern technology (and no firearms), no significant outside interference in interpersonal violence or fertility rates, and no significant access to modern medicine. The chimpanzee data are compiled from all published and unpublished sources of which we are aware and to which we had access (Hill et al. 2001; Kaplan et al. 2000b).
3. Technically, complementarity occurs when marginal rates of substitution along fitness isoclines or indifference curves change as the ratio of the two inputs change, making those curves convex to the origin.

REFERENCES

Allman J, McLaughlin T, Hakeem A (1993) Brain weight and life-span in primate species. *Proceedings of the National Academy of Sciences* 90:118–122.
Alvard M (1995) Intraspecific prey choice by Amazonian hunters. *Current Anthropology* 36:789–818.

Armstrong E, Falk D (Eds) (1982) *Primate Brain Evolution* (New York, Plenum Press).

Austad SN, Fischer KE (1991) Mammalian aging, metabolism, and ecology: evidence from the bats and marsupials. *Journal of Gerontology* 46:47–51.

Austad SN, Fischer KE (1992) Primate longevity: its place in the mammalian scheme. *American Journal of Primatology* 28:251–261.

Barton RA (1999) The evolutionary ecology of the primate brain. In PC Lee (Ed) *Comparative Primate Socioecology* (Cambridge, Cambridge University Press), 167–203.

Barton RA, Dunbar RIM (1997) Evolution of the social brain. In A Whiten, RW Byrne (Eds) *Machiavellian Intelligence II: Extensions and Evaluations* (Cambridge, Cambridge University Press), 240–263.

Bird R (1999) Cooperation and conflict: the behavioral ecology of the sexual division of labor. *Evolutionary Anthropology* 8:65–75.

Blurton Jones N, Hawkes K, O'Connell J (1989) Modeling and measuring the costs of children in two foraging societies. In V Standen, RA Foley (Eds) *Comparative Socioecology of Humans and Other Mammals* (London, Basil Blackwell), 367–390.

Blurton Jones N, Hawkes GK, Draper P (1994) Foraging returns of !Kung adults and children: why didn't !Kung children forage? *Journal of Anthropological Research* 50:217–248.

Blurton Jones N, Hawkes K, O'Connell J (1997) Why do Hadza children forage? In NL Segal, GE Weisfeld, CC Weisfeld (Eds) *Uniting Psychology and Biology: Integrative Perspectives on Human Development* (New York, American Psychological Association), 297–331.

Bock JA (1995) The Determinants of Variation in Children's Activities in a Southern African Community. Ph.D. dissertation (Albuquerque, University of New Mexico).

Boesch C, Boesch H (1999) *The Chimpanzees of the Tai Forest: Behavioural Ecology and Evolution* (Oxford, Oxford University Press).

Byrne R (1995) The smart gorilla's recipe book. *Natural History* (October):12–15.

Byrne R (1996) Machiavellian intelligence. *Evolutionary Anthropology* 5:172–180.

Byrne R (1997a) Machiavellian intelligence. In A Whiten, RW Byrne (Eds) *Machiavellian Intelligence II: Extensions and Evaluations* (Cambridge, Cambridge University Press), 1–23.

Byrne R (1997b) The technical intelligence hypothesis: an additional evolutionary stimulus to intelligence? In A Whiten, RW Byrne (Eds) *Machiavellian Intelligence II: Extensions and Evaluations* (Cambridge, Cambridge University Press), 289–312.

Clutton-Brock TH (1991) *The Evolution of Parental Care* (Princeton, Princeton University Press).

Clutton-Brock TH, Harvey PH (1980) Primates, brains and ecology. *Journal of Zoology* (London) 109:309–323.

Cole LC (1954) The population consequences of life history phenomena. *Quarterly Review of Biology* 29:103–137.

Dunbar RIM (1992) Neocortex size as a constraint on group size in primates. *Journal of Human Evolution* 20:469–493.

Dunbar RIM (1998) The social brain hypothesis. *Evolutionary Anthropology* 6:178–190.

Economos AC (1980) Brain-life span conjecture: a re-evaluation of the evidence. *Gerontology* 26:82–89.

Fleagle JG (1999) *Primate Adaptation and Evolution*, second ed. (New York, Academic Press).

Foley RA, Lee PC (1991) Ecology and energetics of encephalization in human evolution. *Philosophical Transactions of the Royal Society of London,* B 334:63–72.

Gadgil M, Bossert WH (1970) Life historical consequences of natural selection. *American Naturalist* 104:1–24.

Gurven M, Allen-Arane W, Hill K, Hurtado AM (2000) "It's a wonderful life": signaling generosity among the Ache of Paraguay. *Evolution and Human Behavior* 21:263–282.

Gurven M, Hill K, Kaplan H, Hurtado M, Lyles R (2000) Food transfers among Hiwi foragers of Venezuela: tests of reciprocity. *Human Ecology* 28:171–218.

Harcourt AH (1988a) Alliances in contests and social intelligence. In R Byrne, A Whiten (Eds) *Machiavellian Intelligence* (Oxford, Clarendon Press), 132–152.

Harcourt AH (1988b) Cooperation as a competitive strategy in primates and birds. In Y Ito, JL Brown (Eds) *Animal Societies: Theories and Facts* (Tokyo, Scientific Societies Press).

Hawkes K, O'Connell JF, Blurton Jones N (1989) Hardworking Hadza grandmothers. In V Standen, RA Foley (Eds) *Comparative Socioecology of Humans and Other Mammals* (London, Basil Blackwell), 341–366.

Hawkes K, O'Connell JF, Blurton Jones NG, Alvarez H, Charnov EL (1998) Grandmothering, menopause, and the evolution of human life histories. *Proceedings of the National Academy of Science* 95:1336–1339.

Hill K (1988) Macronutrient modifications of optimal foraging theory: an approach using indifference curves applied to some modern foragers. *Human Ecology* 16:157–197.

Hill K, Hurtado AM (1996) *Ache Life History: The Ecology and Demography of a Foraging People* (Hawthorne, New York, Aldine de Gruyter).

Hill K, Boesch C, Goodall J, Pusey A, Williams J, Wrangham R (2001) Mortality rates among wild chimpanzees. *Journal of Human Evolution* 39:1–14.

Hiraiwa-Hasegawa M (1990) The role of food sharing between mother and infant in the ontogeny of feeding behavior. In T Nishida (Ed) *The Chimpanzees of the Mahale Mountains: Sexual and Life History Strategies* (Tokyo, Tokyo University Press), 267–276.

Holliday MA (1978) Body composition and energy needs during growth. In F Faulkner, JM Tanner (Eds) *Human Growth,* vol. 2. (New York, Plenum Press), 117–139.

Hurtado AM, Hawkes K, Hill K, Kaplan H (1985) Female subsistence strategies among Ache hunter-gatherers of eastern Paraguay. *Human Ecology* 13:29–47.

Hurtado AM, Hill K (1992) Paternal effects on child survivorship among Ache and Hiwi hunter-gatherers: implications for modeling pair-bond stability. In B Hewlett (Ed) *Father-Child Relations: Cultural and Biosocial Contexts* (Hawthorne, New York, Aldine de Gruyter), 31–56.

Hurtado AM, Hill K, Kaplan H, Hurtado I (1992) Trade-offs between female food acquisition and childcare among Hiwi and Ache foragers. *Human Nature* 3:185–216.

Hurtado AM, Hill K, Kaplan H, Lancaster J (2000) The origins of the sexual division of labor. Ms. in preparation, Department of Anthropology, University of New Mexico.

Jerison, H (1973) *Evolution of the Brain and Intelligence* (New York, Academic Press).

Jerison HJ (1976) Paleoneurology and the evolution of mind. *Scientific American* 234:90–101.

Kaplan, H (1997) The evolution of the human life course. In K Wachter, C Finch (Eds) *Between Zeus and Salmon: The Biodemography of Aging* (Washington DC, National Academy of Sciences), 175–211.

Kaplan H, Hill K (1985) Food-sharing among Ache foragers: tests of explanatory hypotheses. *Current Anthropology* 26:223–245.

Kaplan H, Robson A (2000a) The coevolution of intelligence and longevity and the emergence of humans. Ms. in the authors' possession.

Kaplan H, Robson A (2000b) The coevolution of intelligence and longevity in hunter-gatherer economies. Ms. in the authors' possession.

Kaplan H, Gangestad S, Mueller TC, Lancaster JB (2000a) The evolution of primate life histories and intelligence. Ms. in the authors' possession.

Kaplan H, Hill K, Lancaster JB, Hurtado AM (2000b) A theory of human life history evolution: diet, intelligence, and longevity. *Evolutionary Anthropology* 9: 156–185.

Kelly R (1995) *The Foraging Spectrum: Diversity in Hunter-Gatherer Lifeways* (Washington DC, Smithsonian Institution Press).

Lack D (1954) *The Natural Regulation of Animal Numbers* (Oxford, Oxford University Press).

Lancaster J, Kaplan H, Hill K, Hurtado AM (2000) The evolution of life history, intelligence and diet among chimpanzees and human foragers. In F Tonneau, NS Thompson (Eds) *Perspectives in Ethology: Evolution, Culture and Behavior*, Vol. 13 (New York, Plenum), 47–72.

Lawrence M, Whitehead RG (1988) Physical activity and total energy expenditure of child-bearing Gambian village women. *European Journal of Clinical Nutrition* 42:145–160.

Leibenberg L (1990) *The Art of Tracking: The Origin of Science* (Cape Town, David Phillip).

Lloyd DG (1987) Selection of offspring size at independence and other size-versus-number strategies. *American Naturalist* 129:800–817.

Marlowe, F (2000) The patriarch hypothesis: an alternative explanation of menopause. *Human Nature* 11:27–42.

Martin RD (1996) Scaling of the mammalian brain: the maternal energy hypothesis. *News in Physiological Sciences* 11:149–156.

Milton K (1981) Distribution patterns of tropical plant foods as an evolutionary stimulus to primate mental development. *American Anthropologist* 83:534–548.

Milton K (1993) Diet and primate evolution. *Scientific American* 269:70–77.

Milton K (1999) A hypothesis to explain the role of meat-eating in human evolution. *Evolutionary Anthropology* 8:11–21.

Milton K, Demment M (1988) Digestive and passage kinetics of chimpanzees fed high and low fiber diets and comparison with human data. *Journal of Nutrition* 118:107.

Parker S, Gibson K (1979) A developmental model for the evolution of language and intelligence in early hominids. *Behavioral and Brain Sciences* 2:367–408.

Partridge L, Harvey P (1985) Costs of reproduction. *Nature* 316:20–21.

Pike IL (1999) Age, reproductive history, seasonality, and maternal body composition during pregnancy for nomadic Turkana of Kenya. *American Journal of Human Biology* 11:658–672.

Poppitt SD, Prentice AM, Jequier E, Schutz Y, Whitehead RG (1993) Evidence of energy sparing in Gambian women during pregnancy: a longitudinal study using whole-body calorimetry. *American Journal of Clinical Nutrition* 57: 353–364.

Silk JB (1978) Patterns of food-sharing among mother and infant chimpanzees at Gombe National Park, Tanzania. *Folia Primatologica* 29:129–141.

Smith CC, Fretwell SD (1974) The optimal balance between size and number of offspring. *American Naturalist* 108:499–506.

Stanford CB (1998) *Chimpanzee and Red Colobus: The Ecology of Predator and Prey* (Cambridge Harvard University Press).

Stiner M (1991) An interspecific perspective on the emergence of the modern human predatory niche. In M Stiner (Ed) *Human Predators and Prey Mortality* (Boulder, Westview Press), 149–185.

Teleki G (1973) *The Predatory Behavior of Wild Chimpanzees* (Lewisburg, PA, Bucknell University Press).

Walters JR, Seyfarth RM (1987) Conflict and cooperation. In BB Smuts, DL Cheney, RM Seyfarth, RW Wrangham, TT Struhsaker (Eds) *Primate Societies* (Chicago, University of Chicago Press), 306–317.

Winterhalder B (1996) Social foraging and the behavioral ecology of intragroup resource transfers. *Evolutionary Anthropology* 5:46–57.

Wrangham R (1975) The Behavioral Ecology of Chimpanzees in Gombe National Park, Tanzania. Ph.D. dissertation (Cambridge University).

Wrangham R (1980) Sex differences in behavioral ecology of chimpanzees in Gombe National Park, Tanzania. *Journal of Reproduction and Fertility* 28(Suppl): 13–31.

Part IV

COMPARATIVE CONTEXT

Part IV

COMPARATIVE CONDUCT

14

Strepsirrhine Reproductive Ecology

PATRICIA L. WHITTEN and DIANE K. BROCKMAN

The lemurs, lorises, and galagos comprise a unique group of primates, termed *strepsirrhines,* that share some features with the earliest primates and diverge in interesting ways from the adaptations of monkeys and apes. Although their regulation of reproduction and energy balance has been portrayed as less flexible and efficient than that of haplorhine primates, recent studies have demonstrated the adaptive nature of their reproductive ecology. This chapter will review strepsirrhine life history and reproduction and discuss the explanations that have been offered to explain their divergence from haplorhine primates. The limitations posed by ecological and social constraints will be reviewed along with regulatory factors. Strepsirrhine reproductive strategies will be compared, and the origins of haplorhine reproductive strategies will be discussed.

THE UNIQUE RADIATIONS OF
STREPSIRRHINE PRIMATES

Traditionally, the Primate order has been divided into two suborders reflecting the degree to which individual species express the derived adaptations of primates or the features that are thought to have character-ized the earliest ancestral primates. The lorises, galagos, lemurs, and tar-siers were grouped together on the basis of morphological and behavioral similarities into the Prosimian grade whereas New and Old World mon-keys and apes, including humans, were considered to belong to the Anthropoid grade of organization. This division does not reflect genetic relationships very well, however, because the tarsiers are actually more closely related to monkeys and apes than they are to the other prosimians. In fact, the nocturnal adaptations and small size of tarsiers appear to be secondarily derived (Martin 1990), and many taxonomists now prefer to classify primates into Strepsirrhines, or moist-nosed primates (lemurs, lorises, and galagos), and Haplorhines, or dry-nosed primates (tarsiers, monkeys, and apes). The distinctive features of strepsirrhines include traits that reflect (1) nocturnality, such as large eyes, a tapetum lucidum, vibrissae, and large mobile ears; (2) a heavy dependence on olfactory signals, such as a moist external nose or rhinarium, tethered cleft upper lip, and anatomical connections between the rhinarium and vomeronasal organ; and (3) specialized features such as the toothcomb.

Strepsirrhine similarities to Eocene primates facilitate their use in reconstructing the ancestral primate niche (Covert 1995; Doyle and Martin 1974). However, these primates are not simply evolutionary holdovers from a more "primitive condition" from which more complex, higher primate adaptations evolved. Both the Eocene and modern strepsirrhines are far from homogeneous groups, comprising markedly diverse arrays of species (Bearder 1999; Covert 1995). Among extant taxa, similar looking species are often quite different in niche, locomotion, and reproductive parameters (Bearder 1999; Harcourt and Nash 1986). Species diversity is especially marked in Madagascar where lemurs have evolved in isolation from anthropoids and many other species.

The tendency to equate "primitive" with "inferior" has been an obstacle to understanding the evolution of mammalian (Lillegraven et al. 1987) and strepsirrhine (Bearder 1999) traits. The presence of more gifted haplorhine primates is often used to explain the relative obscurity of strepsirrhines in Africa and Asia in comparison to Madagascar, but there is little evidence for their exclusion from mainland niches by better adapted monkeys and apes (Bouliere 1974). Strepsirrhines are broadly distributed from about 28° S to 26° N latitude, matching the distribution of most haplorhine primates (Ravosa 1998; Rowe 1996). Only a few macaque and langur species are found at more temperate latitudes. Many of the seemingly primitive habits of strepsirrhines (such as fat storage, seasonal torpor, cathemerality, caecotrophy, low metabolic rates, and specialized locomotor adaptations) are actually highly efficient adaptations to very particular niches that may have constrained the emergence of haplorhine competitors (Bearder 1999; Bouliere 1974). Moreover, compared with other mammals, the extant strepsirrhines are large-brained species with prolonged periods of development, both of which may have facilitated the development of complex social behaviors (Bearder 1999). Even the so-called solitary nocturnal strepsirrhines maintain complex social networks within communities of dispersed individuals (Bearder 1999; Sterling and Richard 1995).

The lemurs are particularly interesting because they result from an adaptive radiation long isolated from those from which monkeys and apes were derived, providing an opportunity to test adaptive models for the evolution of social organization. Although lemurs are "hopelessly stupid toward unknown inanimate objects," scoring dismally on tests of object discrimination, delayed response, and insight problems (Jolly 1966b), their social systems approach the diversity and complexity seen in haplorhine primates (Jolly 1966a; Kappeler 1997b). Like monkeys, lemurs form multi-male, multifemale groups that are unusual among mammals. They exhibit many of the outward signs of social bonds such as close physical contact, grooming, and social play. They appreciate social rank and vie for better position. They differentiate between kin and non-kin in mating, affiliation, and aggression.

Nevertheless, there are significant differences between lemur and haplorhine social systems. Although pair-bonding is rare in mammals, occurring in just 3% of species, and uncommon (13%) in haplorhine primates (Kleiman 1977), it is present in more than a quarter of lemur species (Wright 1999). Longitudinal demographic data available on a few species living in polygynous groups show that while most females are philopatric, as in many haplorhines, the development of matrilines is limited by small group size. Among semi-free-ranging populations, rank does not appear to be matrilineally inherited, and coalitionary aggression is rare, an aspect that has been attributed to poor visual acuity (Pereira 1995). However, visual acuity does not appear to constrain targeted aggression, a coordinated attack and ejection of one individual by multiple group members. Unlike most haplorhines, as well as galagos and lorises, lemurs are monomorphic, with little or no sexual dimorphism in body size or mass (Kappeler 1993). Moreover, lemurs stand in marked contrast to most mammalian species where males are dominant over females (Hrdy 1981; Jolly 1984; Richard 1987). Females in most lemur species are socially dominant to males—dominance/subordinance interactions most commonly occur in the context of feeding. Nevertheless, lemur males compete actively for reproductive access. Rates of physical aggression are generally quite low outside of the breeding season, and male proximity is often surprisingly close by anthropoid standards (Kappeler 1999), but mate guarding and bloody battles between males occur often during the breeding season. Male infanticide has been reported in some populations (Brockman et al. 1998; Wright 1999), although the fitness implications of this reproductive tactic have yet to be determined.

EXPLANATIONS FOR LEMUR ADAPTATIONS

Several hypotheses have been offered to explain the unique features of the Malagasy lemurs (Richard and Dewar 1991; Wright 1999). Some characteristics have been attributed to the retention of traits of ancestral primates. This explanation, however, begs the question of why conservative features may have been adaptive for strepsirrhines and not for haplorhines. The considerable taxonomic diversity of the strepsirrhines demonstrates that evolution has not been stagnant in this suborder, and as will be seen below, many of the seemingly primitive traits of strepsirrhines offer substantial adaptive benefits (Bearder 1999; Richard and Dewar 1991).

An alternative hypothesis suggests that cathemerality, small group size, frequent monogamy, lack of sexual dimorphism, and low metabolic rate are all products of a recent transition to a diurnal lifestyle (Tattersall 1982; van Schaik and Kappeler 1996). According to this hypothesis, diurnal lifestyles emerged in extant Malagasy lemurs only within the past 1,000 years, following the extinction of large-bodied diurnal lemurs (Tattersall 1982) or large diurnal raptors (van Schaik and Kappeler 1996). Whether raptors could have been a selective force against diurnality is dubious because extant raptors prey upon nocturnal as well as diurnal lemurs (Wright 1999). Moreover, some adaptations of diurnal lemurs argue against a recent shift to a diurnal lifestyle. Although diurnal and cathemeral lemurs retain the tapetum lucidum of nocturnal strepsirrhines, they also have genes for both short and medium/long wavelength photopigments, permitting dichromatic and trichromatic color vision (Tan and Li 1999), in contrast to the nocturnal galagos, in which the gene for the short wavelength photopigment is degenerate (Jacobs and Deegan 1993). In fact, polymorphism of the X-linked opsin loci in nocturnal as well as diurnal lemur families (Tan and Li 1999) along with the presence of thalamic neurons specialized to detect red/green color differences in strepsirrhines suggest that the ancestral strepsirrhine may have been diurnal.

Various explanations have been proposed for female dominance, including male efforts to conserve energy for the breeding season (Hrdy 1981), male paternal investment (Pollock 1979), male mating strategies (Pereira 1995), or the energetic stress of female reproduction (Jolly 1984; Richard and Nicoll 1987; Young et al. 1990), but these hypotheses have yet to be empirically tested. Male deferral as an energy conservation strategy seems unlikely since some male lemurs compete with one another in periods of food scarcity as well as during the breeding season (Brockman et al. 1998, 2001). Paternal investment is unlikely because extragroup matings in polygynous species are likely to preclude certainty of paternity (Young et al. 1990). Although it has been argued that most lemur societies are built around a monogamously mated pair (van Schaik and Kappeler 1993), there is as yet no empirical evidence for long-term stable and exclusive male-female associations in wild lemurs (Brockman 1994), and recent studies suggest that these relationships may be more accurately described as affiliations rather than pair bonds (Overdorff 1998; but see Pereira and McGlynn 1997). The notion of energetically stressful reproduction has received the most attention, with stress being attributed to a markedly seasonal environment as well as a high rate of maternal investment (Jolly 1966a, 1984; Richard 1987; Wright 1993; Young et al. 1990). Additionally it has been argued that lemurs have evolved a complex of photoperiodically regulated mechanisms for energy conservation during predictable seasonal food shortages, including seasonal reproduction, torpor, and modulation of metabolism and growth rates (Pereira 1993; Sauther et al. 1999; Wright 1999). However, the costs of reproduction have been debated (Kappeler 1995, 1996; Tilden and Oftedal 1997), as has the degree of seasonality (Richard and Dewar 1991). As discussed below, Madagascar may be an especially challenging environment for primates, but the degree to which its seasonal rigors impact female reproductive success is yet to be demonstrated (Richard and Dewar 1991).

LIFE HISTORIES OF STREPSIRRHINES

Prenatal Development

Interpretation of strepsirrhine life histories is complicated by their broad size range. Although galagos and lorises range in mass from 60 to 1,200 g, with most less than 500 g, the extant Malagasy lemurs, ranging in mass from 80 g to 10 kg, encompass a broader range of sizes than is found within other primate families, and the recently extinct lemurs extend that range to the size of the largest apes (Richard and Dewar 1991). It is important to control for body size when making generalizations about strepsirrhines since the smallest lemurs are among the smallest strepsirrhines, equaled in size only by the tarsiers among the haplorhines, whereas the largest extant lemurs at 1.5–3 kg are larger than most strepsirrhines but smaller than most haplorhines. In fact, 1–3 kg is a rare size among the primates, perhaps because it lies astride the mammalian thresholds for diurnality and folivory.

As in other mammals, strepsirrhine life history parameters such as gestation length, rates of pre- and postnatal growth, and neonatal size vary with maternal body size. Like haplorhine primates, strepsirrhines are precocial mammals, producing one to three well-developed neonates after a prolonged gestation with relatively slow somatic growth (Martin and McLarnon 1985). However, strepsirrhine neonates are smaller, weighing only one third as much as the newborn of a comparably sized haplorhine (Leutenegger 1979). This developmental difference is not due to the duration of gestation; neither the duration of gestation nor the duration of lactation differs in similar-sized strepsirrhines and haplorhines (Martin 1990; Schwartz and Rosenblum 1993). Rather the small infant size of lorises and galagos seems to be the result of a significantly slower rate of fetal growth

(Kappeler 1996; Martin and MacLarnon 1988; Young et al. 1990). Although the less invasive (epithelialchorial) placenta of strepsirrhines was initially thought to be the explanation for this difference, that now seems unlikely because mammals with relatively large neonates like dolphins and ungulates have the same type of placentation (Martin 1990). Moreover, lemurs have rates of prenatal growth that are comparable to those of haplorhine primates (Kappeler 1996; Young et al. 1990), showing that the epithelialchorial placenta does not preclude haplorhine rates of development. Yet in spite of differences in fetal growth, the three groups produce similar-sized infants for maternal body size, a result of shorter gestations in the more rapidly growing species.

These adjustments suggest that small neonatal size may be a developmental strategy. Although strepsirrhine neonates are small in body size, they are relatively precocial, a developmental state reflecting increased central nervous system development (Aboitiz 1996; Sacher and Staffeldt 1974). Strepsirrhine neonates maintain the high brain:body ratio (12%) that distinguishes haplorhine neonates from other mammals where the brain is only 6% of body size at birth (Aboitiz 1996). The proportionally large brains of primates are achieved by reduced fetal body growth in comparison with other mammals (Deacon 1997). Prolonged neurogenesis increases adult brain size by increasing the number of precursor neurons (Finlay and Darlington 1995) and delays subsequent somatic growth (Smith 1997). This pattern appears to apply to strepsirrhines as well as haplorhines. Differences among strepsirrhine taxa show that differences in the duration and pace of gestation are associated with differences in motor development even though relative body size is about the same. Paralleling trends seen in other mammals (Martin 1990), the slow-growing lorises are relatively precocial, with open eyes and the capacity for independent movements at birth whereas galagos require a couple more weeks to develop independent movements (Kappeler 1998). The faster growth rate of lemurs permits the production of precocial infants in spite of brief gestations; the larger lemurs produce open-eyed infants that are capable of independent movement and holding onto the mother at birth (Kappeler 1998). Litter size also affects developmental state; lemur species with more than one offspring and very short gestations like the mouse and dwarf lemurs and the ruffed lemur produce altricial infants that have closed eyes and are incapable of coordinated movement (Kappeler 1998).

Postnatal Development

Prenatal developmental patterns have important implications for postnatal maternal investment. The species with the most altricial neonates keep them in a nest or tree hole for the first few weeks of life. Lemur species with precocial neonates carry them while foraging, but lorises, who might be encumbered while foraging for insects, typically park their infants (Kappeler 1998). Moreover, the high rate of prenatal growth in lemurs may be a significant energetic cost constraining the timing of breeding and rate of reproduction (Young et al. 1990). Although the costs of lactation can be substantially higher than the costs of gestation, there may be stronger selective pressures on gestational energy balance. The prenatal period is the major period of development of the nervous system and other physiological systems, and energy deficits in the prenatal period have a more long-lasting impact on body size, health, and survival than postnatal deficits.

Postnatal growth rates of strepsirrhines are higher than in haplorhines. Lorises grow more slowly than similar sized galagos (Rasmussen and Izard 1988), but lemurs do not appear to differ from galagos and lorises (Kappeler 1996). To the extent that growth rates measure maternal investment, these differences would appear to indicate that lemurs have a more costly reproduction overall, investing at a rate comparable to or greater than that of haplorhine primates throughout the reproductive cycle. However, growth rates provide a less than complete picture of the costs of maternal investment. Galagos and lorises produce very rich milk for primates, with high concentrations of fat and dry matter, and estimated daily and total milk energy output is higher in galagos than in lemurs of similar size (Tilden and Oftedal 1995, 1997). These comparisons suggest that postnatal investment of lorises and galagos may exceed that of lemurs, but they neglect important differences in maternal carriage (Pereira 1993). Whereas most lemurs are in nearly constant contact with their infants, lorises and galagos park their infants during maternal foraging (Tilden and Oftedal 1997), which may explain their richer milk. Fat content is also higher in lemurs like mouse and ruffed lemurs with litters that also are parked. Higher fat content facilitates less frequent suckling of parked infants. The costs of infant carriage are an additional energetic cost of lemur reproduction that should be taken into account (Whitten 1982), although these costs are not likely to raise daily energy requirements by more than 10–15% over basal metabolic rate. Perhaps more important, estimates of investment costs must be assessed in the context of resource abundance. As noted below, the short gestations of the smaller lemurs make it possible to compress the reproductive cycle within the limited Malagasy periods of food abundance. Although the high rate of maternal investment may impose high daily energetic costs, it may not be stressful if it is scheduled during a period of food abundance. However, in the larger lemurs, gestation extends into periods of resource scarcity, and in this context, high investment rates may be energetically stressful.

Thus in general it appears that lorises are characterized by slow reproduction whereas galagos have high postnatal growth rates and lemurs have high fetal growth rates. The ecological basis of these different developmental strategies is unclear. One prediction is that birth rate will be higher in habitats with higher adult mortality (Charnov 1993). Although comparative data on mortality rates are limited, less predictable environments do appear to be associated with higher reproductive rates in galagos and lorises. Galago breeding rate rises with increasing variability in temperature (Nash 1983). Owing to twin births and twice-yearly reproduction, galagos in the seasonally arid parts of South Africa can have three or four infants per year whereas galagos in equatorial habitats have only one infant per year (Bearder 1999). Angwantibos, which exploit short-lived tree-fall zones of tropical forests, have a reproductive potential twice that of pottos living sympatrically in primary forest (Bearder 1999). On the other hand, litter size is higher in lemurs from moist tropical forests than in lemurs from drier, deciduous woodlands (Rasmussen 1985).

SEASONALITY

Like most haplorhine primates, strepsirrhines are restricted in distribution to tropical biomes where they are found primarily in tropical forests (Richard 1985). The dry forests and woodlands of South Africa and southern Madagascar, where winter temperatures may drop below freezing and food may be scarce for a significant portion of the year, mark the limits of their distribution. The eastern Malagasy forests are on the fringe of the tropics and among the most southern of rain forests. Thus Madagascar is a relatively extreme environment for primates, and many of the unique aspects of lemur biology have been attributed to the rigors of its habitats (Jolly 1984; Martin 1972; Pereira 1993; Sauther 1993).

The significance of seasonality has been questioned because the patterning of rainfall in the eastern forests does not appear much different from rainfall patterns in tropical forests elsewhere (Richard and Dewar 1991). Nor does it appear that more seasonal environments prevailed in the past history of Madagascar. However, phenological evidence suggests that lemurs may experience seasonal nutritional stress. In the eastern rain forest of Ranomafana, fruit may be scarce for as much as five months of the year (Overdorff et al. 1999). Seasonality is even more extreme in the dry forests of the south and west, where fruit, leaves, and flowers are scarce for 6–8 months of the year (Curtis et al. 1999; Sauther et al. 1999), but the soils of the west are more fertile and productivity of the dry forests is higher and more predictable than that of the eastern rain forests (Ganzhorn et al. 1999).

How different this patterning is from seasonal variation in African, Asian, or Neotropical forests is difficult to estimate. Frugivores in many rain forest habitats must cope with extended periods of fruit scarcity (Whitten 1999), ranging in duration from 4 to 5 months in the East African rain forests of Kibale (Wrangham et al. 1996) and the Neotropical forests of Coshu Cashu (Terborgh 1983) to 8–10 months in the mast-fruiting forests of Malaysia (Leighton 1993). Is the Malagasy season of scarcity more severe? A comparison of monthly fruit fall records from Ranomafana and Coshu Cashu suggests that fruit productivity is lower in most months in Ranomafana (Wright and Martin 1995), which may be attributable to poorer soils and smaller crown volumes than in other rain forest habitats (Ganzhorn et al. 1999; Wright 1999). However, the duration of fruit scarcity at Coshu Cashu can be as prolonged as that in Ranomafana in some years (see Terborgh 1983), suggesting that more lengthy sampling will be necessary to estimate differences between these variable rain forest habitats accurately. Variability in itself may be an important selective factor. The timing of seasonal peaks in fruit resources varies from year to year owing to drought, cyclones, and irregular fruiting cycles, and this unpredictability, as will be seen below, significantly impacts lemur reproduction (Overdorff et al. 1999; Wright 1999). Variability in fruit availability may be exacerbated by the scarcity of foods like nectar, figs, immature leaves, or palm nuts in the dry season (Curtis et al. 1999; Sauther et al. 1999), resources that primates in Neotropical and Southeast Asian forests rely on when fruit is scarce (Meyers and Wright 1993; Terborgh 1992; Wright and Martin 1995).

BEHAVIORAL MECHANISMS FOR ENERGY CONSERVATION

Thermoregulatory stress may be another important constraint imposed by seasonality (Richard and Dewar 1991). Although there is only about 5°C variation in mean temperature over the year, the diurnal range can be as high as 15°C (Morland 1993; Richard and Dewar 1991), with nighttime lows below the thermoneutral zone for some of the larger lemurs (Curtis et al. 1999; Schmid and Kappeler 1998). Lemurs utilize a variety of behavioral responses to low temperature, such as huddling, sleeping in contact or in holes or nests, and sunning (Curtis et al. 1999; Morland 1993; Richard and Dewar 1991). Although behavioral regulation of temperature was initially taken as evidence of poor physiologic control (Pollock 1989), more recent research suggests that these behaviors are important energy-conserving mechanisms (Curtis et al. 1999). An additional mechanism for coping with seasonally low temperatures may be modification of daily activity patterns. Most strepsirrhines are nocturnal, but many indriids and lemurids are active during the daylight hours (Richard and Dewar 1991).

Eulemur and *Hapalemur* species are cathemeral, active in both the light and dark phases of the 24-hour cycle. This unusual pattern of activity may provide thermoregulatory benefits since increasing activity in the coolest part of the day reduces the energetic cost of homeothermy (Curtis et al. 1999). Alternative explanations for cathemerality are that it is an ancestral pattern, that it is a transitional stage between nocturnality and diurnality, or that it allows the ingestion and processing of fibrous foods by small lemurs that have expanded their diets following the extinction of the Malagasy megafauna (Richard and Dewar 1991).

METABOLIC RATE

Basal metabolic rate (BMR) is lower in strepsirrhines than in most haplorhine primates (Müller 1985; Müller et al. 1985; Richard and Nicoll 1987), with basal heat production falling 20–60% below mass-specific mammalian standards (Müller et al. 1985). The low BMR of strepsirrhines has been attributed to retention of an ancestral condition (Martin 1972), a toxic or low-quality diet (Kurland and Pearson 1986; McNab 1984), or an adaptation to a nocturnal lifestyle (Müller et al. 1985). Cross-species regressions do not support a link between BMR and dietary variation within the primates (Ross 1992). Nor is there a clear relation to nocturnality. Although nocturnal haplorhines (tarsiers, night monkeys) have a relatively low BMR, strepsirrhines have a low BMR whether they are diurnal or nocturnal, suggesting that low BMR may be an ancestral primate trait (Ross 1992). The question remains, however, why the diurnal lemurs have retained a low BMR. It may be that the energy-saving benefits of lowered metabolism are well suited to Madagascar's seasonal environments. Species with a lowered metabolic rate save energy by allowing the body surface to cool during the inactive phase, relying on thick fur and vascular adaptations for counter current heat exchange to maintain core body temperature (Müller et al. 1985). Body cooling is not a result of deficient thermoregulation; slender lorises, slow lorises, and potto are capable of tripling heat production in response to very low ambient temperatures (Müller et al. 1985). A low BMR is well suited to a nocturnal lifestyle because homothermy is relaxed during the warmest part of the day. Reductions in BMR during the inactive phase also have been reported in callitrichids and small rodents (Power 1999). Apparently, daily shifts in metabolic rate are not be limited to strepsirrhines but rather may be a more widespread energetic strategy of small mammals. In fact, it has been suggested that the uniformly low metabolic rates reported for nocturnal primates may reflect the fact that the measurements of nocturnal primates have generally been taken during the inactive phase whereas measurements for diurnal primates were collected during the active phase (Power 1999).

Low BMR may be an initial obstacle to strepsirrhine reproduction since increases in metabolic rate are generally a prerequisite to reproduction, and the proportionate increase in mammals with low BMR is much greater than in species with a higher BMR (Thompson and Nicoll 1986). Field data suggest that BMR is elevated in sifaka females during gestation (Richard and Nicoll 1987). As described above, the smallest lemurs also undergo marked increases in metabolic rate and weight loss during the mating season (Perret et al. 1998; Schmid and Kappeler 1998). Raising metabolic rate could be energetically stressful in a resource-poor environment. However, female mouse lemurs actually put on weight during lactation and weaning (Schmid and Kappeler 1998), suggesting that not only are they not energetically stressed but they also may be taking advantage of a superabundance of resources during the most costly period of reproduction.

SEASONAL TORPOR

Facultative adjustments in metabolism and body temperature are additional energy-saving mechanisms. The dwarf and mouse lemurs exhibit both brief daily bouts of torpor and more prolonged periods of seasonal torpor or lethargy (Ortmann and Heldmaier 1997; Petter 1965; Schmid 1999; Wright and Martin 1995). Marked daily changes in basal metabolic rate and body temperature also have been observed in sportive lemurs (Schmid and Ganzhorn 1996).

Although torpor was originally thought to reflect an imperfect thermoregulation (Pollock 1989), it now appears to be a mechanism for energy conservation in habitats with fluctuating food resources (Geiser 1998). The mouse and dwarf lemurs are the smallest strepsirrhines (25–450 g) and may find it difficult to acquire the energy necessary to maintain homeothermy under conditions of food scarcity. Fruit, the major food of the greater dwarf lemur, is scarce for five months of the year (Wright and Martin 1995). Insects, a major food of mouse lemurs, become inactive or die during cold (Nash 1983) or dry (Butynski 1988) seasons.

Like cathemerality, daily torpor saves energy by making use of daily temperature gradients. Metabolism declines as much as 90% in the early morning hours, and body temperature falls to ambient temperatures over the animal's diurnal resting phase (Aujard et al. 1998; Ortmann and Heldmaier 1997). Body temperature rises passively as ambient temperature climbs over the course of the warm daylight hours. When body temperature surpasses 25°C near the end of the day, metabolic rate returns to the normothermic level, in time for the nocturnal activity phase. The

predictable increase in ambient temperature over the day allows reawak-
ening from torpor without endogenous heat production, providing as
much as a threefold energy savings (Lovegrove et al. 1999). This cycle of
hypothermia reduces daily energy expenditure by as much as 60%. However, torpor can be maintained only as long as ambient temperatures are
below 29°C, a limitation on the duration of torpor that can be moderated
by making use of the insulating properties of tree holes (Schmid 1998).
Further energy savings are achieved by nesting in groups of three or more
animals (Perret 1998).

More prolonged torpor occurs during the dry season when both temperature and rainfall reach their annual nadir. Seasonal torpor may last as
long as 4 months in the greater fat-tailed dwarf lemur (Cheirogaleus major)
and 8–9 months in the fat-tailed dwarf lemur (Cheirogaleus medius) and the
gray mouse lemur (Microcebus murinus) (Schmid and Kappeler 1998;
Wright and Martin 1995). However, mouse lemurs do not enter as profound a torpor as dwarf lemurs, and they become active again every few
days (Richard 1985). Moreover, male mouse lemurs may hibernate for
shorter periods of time or not at all, increasing activity two months before
females to establish territories and hierarchies in preparation for breeding
(Miller 1999; Schmid 1999; Schmid and Kappeler 1998). No seasonal torpor
has been observed in other strepsirrhines (Petter-Rousseaux 1980), but
increased inactivity during the cool, dry season has been reported in a
sportive lemur (Nash 1998).

SEASONAL CHANGES IN BODY MASS

The adaptation for seasonal torpor in the smallest lemurs includes the ability to gain remarkable amounts of weight during the relatively short
period of food abundance (Miller 1999; Wright and Martin 1995). Captive
dwarf lemurs may double their weight in a little over a week. Because they
do not enter torpor in captivity, this excessive weight gain may have fatal
consequences (Lee et al. 1996; Miller 1999). Although daily and seasonal
torpor have been posited as alternative strategies in mouse lemurs
(Schmid 1999) and other mammals (Geiser 1998; Geiser and Ruf 1995),
daily torpor may permit weight gain in preparation for seasonal torpor.
For example, insectivorous bats store fat in the pre-hibernal period
through daily torpor (Speakman and Rowland 1999). Attaining a minimal
mass appears to be essential in order for mouse lemurs to enter seasonal
torpor, and females and juveniles who have not done so may forgo hibernation (Schmid and Kappeler 1998).

Contrary to what one might expect, seasonal torpor does not appear to
promote the storage of fat for pregnancy and lactation. In fact, female

mouse lemurs may actually lose as much as a third of their weight during the period of torpor, regaining weight during the four months of gestation and lactation (Schmid and Kappeler 1998). Thus it appears that seasonal resource abundance supports female reproductive effort, and seasonal torpor functions primarily as a survival mechanism, preventing fitness-compromising weight loss during a period of energetic stress.

Male mouse lemurs, on the other hand, may gain weight during the dry-season months prior to the mating season (Kappeler 1997a; Schmid and Kappeler 1998). How weight gain can occur is unclear, since the majority of males are not in torpor, and in fact males in torpor do not gain or lose weight (Schmid 1999). Weight increases may be due to the anabolic actions of sex steroids, as has been shown for the seasonal fattening of Neotropical squirrel monkeys (Boinski 1987), and appear to be due in large part to the proliferation of testicular tissue (Schmid and Kappeler 1998). Males subsequently lose weight in conjunction with male-male competition during the breeding season.

Seasonal weight changes are not limited to diminutive lemurs. Weight gain prior to the mating season also has been reported in captive ringtailed lemur males and females, which is lost over the mating season (Pereira 1993). Captive females provisioned with an abundant diet also show a marked increase in weight early in lactation whereas females on a low provisioned diet lost weight over the same period, suggesting a change in metabolism or foraging behavior. Sifaka, on the other hand, lose weight at the end of the mating season, but at the same time as ringtailed lemurs, in the late dry season. Longitudinal data from the dry forest habitat of Beza Mahafaly in southwestern Madagascar show that sifaka females of reproductive age lose significantly more mass during the dry season than males, especially in drought years (Richard et al. 2000). Females may lose 12–21% of body mass whereas males lose 6–12% by the end of the dry season. More marked losses in drought years suggest that these fluctuations in body mass are related to resource availability, but mass changes are not restricted to lemurs in dry forests. In the rain forest habitat of Ranomafana, mass losses of 12% have been reported over the year in sifaka and losses of 5–9% have been observed over three-month periods in rufous and red-bellied lemurs (Glander et al. 1992).

Photoperiod-mediated changes in metabolism also may play a role in seasonal mass changes. Mass gain begins after the summer solstice in captive female ringtailed lemurs and just before the autumnal equinox in males (Pereira 1993). Experimental studies in mouse and dwarf lemurs show that changes in male body mass are produced by photoperiod-regulated changes in metabolic rate and activity levels (Aujard et al. 1998; Perret et al. 1998). Short days, which herald the cool, dry austral winter in Madagascar, suppress resting metabolic rate and water loss in mouse lemur males, resulting in mass gain, whereas long days stimulate increases in metabolic rate and activity, causing mass loss (Perret et al. 1998). The proximate mechanisms regulating female activity have not been examined in mouse lemurs, but increases in day length have been shown to stimulate activity levels in female as well as male dwarf lemurs (Foerg and Hoffmann 1982).

REPRODUCTIVE SCHEDULES

About 80% of ringtail lemur females (Sauther et al. 1999) and 52–60% of red-fronted lemur females (Overdorff et al. 1999) give birth each year. In contrast, only 48% of sifaka in southwestern Madagascar give birth each year (Richard et al. 1991; Richard in press). In spite of this variation in fertility, all three species have high infant mortality rates in comparison with haplorhine rates (Wright 1999), averaging 30–50% in ringtail lemurs (Sauther et al. 1999), 41% in red-fronted lemurs (Overdorff et al. 1990), and 48% in sifaka (Richard in press). Demographic data from sifaka at Beza Mahafaly show that these rates can vary markedly in times of drought or food abundance, with the percentage of females giving birth ranging from 27% to 65% and infant mortality ranging from 30% to 70% in any given year. Individual females also vary in reproductive success as a function of age, rank, or body condition. In red-fronted lemurs and Milne-Edward's sifaka, one female in each group may be responsible for the majority of successful births (Overdorff and Erhart 1998; Overdorff et al. 1999). In ringtailed lemurs, young and prime-aged females have higher survival rates than older females (Sauther et al. 1999) whereas in red-fronted lemurs it is the older females, who are generally heavier and have feeding priority over younger females, that have higher cumulative reproductive success (Overdorff et al. 1999). In Verreaux's sifaka, older, higher-ranking females also outreproduce younger females when groups are large (Kubzdela 1997). Moreover, longitudinal data from Beza Mahafaly show that sifaka females who are heavier at the onset of the mating season are more likely to give birth the following birth season (Richard et al. 2000).

The consequences of reproductive effort for future fertility appear to vary across species. In red-fronted lemurs, interbirth intervals are 1–2 years longer after a surviving infant (Overdorff et al. 1999). In sifaka, on the other hand, females with surviving infants actually have a higher probability of giving birth in the subsequent year, and successful reproduction does not reduce the likelihood of maternal or infant survival (Richard, in prep.). Moreover, some smaller-bodied strepsirrhines can reproduce as often as twice per year because of a postpartum estrus or a very brief lactation (Bearder 1987; Lindburg 1987; MacKinnon and MacKinnon 1980; Martin

1972; Nash 1983; Roberts 1994; Zimmerman 1989). Species with twice-yearly reproduction include the angwantibo and slender loris, and the smaller galago species (Nash 1983), all weighing 300 g or less. In captivity, mouse lemurs also may produce a second litter from a postpartum estrus (Andriantsiferana et al. 1974), but field data suggest that second litters rarely if ever occur in free-ranging mouse lemurs (Atsalis, 1998).

The costs of reproduction are borne almost solely by females. Paternal investment is limited in strepsirrhines. The intensive infant care observed for males of small-bodied monogamous or polyandrous haplorhines like the callitrichids has not been observed in monogamous strepsirrhines like indri or avahi or in species with relatively large neonates (Miller 1999). It has been suggested that females in these species may cache or park their infants owing to the lack of paternal care (Miller 1999; Wright 1990), but these neonates are considerably smaller than the 22% or more of maternal body weight typical of the monkeys with paternal carrying (Whitten 1987). Male fat-tailed dwarf lemurs do assist in babysitting, which appears to be crucial for successful rearing of offspring (Fietz 1999).

BREEDING SEASONS

Although reproduction is somewhat seasonal in most strepsirrhines, the degree of reproductive seasonality varies with climatic seasonality. In equatorial West Africa, where there are two 4–5 month rainy seasons per year, nonseasonal breeding with birth peaks appears to be the norm for angwantibos, the needle-clawed galago, Demidoff's galago, and Allen's galago, whereas sympatric pottos give birth in a distinct season (Charles-Dominique 1977; Nash 1983). The difference in breeding schedules may be related to allometric differences in maturation rates. The 2–3 month lactation periods of the tiny (60–300 g) galagos can be contained within a single wet season whereas the seven-month lactation periods of the 1,200 g potto, extending over both wet and dry seasons, require more precise scheduling. The galagos of the more seasonal habitats of East and Southern Africa breed more seasonally, giving birth within three-month birth seasons. The Zanzibar bushbaby takes advantage of the two rainy seasons of East Africa, giving birth just after the short rains, as does its larger sympatric congener, but giving birth again one gestation period later, just before the start of the long rains (Nash 1983). The southern lesser bushbaby in Southern Africa and the gray mouse lemur in western Madagascar, both weighing less than 200 g, manage to squeeze two reproductive cycles into their brief four-month rainy seasons (Nash 1983; Schmid and Kappeler 1998). Less is known about breeding seasonality in the Southeast Asian lorises. Slow lorises may be nonseasonal (Lindburg 1987), whereas

slender lorises in India have two birth seasons per year, at the beginning
and end of the rainy season (MacKinnon and MacKinnon 1980; Roonwal
and Mohnot 1977).

Two lemur species, the aye-aye and the crowned lemur, appear to be
nonseasonal breeders (Sterling 1994), but all other lemurs appear to be
highly seasonal, giving birth within a period of 1–3 months whether in rain
forest or dry forest habitats (Richard and Dewar 1991; Sterling 1994),
although birth seasonality is relaxed in some species in captivity. For example, 96% of Verreaux's sifaka births ($n = 166$) are confined to the austral winter months of July and August in southwest Madagascar, whereas 86% of
Coquerel's sifaka births ($n = 55$) are spread over the months of December
through March in the captive environs of North Carolina (Brockman, in
prep.). Although the exact timing of births varies across species (Sterling
1994; Wright 1999), births are highly synchronized within lemur populations. Captive breeding records for six lemur species indicate a bimodal
pattern with clusters of births approximately one month apart (Rasmussen
1985), a patterning suggestive of estrus synchrony. Mating is clustered
within a one- to three-week period within ringtailed and rufous lemur
groups (Overdorff 1998; Sauther et al. 1999). However, fecal steroid data
from free-ranging sifaka have shown that both behavioral and hormonal
estrus spans a broader period of time than previously thought (Brockman
and Whitten 1996). Relative to primates as a whole, lemur reproduction is
quite seasonal, but it is not as remarkable as is often implied. Anthropoids
as well as strepsirrhines may have highly seasonal births in very seasonal
environments. For example, guenons have birth seasons of 2–3 months in
areas with a single wet season, often with the majority of births occurring
within a 2-week period (Butynski 1988), and squirrel monkeys and a number of macaque species have birth seasons of 2–4 months (Lindburg 1987).

ULTIMATE EXPLANATIONS FOR
BREEDING SEASONALITY

Like all primates, strepsirrhines must cope with prolonged periods of gestation (2–6.5 months) and lactation (1.5–12 months), which generally confine a portion of the reproductive cycle to a less than optimal season. Only
the tiny mouse and dwarf lemurs, with a period of 3–4 months for gestation and lactation combined (Roberts 1994), are able to fit the entire reproductive cycle into a single rainy season (Schmid and Kappeler 1998).
Similar sized galagos have a more extended period of maternal investment (5–8 months). For example, Demidoff's galago, even tinier than the
dwarf and mouse lemurs at just 63 g, has a lactation period as short but has
a 1.5-month-longer gestation (Roberts 1994). However, the availability of

two long rainy seasons (Nash 1983) makes it possible for this West African galago to locate most of its maternal investment within a season of food abundance. The lesser South African galago is less fortunate. Half the size of the greater dwarf lemur, this galago has gestation and lactation periods that are twice as long (Roberts 1994), resulting in an eight-month reproductive cycle that cannot be contained within the single four-month rainy season. Lorises and the larger lemurs have even longer, 8–11 month, periods of investment (Roberts 1994), also necessitating the scheduling of some part of the reproductive cycle during suboptimal periods. Gestation extends into dry season periods of low food availability in most of these species (MacKinnon and MacKinnon 1980; Nash 1983; Roonwal and Mohnot 1977; Wright 1999). Among the lemurs, the interval from the birth season to the onset of the rainy season increases with body size, suggesting that the timing of conception is adjusted so that lactation and weaning occur when food is most abundant, nutritious, and obtainable (Martin 1972; Rasmussen 1985; Wright 1999). Rapid infant growth in ringtailed lemurs, with weight gains of 4–8 g/day in the first seven months of life, helps to compress infant maturation into the period of resource abundance (Pereira 1993). Growth slows markedly after the autumnal equinox, a pattern that also has been reported in mouse and dwarf lemur infants (Pereira 1993). In ringtailed lemurs of Beza Mahafaly in southwestern Madagascar, birth occurs in October, a time of a peak of flower production. Early lactation and weaning in ringtailed lemurs coincide with peaks in fruit availability in October and February, and the entire lactation and weaning period occurs during a period of young leaf availability (Sauther et al. 1999). In contrast, the larger sympatric Verreaux's sifaka must conceive by March and give birth in July–September, when food is scarcest, in order to wean their infants during the December–January onset of summer rains when the breeding season commences and new leaves become most abundant.

Lactation also falls during a period of peak fruit availability in redfronted lemurs and black-and-white ruffed lemurs, but rain forest populations of both species experience considerable year-to-year variability in the timing of fruiting peaks (Overdorff et al. 1999; Sterling 1994). Both greater and lesser galagos in South Africa also appear to be optimizing the availability of weaning foods, weaning infants at the middle or end of the rainy season when food is plentiful for some time so that infants are close to adult size by the end of the period of plenty (Martin 1990; Nash 1983). The same does not appear to apply to East African galagos, who give birth in a dry season and wean before or after periods when food supplies are lowest (Nash 1983).

Although limited, there is some evidence for selective pressure on the timing of lactation. Infant mortality is higher in rufous lemurs when resource availability peaks in late gestation and early lactation than when peak fruit availability occurs mid-lactation (Overdorff et al. 1999).

Proximate Stimuli

There is good evidence that photoperiod regulates the seasonal onset of mating in many strepsirrhines. Northern hemisphere colonies of Malagasy primates show a six-month reversal in the timing of reproduction from that observed in Madagascar, and the modal date of mating is correlated with the latitude of the species range in Madagascar (Lindburg 1987; Rasmussen 1985). The timing of breeding varies with taxonomic group. The lemurs are short-day breeders, mating during decreasing day length 1–2 months before the winter solstice, whereas the dwarf and mouse lemurs and indriids are long-day breeders, mating during increasing day length prior to or at the summer solstice (Rasmussen 1985; Sterling 1994). The seasonally breeding galagos also are short-day breeders, conceiving in the declining days after the autumnal equinox, but the lesser galagos can conceive again during the lengthening days following the vernal equinox, when day length is approximately the same.

Experimental studies have shown that these patterns are regulated photoperiodically. In ringtailed lemurs mating is inhibited by long-day photoperiods, and short-day photoperiods are required for reversal of photoinhibition (Reynolds and van Horn 1977; van Horn 1975). Mouse lemurs and dwarf lemurs, on the other hand, are stimulated to mate by long days and inhibited by short-day photoperiods (Foerg 1982; Petter-Rousseaux 1974).

Males begin preparation for reproductive activity several months before females. Weight gain, testicular enlargement, and elevations in testosterone begin 2–3 months prior to the onset of female sexual receptivity in lesser mouse lemurs (Schmid and Kappeler 1998), Coquerel's mouse lemurs (Kappeler 1997a), ruffed lemurs (Foerg 1982), golden bamboo lemurs (Glander et al. 1992), and Verreaux's sifaka (Brockman et al. 1998; Kraus et al. 1999). This may mean that males are stimulated by different photoperiods than are females or that females require a longer period of time to awaken ovarian function. The need for a warm-up period is suggested by experimental studies showing that 1–3 months may elapse between the onset of short-day photoperiods and the appearance of estrus in ringtailed lemurs (Rasmussen 1985).

Short days stimulate male weight gain in both ringtailed and mouse lemurs in spite of the fact that they reproduce at opposite periods of the year. In lesser and Coquerel's mouse lemurs, body mass and testes size increase during the short days (10–12 hours of light) between the winter solstice and the spring equinox, reaching peak size just before the mating season (Kappeler 1997a; Perret 1977; Schmid and Kappeler 1998). As reviewed above, weight gains occur during the dry season period of food scarcity and appear to be mediated through a short-day-stimulated reduction in resting metabolic rate (Perret et al. 1998). Resting metabolic rate increases during the mating season in response to lengthening days, resulting in weight loss (Perret 1998; Perret et al. 1998). Increased metabolic rate allows increased activity levels, which may be spent in home range establishment and defense. For example, Coquerel's mouse lemur males quadruple their home range size in mating season, covering more than ten females' home ranges (Kappeler 1997b). In captive ringtailed lemurs, male weight gain also occurs between the winter solstice and the spring equinox, but it commences again between the summer solstice and the fall equinox when testicular enlargement and mating occur (Pereira 1993; Rasmussen 1985). This bimodal pattern of weight gain suggests that seasonal changes in body weight may be mediated by several mechanisms, including perhaps thyroid-hormone-mediated changes in metabolism as well as gonadal steroid effects.

Gonadal steroid regulation of breeding season events has been examined in detail in wild and captive sifaka (Brockman 1994, 1999; Brockman and Whitten 1996, 1999; Brockman et al. 1995, 1998, 2001). Fecal steroid profiles show that male testosterone levels are elevated 1–3 months prior to the start of mating activity (Brockman et al. 1995; Kraus et al. 1999). Some females exhibit signs of ovarian activity during this period; elevations in estradiol, but not progesterone, can be seen in some females 1–2 months prior to an ovulatory cycle and behavioral estrus (Brockman and Whitten 1996; Brockman et al. 1995). Mounts, but not completed copulations, may occur in conjunction with these earlier estradiol peaks. These data suggest that gonadal recrudescence generally begins earlier in males than in females but that some females may initiate ovarian steroidogenesis early in the breeding season. The picture is complicated, however, by the fact that some males maintain elevated testosterone levels beyond the breeding season in response to male dispersal or group instability (Brockman and Whitten 1999; Brockman et al. 1998, 2001). Thus social events may modulate the schedules imposed by photoperiodic stimuli (Izard 1990).

Reproductive Suppression

Seasonal testicular enlargement is more marked in dominant males in mouse lemurs (Izard 1990) and sifaka (Kraus et al. 1999), and dominant sifaka males may maintain elevated testosterone levels throughout the year (Brockman et al. 1998, 2001). Grouping of male mouse lemurs results in suppression of seasonal testicular enlargement in all but the dominant male (Izard 1990). Similar results have been obtained with scent marks, or volatile components of the urine of other males, suggesting the importance of olfactory signals in these effects. Whether the rank-related differences in sifaka testicular function represent reproductive suppression in subordinate males (Kraus et al. 1999) or the overriding of photoperiodic stimuli by dominant males remains to be determined.

Suppression of reproductive cycles by other females also has been reported. In mouse lemurs, luteal phase plasma progesterone concentrations in isolated females are double those seen in females housed with other females (Perret 1986). Similar reductions in ovarian steroid concentrations have been observed in young adult daughters in the presence of cycling mothers among captive sifaka (Brockman, unpublished data).

Situation-Dependent Receptivity

The expanded and situation-dependent receptivity of many catarrhine primates provides an evolutionary link to the continuous sexual receptivity that is a hallmark of the human condition (Hrdy and Whitten 1987). In contrast, the brief, hormonally delimited estrous periods of strepsirrhine primates have generally been presented as examples of the generalized mammalian pattern of strictly circumscribed estrus (Hrdy and Whitten 1987). However, there is considerable evidence for social mediation of sexual behavior in strepsirrhine primates.

For example, male-female interactions can have a significant effect on the timing and duration of estrus. Physical proximity to a novel male appears to stimulate aggression-related ovarian activity and subsequent mating in captive sifaka (Brockman, in prep.), and social interaction with a male can induce ovarian cycles in photoperiod-inhibited female ring-tailed lemurs (van Horn 1975, 1980). Coital stimulation has been shown to shorten the period of sexual receptivity or vaginal cornification in small-eared galagos and ringtailed lemurs (Dixson 1995). Housing with an adult male reduces the age of first estrus in small-eared greater galagos and southern lesser galagos, although it has no effect in large-eared greater galagos (Izard 1990). Even in galagos, where cyclical fusion of the vagina would appear to confine copulation to estrus, the duration of sexual receptivity is longer (1–10 days) in nongregarious than in gregarious strepsirrhines (2–24 hours) (Hrdy and Whitten 1987).

In wild multifemale sifaka social groups, behavioral receptivity is associated with 10–15 day elevations in fecal estradiol (Brockman and Whitten 1996), but in captive single-female groups, hormonal estrus is reduced to just five days. Although mating generally occurs in conjunction with elevations in fecal estradiol in sifaka females, some matings may occur in the absence of elevated estrogen. For example, following the immigration of a new resident male, a substantial proportion of sexual presents and matings occurred in the absence of estradiol elevations (Brockman and Whitten 1996).

Female-female interactions also may influence the onset of estrus. Estrous synchrony in lemurs was first reported by Jolly (1966b), who observed that all nine females in a free-ranging group of ringtailed lemurs underwent genital swelling and coloration within a ten-day period; subsequent research has shown that ringtailed females in the same group come into estrus within 1–3 weeks of one another (Sauther et al. 1999), similar to that observed in sympatric sifaka (Brockman and Whitten 1996). The close conjunction of behavioral estrus within social groups has also been reported in ruffed and red-fronted lemurs and sifaka, as well as greater thick-tailed galagos (Izard 1990; Brockman 1994).

Hormonal profiles from wild sifaka show that the patterning of estrus can be quite complex, however, with both synchronous and asynchronous patterning of periovulatory periods, asynchronous mating in spite of ovulatory synchrony, and intense female-female competition during synchronous periovulatory periods (Brockman and Whitten 1996). Moreover, matings with multiple males are not required for fertilization, and estrous synchrony does not appear to prevent females from mating with multiple resident and nonresident males.

Recent evidence suggests that situation-dependent receptivity may be an ancestral, rather than derived, property of the Primate order. Social regulation of estrus is the rule in some shrews, mammals that are thought to be closely related to primates. For example, sexual activity in musk shrews is independent of ovulation and may occur during pregnancy or lactation (Rissman et al. 1988). There is no estrous cycle, and mating occurs prior to estrogen secretion and follicular development (Dryden 1969; Rissman et al. 1988). Female sexual behavior is activated by plasma testosterone aromatized centrally to estradiol (Rissman 1991; Sharma and Rissman 1994), and aggressive interactions with a male are required to initiate sexual receptivity (Rissman 1987). Progesterone and cortisol increase when females begin to display receptive behavior (Rissman and Crews 1988; Rissman et al. 1997). These precopulatory interactions stimulate the release of Gn-RH peptide from the medial septum and preoptic, a response that may stimulate LH production and initiate follicular development and estradiol production (Fortune et al. 1992; Tai et al. 1997), and repeated matings over 24 or more hours stimulate ovulation (Rissman 1992). This socially mediated estrus may be a better model for ancestral primate sexuality than the hormonally circumscribed estrus of rodents.

DISCUSSION

Sharing the large brains, long lifespan, and high reproductive investment of haplorhine primates, strepsirrhine primates provide a unique opportunity to examine the ecological significance of some of the most basic attributes of primates. This review has compared the life history, energetics, and reproductive seasonality of lemurs, galagos, and lorises and raised some questions about their adaptive significance.

Developmental patterns of strepsirrhines provide insight into the evolution of primate life history. The relatively small mass of strepsirrhine neonates may be a consequence of investment in prolonged neurogenesis, reflecting the evolution of primate brain:body ratios. How haplorhine primates are able to maintain the same brain:body ratio in spite of greater investment in somatic growth during gestation is unclear, but the rapid fetal growth rates of lemurs may provide some clues to mechanisms. Although lemur fetal growth equals haplorhine rates, shorter gestations result in strepsirrhine-sized neonates. Brief gestation in the smallest lemurs and galagos makes it possible to compress the reproductive cycle into the period of food abundance. This is not possible in the larger strepsirrhines, where gestation lasts 4–6 months. In these species, conceptions appear to be timed so that peak lactation and weaning coincide with the period of greatest food abundance. Interspecific variation in the duration of gestation and lactation appears to be related to degree of precociality and patterns of postnatal care, but the relative roles of ecological constraints and life history factors in the evolution of gestation and lactation lengths need to be examined in greater detail.

Seasonality may have been an important selective factor in the evolution of lemur physiology and behavior. A number of lemur traits, such as low metabolic rate, cathemeral activity patterns, diurnal and seasonal torpor, and seasonal modulation of metabolism and growth, appear to minimize energetic expense during periods of resource scarcity. These traits may be adaptations to prolonged Malagasy dry periods as well as to seasonally cold temperatures and unpredictable resources. How different Madagascar is from other strepsirrhine habitats, however, needs to be more carefully documented; recent work indicates that there are some significant differences (Richard et al., submitted; Wright 1999).

There is good evidence that strepsirrhines rely on photoperiodic cues to schedule reproduction and seasonal adjustments in metabolism, growth, and body mass. Reliance on photoperiodic cues may have been a constraint in the evolution of gestation length, since the periods of the year when day length varies substantially from 12 hours per day are limited in the tropics (Spinage 1973). Lemur reliance on photoperiodic cuing is surprising in light of the evidence for resource unpredictability in Madagascar. Photoperiod may provide adequate cueing when averaged over the long reproductive lifespans of lemurs, however, and may be the only cue capable of synchronizing weaning with the optimal season through the scheduling of conception (Bronson 1989). Moreover, it appears that other cues help to fine-tune lemur responses to local conditions. Mating season body mass significantly influences a sifaka female's likelihood of giving birth the following birth season (Richard et al., submitted), which could reflect nutritionally mediated attractiveness, anovulation, or conceptive loss. Lemur males also undergo seasonal changes in body mass, but these changes appear to reflect the anabolic actions of sex steroids as well as resource availability. Little is known about how body mass or nutrition affect male reproductive success in any strepsirrhine.

Further fine-tuning may occur through social interactions. In both lemurs and galagos, interactions with a male can help to initiate ovarian cycles and behavioral estrus. Gonadal development begins earlier in lemur males, and their reproductive condition is likely to reflect current environmental conditions as well as social stability. Interactions with other females can increase the synchrony or duration of behavioral estrus or suppress ovulatory cycles. These interactions may help to mediate female reproductive competition in small lemur groups where only one or two females give birth each year and few females are able to reproduce yearly. Flexible sexuality appears to be an important aspect of strepsirrhine reproduction and may be a more ancestral feature of primates than commonly thought.

This review shows that strepsirrhine traits are not evolutionary anachronisms but rather adaptations to schedule activity and reproduction in highly seasonal environments. In fact, the features we tend to consider most derived in primates—large brains, slow reproduction, and flexible sexuality—are distinctive features of strepsirrhine primates. Comparative studies of strepsirrhines are likely to provide new insights into the mechanisms and adaptive significance of the patterning of maternal investment, scheduling of reproduction, and social regulation of sexuality in primates.

REFERENCES

Aboitiz F (1996) Does bigger mean better? Evolutionary determinants of brain size and structure. *Brain Behavior and Evolution* 47:225–245.

Andriantsiferana R, Rarijaona Y, Randrianaivo A (1974) Observations sur la reproduction du Microcebe (*Microcebus murinus*, Miller 1777) en captivite a Tananarive. *Mammalia* 38:234–243.

Atsalis S (1998) Feeding Ecology and Aspects of Life History in *Microcebus rufus* (Family: Cheirogaleidae, Order: Primates). PhD dissertation (City University of New York).

Aujard F, Perret M, Vannier G (1998) Thermoregulatory responses to variations of photoperiod and ambient temperature in the male lesser mouse lemur: a primitive or an advanced adaptive character? *Journal of Comparative Physiology*, B: Biochemical, Systemic, and Environmental Physiology 168:540–548.

Bearder SK (1987) Lorises, bushbabies, and tarsiers: diverse societies in solitary foragers. In BB Smuts, DL Cheney, RM Seyfarth, RW Wrangham, TT Struhsaker (Eds) *Primate Societies* (Chicago, University of Chicago Press), 11–24.

Bearder SK (1999) Physical and social diversity among nocturnal primates: a new view based on long-term research. *Primates* 40:267–282.

Boinski S (1987) Mating patterns in squirrel monkeys *(Saimiri oerstedi):* implications for seasonal sexual dimorphism. *Behavioral Ecology and Sociobiology* 21:13–21.

Bourliere F (1974) How to remain prosimian in a simian world. In RD Martin, GA Doyle, AC Walker (Eds) *Prosimian Biology* (Pittsburgh, University of Pittsburgh Press), 17–22.

Brockman DK (1994) Reproduction and mating system of Verreaux's sifaka, *Propithecus verreauxi*, at Beza Mahafaly, Madagascar. PhD dissertation (New Haven, Yale University).

Brockman DK (1999) Reproductive behavior of female *Propithecus verreauxi* at Beza Mahafaly, Madagascar. *International Journal of Primatology* 20:375–398.

Brockman DK, Whitten PL (1996) Reproduction in free-ranging *Propithecus verreauxi:* estrus and the relationship between multiple partner matings and fertilization. *American Journal of Physical Anthropology* 100:57–69.

Brockman DK, Whitten PL (1999) Group transfer and male competition in *Propithecus verreauxi:* insights into factors mediating male infanticide in a seasonally breeding primate. *American Journal of Physical Anthropology* 28(Suppl):98.

Brockman DK, Whitten PL, Richard AF, Schneider A (1998) Reproduction in free-ranging male *Propithecus verreauxi:* hormonal correlates of mating and aggression. *American Journal of Physical Anthropology* 105:137–151.

Brockman DK, Whitten PL, Russell E, Richard AF, Izard MK (1995) Application of fecal steroid techniques to the reproductive endocrinology of female Verreaux's sifaka, *Propithecus verreauxi. American Journal of Primatology* 36:313–325.

Brockman DK, Whitten PL, Richard AF, Benander B (2001) Birth season testosterone levels in male Verreaux's sifaka, *Propithecus verreauxi:* insights into sociodemographic factors mediating seasonal testicular function. *Behavioral Ecology and Sociobiology* 49:117–127.

Bronson FH (1989) *Mammalian Reproductive Biology* (Chicago, University of Chicago Press).

Butynski TM (1988) Guenon birth seasons and correlates with rainfall and food. In A Gautier-Hion, F Bourliere, JP Gautier, J Kingdon (Eds) *A Primate Radiation: Evolutionary Biology of the African Guenons* (Cambridge, Cambridge University Press), 284–322.

Charles-Dominique P (1977) *Ecology and Behaviour of Nocturnal Prosimians* (London, Duckworth).

Charnov EL (1993) *Life History Invariants: Some Explorations of Symmetry in Evolutionary Ecology* (Oxford, Oxford University Press).

Covert HH (1995) Locomotor adaptations of Eocene primates: adaptive diversity in the earliest prosimians. In L Alternman, GA Doyle, MK Izard (Eds) *Creatures of the Dark: The Nocturnal Prosimians* (New York), 495–509.

Curtis DJ, Zaramody A, Martin RD (1999) Cathemerality in the mongoose lemur, *Eulemur mongoz. American Journal of Primatology* 47:279–298.

Deacon TW (1997) *The Symbolic Species: The Co-evolution of Language and the Brain* (New York, WW Norton).

Dixson AF (1995) Sexual selection and the evolution of copulatory behavior in nocturnal prosimians. In L Alternman, GA Doyle, MK Izard (Eds) *Creatures of the Dark: The Nocturnal Prosimians* (New York, Plenum Press), 93–118.

Doyle GA, Martin RD (1974) The study of prosimian behaviour. In RD Martin, GA Doyle, AC Walker (Eds) *Prosimian Biology* (Pittsburgh, University of Pittsburgh Press), 4–14.

Dryden GL (1969) Reproduction in *Suncus murinus*. *Journal of Reproduction and Fertility* Supplement 6:377–396.

Fietz J (1999) Monogamy as a rule rather than exception in nocturnal lemurs: the case of the fat-tailed dwarf lemur, *Cheirogaleus medius*. *Ethology* 10:259–272.

Finlay BL, Darlington RB (1995) Linked regularities in the development and evolution of mammalian brain. *Science* 268:1578–1584.

Foerg R (1982) Reproduction in *Cheirogaleus medius*. *Folia Primatologica* 39:49–69.

Foerg R, Hoffmann R (1982) Seasonal and daily activity changes in captive *Cheirogaleus medius*. *Folia Primatologica* 38:259–268.

Fortune JE, Eppig JJ, Rissman EF (1992) Mating stimulates estradiol production by ovaries of the musk shrew *(Suncus murinus)*. *Biology of Reproduction* 46:885–891.

Ganzhorn JU, Wright PC, Ratsimbazafy HJ (1999) Primate communities: Madagascar. In JG Fleagle, CH Janson, K Reed (Eds) *Primate Communities* (Cambridge, Cambridge University Press), 75–89.

Geiser F (1998) Evolution of daily torpor and hibernation in birds and mammals: importance of body size. *Clinical and Experimental Pharmacology and Physiology* 25:736–739.

Geiser F, Ruf T (1995) Hibernation versus daily torpor in mammals and birds—physiological variables and classification of torpor patterns. *Physiological Zoology* 68:935–966.

Glander KE, Wright PC, Daniels PS, Merenlender AM (1992) Morphometrics and testicle size in rain forest lemur species from southwestern Madagascar. *Journal of Human Evolution* 92:1–17.

Harcourt CS, Nash LT (1986) Species differences in substrate use and diet between sympatric galagos in two Kenyan coastal forests. *Primates* 27:41–45.

Hrdy SB (1981) *The Woman That Never Evolved* (Cambridge, Harvard University Press).

Hrdy SB, Whitten PL (1987) The patterning of sexual activity. In BB Smuts, DL Cheney, RM Seyfarth, RW Wrangham, TT Struhsaker (Eds) *Primate Societies* (Chicago, University of Chicago Press, 370–384.

Izard MK (1990) Social influences on the reproductive success and reproductive endocrinology of prosimian primates. In F Bercovitch, T Ziegler (Eds) *Socioendocrinology of Primate Reproduction* (New York, Wiley-Liss), 159–186.

Jacobs GH, Deegan JF II (1993) Photopigments underlying color vision in ringtail lemurs *(Lemur catta)* and brown lemurs *(Eulemur fulvus)*. *American Journal of Primatology* 30:243–256.

Jolly A (1966a) Lemur social behaviour and primate intelligence. *Science* 153: 501–506.

Jolly A (1966b) *Lemur Behaviour: A Madagascar Field Study* (Chicago, University of Chicago Press).

Jolly A (1984) The puzzle of female feeding priority. In M Small (Ed) *Female Primates: Studies by Women Primatologists* (New York, Alan R Liss), 197–215.

Kappeler PM (1993) Sexual selection and lemur social systems. In PM Kappeler, JU Ganzhorn (Eds) *Lemur Social Systems and Their Ecological Basis* (New York, Plenum), 223–240.

Kappeler PM (1995) Causes and consequences of life history variation among strepsirrhine primates. *American Naturalist* 148:868–891.

Kappeler PM (1996) Life history variation among nocturnal prosimians. In L

Alternman, GA Doyle, MK Izard (Eds) *Creatures of the Dark: The Nocturnal Prosimians* (New York, Plenum Press), 75–92.

Kappeler PM (1997a) Intrasexual selection in *Mirza coquereli:* evidence for scramble competition polygyny in a solitary primate. *Behavioral Ecology and Sociobiology* 45:115–127.

Kappeler PM (1997b) Determinants of primate social organization: comparative evidence and new insights from Malagasy lemurs. *Biological Review* 72:111–151.

Kappeler PM (1998) Nests, tree holes, and the evolution of primate life histories. *American Journal of Primatology* 46:7–33.

Kappeler PM (1999) Lemur social structure and convergence in primate socioecology. In PC Lee (Ed) *Comparative Primate Socioecology* (New York, Cambridge University Press), 273–299.

Kleiman DG (1977) Monogamy in mammals. *Quarterly Review of Biology* 52:39–69.

Kraus C, Heistermann M, Kappeler PM (1999) Physiological suppression of sexual function of subordinate males: a subtle form of intrasexual competition among male sifakas *(Propithecus verreauxi)? Physiology and Behavior* 66:855–861.

Kubzdela KS (1997) Social relations in *Propithecus verreauxi* at Beza Mahafaly, Madagascar. PhD dissertation (Chicago, University of Chicago).

Kurland JA, Pearson JD (1986) Ecological significance of hypometabolism in nonhuman primates: allometry, adaptation, and deviant diets. *American Journal of Physical Anthropology* 71:445–457.

Lee JT, Miller CA, McDonald CT, Allman JM. (1996) Xanthogranuloma of the choroid plexus in the fat-tailed dwarf lemur *(Cheirogaleus medius). American Journal of Primatology* 38:349–355.

Leighton M (1993) Modeling dietary selectivity by Bornean organutans: evidence for integration of multiple criteria in fruit selection. *International Journal of Primatology* 14:257–313.

Leutenegger W (1979) Evolution of litter size in primates. *American Naturalist* 114:525–531.

Lillegraven JA, Thompson SD, McNab BK, Patton JL (1987) The origin of eutherian mammals. *Biological Journal of the Linnean Society* 32:281–336.

Lindburg DG (1987) Seasonality of reproduction in primates. In J Erwin, GD Mitchell (Eds) *Comparative Primate Biology*, Vol. 2B: Behavior, Cognition, and Motivation (New York, Alan R Liss), 167–218.

Lovegrove BG, Kortner G, Geiser F (1999) The energetic cost of arousal from torpor in the marsupial *Sminthopsis macroura:* benefits of summer ambient temperature cycles. *Journal of Comparative Physiology, B: Biochemical, Systemic, and Environmental Physiology* 169:11–18.

MacKinnon J, MacKinnon K (1980) The behavior of wild spectral tarsiers. *International Journal of Primatology* 1:361–379.

McNab BK (1984) Basal metabolic rate and the intrinsic rate of natural increase: an empirical and theoretical reexamination. *Œcological* 64:419–424.

Martin RD (1972) Adaptive radiation and behavior of the Malagasy lemurs. *Philosophical Transactions of the Royal Society of London*, Series B 264:295–353.

Martin RD (1990) *Primate Origins and Evolution* (London, Chapman Hall).

Martin RD, MacLarnon AM (1985) Gestation period, neonatal size and maternal investment in placental mammals. *Nature* 313:220–223.

Martin RD, MacLarnon AM (1988) Comparative quantitative studies of growth and reproduction. *Symposia of the Zoological Society of London* 60:39–80.

Meyers DM, Wright PC (1993) Resource tracking, food availability and *Propithecus* seasonal reproduction. In PM Kappeler, JU Ganzhorn (Eds) *Lemur Social Systems and Their Ecological Basis* (New York, Plenum Press), 179–192.

Miller AE (1999) Aspects of social life in the fat-tailed dwarf lemur *(Cheirogaleus medius)*: inferences from body weights and trapping data. *American Journal of Primatology* 49:265–280.

Morland HS (1993) Seasonal behavioral variation and its relationship to thermoregulation in ruffed lemurs *(Varecia variegata variegata)*. In PM Kappeler, JU Ganzhorn (Eds) *Lemur Social Systems and Their Ecological Basis* (New York, Plenum Press), 193–204.

Müller EF (1985) Basal metabolic rates in primates—the possible role of phylogenetic and ecological factors. *Comparative Biochemistry and Physiology, A: Molecular and Integrative Physiology* 81:707–711.

Müller EF, Nieschalk U, Meier B (1985) Thermoregulation in the slender loris *(Loris tardigradus)*. *Folia Primatologica* 44:216–226.

Nash LT (1983) Reproductive patterns in galagos *(Galago zanzibaricus* and *Galago garnettii)* in relation to climatic variability. *American Journal of Primatology* 5:181–196.

Nash LT (1998) Vertical clingers and sleepers: seasonal influences on the activities and substrate use of *Lepilemur leucopus* at Beza Mahafaly Special Reserve, Madagascar. *Folia Primatologica* 69:204–217.

Ortmann S, Heldmaier G (1997) Spontaneous daily torpor in Malagasy mouse lemurs. *Naturwissenschaften* 84:28–32.

Overdorff DJ (1998) Are Eulemur species pair-bonded? Social organization and mating strategies in *Eulemur fulvus rufus* from 1988–1995 in southeast Madagascar. *American Journal of Physical Anthropology* 105:153–166.

Overdorff DJ, Erhart EM (1998) Group movements in wild *Propithecus diadema edwardsi* and *Eulemur fulvus rufus*. *American Journal of Primatology* 45:198.

Overdorff DJ, Merenlender AM, Talata P, Telo A, Forward ZA (1999) Life history of *Eulemur fulvus rufus* from 1988–1998 in southeastern Madagascar. *American Journal of Physical Anthropology* 108:295–310.

Pereira M (1993) Seasonal adjustment of growth rate and adult body weight in ringtailed lemurs. In PM Kappeler, JU Ganzhorn (Eds) *Lemur Social Systems and Their Ecological Basis* (New York, Plenum Press), 205–221.

Pereira M (1995) Development and social dominance among group-living primates. *American Journal of Primatology* 37:143–175.

Pereira M, McGlynn CA (1997) Special relationships instead of female dominance for red-fronted lemurs, *Eulemur fulvus rufus*. *American Journal of Primatology* 43:239–258.

Perret M (1977) Influence du groupement social sur l'activation sexuelle saisonnière chez le mâle de *Microcebus murinus* (Miller 1777). *Zeitschrift für Tierpsychologie* 43:159–179.

Perret M (1986) Social influences on oestrous cycle length and plasma progesterone concentrations in the female lesser mouse lemur *(Microcebus murinus)*. *Journal of Reproduction and Fertility* 77:303–311.

Perret M (1998) Energetic advantage of nesting sharing in a solitary primate, the lesser mouse lemur. *Journal of Mammalogy* 79:1093–1102.

Perret M, Aujard F, Vannier G (1998) Influence of daylength on metabolic rate and daily water loss in the male prosimian primate *Microcebus murinus*. *Comparative Biochemistry and Physiology, A: Molecular and Integrative Physiology* 119:981–989.

Petter JJ (1965) The lemurs of Madagascar. In I DeVore (Ed) *Primate Behavior* (New York, Holt, Rinehart, Winston), 292–319.

Petter-Rousseaux A (1974) Seasonal activity rhythms, reproduction, and body weight variations of *Microcebus murinus* (Miller 1777). In RD Martin, GA

Doyle, AC Walker (Ed) *Prosimian Biology* (Pittsburgh, University of Pittsburgh Press), 365–373.

Petter-Rousseaux A (1980) Seasonal activity rhythms, reproduction, and body weight variations in five sympatric nocturnal prosimians in simulated light and climatic conditions. In P Charles-Dominique, M Cooper, A Hladik, CM Hladik, E Pages, A Petter-Rousseaux, A Schilling (Eds) *Nocturnal Malagasy Prosimians: Ecology, Physiology, and Behavior* (New York, Academic Press), 137–152.

Pollock JI (1979) Female dominance in *Indri indri. Folia Primatologica* 31:143–164.

Pollock JI (1989) Intersexual relationshps amongst prosimians. *Human Evolution* 4:133–143.

Power ML (1999) Aspects of energy expenditure of callitrichid primate: physiology and behavior. In P Dolhinow, A Fuentes (Eds) *The Nonhuman Primates* (Mountain View, CA, Mayfield), 225–230.

Rasmussen DT (1985) A comparative study of breeding seasonality and litter size in eleven taxa of captive lemurs (*Lemur* and *Varecia*). *International Journal of Primatology* 6:501–517.

Rasmussen DT, Izard MK (1988) Scaling of growth and life history traits relative to body size, brain size, and metabolic rate in lorises and galagos (Lorisidae, Primates). *American Journal of Physical Anthropology* 75:357–367.

Ravosa MJ (1998) Cranial allometry and geographical variation in slow loris (*Nycticebus*). *American Journal of Primatology* 45:225–243.

Reynolds RL, van Horn RN (1977) Induction of estrus in intact *Lemur catta* under photoinhibition of ovarian cycles. *Physiology and Behavior* 18:693–700.

Richard AF (1985) *Primates in Nature* (New York, WH Freeman).

Richard AF (1987) Malagasy prosimians. In BB Smuts, DL Cheney, RM Seyfarth, RW Wrangham, TT Struhsaker (Eds) *Primate Societies* (Chicago, University of Chicago Press), 25–33.

Richard AF (in press) Life in the slow lane? Demography and life histories of male and female sifaka (*Propithecus verreauxi verreauxi*). *Journal of Zoology*.

Richard AF, Dewar RE (1991) Lemur ecology. *Annual Review of Ecology and Systematics* 22:145–175.

Richard AF, Nicoll ME (1987) Female social dominance and basal metabolism in a Malagasy primate, *Propithecus verreauxi. American Journal of Primatology* 12:309–314.

Richard AF, Dewar RE, Schwartz M, Ratsirarson J (2000) Mass change, environmental variability and female fertility in wild *Propithecus verreauxi. Journal of Human Evolution* 39:381–391.

Richard AF, Rakotomanga P, Schwartz M (1991) Demography of *Propithecus verreauxi* at Beza Mahafaly Madagascar: sex ratio, survival and fertility. *American Journal of Physical Anthropology* 84:307–322.

Rissman EF (1987) Gonadal influences on sexual behavior in the male musk shrew (*Suncus murinus*). *Hormones and Behavior* 21:132–136.

Rissman EF (1991) Evidence that neural aromatization of androgen regulates the expression of sexual behavior in female musk shrews. *Journal of Neuroendocrinology* 3:441–448.

Rissman EF (1992) Mating induces puberty in the musk shrew. *Biology of Reproduction* 47:473–477.

Rissman EF, Crews D (1988) Hormonal correlates of sexual behavior in the female musk shrew: the role of estradiol. *Physiology and Behavior* 44:1–7.

Rissman EF, Silveira J, Bronson FH (1988) Patterns of sexual receptivity in the female musk shrew (*Suncus murinus*). *Hormones and Behavior* 22:186–193.

Rissman EF, Li X, King JA, Millar RP (1997) Behavioral regulation of gonadotropin-releasing hormone production. *Brain Research Bulletin* 44:459–464.

Roberts M (1994) Growth, development, and parental care in the western tarsier *(Tarsius bancanus)* in captivity: evidence for a "slow" life-history and non-monogamous mating system. *International Journal of Primatology* 15:1–28.

Roonwal ML, Mohnot SM (1977) *Primates of South Asia* (Cambridge, Harvard University Press).

Ross C (1992) Basal metabolic rate, body weight and diet in primates: an evaluation of the evidence. *Folia Primatologica* 58:7–23.

Rowe N (1996) *The Pictoral Guide to the Living Primates* (East Hampton, NY, Pogonias Press).

Sacher GA, Staffeldt EF (1974) Relation of gestation time to brain weight for placental mammals: implications for the theory of vertebrate growth. *American Naturalist* 108:593–615.

Sauther ML (1993) Resource competition in wild populations of ring-tailed lemurs *(Lemur catta)*. In PM Kappeler, JU Ganzhorn (Eds) *Lemur Social Systems and Their Ecological Basis* (New York, Plenum), 135–152.

Sauther ML, Sussman RW, Gould L (1999) The socioecology of the ringtailed lemur: 35 years of research. *Evolutionary Anthropology* 8:120–132.

Schmid J (1998) Tree holes used for resting by gray mouse lemurs *(Microcebus murinus)* in Madagascar: insulation capacities and energetic consequences. *International Journal of Primatology* 19:797–809.

Schmid J (1999) Sex-specific differences in activity patterns and fattening in the gray mouse lemur *(Microcebus murinus)* in Madagascar. *Journal of Mammalogy* 80:749–757.

Schmid J, Ganzhorn JU (1996) Resting metabolic rate of *Lepilemur ruficaudatus. American Journal of Primatology* 38:169–174.

Schmid J, Kappeler PM (1998) Fluctuating sexual dimorphism and differential hibernation by sex in a primate, the gray mouse lemur *(Microcebus murinus). Behavioral Ecology and Sociobiology* 43:125–132.

Schwartz GG, Rosenblum LA (1993) Allometric influences on primate mothers and infants. In LA Rosenblum, H Moltz (Eds) *Symbiosis in Parent-Offspring Interactions* (New York, Plenum Press), 215–248.

Sharma UR, Rissman EF (1994)Testosterone implants in specific neural sites activate female sexual behavior. *Journal of Neuroendocrinology* 6:423–432.

Smith KK (1997) Comparative patterns of craniofacial development in eutherian and metatherian mammals. *Evolution* 51:1663–1678.

Speakman JR, Rowland A (1999) Preparing for inactivity: how insectivorous bats deposit a fat store for inactivity. *Proceedings of the Nutrition Society* 58:123–131.

Spinage CA (1973) The role of photoperiodism in the seasonal breeding of tropical African ungulates. *Mammal Review* 3:71–84.

Sterling EJ (1994) Evidence for nonseasonal reproduction in wild aye-ayes *(Daubentonia madagascarensis). Folia Primatologica* 62:46–53.

Sterling EJ, Richard AF (1995) Social organization in the aye-aye *(Daubentonia madagascariensis)* and the perceived distinctiveness of nocturnal primates. In L Alterman, GA Doyle, MK Izard (Eds) *Creatures of the Dark: The Nocturnal Prosimians* (New York, Plenum Press), 439–445.

Tai VC, Schiml PA, Li X, Rissman EF (1997) Behavioral interactions have rapid effects on immunoreactivity of prohormone and gonadotropin-releasing hormone peptide. *Brain Research* 772:87–94.

Tan Y, Li W-H (1999) Trichromatic vision in prosimians. *Nature* 402:36.

Tattersall I (1982) *The Primates of Madagascar* (New York, Columbia University Press).

Terborgh J (1983) *Five New World Primates: A Study in Comparative Ecology* (Princeton, Princeton University Press.

Terborgh J (1992) *Diversity and the Tropical Rainforest* (New York, Scientific American Library, WH Freeman).

Thompson SD, Nicoll ME (1986) Basal metabolic rate and energetics of reproduction in therian mammals. *Nature* 321:690–693.

Tilden CD, Oftedal OT (1995) The bioenergetics of reproduction in prosimian primates: is it related to female dominance? In L Alternman, GA Doyle, MK Izard (Eds) *Creatures of the Dark: The Nocturnal Prosimians* (New York, Plenum Press), 119–131.

Tilden CD, Oftedal OT (1997) Milk composition reflects pattern of maternal care in prosimian primates. *American Journal of Primatology* 41:195–211.

van Horn RN (1975) Primate breeding season: photoperiodic regulation in captive *Lemur catta. Folia Primatologica* 24:203–220.

van Horn RN (1980) Seasonal reproductive patterns in primates. *Progress in Reproductive Biology* 5:181–221.

van Schaik CP, Kappeler PM (1993) Life history, activity period, and lemur social systems. In PM Kappler, JU Ganzhorn (Eds) *Lemur Social Systems and Their Ecological Basis* (New York, Plenum Press), 241–260.

van Schaik CP, Kappeler PM (1996) The social systems of gregarious lemurs: lack of convergence with anthropoids due to evolutionary disequilibrium? *Ethology* 102:915–941.

Whitten PL (1982) Female reproductive strategies in vervet monkeys. PhD dissertation (Cambridge, Harvard University).

Whitten PL (1987) Primate males and infants. In BB Smuts, DL Cheney, RM Seyfarth, RW Wrangham, TT Struhsaker (Eds) *Primate Societies* (Chicago, University of Chicago Press), 343–357.

Whitten PL (1999) Diet, hormones, and health: an evolutionary-ecological perspective. In C Panter-Brick, CM Worthman (Eds) *Hormones, Health, and Behavior: A Socioecological and Lifespan Perspective* (New York, Cambridge University Press), 210–243.

Wrangham RW, Chapman CA, Clark-Arcadi AP, Isabirye-Basuta G (1996) Social ecology of Kanyawara chimpanzees: implications for understanding the costs of Great Ape groups. In WC McGrew, LF Marchant, T Nishida (Eds) *Great Ape Societies* (New York, Cambridge Unversity Press), 45–57.

Wright PC (1990) Patterns of paternal care in primates. *International Journal of Primatology* 11:89–102.

Wright PC (1993) The evolution of female dominance and biparental care among non-human primates. In B Miller (Ed) *Sex and Gender Hierarchies* (Cambridge, Cambridge University Press), 127–147.

Wright PC (1999) Lemur traits and Madagascar ecology: coping with an island environment. *Yearbook of Physical Anthropology* 42:31–72.

Wright PC, Martin LB (1995) Predation, pollination and torpor in two nocturnal prosimians: *Cheirogaleus major* and *Microcebus rufus* in the rain forest of Madagascar. In L Alternman, GA Doyle, MK Izard (Eds) *Creatures of the Dark: The Nocturnal Prosimians* (New York, Plenum Press), 45–59.

Young AL, Richard AF, Aiello LC (1990) Female dominance and maternal investment in strepsirrhine primates. *American Naturalist* 135:473–488.

Zimmermann E (1989) Aspects of reproduction and behavioral and vocal development in Senegal bushbabies *(Galago senegalensis). International Journal of Primatology* 10:1–16.

15

Reproductive Ecology of New World Monkeys

KAREN B. STRIER

The New World monkeys, or platyrrhines, are divided into two families, the Callitrichidae and Cebidae, with a total of 16 genera and from 98 to 202 recognized species and subspecies (Rylands et al. 1997). Platyrrhines are found from southern Mexico through northern Argentina across an immense diversity of habitat types. Some genera, such as the howler monkeys *(Alouatta)* and capuchin monkeys *(Cebus)*, are widely distributed from the equator to more seasonal latitudes extending beyond the Tropic of Cancer. Most genera, and some species of common genera, have much more restricted distributions, with high levels of endemism and correspondingly high risks of extinction.

Platyrrhine body sizes range from the tiny 160 gram pygmy marmoset *(Cebuella pygmae)* to the impressive 9+ kg muriqui *(Brachyteles arachnoides)*. Yet, both the diets (Ford and Davis 1992) and reproductive rates (Ross 1991) of many platyrrhines deviate from predictions based on body size energetics derived from other primates. At one extreme are the callitrichids, whose capacity for producing litters of two or more infants up to twice each year with the help of nonmaternal infant caretakers have earned them the distinction of having both the fastest reproductive rates and the most cooperative reproductive system of any primate. At the other extreme are the atelins (muriquis, spider monkeys [*Ateles*], and woolly monkeys [*Lagothrix*]), whose delayed sexual maturation and production of single offspring at 3-year intervals make their reproductive rates more similar to those of apes than to Old World monkeys of similar body size (Ross 1991; Strier 1999a).

The other well-studied platyrrhines, such as capuchin monkeys, squirrel monkeys *(Saimiri)*, and howler monkeys, give birth to single offspring at 1–2 year intervals. Among these genera, the relatively slow reproductive rates of capuchin monkeys have been attributed to their relatively large brains (Fedigan and Rose 1995; Hartwig 1996). Thus, from the intensive alloparental care that minimizes interbirth intervals in callitrichids to

351

the apelike life histories of atelins to the developmental constraints of large brains in capuchin monkeys, platyrrhines provide some of the best comparative models for understanding the evolutionary forces that have shaped the reproductive ecology of humans.

Despite the potential insights that platyrrhines provide into other primates, including humans, comparative analyses are still hampered by the paucity of relevant knowledge on all but a very small number of species. For instance, although detailed studies have been conducted on the reproductive physiology of captive marmosets (*Callithrix*), tamarins (*Saguinus* and *Leontopithecus*), and squirrel monkeys, field studies on the physiology of wild subjects are only now underway. Conversely, although long-term field studies of particular study groups and censused populations of callitrichids as well as the three atelin genera, howler monkeys, capuchin monkeys, and squirrel monkeys, have yielded important information about their behavioral and reproductive ecology, corresponding physiological data on most wild subjects are still rare.

Advances in the development of noninvasive fecal steroid assays have encouraged their widespread adoption in field studies, offering tantalizing prospects for understanding the physiological basis of platyrrhine reproductive ecology. Fecal hormone studies conducted on one population of wild muriquis, which has been monitored for more than 18 years (Strier 1999b; Strier and Ziegler 1994, 1997, in press; Strier et al. 1999; Ziegler et al. 1997), have revealed intriguing insights into the interacting effects of behavioral, ecological, and demographic variables on muriqui reproductive physiology and highlight the need for comparable physiological data from other wild platyrrhines.

In this chapter I review the available literature on New World monkey reproductive patterns, focusing on evidence for the ways in which dispersal and other behavioral patterns interact with ecology and demography to affect platyrrhine life histories and reproduction. Physiological data from various captive studies and from wild muriquis provide insights into some of the mechanisms that regulate reproductive patterns and suggest compelling directions for future field research.

PLATYRRHINE PATTERNS

Contrasts in the reproductive biology and behavior of callitrichids and atelins are useful in establishing the fast and slow extremes of the reproductive continuum along which most of the other known platyrrhines fall. In general, the rapid reproductive rates of callitrichids and the slow reproductive rates of atelins can be distinguished by three interrelated variables: (*a*) age at puberty and first reproduction, which need not be the same; *(b)* interbirth intervals, which have multiple, and not necessarily mutually exclusive, components; and *(c)* maternal investment strategies, which have predictable effects on infant mortality and therefore influence interbirth intervals. Underlying these variables are life history, behavioral, ecological, and demographic constraints, which affect both females and males, and which differ to varying degrees across populations of the same and closely related species.

Life History Patterns

Life histories encompass a range of variables, including age at first reproduction and interbirth intervals, that affect female reproductive rates (DeRousseau 1990; Fedigan 1997; Ross 1991). Not surprisingly, age at first reproduction and interbirth intervals tend to be positively related, and they set the upper and lower boundaries of each species' intrinsic reproductive rates. For example, callitrichid females can reach sexual maturity and begin to ovulate as early as 12–18 months of age, and give birth to their first infants at 12–24 months. Atelin females, by contrast, give birth to their first infants at 6–9 years of age (reviewed in Strier 1999a). In muriquis, age at first birth is delayed by an extended period of adolescent infertility, during which time females experience hormonally normal ovarian cycles and mate, but nonetheless fail to conceive (Strier and Ziegler 2000). Early puberty in callitrichids, together with their short interbirth intervals, are responsible for their high reproductive potential, whereas delayed puberty and long interbirth intervals in atelins inevitably result in their much lower reproductive potential.

Despite differences in female body size, the other well-studied platyr-rhines (e.g., squirrel monkeys, howler monkeys, and capuchin monkeys) have comparable 1–2 year interbirth intervals. Consequently, most of the variation in their reproductive rates can be attributed to differences in female age at first reproduction and the degree to which reproductive sea-sonality constrains interbirth intervals. Age at first reproduction in these platyrrhines ranges from 2–3 years in squirrel monkeys to 3–6 years in both capuchins and howler monkeys. Female capuchin monkeys are much smaller in body mass than their howler monkey counterparts, suggesting that their relatively late maturation, like their relatively long interbirth intervals, reflect developmental constraints of their large brains (Fedigan and Rose 1995; Hartwig 1996).

Phylogenetic and Ecological Constraints

While large brains may account for the relatively delayed maturation and long interbirth intervals in capuchin monkeys, neither brain size nor body size explains the slow reproductive rates of atelins. Instead, phylogenetic relationships appear to be the strongest predictors of the life history traits that affect their reproductive rates. For example, although female woolly monkeys are more similar in body mass to female howler monkeys than to female spider monkeys or muriquis, their age at first reproduction and interbirth intervals more closely resemble those of spider monkeys and muriquis. The similarities among the three atelin genera imply that phylogeny is a stronger predictor of their life histories than the energetics of body size alone (Strier 1999a, 1999c).

Complementary ecological and phylogenetic considerations figure prominently in efforts to understand the unusual range of platyrrhine reproductive patterns and the divergent life histories of New World and Old World monkeys. Ecological explanations have focused on the possible evolutionary histories of primates adapted to inhabiting primary forests (Ross 1991) and on the cognitive requirements that locating patchy fruit resources and extractive foraging techniques might place on rates of neural development and corresponding maturation rates (Fedigan 1993; Fedigan and Rose 1995; Gibson 1986). Phylogenetic explanations have emphasized the associations between slow life histories and female dispersal patterns, which coincide with the ways in which Cebidae reproductive patterns resemble those of apes instead of Old World monkeys (Strier 1999a, 1999c). Indeed, dispersal patterns may play a key role in mitigating the ecological constraints on puberty in callitrichids as well.

Puberty and Age at First Reproduction

Delayed maturation can reflect a variety of selection pressures, including the time needed to compensate for low neonatal-to-maternal brain weights and the adaptive value of postponing direct competition with full-grown adults over food (Charnov and Berrigan 1993; Janson and van Schaik 1993; Pagel and Harvey 1993). However, delayed maturation can also be a facultative response to demographic and social conditions that restrict individual reproductive opportunities, or that necessitate risky or high energetic expenditures.

Reproductive suppression. Captive studies have demonstrated that ovulation is suppressed in subordinate female marmosets (Abbott et al. 1993) and tamarins (Ziegler 1987) housed in family groups with their reproductively active mothers. These females are old enough to ovulate, and do so within days when they are released from the behavioral and chemical cues emitted by their mothers and, to a lesser degree, fathers (Widowski et al. 1990, 1992).

In the wild, subordinate female callitrichids can theoretically escape from reproductive suppression by dispersing from their natal groups. Yet, many subordinate females fail to do so. Instead, they remain as nonreproductive members of their natal groups where they help their dominant mothers to rear successive litters of siblings by carrying them. If habitat saturation makes it difficult for young females to establish their own reproductive groups, then accepting subordinate, nonreproductive status in their natal group might be preferable to dispersing (Ferrari and Digby 1996). By doing so, daughters not only contribute to the successful rearing of siblings, with whom they share some of their genes, but they can also gain valuable parenting experience and thus increase the survival of their own infants should future reproductive opportunities arise. The fact that infants born to inexperienced callitrichid mothers suffer higher mortality than the infants of experienced mothers reinforces the benefits of gaining parenting skills prior to reproducing themselves (Epple 1978; Tardif et al. 1984). Moreover, because the number of helpers increases infant survivorship, dominant mothers also benefit by permitting their daughters to remain in their natal groups instead of expelling them (Savage et al. 1996a).

Although the presence of two or more reproductive females has now been documented in a number of wild callitrichid groups (e.g., saddlebacked tamarins: Goldizen et al. 1996; cotton-top tamarins: Savage et al. 1996b, 1997; buffy-tufted-ear marmosets: Coutinho and Corrêa 1995; common marmosets: Digby and Ferrari 1994; buffy-headed marmosets: Guimarães 1998; Ferrari et al. 1996; golden lion tamarins: Baker et al. 1993; Dietz and Baker 1993), reproductive subordinates are still compromised relative to their dominant counterparts. For example, in wild cotton-top tamarins, subordinate females with palpable pregnancies did not give birth (Savage et al. 1996b). In both buffy-headed marmosets and common marmosets, parturitions by subordinate females occurred after those of the dominant female in their respective groups, and subordinate mothers did not receive help from group males in carrying their infants (Digby and Ferrari 1994; Guimarães 1998). In one common marmoset group, the dominant female targeted aggression toward the subordinate female and her infant, resulting in the death of the infant (Digby 1995).

How these subordinate females override the inhibitory cues that lead to reproductive suppression in captive callitrichids without dispersing is not clear. It is possible that chemical and behavioral cues are diluted by the greater interindividual distances that can be maintained in the wild, or that some of the reproductive subordinates are females who have immigrated from neighboring groups after ovulating or conceiving (Digby and Ferrari 1994). In either case, it is clear that the physiological suppression of ovulation in callitrichids can result in the facultative delay of reproduction in subordinate females.

Effects of dispersal. Reproductive suppression does not appear to be responsible for the delayed onset of puberty in wild muriqui females, which typically transfer out of their natal groups between 5 and 7 years of age (Strier 1996a). Analyses of fecal hormones collected from adolescent females up to 30 months prior to their emigrations, and up to 12 months after their immigrations, indicate stable, baseline estrogen levels and much lower peaks in progesterone levels than are found in cycling adult females (Strier and Ziegler 2000). Instead, the long latencies between intergroup transfer, the onset of normal ovarian cycling, and the timing of first reproduction in female muriquis are consistent with the hypothesis that dispersal and puberty in this, and perhaps other, platyrrhine species are regulated by energetic and nutritional constraints (Bronson and Rissman 1986).

Unlike in most prosimians and cercopithecine monkeys, female dispersal is common among platyrrhines (Strier 1994, 1999c). In some genera, such as howler monkeys and the callitrichids, males as well as females disperse from their natal groups. In others, such as the three atelins, dispersal patterns are clearly female-biased with male philopatry. The three species of squirrel monkeys exhibit varying dispersal patterns, ranging from female-biased dispersal with male philopatry in Costa Rican *Saimiri oerstedi* and probably Suriname *S. sciureus* to male cohort dispersal and female philopatry in Peruvian *S. boliviensus* (Boinski 1999). In fact, capuchin monkeys are the only genus of platyrrhines characterized by male-biased dispersal and female philopatry.

The prevalence of female dispersal among platyrrhines raises the intriguing suggestion that it is responsible for delaying reproductive maturity. The effects of female dispersal on platyrrhine puberty appear to differ from those on hominoids such as chimpanzees, which often show sexual swellings indicative of ovarian cycling while still residing in their natal communities, and which sometimes transfer after they have become sexually active, conceived, or even given birth (Wallis 1997). Like muriquis, however, other female platyrrhines, including Costa Rican squirrel monkeys and Venezuelan red howler monkeys, disperse prior to the onset of mating and presumably puberty (Crockett and Pope 1993; Boinski 1999).

Red howler monkey females expelled from their natal groups reproduce later than females permitted to stay (Crockett and Pope 1993). Yet even among muriquis, for which there is no evidence of young natal muriquis being expelled from their natal groups, and immigrant females appear to be fully integrated into the peaceful societies of their new groups within a few months (Printes and Strier 1999), female dispersal still appears to coincide with delayed puberty. For example, the sole female muriqui known to reproduce in her natal group did so at 7½ years of age, or roughly one year earlier than the age at which immigrant females are estimated to give birth to their first infants (Strier and Ziegler 2000).

Although females tolerated in their natal groups can begin their reproductive careers sooner than dispersing females, the potential benefits of dispersing prior to puberty may override the immediate reproductive costs. For instance, dispersing prepubertal females avoid the risks of close inbreeding with related natal males and minimize the risks of incurring additional energetic costs while pregnant or lactating. Locating suitable habitats in which to establish a new breeding group can require long distance travel in saturated habitats (Crockett 1996), and females migrating into established neighboring groups can suffer from reduced access to food owing to social peripheralization or targeted aggression from established resident females (Jones 1980; Zucker and Clarke 1998). That Costa Rican squirrel monkeys emigrate prior to their first mating season in their natal groups (Boinski 1999) and adolescent muriquis emigrate prior to the onset of ovarian cycling (Strier and Ziegler 2000) is consistent with the avoidance of close inbreeding with philopatric males in their natal groups, and with the potential energetic and social costs associated with dispersal and social integration.

There is no evidence yet with which to evaluate whether female squirrel monkeys disperse to avoid reproductive suppression in their natal groups or whether they experience delayed reproduction as a result of dispersal. In muriquis, however, the long delay in the onset of ovarian cycling among immigrants, especially during the mating season when mature resident females are cycling and sexually active, implies that contrary to the case among callitrichids, release from reproductive suppression is not a stimulus for natal group dispersal by female muriquis (Strier and Ziegler 2000). However, the coincidence of female dispersal and delayed maturation in both platyrrhines and hominoids suggests that the interactions between behavior and life history strategies are important considerations in understanding the reproductive ecology of other primates, including humans.

Interbirth Intervals

Interbirth intervals can be divided into three components: gestation, lactation, and weaning-to-conception intervals (Fedigan and Rose 1995). In most mammals, and nearly all primates, gestation and lactation are temporally distinct components of interbirth intervals. This mutual incompatibility results from the hormonal inhibition of ovulation during pregnancy and lactation (Bronson 1989). Unless ovarian cycling and breeding are regulated by strong seasonal cues (see below), embryonic or fetal loss or infant mortality tends to result in the rapid resumption of fertile ovarian cycling.

Callitrichids are exceptions to this mammalian pattern because lactating females ovulate and conceive again within days of giving birth. Although mothers continue to nurse their infants during most of their subsequent pregnancies, males and subordinate females take over nearly all other aspects of infant care, including the heavy energetic burden of carrying dependent infants (Snowdon 1996). Subordinate mothers that manage to reproduce receive little, if any, help with infant carrying, and not surprisingly, they also fail to exhibit the postpartum estrus and correspondingly short interbirth intervals that characterize dominant reproductive females in their groups. Subordinate callitrichid mothers, like most other platyrrhines, bear the energetic costs of reproduction by themselves.

Components. Gestation length is generally considered to be the least variable of the multiple components of interbirth intervals within species (Fedigan and Rose 1995). Gestation lengths determined from fecal steroids for five wild muriquis averaged 216.4 ± 1.5 days (Strier and Ziegler 1997). Although comparable hormonal data on the variation in gestation length from other wild platyrrhines are not available, mean or median gestation lengths tend to correspond more closely with neonatal brain mass than with maternal body weights (Lee 1999). Thus, deviations from expected interbirth intervals can usually be attributed to the duration of lactation and weaning-to-conception phases.

In other primates, these two components of the interbirth interval tend to correspond with maternal body mass (Lee 1999), but in cebids, they appear to correspond with brain size. In comparisons among sympatric capuchin monkeys, howler monkeys, and spider monkeys in Costa Rica, Fedigan and Rose (1995) found that the longer median interbirth interval (26.4 months) of capuchin monkeys relative to howler monkeys (19.9 months) was consistent with their relative brain weights, but not body weights. However, although capuchins have shorter interbirth intervals than the much larger spider monkeys (34.7 months), gestation accounted for a similarly lower proportion (20–22%) of their respective interbirth intervals than howler monkeys (31%). Thus, the relatively long interbirth intervals of large-brained capuchin monkeys are the result of extended postpartum, rather than prenatal, maternal investment.

Maternal investment and infant mortality. Maternal investment strategies can be dichotomized into those that involve investing in present offspring versus investing in maternal survival for future offspring (Stearns 1992). Investing in present offspring means that mothers minimize the risks of infant mortality by delaying weaning and postweaning conception with the result of lengthening the interval between births. Shorter interbirth intervals owing to earlier weaning and rapid postweaning conceptions correspond to maternal strategies aimed at maximizing opportunities to produce additional offspring. Rates of infant mortality tend to be higher when maternal investment strategies favor future offspring unless other group members compensate for minimal maternal care by caring for infants themselves.

Among callitrichids, such allomaternal care results in high offspring survival without reducing maternal reproductive output. Evidence of the role of infant carrying by nonmothers in wild callitrichid groups includes a positive relationship between the number of helpers and infant survival in wild cotton-top tamarins (Savage et al. 1996a) and higher survival of infants produced by dominant female common marmosets with helpers relative to survival rates of infants produced by subordinate females, who receive little if any help caring for their infants from other group members (Digby 1995; Digby and Ferrari 1994).

Extended lactation with delayed weaning is generally associated with high maternal investment and infant survival. Yet weaning is also known to be a gradual process, and distinguishing between the end of lactation and the resumption of ovarian cycling is difficult without accompanying hormonal data (Lee 1996). For example, muriqui mothers, like many other primate mothers, continue to provide rides for and to sleep with their infants until their next parturitions, even though infants devote nearly 72% of their feeding time to solid food by 7–12 months of age (Odalia Rímoli 1998). Hormonal data indicate that mothers experience from 3 to 6 ovulatory cycles between their first postweaning cycle and conception (Strier and Ziegler 1997), accounting for roughly 8–16% of their interbirth interval. With gestation accounting for 19% of the interbirth interval, the remaining 27–35% is therefore devoted to their extended lactation and what appears to be is a postweaning anovulatory phase linked to the recovery of maternal energetic reserves (Strier and Ziegler 1997).

Investment strategies that deplete maternal energy reserves to the extent we suspect may occur in muriquis contrast sharply with those of dominant female callitrichids, whose energy reserves are conserved by the redistribution of carrying infants among other group members. Variation in the weaning-to-conception phase of interbirth intervals in other wild platyrrhines remains poorly understood. For example, both captive and wild female squirrel monkeys appear to conceive by their first or, more rarely, second postweaning ovulation (Schiml et al. 1996). However, squirrel monkeys also have limited breeding seasons that are no more than 2 months long (Boinski 1999). Differences in postweaning maternal investment strategies may therefore be linked to ecological constraints imposed by the length of the breeding seasons rather than by the energetic requirements of mothers.

Reproductive Seasonality

Identifying the interacting effects of postpartum energetics and ecology on maternal investment strategies, interbirth intervals, and reproductive patterns is confounded by the difficulties of measuring seasonality. For example, reproductive seasonality is usually characterized by the degree of clustering of births or breeding patterns over an annual cycle (Lindburg 1987). Both methods have flaws, however, because not all pregnancies result in documented births, and many primates copulate at times when the probability of conception is low. Platyrrhines lack the perineal swellings and color changes that signal ovulation and pregnancy in some cercopithecines and hominoids, making it difficult for observers to distinguish these reproductive states from anovulatory phases based on visual cues alone (Dixson 1983). In muriquis, for example, infant mortality results in the rapid resumption of ovarian cycling and copulation irrespective of time of year. However, the dry season peak in muriqui births implies that seasonal ecological cues or nutritional condition in one or both partners may be necessary for the matings to lead to successful conceptions (Strier et al. 1999). Thus, muriqui fertility, but not ovarian cycling or sexual activity, appears to be regulated by seasonal cues. These findings emphasize the importance of distinguishing between mating and actual breeding seasons in comparative analyses of reproductive ecology and other behavioral patterns.

In addition to distinguishing mating from breeding seasons, it is necessary to distinguish fertile from nonfertile matings. In muriquis, for example, nearly 50% of copulations by cycling females during the so-called breeding season occurred outside of their hormonally detected periovulatory periods (Strier and Ziegler 1997; Strier 2001). It is not clear whether males can distinguish fertile from nonfertile matings and alter their behavior accordingly, but these possibilities dictate caution in analyses that link behavior to any estimates of female breeding synchrony (Nunn 1999).

Benefits. Several potential benefits have been associated with seasonal reproduction, including synchronizing births to swamp predators, as has been suggested for Costa Rican squirrel monkeys (Boinski 1987a), and timing the periods of greatest maternal energetic and nutritional requirements or weaning food requirements to coincide with periods when appropriate high-quality foods are most abundant (Chapman and Chapman 1990; Crockett and Rudran 1987). However, because conceptions occur prior to the optimal ecological conditions, even predictable cues, such as photoperiod, may be unreliable from one year to the next.

Presumably, short breeding seasons reflect both more extreme ecological conditions between seasons and greater year-to-year predictability in seasonal ecological conditions than long breeding seasons. However, there are few data with which to evaluate these predictions for platyrrhines. For example, the higher survivorship of infants produced by dominant female marmosets (Digby 1995) or the higher reproductive rates of large capuchin monkey groups (Robinson 1988) could reflect better maternal condition resulting from priority of access to foods during gestation and lactation, greater contributions from helpers, or fewer direct threats from conspecifics, as well as variability in the timing of conceptions, parturition, or weaning among mothers.

Platyrrhines differ in their sensitivity to ecological factors that affect reproductive seasonality. It is not uncommon to find dramatic divergence in the timing of births among either sympatric species with high dietary overlap or populations of the same or closely related species living in different habitats. For example, in one seasonal Atlantic forest community in southeastern Brazil, births of muriquis tend to be clustered during the dry season months (Strier 1996a, 1999d), whereas those of brown capuchin monkeys appear to cluster during the rainy season months (Lynch 1998; Rímoli and Lynch 1999) and those of brown howler monkeys show little, if any, seasonality (Mendes and Santos 1999). In a seasonal Costa Rican forest, by contrast, births of white-fronted capuchins, like those of sympatric spider monkeys and mantled howler monkeys, were similarly clustered during the dry season (Fedigan and Rose 1995).

Maternal investment strategies aimed at maximizing reproductive output should be more sensitive to ecological factors that favor early weaning and rapid postweaning cycling and conception. Conversely, intensive maternal investment in current offspring should buffer mothers and infants alike from seasonal scarcity in food availability. Among atelins, for example, the seasonal clustering of births with prolonged lactation and especially delayed weaning-to-conception phases may reflect more about maternal abilities to replenish their energy reserves prior to conceiving again than about reducing interbirth intervals to maximize reproductive output. By contrast, the shorter birth seasons of Peruvian brown capuchin monkeys compared with Costa Rican white-fronted capuchins, or of Costa Rican and Suriname squirrel monkeys compared with Peruvian squirrel monkeys, might result in higher infant mortality as mothers reduce their postpartum investment in offspring so as not to risk missing the narrow window of reproductive opportunity.

The case of howler monkeys is enigmatic among platyrrhines, for although their investment strategies favor future offspring over intense investment in present offspring (Jones 1997), they are also the most folivorous platyrrhines, defined by the proportion of leaves in their annual diets relative to that of sympatric atelins (Strier 1992). It is therefore possible that their relatively low quality diets impose additional energetic constraints on maternal investment strategies that platyrrhines with higher quality frugivorous and insectivorous diets can avoid.

Effects on males. The degree of reproductive seasonality, together with variance in female life history strategies, influences the degree to which males can alter female reproductive rates and therefore affects male behavioral strategies (Strier 1996b). Thus, by helping to bear the energetic burden of carrying infants, male marmosets and tamarins reduce female interbirth intervals. Captive studies of both common marmosets and cotton-top tamarins indicate postpartum elevations in prolactin in both male and female helpers (Dixson and George 1982; Ziegler et al. 1996; Mota and Sousa 2000; Ziegler 2000). By contrast, male aggression that results in infant mortality will shorten interbirth intervals in other primates unless, as among Costa Rican squirrel monkeys, short (2-week) annual breeding seasons mean that males cannot reduce the length of interbirth intervals. The longer breeding seasons (2 months) and interbirth intervals (2 years) of Peruvian squirrel monkeys correspond with predictably higher levels of aggression among males (Boinski 1999).

The fact that longer breeding seasons and longer (>1 year) interbirth intervals do not always favor high levels of male competition suggests that additional physiological factors may be involved. For example, captive male squirrel monkeys exhibit a pre-breeding-season rise in their cortisol levels prior to the elevation of testosterone at the onset of the breeding season (Schiml et al. 1996; Wiebe et al. 1988). Seasonal cortisol elevations have been attributed to seasonal fat storage, which provides well-nourished males with energy reserves to draw on during the competitive conditions that arise during their short breeding season (Bercovitch 1992). In wild male muriquis, by contrast, neither pre-breeding-season elevations in cortisol nor breeding-season elevations in testosterone were evident. Instead, twofold increases in male cortisol levels occurred around the middle of the mating season, both when high quality fruits tend to be most abundant and when most conceptions occur (Strier et al. 1999).

Muriquis differ from most other platyrrhines in their low levels of aggression and the egalitarian relationships philopatric males maintain with one another and with females (Strier 1990). Indeed, the only other platyrrhines that approach the tolerance exhibited by male muriquis are male Costa Rican squirrel monkeys, which maintain peaceful relationships except during the brief annual breeding season when they compete with one another for mating opportunities (Boinski 1987b, 1994). Thus, comparisons of male platyrrhine reproductive physiology must be sensitive to differences in their social relationships as well as their relationships with females.

REPRODUCTIVE ECOLOGY AND DEMOGRAPHY

It is tempting to classify the reproductive ecology of platyrrhines, or any other primates, along simple dimensions based on recurrent patterns and detectable correlations between behavioral and ecological variables. However, it is also important to recognize that demographic fluctuations can play a powerful role in the interpretations of reproductive patterns. For example, annual deviations from typical breeding and birth seasons can often be attributed to year-to-year fluctuations in rainfall and its effects on the availability of food (Lindburg 1987). Yet, in muriquis, independent of rainfall, the duration of annual birth seasons was positively related to the number of sexually active females each year (Strier 1999d).

Similar demographic effects are likely to be compounded in comparative analyses of primate reproductive ecology that neglect to control for differences in intra- and interspecific group sizes, dispersal patterns, and life histories. For example, a group with twice the number of sexually active females as another might be expected to have a correspondingly long breeding season (Nunn 1999), even under identical ecological conditions. Species and population differences in whether breeding females are recruited from within their natal groups or through dispersal can affect the age at first reproduction, and thus reproductive rates as well as the number of reproductively active females present at any time. Even differences in the degree of habitat saturation, which reflects population density, can affect dispersal opportunities, and therefore the prevalence of reproductive suppression or delayed maturation and the number of reproductively active females.

The ecology and demography of many platyrrhine populations have been altered by habitat disturbances and hunting pressures in the past 50 years. Yet, the effects of these alterations on platyrrhine reproductive ecology are still poorly understood. For example, habitat disturbances, including the elimination of natural predators and the creation of regenerating edges, can lead to artificially high population densities that affect different primates in different ways (Strier 2000) and, as such, serve as natural experiments into the ways in which primates modify their reproductive patterns in response to fluctuations in local ecological and demographic conditions. The continued monitoring of long-term reproductive patterns in disturbed as well as undisturbed populations is thus critical to understanding platyrrhine reproductive ecologies from a comparative evolutionary perspective.

I am grateful to the Brazilian CNPq, sponsors and funding agencies, students, and collaborators who have made long-term muriqui research possible, and to Peter Ellison for inviting me to contribute to this volume.

REFERENCES

Abbott DH, Barrett J, George LM (1993) Comparative aspects of the social suppression of reproduction in female marmosets and tamarins. In AB Rylands (Ed) *Marmosets and Tamarins: Systematics, Ecology and Behavior* (Oxford, Oxford University Press), 152–163.

Baker AJ, Dietz JM, Kleiman DG (1993) Behavioural evidence for monopolization of paternity in multi-male groups of golden lion tamarins. *Animal Behavior* 46:1091–1103.

Bercovitch FB (1992) Estradiol concentrations, fat deposits, and reproductive strategies in male rhesus macaques. *Hormones and Behavior* 26:272–282.

Boinski S (1987a) Birth synchrony in squirrel monkeys *(Saimiri oerstedi)*. *Behavioral Ecology and Sociobiology* 21:393–400.

Boinski S (1987b) Mating patterns in squirrel monkeys *(Saimiri oerstedi)*. *Behavioral Ecology and Sociobiology* 21:13–21.

Boinski S (1994) Affiliation patterns among male Costa Rican squirrel monkeys. *Behaviour* 130:191– 209.

Boinski S (1999) The social organizations of squirrel monkeys: implications for ecological models of social evolution. *Evolutionary Anthropology* 8:101–112.

Bronson FH (1989) *Mammalian Reproductive Biology* (Chicago, University of Chicago Press).

Bronson FH, Rissman EF (1986) The biology of puberty. *Biological Reviews* 61: 157–195.

Chapman CA, Chapman LJ (1990) Reproductive biology of captive and free-ranging spider monkeys. *Zoo Biology* 9:1–9.

Charnov EL, Berrigan D (1993) Why do female primates have such long lifespans and so few babies? Or, life in the slow lane. *Evolutionary Anthropology* 1:191–194.

Coutinho PEG, Corrêa HKM (1995) Polygyny in free-ranging group of buffy tufted-ear marmosets, *Callithrix aurita*. *Folia Primatologia* 65:25–29.

Crockett CM (1996) The relation between red howler monkey *(Alouatta seniculus)* troop size and population growth in two habitats. In MA Norconk, AL Rosenberger, PA Garber (Eds) *Adaptive Radiations of Neotropical Primates* (New York, Plenum Press), 489–510.

Crockett CM, Pope TR (1993) Consequences of sex differences in dispersal for juvenile red howler monkeys. In ME Pereira, LA Fairbanks (Eds) *Juvenile Primates: Life History, Development, and Behavior* (New York, Oxford University Press), 104–118.

Crockett CM, Rudran R (1987) Red howler monkey birth data, I: seasonal variation. *American Journal of Primatology* 13:347–368.

DeRousseau CJ (1990) Life-history thinking in perspective. In CJ DeRousseau (Ed) *Primate Life History and Evolution* (New York, Wiley-Liss), 1–13.

Dietz JM, Baker AJ (1993) Polygyny and female reproductive success in golden lion tamarin *(Leontopithecus rosalia)*. *Animal Behavior* 46:1067–1078.

Digby L (1995) Infant care, infanticide, and female reproductive strategies in polygynous groups of common marmosets *(Callithrix jacchus)*. *Behavioral Ecology and Sociobiology* 37:51–61.

Digby LJ, Ferrari SF (1994) Multiple breeding females in free-ranging groups of *Callithrix jaccus*. *International Journal of Primatology* 15:389–397.

Dixson AF (1983) Observations on the evolution and behavioral significance of "sexual skin" in female primates. *Advances in the Study of Behaviour* 13:63–106.

Dixson AF, George L (1982) Prolactin and parental behaviour in a male New World primate. *Nature* 299:551–553.

Epple G (1978) Reproductive and social behavior of marmosets with special reference to captive breeding. In N Gengozian, F Diehards (Eds) *Primates in Medicine*, vol. 10 (Basel, Karger), 50–62.

Fedigan L (1993) Sex differences and intersexual relations in adult white-faced capuchins *(Cebus capucinus)*. *International Journal of Primatology* 14:853–878.

Fedigan LM (1997) Changing views of female life histories. In ME Morbeck, A Galloway, AL Zihlman (Eds) *The Evolving Female* (Princeton, Princeton University Press), 15–26.

Fedigan LM, Rose LM (1995) Interbirth interval variation in three sympatric species of Neotropical monkey. *American Journal of Primatology* 37:9–24.

Ferrari SF, Digby LJ (1996) Wild *Callithrix* groups: stable extended families? *American Journal of Primatology* 38:19–27.

Ferrari SF, Correa HKM, Coutinho PEG (1996) Ecology of the "southern" marmosets (*Callithrix aurita* and *Callithrix flaviceps*): how different, how similar? In MA Norconk, AL Rosenberger, PA Garber (Eds) *Adaptive Radiations of Neotropical Primates* (New York, Plenum Press), 157–171.

Ford SM, Davis LC (1992) Systematics and body size: implications for feeding adaptations in New World monkeys. *American Journal of Physical Anthropology* 88:415–468.

Gibson KR (1986) Cognition, brain size and the extraction of embedded food resources. In J Else, PC Lee (Eds) *Primate Ontogeny, Cognition and Social Behaviour* (Cambridge, Cambridge University Press), 93–104.

Goldizen AW, Mendelson J, van Vlaardingen M, Terborgh J (1996) Saddle-back tamarin (*Saguinus fuscicollis*) reproductive strategies: evidence from a thirteen-year study of a marked population. *American Journal of Primatology* 38:57–83.

Guimarães A (1998) *Comportamento Reprodutivo e Marcacao de Cheiro em um Grupo Silvestre de* Callithrix flaviceps. Masters thesis, Universidade Federal de Minas Gerais.

Hartwig WC (1996) Perinatal life history traits in New World monkeys. *American Journal of Primatology* 40:99–130.

Janson CH, van Schaik CP (1993) Ecological risk aversion in juvenile primates: slow and steady wins the race. In ME Pereira, LA Fairbanks (Eds) *Juvenile Primates: Life History, Development, and Behavior* (New York, Oxford University Press), 57–74.

Jones CB (1980) The functions of status in the mantled howler monkey, *Alouatta palliata* Gray: intraspecific competition for group membership in a folivorous Neotropical primate. *Primates* 21:389–405.

Jones CB (1997) Life history patterns of howler monkeys in a time-varying environment. *Boletin Primatologico Latinamericano* 6:1–8.

Lee PC (1996) The meanings of weaning: growth, lactation and life history. *Evolutionary Anthropology* 5:87–96.

Lee PC (1999) Comparative ecology of postnatal growth and weaning among haplorhine primates. In PC Lee (Ed) *Comparative Primate Socioecology* (Cambridge, Cambridge University Press), 111–136.

Lindburg DG (1987) Seasonality of reproduction in primates. In G Mitchell, J Erwin (Eds) *Comparative Primate Biology*, Vol. 2B: Behavior, Cognition, and Motivation (New York, Alan R. Liss), 167–218.

Lynch JW (1998) Mating behavior in wild tufted capuchins (*Cebus apella nigritus*) in Brazil's Atlantic forest. *American Journal of Physical Anthropology* 26 (Suppl):153.

Mendes SL, Santos RR (1999) Nascimentos de *Alouatta fusca* (Primates: Atelidae) na Estação Biológica de Caratinga, Minas Gerais. *Livro de Resumos, IX Congresso Brasileiro de Primatologia*, 72–73.

Mota MT, Sousa MBC (2000) Prolactin levels of fathers and helpers related to alloparental care in common marmosets, *Callithrix jacchus*. *Folia Primatologia* 71:22–26.

Nunn CL (1999) The number of males in primate social groups: a comparative test of the socioecological model. *Behavioral Ecology and Sociobiology* 46:1–13.

Odalia Rímoli A (1998) *Desenvolvimento Comportamental do Muriuqi* (Brachyteles arachnoides) *na Estação Biológica de Caratinga, Minas Gerais.* PhD dissertation (Universidade de São Paulo).

Pagel MD, Harvey PH (1993) Evolution of the juvenile period in mammals. In ME Pereira, LA Fairbanks (Eds) *Juvenile Primates: Life History, Development, and Behavior* (New York, Oxford University Press), 28–37.

Printes RC, Strier KB (1999) Behavioral correlates of dispersal in female muriquis *(Brachyteles arachnoides). International Journal of Primatology* 20:941–960.

Rímoli J, Lynch JW (1999) Demografia de um grupo de macacos pregos *(Cebus apella nigritus,* Primates: Cebidae) na Estação Biológica de Caratinga, Minas Gerais. *Livro de Resumos, IX Congresso Brasileiro de Primatologia,* 71.

Robinson JG (1988) Group size in wedge-capped capuchin monkeys *Cebus olivaceus* and the reproductive success of males and females. *Behavioral Ecology and Sociobiology* 23:187–197.

Ross C (1991) Life history patterns of New World monkeys. *International Journal of Primatology* 12:481–502.

Rylands AB, Mittermeier RA, Luna ER (1997) Conservation of Neotropical primates: threatened species and an analysis of primate diversity by country and region. *Folia Primatologia* 68:134–169.

Savage A, Snowdon CT, Giraldo LH, Soto LH (1996a) Parental care patterns and vigilance in wild cotton-top tamarins *(Saguinus oedipus).* In MA Norconk, AL Rosenberger, PA Garber (Eds) *Adaptive Radiations of Neotropical Primates* (New York, Plenum Press), 187–199.

Savage A, Giraldo LH, Soto LH, Snowdon CT (1996b) Demography, group composition, and dispersal in wild cotton-top tamarin *(Saguinus oedipus)* groups. *American Journal of Primatology* 38:85–100.

Savage A, Shideler SE, Soto LH, Causado J, Giraldo LH, Lasley BL, Snowdon CT (1997) Reproductive events of wild cotton-top tamarins *(Saguinus oedipus)* in Colombia. *American Journal of Primatology* 43:329–337.

Schiml PA, Mendoza SP, Saltzman W, Lyons DM, Mason WA (1996) Seasonality in squirrel monkeys *(Saimiri sciureus). Physiology and Behavior* 60:1105–1113.

Snowdon CT (1996) Infant care in cooperatively breeding species. In JS Rosenblatt, CT Snowdon (Eds) *Parental Care: Evolution, Mechanisms, and Adaptive Significance* (San Diego, Academic Press), 643–689.

Stearns SC (1992) *The Evolution of Life Histories* (Oxford, Oxford University Press).

Strier KB (1990) New World primates, new frontiers: insights from the wooly spider monkey, or muriqui *(Brachyteles arachnoides). International Journal of Primatology* 11:7–19.

Strier KB (1992) Atelinae adaptations: behavioral strategies and ecological constraints. *American Journal of Physical Anthropology* 88:515–524.

Strier KB (1994) Myth of the typical primate. *Yearbook of Physical Anthropology* 37:233–271.

Strier KB (1996a) Reproductive ecology of female muriquis. In M Norconk, A Rosenberger, P Garber (Eds) *Adaptive Radiations of Neotropical Primates* (New York, Plenum Press), 511–532.

Strier KB (1996b) Male reproductive strategies in New World primates. *Human Nature* 7:105–123.

Strier KB (1999a) The atelines. In A Fuentes, P Dolhinow (Eds) *Comparative Primate Behavior* (New York, McGraw Hill), 109–114.

Strier KB (1999b) *Faces in the Forest: The Endangered Muriqui Monkeys of Brazil* (Cambridge, Harvard University Press).

Strier KB (1999c) Why is female kin bonding so rare? Comparative sociality of New World primates. In PC Lee (Ed) *Comparative Primate Socioecology* (Cambridge, Cambridge University Press), 300– 319.

Strier KB (1999d) Predicting primate responses to "stochastic" demographic events. *Primates* 40:131–142.

Strier KB (2000) Population viabilities and conservation implications for muriquis *(Brachyteles arachnoides)* in Brazil's Atlantic forest. *Biotropica.* 32:903–913.

Strier KB (2001) Beyond the apes: the primate continuum. In FBM de Waal (Ed) *Tree of Origin* (Cambridge, Harvard University Press), 69–93.

Strier KB, Ziegler TE (1994) Insights into ovarian function in wild muriqui monkeys *(Brachyteles arachnoides). American Journal of Primatology* 32:31–40.

Strier KB, Ziegler TE (1997) Behavioral and endocrine characteristics of the reproductive cycle in wild muriqui monkeys, *Brachyteles arachnoides. American Journal of Primatology* 42:299–310.

Strier KB, Ziegler TE (2000) Lack of pubertal influences on female dispersal in muriqui monkeys *(Brachyteles arachnoides). Animal Behaviour* 49:849–860.

Strier KB, Ziegler TE, Wittwer D (1999) Seasonal and social correlates of fecal testosterone and cortisol levels in wild male muriquis *(Brachyteles arachnoides). Hormones and Behavior* 35:125–134.

Tardif SD, Richter CB, Carson RL (1984) Effects of sibling experience on future reproductive success in two species of Callitrichidae. *American Journal of Primatology* 6:377–380.

Wallis J (1997) A survey of reproductive parameters in the free-ranging chimpanzees of Gombe National Park. *Journal of Reproduction and Fertility* 109: 297–307.

Widowski TM, Ziegler TE, Elowson AM, Snowdon CT (1990) The role of males in the stimulation of reproductive function in female cotton-top tamarins, *Saguinus o. oedipus. Animal Behavior* 40:731–741.

Widowski TM, Porter TA, Ziegler TE, Snowdon CT (1992) The stimulatory effect of males on the initiation but not the maintenance of ovarian cycling in cotton-top tamarins *(Saguinus oedipus). American Journal of Primatology* 26:97–108.

Wiebe RH, Wiliams LE, Abee CR, Yeoman RR, Diamond EJ (1988) Seasonal changes in serum dehydroepiandrosterone, androstenedione, and testosterone levels in the squirrel monkey *(Saimiri boliviensis boliviensis). American Journal of Primatology* 14:285–291.

Ziegler TE (1987) The endocrinology of puberty and reproductive functioning in female cotton-top tamarins *(Saguinus oedipus)* under varying conditions. *Biology of Reproduction* 37:618–627.

Ziegler TE (2000) Hormones associated with non-maternal infant care: a review of mammalian and avian studies. *Folia Primatologia* 71:6–21.

Ziegler TE, Wegner FH, Snowdon CT (1996) Hormonal responses to parental and nonparental conditions in male cotton-top tamarins, *Saguinus oedipus*, a New World primate. *Hormones and Behavior* 30:287–297.

Ziegler TE, Santos CV, Pissinatti A, Strier KB (1997) Steroid excretion during the ovarian cycle in captive and wild muriquis, *Brachyteles arachnoides. American Journal of Primatology* 42:311–321.

Zucker EL, Clarke MR (1998) Agonistic and affiliative relationships of adult female howlers *(Alouatta palliata)* in Costa Rica over a 4-year period. *International Journal of Primatology* 19:433–449.

16

Reproductive Ecology of Old World Monkeys

FRED B. BERCOVITCH

Feeding strategies are an integral component of reproductive strategies (Bercovitch 1992). In the South American bloodsucking bug, *Rhodnius,* molt is stimulated by release of the hormone ecdysone, which is stimulated by body distension resulting from feasting on blood (Schmidt-Nielson 1997). Following successive molts, animals are capable of reproduction. In Old World monkeys, the linkage between dietary input and hormone output is more complicated but driven by a single neurobiological foundation. The hypothalamus is the crucial brain region that regulates both food ingestion and neuroendocrine profiles. Neuronal connections within the hypothalamus link satiety and endocrine state by conveying metabolic cues regarding energy balance.

Old World monkeys subsist on a diverse array of dietary items, and most reside in multimale-multifemale social systems. When traveling in groups composed of a range of age/sex classes, individuals need to engage in foraging strategies designed to promote their own growth, development, and reproductive success, but such strategies are often different from those of conspecifics resident in the same troop. In general, male mammals expend more reproductive energy on mating effort, while females concentrate on rearing effort (Trivers 1972). For example, prior to the mating season, male rhesus macaques, *Macaca mulatta,* accumulate fat reserves that boost body weight by about 10%, which enables them to forgo feeding and concentrate on reproductive activity during the mating season (Bercovitch 1992, 1997). Pre-mating-season adipose tissue levels are predictive of progeny production within a season (Bercovitch and Nürnberg 1996). In contrast, female savanna baboons, *Papio cynocephalus,* experience the greatest energetic costs to reproduction not during mating activity but while lactating, when their body weight declines by about 7% (Bercovitch 1987). Reaccumulation of sufficient body reserves seems to be a prerequisite to resumption of postlactational cycling.

Recognizing how social and ecological factors regulate reproductive processes in Old World monkeys can generate insights into human reproductive ecology. Human reproductive functions are constrained by evolutionary rules guiding phylogenetic potential in specific socioecological circumstances. The goals of this contribution are to explain how sexual selection molds the reproductive ecology of Old World monkeys in three realms (sexual bimaturism, sexual advertisements, maternal investment) and to explore the implications of these patterns for understanding the evolution of human reproductive ecology.

SEXUAL BIMATURISM

Sex differences in age at first breeding evolve when prolonged growth enhances the size of one sex, which increases the prospects for reproduction in that sex (Wiley 1974). Sexual bimaturism is most often witnessed in the larger size, and later development, of males residing in polygynous societies, a pattern frequently attributed to sexual selection favoring male competitive ability (Andersson 1994; Wiley 1974; Wilson 1975). Reproductive maturation among Old World monkey males begins at later ages than among females (Figure 16.1), requires more time to complete, and is more variable in duration (Bercovitch 2000). Reproductive energetics among males augment growth in body size as a mechanism enhancing both agonistic competition and endurance rivalry, while reproductive energetics among females suppress growth in body size in favor of allocating resources to gestation and lactation (Bercovitch 1997, 2000; Demment 1983; Martin et al. 1994). Body-size dimorphism can promote sex differences in foraging strategies (Bean 1999; Selander 1972), which reduce the costs of cohabitation in mixed-sex social groups.

Sexual bimaturism in Old World monkeys raises an evolutionary irony because retarded development could be advantageous to females while accelerated development could be beneficial to males. Rapid reproductive maturation among female Old World monkeys is disassociated from lifetime reproductive success, so an early age at first birth is not synonymous with increased fitness (Bercovitch and Berard 1993; Fedigan et al. 1986; Packer et al. 1995). Delayed reproductive maturation would benefit females if those producing first progeny at later ages experience reduced rates of infant loss compared with peers producing first offspring at younger ages (Paul and Kuester 1996; Sade 1990). If learning to mother is vital to female success at rearing offspring, then one might expect that females would delay progeny production in order to learn the nuances of motherhood.

Progeny loss among primiparous females is about twice that of multiparous females (Bercovitch et al. 1998). Although primiparous mothers are

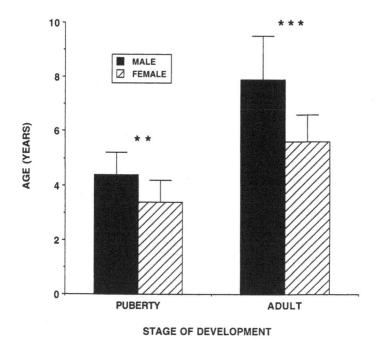

Figure 16.1. Sexual bimaturism in Old World monkeys. Histogram bars plot the mean + s.d. of developmental milestones reported for fourteen cercopithecine species (see Bercovitch 2000). Comparisons between sexes were analyzed using a paired *t*-test for male and female values within a species. ** p < 0.01; *** p < 0.001.

clumsy and awkward when handling newborns, maternal competence improves within a matter of days (Altmann 1980; Chism 1986; Hiraiwa 1981). Reduced survivorship of firstborns is probably a consequence of age-related developmental changes associated with alterations in sensitivity of the hypothalamic-pituitary-ovarian axis to suckling stimuli (Bercovitch et al. 1998). Limited milk yield among primiparous mothers is likely to promote frequent suckling, which drains resources from maternal reserves (Gomendio 1989). Neonatal mortality among primiparous females probably arises from the imposition of large energetic demands on an organism striving to partition resources into both growth and reproduction (Lancaster 1986; Lee and Bowman 1995). Physiological constraints impose a ceiling on female size because pregnant and lactating females need to ingest sufficient resources during their daily travels to nurture two individuals.

Successful reproduction requires adequate foraging to maintain energetic balance. Pregnant and lactating female savanna baboons spend more time feeding, and feed for more time on more nutritious foods, than cycling females (Muruthi et al. 1991). During peak nursing periods, lactating female gelada monkeys, *Theropithecus gelada*, devote about 70% of their daily time budget to feeding activity (Dunbar and Dunbar 1988). Under conditions of food scarcity, infant mortality increases and growth rates decrease because nursing capabilities and daily metabolic requirements are compromised (Richard 1985). Ecological conditions impose a ceiling on female size because individuals must ingest enough resources within set daylight hours to nurture themselves and their dependent young while traveling with a social group. The process of reproductive maturation among Old World monkey females is compressed compared with that of males, but the tempo of reproductive maturation is delayed until females have transcended an adequate size threshold, either involving pelvic dimensions (Ellison 1990) or body mass (Bercovitch et al. 1998), necessary to produce and nurture offspring.

Deferred breeding in males is favored when male longevity exceeds that of females (Wiley 1974), but the life history profile of Old World monkeys is opposite to this characteristic (Dunbar 1987). Sons of high-ranking female rhesus macaques (Bercovitch et al. 2000), Barbary macaques, *M. sylvanus* (Paul and Kuester 1996), and longtail macaques, *M. fascicularis* (van Noordwijk and van Schaik 1999) initiate their reproductive careers at younger ages than sons of low-ranking females, with dominance rank contributing to more rapid growth among males (Bercovitch 1993; Dixson and Nevison 1997). Males could benefit by reproducing in their natal troop as young adults prior to embarking on the potentially costly activity of natal dispersal. A lengthy adolescent phase provides a life history stage that enables males to grow larger than females, as well as extending the time frame for refining their social and competitive skills (Bercovitch 2000; Bronson 1989; Leigh 1995).

Body size among males accounts for only a fraction of the variance in progeny production. For example, the outcome of aggressive competition is independent of body weight in both savanna baboons (Bercovitch 1989) and gelada monkeys (Dunbar 1984). In longtail macaques, males abandon their natal troop and live a solitary lifestyle for a few years while augmenting size prior to immigration and challenging the resident males for the alpha position (van Noordwijk and van Schaik 1985). Genetic analysis of paternity reveals that the alpha male is responsible for siring most offspring in a troop, but the relative proportion of progeny produced is inversely related to the number of adult males in the troop (de Ruiter et al. 1992). Among rhesus macaques, paternity analysis revealed that body weight explained 25% of the variance in progeny production, but, among sires, the number of offspring produced was independent of body weight (Bercovitch and Nürnberg 1996).

Tactical reproductive maneuvers can overcome size deficits in male competitive interactions. For example, in savanna baboons, lighter males with strong affiliative bonds to females have comparable consort success to heavier males (Strum 1994). A classic example of the unreliability of predicting winners based only on size occured during the heavyweight title match on 4 July 1919, when Jack Dempsey (6'1"; 191 lbs) knocked out Jess Willard (6'6.25"; 252 lbs) in three rounds. The salient issue is identifying the evolutionary dynamics responsible for patterns of sex differences in rates of growth culminating in size dimorphism. Energetic constraints on reproductive effort promote progeny production in females by limiting body size, while development of complex mating strategies requiring social skills in males operates in conjunction with enlarged body size to maximize progeny production. Contrary to popular perception, males are not brain dead during adolescence; they are scheming about tactics to adopt to try to copulate with females.

Resource availability has more impact on the timing of sexual maturation among females than among males. Food restriction suppresses steroidogenesis and LH output, which generates strong negative effects on ovulation but has little influence on spermatogenesis (Bronson 1989). Male access to food resources influences the pace of reproductive development, but male reproductive success depends more on complex social strategies than on large size (Bercovitch 1991; Clutton-Brock 1994; Strum 1994). Abundant rainfall correlates with adult male size across populations of savanna baboons (Dunbar 1990; Strum 1994), but age at testicular enlargement is independent of rainfall quantity preceding testes growth (Alberts and Altmann 1995). On the other hand, age at first sexual swelling among female savanna baboons depends upon resource availability during the six months preceding the onset of sexual swelling (Bercovitch and Strum 1993). Among savanna baboons, the number of cycles to conception is inversely related to amount of rainfall (Bercovitch 1987), and, although savanna baboons do not reproduce on a seasonal basis, conceptions tend to cluster during the wet season (Bercovitch and Harding 1993; Wasser and Norton 1993). In Hanuman langurs, *Semnopithecus entellus*, plentiful resources improve female condition and increase the chances of conception (Koenig et al. 1997).

The key determinants of sexual bimaturism in Old World monkeys are physiological constraints that telescope female maturation into a condensed period and social and competitive complexity that stretches male maturation into an expanded period of growth. Reproductive maturation is molded by ecological factors, but social forces can exert an impact on the pace of reproductive maturation by modifying access to food resources vital to growth and development. Among human primates, females attain reproductive potential at younger ages than males, while cessation of growth in males occurs at later ages than in females. Reproductive energetics have an impact on profiles and patterns of sexual bimaturism in people.

SEXUAL ADVERTISEMENTS

Copulations often result in the emission of high-pitched squeals by male rhesus macaques (Hauser 1993), and proximity to ovulation is pronounced by protuberant sexual skin swellings among savanna baboons (Bercovitch 1987, 1999). Sexual advertisements are transmitted using multiple sensory channels and include not only vocalizations, ornaments, and odors broadcasting reproductive status, but also behavioral cues indicating sexual state. Signal conspicuousness is beneficial when it attracts mates, but costly when it invites predation or incites competition. Signal transmission tends to be endocrine-dependent (Bercovitch 1999; Dixson 1990, 1998; Wallen 1990), but whether differences in signal perception are also endocrine-dependent has not been satisfactorily studied.

Advertisements are mechanisms adopted to sway individuals in their choice of options when intended recipients have the potential to exercise a preference. The Marlboro Man could ride off into the sunset were it not for Joe Camel. Advertisements are superfluous when alternatives are nonexistent. Sexual selection promotes the expression of secondary sexual traits because they function in the context of choice of mate(s) (Darwin 1871). In Old World monkeys, studies of mate choice concentrate on females (see Keddy-Hector 1992; Small 1993), but male choice is expected when the costs of mating with multiple females are extensive, when females exhibit large differences in reproductive quality, when males must defend females over prolonged periods, and when male rearing effort improves survivorship prospects of progeny (Bercovitch 1978, 1985; Cunningham and Birkhead 1998; Darwin 1871; Pagel 1994; Parker 1983). Regardless of whether one sex or both have a more potent role in mate choice, sexual signals convey information about reproductive capability, which is a function of "quality" (see Johnstone 1995).

One aspect of quality is reproductive value, which provides an estimate of prospects for future offspring production (Fisher 1930). Late adolescence/young adulthood corresponds with the cusp in female reproductive value, so nulliparous females transcending the reproductive capability threshold should discharge the most pungent odors, display the most colossal visual banners, deliver the most thundering or mellifluous vocalizations, and demonstrate the most active pursuit of males. The age-dependent expression of secondary sexual traits in males is often regarded as an indicator mechanism broadcasting quality (Andersson 1994), but little research has been undertaken either on age-dependent expression of secondary sexual traits or on reproductive tactics in female Old World monkeys. Increasing sexual attractiveness to males can generate conditions conducive to subsequent female mate choice (Clutton-Brock and Harvey 1976; Wiley and Poston 1996) or male mate choice (Bercovitch 1978, 1985; Pagel 1994). For example, young adolescent female rhesus macaques are more likely than adult females to exuberantly solicit males, but they are also more likely to be ignored or rejected by adult males (Lindburg 1971). Sexual signals vary with age in rhesus macaques (Rowell 1967), gelada monkeys (Dunbar 1977), patas monkeys, *Erythrocebus patas* (Rowell 1977), Barbary macaques (Kuester and Paul 1984), and guinea baboons, *Papio papio* (Gauthier 1999), but the prime example of a connection between female age and sexual advertisements among Old World monkeys involves sexual skin swellings in savanna baboons.

The sex skin is a secondary sexual trait consisting of a specialized region in the perineal area that alters in appearance concurrent with fluctuations in ovarian steroid concentrations. In savanna baboons, the sex skin swelling reaches its zenith on the final few days of the follicular phase (Bercovitch 1999). The size of sex skin expansion does not precisely mirror steroid hormone levels, but rising estrogen concentrations foster growth of the sex skin, whereas elevations in progesterone counteract this effect (Gillman 1940, 1942; Parkes and Zuckerman 1931). When estrogen is administered to juvenile rhesus macaques, hypertrophy of the sex skin develops, but the treatment has no effect on GnRH output (Dierschke et al. 1974). The ballooning of the sex skin reflects increases in estradiol levels, which generally peak immediately prior to ovulation, rather than a linkage to actual ovulation; hence, enlarged sex skin swellings provide cues regarding the probability of ovulation.

Female "quality" for reproductive purposes peaks when the probability of ovulation is greatest. Copulating with good-quality partners is more likely to be productive than coition with wretched companions, and male mate selectivity has been widely documented in savanna baboons (Hausfater 1975; Packer 1979; Smuts 1985). Male savanna baboons are more likely to engage in aggressive reproductive strategies, and establish coalitions with other males, on the two most probable days of ovulation, when the size of sex skin swelling is maximal (Bercovitch 1988, 1989).

The display of sexual advertisements is a courtship mechanism designed to entice the opposite sex to mate (Andersson 1994; Darwin 1871), and enlarged sexual skin swellings correspond with the period of greatest sexual arousal and activity in males (Bercovitch 1988; Bielert and van der Walt 1982). Late adolescent females produce more bloated sex skin

swellings than other age classes (Altmann et al. 1988; Bercovitch 1999; Bielert et al. 1986; Scott 1984). Age differences in sex skin attributes could arise
from two primary pathways: either endocrine concentrations alter with
age or frequent steroid stimulation of the sex skin during life reduces the
responsiveness or number of steroid receptors in the sex skin and results
in diminished growth with age—in other words, downregulation. The
degree of sex skin hypertrophy at maximum turgescence is a reliable indicator of both the reproductive value of females (Figure 16.2) and proximity to ovulation (Bercovitch 1985, 1999). When females have more
conspicuous secondary sexual traits than males, such as sex skin
swellings, and when females flaunt their flamboyant features to foster
mating, then the most plausible evolutionary mechanism responsible for
development of the sexual advertisement is male mate choice (Darwin
1871).

Quality has been linked with sexual advertisements in nonprimates by
scrutinizing patterns of fluctuating asymmetry and disease resistance, but

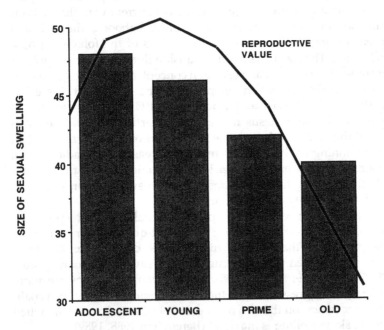

Figure 16.2. Sex skin swelling size and reproductive value in savanna baboons.
Size of sex skin was recorded on a 50-point scale during a lengthy field study in
Kenya (see Bercovitch 1985, 1999). Histogram bars plot the maximum size
obtained by females within the four age classes when they were most likely to
ovulate. The curve approximating the reproductive value was estimated from
data in Strum and Western 1982.

few studies of Old World monkeys have attempted to ascertain whether either factor is associated with variation in display of sexual advertisements. Fluctuating asymmetry refers to the nonidentical development of bilateral traits in an organism, with no consistent tendency to favor one side or the other (Palmer and Strobeck 1986; Van Valen 1962). Good-quality animals are expected to be buffered against socioecological disruptions to developmental stability and emerge as adults with less fluctuating asymmetry than poor-quality individuals (Livshits and Kobyliansky 1991; Parsons 1992). As a consequence, limited fluctuating asymmetry in secondary sexual traits is presumed to reflect genetic quality, and traits that are honest signals of genetic quality have been reasoned to be favored by sexual selection (Grafen 1990; Kodric-Brown and Brown 1984). Research on nonprimates has produced conflicting results (see, e.g., Balmford et al. 1993; Kieser and Groeneveld 1991; Møller 1990; Novack et al. 1993), and studies of fluctuating asymmetry and reproductive performance in Old World monkeys are lacking.

In pigtail macaques, *M. nemestrina*, the fluctuating asymmetry of dermatoglyphic traits was greater in the offspring of prenatally stressed mothers (Newall-Morris et al. 1989), revealing an association between developmental stability and environmental perturbation but demonstrating nothing about the impact of dermatoglyphic asymmetry on reproductive success. In male rhesus macaques, absolute canine size is not correlated with number of progeny produced within a season (Bercovitch and Nürnberg 1996), but longer canines are associated with less fluctuating asymmetry (Figure 16.3). However, fluctuating asymmetry in canine size was indistinguishable between sires and non-sires (Figure 16.3). One might even reason that more fluctuating asymmetry in secondary sexual traits, such as canines, would be present in successful males if their reproductive output derived from physical confrontations that damaged canines or inflicted facial scars distorting symmetry. To date, no evidence has been published linking improved reproductive success with reduced fluctuating asymmetry in secondary sexual traits in Old World monkeys, and such a relationship is unlikely to characterize species in which morphological attributes only account for a small fraction of the variance in reproductive success.

The concept of disease resistance as an indicator of quality has been developed into the Immunocompetence Model (Folstad and Karter 1992; Zahavi and Zahavi 1997; Zuk 1994). Massive parasite loads are expected to diminish the ability to display ostentatious sexual advertisements, which then reduces male attractiveness and reproductive success. Because sexual advertisements in males are testosterone-dependent, and testosterone depresses immune function, only good-quality males should be capable of simultaneously maintaining high testosterone titers while flaunting

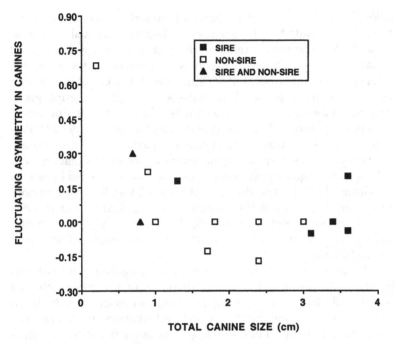

Figure 16.3. Fluctuating asymmetry in canine size and sirehood among rhesus macaques. Canine size was measured from gingiva to apex and sirehood was determined with DNA fingerprinting and STR marker typing (see Bercovitch and Nürnberg 1996). Fluctuating asymmetry was calculated as $(R - L) / [(R + L) / 2]$. Sample size ($n = 21$) was greater than indicated owing to overlap among individuals. Longer canines correlated with reduced levels of fluctuating asymmetry ($r_s = -0.531$, $p < 0.05$), but fluctuating asymmetry in canine size was indistinguishable between sires and non-sires (Mann-Whitney U = 65, $n_1 = 8$, $n_2 = 13$, $p > 0.20$). Data from Bercovitch and Nürnberg (unpublished).

pronounced sexual advertisements. Investigations aimed at testing whether sexual advertisements, immunocompetence, and reproductive output are connected have yielded inconsistent results (see, e.g., Braude et al. 1999; Hasselquist et al. 1999; Saino and Møller 1994; Zuk et al. 1995).

In the rhesus macaques on Cayo Santiago, parasite load is significantly higher in males than in females, but parasite load declines with age, is independent of dominance rank, and has no measurable impact on female reproductive performance (File and Kessler 1989; Knezevich 1998). However, if parasite saturation induces lethargy and weight loss in males, then their endurance rivalry would be compromised, which would diminish reproductive potential. Although secondary sexual traits such as canine size are not affected by suppressed immune function, male body mass and reproductive tactics could be handicapped under conditions of severe parasite infestation. Therefore, male fertility could be indirectly influenced by parasite load if it modifies male capability to gain and retain sexually receptive females. Among adult male savanna baboons, the number of parasite ova per gram of feces is positively correlated with dominance rank (Hausfater and Watson 1976), which in turn is positively correlated with relative reproductive output (Altmann et al. 1996; Hausfater 1975), providing circumstantial evidence that the effects of a high parasite load can be suppressed by dominant males. However, fecal parasite level could reflect host resistance ability or extent and duration of exposure. To date, no evidence has been published testing the Immunocompetence Model in Old World monkeys, but male reproductive success is likely to be influenced by parasite infestation and immune function.

Sexual advertisements are expected to broadcast "quality." From an evolutionary vantage point, quality ought to coincide with viability or fertility, and from a physiological perspective quality is expected to vary with age, and health. Socioecological conditions influence reproductive maturation and mediate reproductive success in Old World monkeys by entraining ovarian cyclicity with resource acquisition and by promoting sexual advertisements that encourage mate choice. In human primates, sexual advertisements, such as protuberant female bosoms, reflect reproductive value and can be attributed to male mate choice.

MATERNAL INVESTMENT

Energy transfer of milk from mother to infant is the cornerstone of maternal investment because duration of lactation directly influences interbirth interval (Lee 1987). Maternal investment involves costs to the mother that entail negative reproductive consequences, as well as benefits to the infant by increasing the probability of survival (Trivers 1972). Although maternal investment has been expanded in scope to include maternal support of mature offspring, care or support of independent offspring that does not involve fitness costs does not fall under the rubric of maternal investment. Maternal investment alters with resource availability, mortality risk, maternal and offspring condition, parity, infant growth rate, birth order, and age (Berman 1992; Fairbanks and McGuire 1995; Hauser 1988; Hauser and Fairbanks 1988; Hrdy 1987; Lee 1984; Lee et al. 1991).

Natural selection is expected to yield organisms that have an ability to invest unequally in sons and daughters based upon the expected reproductive consequences of differential expenditure (Clutton-Brock 1991; Fisher 1930; Maynard Smith 1980; Trivers and Willard 1973). Each sex supplies half the ancestry to future generations, so the total reproductive value of males in one generation must equal that of females of the same generation (Fisher 1930). As a result, a numerical excess of one sex over the other at the end of the period of parental expenditure is expected to be compensated for by reduced investment in that sex so that expenditure in both sexes is comparable. When species exhibit prolonged periods of parental investment, and when offspring survivorship, not production, is the critical component regulating differential reproduction, then one is less likely to encounter sex biases in the production of offspring, and more likely to observe sex-biased maternal resource distribution to offspring (Fisher 1930; Hrdy 1987; Trivers and Willard 1973; Wasser and Norton 1993). Mothers are predicted to partition resources according to sex of progeny when such investment patterns have an impact on characteristics related to variation in offspring reproductive success.

Maternal investment is problematic to quantify (see Clutton-Brock 1991), and subject to adjustment depending upon socioecological surroundings, but is expected to vary with sex of offspring when mothers reap reproductive rewards from sex-biased patterns of investment. In polygynous Old World monkeys, determining reproductive consequences of maternal investment in sons is considerably complicated owing to male dispersal strategies and paternal uncertainty in the absence of genetic analysis. In addition, academic disputes in the area of maternal investment and sex ratio manipulation are as relentless, unremitting, and innovative as are Wile E. Coyote's uses of Acme products to catch the Roadrunner (e.g., Clutton-Brock and Iason 1986; Festa-Bianchet 1996; Hardy 1997; Krackow 1995; van Hooff 1997; van Schaik and Hrdy 1991). Only limited sex-biased maternal investment is expected when sex differences in mortality to the age of independence are small, when maternal investment aimed at augmenting infant male size has modest effects on adult size, and when adult male size accounts for a fraction of the variance in male reproductive success. When adult male size is subject to socioecological determinants, and when adult size is only minimally dependent on extraction of maternal resources, then one does not expect enormous sex differences in maternal investment. Such conditions characterize Old World monkeys.

Among Old World monkeys, the prevalent mode is unbiased birth sex ratios that are accompanied by profiles of sexual bimaturism *beginning at birth* that align with a profile of greater maternal investment in sons. The seeds stimulating sexual size dimorphism are sown before the pronounced adolescent male growth spurt. Across primates, neonatal body mass dimorphism correlates with degree of adult body mass dimorphism (Smith and Leigh 1998). Males are often heavier than females at birth, with size dimorphism increasing during the first year of life (Figure 16.4), suggesting elevated prenatal and postnatal partitioning of maternal resources

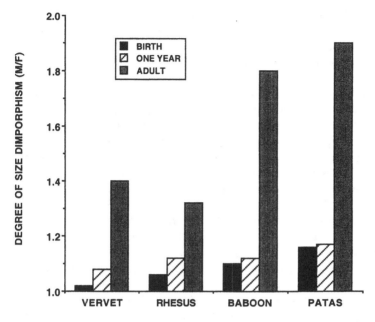

Figure 16.4. The ontogeny of sexual size dimorphism in four species of Old World monkeys. Relative dimorphism was calculated as the extent to which male mass at three different ages (birth, infancy, adulthood) exceeds female mass. Data from Harvey et al. (1987), Smith and Jungers (1997), Debbie Pollack, Lynn Fairbanks, and Mike McGuire, UCLA Department of Psychiatry and Biobehavioral Sciences, personal communication (vervets); Bercovitch et al. (2000), Bercovitch, unpublished data (rhesus macaques); Bercovitch 1989, Coehlo 1985, Dunbar 1990, Glassman et al. 1984, McMahon et al. 1976 (savanna baboons); Sly et al. 1983, Harvey et al. 1987, Bercovitch 1996, unpublished data (patas monkeys).

to sons. However, whether sex-biased allocation of resources results in greater reproductive costs by increasing interbirth interval or reducing son's survivorship is not clear.

In vervet monkeys, *Cercopithecus aethiops* (Cheney et al. 1988), savanna baboons (Altmann 1980; Smuts and Nicolson 1989), and rhesus monkeys (Drickamer 1974; but see Meikle and Vessey 1988), infant survivorship is comparable for sons and daughters. In savanna baboons, the interbirth interval following successful rearing of sons is comparable to that following successful rearing of daughters (Smuts and Nicolson 1989), but in the rhesus monkeys on Cayo Santiago, mothers who successfully raise sons are more likely to delay subsequent conception than are mothers who rear daughters (Bercovitch and Berard 1993; Berman 1988). The greater energetic investment involved in rearing sons could fail to impose a fitness cost if mothers have compensatory mechanisms to meet male demands by modifying feeding behavior or activity levels that offset the enegetic costs. In Old World monkeys, strong familial bonds promote infant handling by non-mothers (Maestripieri 1994; Paul 1999; Ross and MacLarnon 1995; Silk 1999), which diminishes the metabolic expenditures essential for rearing heavier male than female progeny. Sex differences in immature growth rates could accrue from sex diffferences in metabolic efficiency, rather than from differences in maternal investment patterns (Birgersson et al. 1998; Clutton-Brock 1991, 1994; Moses et al. 1998). Energy transfer from mothers to progeny during lactation seems to accelerate male growth but, in the absence of fitness costs, falls outside the domain of maternal investment.

Biased sex ratios have also been examined as a form of maternal investment and seem most likely to emerge when competition among females is intense (Hiraiwa-Hasegawa 1993; Johnson 1988; van Schaik and Hrdy 1991). When females find themselves in harsh conditions, owing to either restricted food resources or confined space, then reproductive endocrinology should be adjusted to favor production of the cheaper sex. Because infant weight is dependent on maternal weight (Bowman and Lee 1995; Lee 1999), and females weigh less than males at birth, daughters should be the less expensive sex to produce. However, larger infants are a smaller proportion of maternal mass than are smaller infants (Bowman and Lee 1995; Lee 1999), so a hefty mother producing a son could sustain less energetic costs than a petite mother producing a daughter. In addition, maternal weight could be a consequence of sex of fetus. Passive diffusion of fetal hormones through the placenta can inform the mother of the sex of the womb's occupant. Upon receiving signals that she is carrying a male, her body might adjust its metabolism and fat storage to prepare for nursing a son. Prenatal androgen injections to pregnant females cross the placenta and influence both the behavior and morphology of daughters (Goy et al. 1988), so fetal androgens could enter maternal circulation. In rhesus macaques, fetal testosterone begins to circulate by 40 to 50 days postconception (Resko and Ellinwood 1981), and testosterone is the precursor to estrogen, which encourages adipose tissue deposition (Norman and Litwack 1997). Elevated expenses incurred in producing sons could be offset by fetal manipulation of maternal condition.

The premise of sex-biased maternal investment is that reproductive rewards to mothers are a direct consequence of differential levels of resource distribution to sons and daughters (Frank 1990; Maynard Smith 1980; Trivers 1972), which probably varies with the dominance position of the mother (Altmann 1980; Silk 1983). However, among Old World monkeys living in natural surroundings, dominance rank rarely influences secondary sex ratio. Dominant female savanna baboons at Amboseli National Park, Kenya, produce a surfeit of daughters (Altmann 1980), but rank effects on sex ratio at birth are absent among the savanna baboons at

Mikumi National Park, Tanzania (Rhine et al. 1992; Wasser and Norton 1993), and at Gilgil, Kenya (Smuts and Nicolson 1989). Only three field studies of Old World monkeys, other than baboons, that examine the rank effects on secondary sex ratios could be located, and none found that dominance status influenced sex of progeny (Cheney et al. 1988; Dunbar 1984; van Noordwijk and van Schaik 1999). In three macaque species, a rank-biased secondary sex ratio was recorded in captivity, but not in wild or semi-free-ranging populations (*M. mulatta*, cf. Simpson and Simpson 1982 with Berman 1988; *M. fascicularis*, cf. van Schaik et al. 1989 with van Noordwijk and van Schaik 1999; *M. fuscata*, cf. Aureli et al. 1990 with Koyama et al. 1992). Hence, dominance rank in Old World monkeys seems to influence the secondary sex ratio only under unusual circumstances.

Facultative adjustment of maternal resources devoted to nurturing offspring is not a unique adaptation, but an expansion of a physiological system that has evolved the capacity to maximize reproductive output by partitioning investment in growth, maintenance, and reproduction in terms of probable payoffs given current socioecological constraints. Levels of maternal investment form a continuum from abortion or stillbirth when conditions, either physiological or ecological, are poor to pouring resources into a son's growth when conditions, either physiological or ecological, are rich. Female reproductive flexibility results in a diversity of investment patterns as mechanisms strive to achieve the greatest reproductive returns with the minimum reproductive costs. In human primates, evolution of a capacious cranium extracted considerable maternal resources and set the stage for limits to size dimorphism.

EVOLUTION OF HUMAN REPRODUCTIVE ECOLOGY

A life history diorama of human reproductive ecology commences at parturition. Boys weigh about 1.05 times as much as girls at birth (ca. 3.4 vs. 3.25 kg; Sinclair 1973), a ratio midway between that of vervets and rhesus monkeys (see Figure 16.4). However, whereas the weight dimorphism of these latter two species amplifies to 130–140%, men weigh only about 116% as much as women, or about the same proportion as among one-year-old patas monkeys (see Figure 16.4). The culprit limiting size dimorphism in human beings is physiological restrictions imposed upon levels of maternal investment.

Among human primates, birth weight is correlated with maternal weight (Stock and Metcalfe 1994). Low birth weight is a high risk factor for infant mortality (Martorell and Gonzalez-Cossio 1987; Shapiro et al. 1968), but larger babies increase the prospects of dystocia. Although adult stature is not reliably predicted from birth size, estimates of adult size generated from stature at two years of age are fairly dependable (Sinclair 1973). Size dimorphism among adults is a function of size dimorphism at independence, which depends on maternal ability to channel resources into infant growth because growth trajectories are greatest during the dependent period of life. By one year of age, boys weigh close to 20% of their mother's weight. Time budgets will limit the degree to which hominids can nurture dependent offspring, while the pelvic canal will limit size of progeny at birth. In primates, the size of the maternal pelvic ring corresponds with the size of the newborn head, and both Old World monkeys and women experience a tighter squeeze at birth than occurs among apes (Schultz 1949, 1969). The upper boundary to birth size will depend upon maximum head size because neonatal brain weight, or head size, is correlated with neonatal body weight, or birth size (Martin 1990), and human babies have gargantuan heads. In human primates, unlike Old World monkeys, the head at birth is often turned sideways to facilitate passage through the birth canal because the pelvic sagittal diameter is smaller than the transverse diameter as a consequence of the evolution of bipedalism (Schultz 1969). While neonatal head size relative to body size at birth among people is *larger* than in most primates, neonatal weight relative to maternal weight at birth among people is *smaller* (ca. 5.5%) than in most nonhominoid primates (ca. 7%; see Lee 1999; Schultz 1969).

Maternal ability to nourish infant brain growth regulates the tempo of development and is a consequence of maternal metabolic efficiency (Martin 1981, 1996; Martin and MacLarnon 1985). Lactation is the most metabolically expensive reproductive state, but maternal metabolic adjustments during the reproductive cycle minimize the energetic costs of producing and rearing progeny (Stock and Metcalfe 1994). Maternal capacity to deliver milk to dependent young not only guides the duration of lactation and interbirth intervals but establishes the foundation for regulating size dimorphism among adults. Reproductive energetics will curtail sexual dimorphism in people because mothers are limited in the amount of resources that they can transfer to a dependent offspring with a metabolically expensive head (see also Smith and Leigh 1998). Head size at two years of age is already 60% that of adult size (Sinclair 1973). Adult stature is a function of infant body size, which is associated with neonatal head size, and which in turn is curbed by restrictions imposed by the dimensions of the pelvic canal. Regardless of the evolutionary explanation for the emergence of a megacephalic hominid, the development brought an albatross-around-the-neck that siphons prodigious amounts of maternal resources.

The limited size dimorphism of people implies a polygynous past, but one in which levels of male-male competition either were not severe enough to promote bulky bodies or were mediated using nonmorphological traits, such as weaponry. Men are not unique in possessing facial hair, since other mammals display similar secondary sexual traits, and human beings are not unique in using tools, because chimpanzees use stones to crack walnut-like fruits for food (Darwin 1871). However, the ability of men to "throw a stone or spear [with accuracy] . . . demands the perfect co-adaptation of numerous muscles" (Darwin 1871:432) and is a unique evolutionary development. Sexual bimaturism among people not only enables men to accumulate added muscular bulk, it provides time to develop both social skills that mediate mate acquisition and physical skills that mediate armament use in male-male competition. A crucial stage in hominid evolution was not development of the ability to make tools, but development of the ability to manufacture weapons for settling male-male competitive bouts.

Production and use of weapons required neurobiological modifications along with morphological refinements. The most widely documented sexual dimorphisms in neural abilities in people are female superiority in verbal tasks and male superiority in visuospatial tasks (Hampson and Kimura 1992; Hedges and Nowell 1995). Right hemisphere specialization in spatial tasks occurs among children as young as six years of age (Witelson 1976). The enhanced visuospatial ability of men, and the development of upper body strength, can be considered adaptations that emerged not as a means of pursuing big game, but because they were beneficial in confrontations over access to female mates. The rotary motion of the hominoid shoulder provided a basis for development of the overhand throw, which was capitalized on by men in the context of male-male competition. Despite profound differences in pelvic structure, men and women differ little in speed or endurance, but substantial differences are apparent in upper torso strength.

The Olympic record in the 100 m dash for women is about 7% slower than that for men (10.54 vs. 9.84 sec.) and the marathon record is 12% slower (2:24:52 vs. 2:09:21). But the Olympic record in the javelin throw is 27% greater for men than for women (94.6 vs. 74.7 m). Darwin (1871:872) remarked that "There can be little doubt that the greater size and strength of man, in comparison with woman, together with his broader shoulders, more developed muscles, rugged outline of body, his greater courage and pugnacity, are all due in chief part to inheritance from his half-human male ancestors. These characters would, however, have been preserved . . . by the success of the strongest and boldest men, both in the general struggle for life and *in their contests for wives; a success which would have ensured their leaving a more numerous progeny than their less favoured brethren*" [emphasis added]. Men have retained a fairly primitive apelike physique with a crucial element of sexual selection not involving display of facial hair or enormous increases in body mass, but development of the neurobiological and morphological capacity to construct and use weapons in the context of male competitive interactions for mates.

On the other hand, women are possessed of a derived, novel physique with a crucial element of sexual selection involving major alterations in morphology and appearance as means to attract mates. The near depilation of the body, and the development of pendulous breasts, are secondary traits that emerged as sexual advertisements promoting male mate choice and improving female reproductive success. Alternative evolutionary explanations include female competition, with breasts being designed to deceive males about female quality (Low 1990); female choice, with breasts being designed to reliably signal males about female quality (Cant 1981; Reynolds 1991); and natural selection, with increased breast size boosting nutritional reserves for lactation (Caro and Sellen 1990). If protuberant breasts evolved as sexual advertisements, then one would expect that the structural appearance of the bosoms reflects the reproductive value of the organism, which indicates fertility potential and attracts mates. If the primary evolutionary advantage of body hair thinning were heat dispersion and sweating while charging around the African savanna hunting big game, then one would expect that men would have evolved with less body hair than women. But the opposite pattern has evolved among hominids. The smooth skin of women may have originated as a mechanism to maximize exposure of enlarged breasts. Adipose tissue accumulates in mammals in association with growth of the mammary gland, but the pronounced development of human breasts prior to first ovulation is an unusual pattern of fat deposition (Hrdy 1988; Pond 1978; Short 1976).

The first sign of impending reproductive capacity in girls is the appearance of breast buds about two years before menarche and three years prior to first ovulation (Edwards 1980; Jones 1997). First ovulation is followed by a phase of intermittent ovulatory cycles, with regular ovulatory cyclicity occurring in about half the population by the early twenties (Edwards 1980). At about the same age, maximum nulliparous breast size is attained. The peak reproductive value among women occurs at approximately 18.5 years of age (Fisher 1930), indicating that a loose concordance between achievement of complete breast development and arrival at the summit in reproductive value characterizes human females in their late teens and early twenties. For mate selection to track reproductive value, partner preferences should be predicated on future reproductive prospects, not prior reproductive performance, whereas the opposite situation should occur if mate selection targets fitness, because older individuals with a lower reproductive value are the ones most likely to have the greatest fitness. Protuberant breasts provide men with clues about female reproductive value, but the svelte, Barbie doll, nymphette morphotype is unlikely to have been the archetypical female of choice during human evolution. The oldest example of a female figure in art is the Venus limestone carvings found at Laussal, France, dating to 20–25,000 years ago, which depict someone with pendulant breasts and a rotund body (see Figure 3 in Ucko and Rosenfeld 1967), similar to the women found in Renaissance paintings.

The proposed evolutionary scenario does not imply that men evolved as sex-craved, primitive, violent, weapons-wielding creatures fighting to obtain the flirtatious, nubile, hairless, buxom females who were enticing men to battle by displaying their assets in order to conceive children by the most skillfully endowed males. The proposed scenario reasons that features unique to each sex, and to the emergence of modern hominids, evolved as an outcome of sexual selection that was channeled into a novel path regulated by restrictions imposed upon maternal investment owing to the origin of a megacephalic hominid. The focus on male mate choice and male-male competition does not indicate that female mate choice and female-female competition were unimportant in hominid evolution, only that the former two processes of sexual selection have made a substantial contribution to the origin of some unique hominid features.

Sexual advertisements in the form of bulging bosoms are unique to human beings, probably originated coincident with thinning of body hair, and reflect reproductive value. Males seized upon these clues to enhance their reproductive success and developed the ability to aim armaments with accuracy at opponents seeking the same mate. The ability to nurture young and to attract male mates was a factor responsible for the evolution of the female physique, but differential reproductive success among women today is not a function of breast size any more than differential reproductive success among men is a function of speed and accuracy of spear-throwing.

As with Old World monkeys, indices of "quality" promoting mate attraction are likely to involve features demonstrating health and reproductive value. For example, Tovée et al. (1999) have contested the suggestion that a low waist-to-hip ratio—in other words, a curvaceous body—is a central feature of female sexual attractivity, demonstrating instead that the primary determinant of female attractiveness is the body mass index, a reflection of condition. In *The Descent of Man and Selection in Relation to Sex*, Darwin (1871:890) wrote "It is certainly not true that there is in the mind of man any universal standard of beauty with respect to the human body." He reasoned that worldwide practices of body painting, tatooing, scarification, removing or filing teeth, and body piercing, as well as "the almost universal habits of dancing, masquerading, and making rude pictures" (p. 889) were the outcome of mate choice molded by the social environment. Although the form of sexual advertisements will differ across populations, and the importance attached to advertisements will vary with socioecological surroundings, sexual advertisements in people are expected to reflect quality in order to attract mating partners.

Sexual selection has had an impact on the evolution of human physiology and behavior. Human reproductive ecology is based upon the evolution of life history strategies molded by maternal investment, sexual bimaturism, and sexual advertisements. In human primates, as in Old World monkeys, feeding strategies regulate reproductive strategies because energy balance will influence the degree to which mothers can produce and nurture their young. Hominids, like Old World monkeys, have evolved a physiological flexibility that maximizes reproductive success by governing reproductive strategies in a fashion commensurate with socioecological conditions that are encountered by individuals. The central feature in the evolution of modern hominids is the emergence of an exceedingly large head, and the origin of this unique trait had life history consequences resulting in a limited size dimorphism because of constraints imposed on maternal investment. And the limited size dimorphism was accompanied by development of some unusual secondary sexual traits operating in the context of male mate choice and male-male competition within a polygynous social system.

REFERENCES

Alberts SC, Altmann J (1995) Preparation and activation: determinants of age at reproductive maturity in male baboons. *Behavioral Ecology and Sociobiology* 36:397–406.

Altmann, J (1980) *Baboon Mothers and Infants* (Cambridge, Harvard University Press).

Altmann J, Altmann SA, Hausfater G (1988) Physical maturation and age estimates of yellow baboons, *Papio cynocephalus*, in Amboseli National Park, Kenya. *American Journal of Primatology* 1:389–399.

Altmann J, Alberts SC, Haines SA, Dubach J, Muruthi P, Coote T, Geffen E, Cheesman DJ, Mututua RS, Saiyael SN, Wayne RK, Lacy RC, Bruford MW (1996) Behavior predicts genetic structure in a wild primate group. *Proceedings of the National Academy of Sciences* 93:5797–5801.

Andersson M (1994) *Sexual Selection* (Princeton, Princeton University Press).

Aureli F, Schino G, Cordischi C, Cozzolini R, Scucchi S, van Schaik CP (1990) Social factors affect the secondary sex ratio in captive Japanese macaques. *Folia Primatologica* 55:176–180.

Balmford A, Jones IL, Thomas ALR (1993) On avian asymmetry: evidence of natural selection for symmetrical tails and wings in birds. *Proceedings of the Royal Society of London, B* 252:245–251.

Bean A (1999) Ecology of sex differences in great ape foraging. In PC Lee (Ed) *Comparative Primate Socioecology* (Cambridge, CambridgeUniversity Press), 339–362.

Bercovitch FB (1978) Mate selection and sexual selection in nonhuman primates. *California Anthropologist* 7:9–12.

Bercovitch FB (1985) *Reproductive Tactics in Adult Female and Adult Male Olive Baboons.* PhD dissertation (University of California).

Bercovitch FB (1987) Female weight and reproductive condition in a population of olive baboons (*Papio anubis*). *American Journal of Primatology* 12:189–195.

Bercovitch FB (1988) Coalitions, cooperation, and reproductive tactics in savanna baboons. *Animal Behavior* 36:1198–1209.

Bercovitch FB (1989) Body size, sperm competition, and determinants of male reproductive success in savanna baboons. *Evolution* 43:1507–1521.

Bercovitch FB (1991) Social stratification, social strategies, and reproductive success in primates. *Ethology and Sociobiology* 12:315–333.

Bercovitch FB (1992) Estradiol concentrations, fat deposits, and reproductive strategies in male rhesus macaques. *Hormones and Behavior* 26:272–282.

Bercovitch FB (1993) Dominance rank and reproductive maturation in male rhesus macaques *(Macaca mulatta). Journal of Reproduction and Fertility* 99:113–120.

Bercovitch FB (1996) Testicular function and scrotal coloration in patas monkeys. *Journal of Zoology* 239:93–100.

Bercovitch FB (1997) Reproductive strategies of rhesus macaques. *Primates* 38:247–263.

Bercovitch FB (1999) Sex skin. In E Knobil, JD Neill (Eds) *Encyclopedia of Reproduction* (San Diego, Academic Press), 437–443.

Bercovitch FB (2000) Behavioral ecology and socioendocrinology of reproductive maturation in cercopithecines. In PF Whitehead, CJ Jolly (Eds) *Old World Monkeys* (Cambridge, Cambridge University Press), 298–320.

Bercovitch FB, Berard JD (1993) Life history costs and consequences of rapid reproductive maturation in female rhesus macaques. *Behavioral Ecology and Sociobiology* 32:103–109.

Bercovitch FB, Harding RSO (1993) Annual birth patterns of savanna baboons over a ten year period at Gilgil, Kenya. *Folia Primatologica* 61:115–122.

Bercovitch FB, Nürnberg P (1996) Socioendocrine and morphological correlates of paternity in rhesus macaques. *Journal of Reproduction and Fertility* 107:59–68.

Bercovitch FB, Strum SC (1993) Dominance rank, resource availability, and reproductive maturation among female savanna baboons. *Behavioral Ecology and Sociobiology* 33:313–318.

Bercovitch FB, Lebron MR, Martinez HS, Kessler MJ (1998) Primigravidity, body weight, and costs of rearing first offspring in rhesus macaques. *American Journal of Primatology* 46:135–144.

Bercovitch FB, Widdig A, Nürnberg P (2000) Maternal investment and reproductive success of sons in rhesus macaques. *Behavioral Ecology and Sociobiology* 48:1–11.

Berman CM (1988) Maternal condition and offspring sex ratio in a group of free-ranging rhesus monkeys: An eleven year study. *American Naturalist* 131:307–328.

Berman CM (1992) Immature siblings and mother-infant relationships among free-ranging rhesus monkeys on Cayo Santiago. *Animal Behavior* 44:247–258.

Bielert C, van der Walt MA (1982) Male chacma baboon *(Papio ursinus)* sexual arousal: mediation by visual cues from female conspecifics. *Psychoneuroendocrinology* 7:31–48.

Bielert C, Girolami L, Anderson CM (1986) Male chacma baboon *(Papio ursinus)* sexual arousal: studies with adolescent and adult females as visual stimuli. *Developmental Psychobiology* 19:369–383.

Birgersson B, Tillbom M, Ekvall K (1998) Male-biased investment in fallow deer: an experimental study. *Animal Behavior* 56:301–307.

Bowman JE, Lee PC (1995) Growth and threshold weaning weights among captive rhesus macaques. *American Journal of Physical Anthropology* 96:159–175.

Braude S, Tang-Martinez Z, Taylor GT (1999) Stress, testosterone, and the immunoredistribution hypothesis. *Behavioral Ecology* 10:345–350.

Bronson FH (1989) *Mammalian Reproductive Biology* (Chicago, University of Chicago Press).

Cant JGH (1981) Hypothesis for the evolution of human breasts and buttocks. *American Naturalist* 117:119–204.

Caro TM, Sellen DW (1990) The reproductive advantages of fat in women. *Ethology and Sociobiology* 11:51–66.

Cheney DL, Seyfarth RM, Andelman SJ, Lee PC (1988) Reproductive success in vervet monkeys. In TH Clutton-Brock (Ed) *Reproductive Success* (Chicago, University of Chicago Press), 384–402.

Chism J (1986) Development and mother-infant relations among captive patas monkeys. *International Journal of Primatology* 7:49–81.

Clutton-Brock TH (1991) *The Evolution of Parental Care* (Princeton, Princeton University Press).

Clutton-Brock TH (1994) The costs of sex. In RV Short, E Balaban (Eds) *The Differences between the Sexes* (Cambridge, Cambridge University Press), 347–362.

Clutton-Brock TH, Harvey PH (1976) Evolutionary rules and primate societies. In PPG Bateson, RA Hinde (Eds) *Growing Points in Ethology* (Cambridge, Cambridge University Press), 195–237.

Clutton-Brock TH, Iason GR (1986) Sex ratio variation in mammals. *Quarterly Review of Biology* 61:339–374.

Coelho AM, Jr. (1985) Baboon dimorphism: growth in weight, length and adiposity from birth to 8 years of age. In ES Watts (Ed) *Nonhuman Primate Models for Human Growth and Development* (New York, Alan R. Liss), 125–159.

Cunningham EJA, Birkhead TR (1998) Sex roles and sexual selection. *Animal Behavior* 56:1311–1321.

Darwin CR (1871) *The Descent of Man and Selection in Relation to Sex* (London, John Murray).

Demment MW (1983) Feeding ecology and the evolution of body size of baboons. *African Journal of Ecology* 21:219–233.

de Ruiter JR, Scheffrahn W, Trommelen GJJM, Uitterlinden AG, Martin RD, van Hooff JARAM (1992) Male social rank and reproductive success in wild long-tailed macaques: paternity exclusions by blood protein naalysis and DNA fingerprinting. In RD Martin, AF Dixson, EJ Wickings (Eds) *Paternity in Primates: Genetic Tests and Theories* (Basel, Karger), 175–191.

Dierschke DJ, Weiss G, Knobil E (1974) Sexual maturation in the female rhesus monkey and the development of estrogen-induced gonadotropic hormone release. *Endocrinology* 94:198–206.

Dixson AF (1990) The neuroendocrine regulation of sexual behaviour in female primates. *Annual Review of Sex Research* 1:197–226.

Dixson AF (1998) *Primate Sexuality* (Oxford, Oxford University Press).

Dixson AF, Nevison CM (1997) The socioendocrinology of adolescent development in male rhesus monkeys (*Macaca mulatta*). *Hormones and Behavior* 31:126–135.

Drickamer LC (1974) A ten-year summary of reproductive data for free-ranging *Macaca mulatta. Folia Primatologica* 21:61–80.

Dunbar RIM (1977) Age-dependent changes in sexual skin colour and associated phenomena of female gelada baboons. *Journal of Human Evolution* 6:667–672.

Dunbar RIM (1984) *Reproductive Decisions* (Princeton, Princeton University Press).

Dunbar RIM (1987) Demography and reproduction. In BB Smuts, DL Cheney, RM Seyfarth, RW Wrangham, TT Struhsaker (Eds) *Primate Societies* (Chicago, University of Chicago Press), 240–249.

Dunbar RIM (1988) *Primate Social Systems* (Ithaca, New York, Comstock Press).

Dunbar RIM (1990) Environmental determinants of intraspecific variation in body weight in baboons (*Papio* spp.). *Journal of Zoology* 220:157–169.

Dunbar RIM, Dunbar P (1988) Maternal time budgets of gelada baboons. *Animal Behavior* 36:970–980.

Edwards RG (1980) *Conception in the Human Female* (New York, Academic Press).

Ellison PT (1990) Human ovarian function and reproductive ecology: new hypotheses. *American Anthropologist* 92:933–952.

Fairbanks LA, McGuire MT (1995) Maternal condition and the quality of maternal care in vervet monkeys. *Behaviour* 132:733–754.

Fedigan LM, Fedigan L, Gouzoules S, Gouzoules H, Koyama N (1986) Lifetime reproductive success in female Japanese macaques. *Folia Primatologica* 47: 143–157.

Festa-Bianchet M (1996) Offspring sex ratio studies of mammals: does publication depend upon the quality of the research or the direction of the results? *Ecoscience* 3:42–44.

File S, Kessler MJ (1989) Parasites of free-ranging Cayo Santiago macaques after 46 years of isolation. *American Journal of Primatology* 18:231–236.

Fisher RA (1930) *The Genetical Theory of Natural Selection* (Oxford, Clarendon).

Folstad I, Karter AJ (1992) Parasites, bright males and the immunocompetence handicap. *American Naturalist* 139:603–622.

Frank SA (1990) Sex allocation theory for birds and mammals. *Annual Review of Ecology and Systematics* 21:13–55.

Gauthier C-A (1999) Reproductive parameters and paracallosal skin color changes in captive female guinea baboons, *Papio papio*. *American Journal of Primatology* 47:67–74.

Gillman J (1940) The effect of multiple injections of progesterone on the turgescent perineum of the baboon *(Papio porcarius)*. *Endocrinology* 26:1072–1077.

Gillman J (1942) Effects on the perineal swelling and on the menstrual cycle of single injections of combinations of estradiol benzoate and progesterone given to baboons in the first part of the cycle. *Endocrinology* 30:54–60.

Glassman DK, Coelho AM, Jr, Carey KD, Bramblett CA (1984) Weight growth in savannah baboons: a longitudinal study from birth to adulthood. *Growth* 48:425–433.

Gomendio M (1989) differences in fertility and suckling patterns between primiparous and multiparous rhesus monkeys *(Macaca mulatta)*. *Journal of Reproduction and Fertility* 87:529–542.

Goy RW, Bercovitch FB, McBrair MC (1988) Behavioral masculinization is independent of genital masculinization in prenatally androgenized female rhesus macaques. *Hormones and Behavior* 22:552–571.

Grafen A (1990) Biological signals as handicaps. *Journal of Theoretical Biology* 144:517–546.

Hampson E, Kimura D (1992) Sex differences and hormonal influences on cognitive function in humans. In JB Becker, SM Breedlove, D Crews (Eds) *Behavioral Endocrinology* (Cambridge, Massachusetts, MIT Press), 357–398.

Hardy ICW (1997) Possible factors influencing vertebrate sex ratios: an introductory overview. *Applied Animal Behavior Science* 51:217–241.

Harvey PH, Martin RD, Clutton-Brock TH (1987) Life histories in a comparative perspective. In BB Smuts, DL Cheney, RM Seyfarth, RW Wrangham, TT Struhsaker (Eds) *Primate Societies* (Chicago, University of Chicago Press), 181–196.

Hasselquist D, Marsh JA, Sherman PW, Wingfield JC (1999) Is avian humoral immunocompetence suppressed by testosterone? *Behavioral Ecology and Sociobiology* 45:167–175.

Hauser MD (1988) Variation in maternal responsiveness in free-ranging vervet monkeys: a response to infant mortality risk? *American Naturalist* 131:573–587.

Hauser MD (1993) Rhesus monkey copulation calls: honest signals for female choice? *Proceedings of the Royal Society of London* B 254:93–96.

Hauser MD, Fairbanks LA (1988) Mother-offspring conflict in vervet monkeys: variation in response to ecological conditions. *Animal Behavior* 36:802–813.

Hausfater G (1975) *Dominance and Reproduction in Baboons* (Papio cynocephalus) (Basel, Karger).

Hausfater G, Watson DF (1976) Social and reproductive correlates of parasite ova emissions by baboons. *Nature* 262:688–689.

Hedges LV, Nowell A (1995) Sex differences in mental test scores, variability, and numbers of high-scoring individuals. *Science* 269:41–45.

Hiraiwa M (1981) Maternal and alloparental care in a troop of free-ranging Japanese macaques. *Primates* 22:309–329.

Hiraiwa-Hasegawa M (1993) Skewed birth sex ratios in primates: should high ranking mothers have daughters? *Trends in Ecology and Evolution* 8:395–400.

Hrdy SB (1987) Sex-biased parental investment among primates and other mammals: a critical evaluation of the Trivers-Willard hypothesis. In R Gelles, JB Lancaster (Eds) *Child Abuse and Neglect: Biosocial Dimensions* (New York, Aldine), 97–147.

Hrdy SB (1988) The primate origins of human sexuality. In R Bellig, G Stevens (Eds) *The Evolution of Sex* (New York, Harper and Row), 101–136.

Johnson CN (1988) Dispersal and the sex ratio at birth in primates. *Nature* 332:726–728.

Johnstone RA (1995) Sexual selection, honest advertisement and the handicap principle: reviewing the evidence. *Biological Reviews* 70:1–65.

Jones RE (1997) *Human Reproductive Biology* (San Diego, Academic Press).

Kieser JA, Groeneveld HT (1991) Fluctuating asymmetry, morphological variability, and genetic monomorphism in the cheetah *Acinonyx jubatus*. *Evolution* 45:1175–1183.

Keddy-Hector AC (1992) Mate choice in non-human primates. *American Zoologist* 32:62–70.

Knezevich M (1998) Geophagy as a therapeutic mediator of endoparasitism in a free-ranging group of rhesus macaques *(Macaca mulatta)*. *American Journal of Primatology* 44:71–82.

Kodric-Brown A, Brown JH (1984) Truth in advertising: the kinds of traits favored by sexual selection. *American Naturalist* 124:309–323.

Koenig A, Borries C, Chalise MK, Winkler P (1997) Ecology, nutrition, and timing of reproductive events in an Asian primate, the Hanuman langur *(Presbytis entellus)*. *Journal of Zoology* 243:215–235.

Koyama N, Takahata Y, Huffman M, Norikoshi N, Suzuki H (1992) Reproductive parameters of female Japanese macaques: thirty years of data from the Arashiyama troops. *Primates* 33:33–47.

Krackow S (1995) Potential mechanisms for sex ratio adjustment in mammals and birds. *Biological Reviews* 70:225–241.

Küster J, Paul A (1984) Female reproductive characteristics in semifree-ranging Barbary macaques *(Macaca sylvanus* L. 1758). *Folia Primatologica* 43:69–83.

Lancaster JB (1986) Human adolescence and reproduction: an evolutionary perspective. In JB Lancaster, BA Hamburg (Eds) *School-Age Pregnancy and Parenthood: Biosocial Dimensions* (New York, Aldine de Gruyter), 17–37.

Lee PC (1984) Ecological constraints on the social development of vervet monkeys. *Behaviour* 91:245–262.

Lee PC (1987) Nutrition, fertility and maternal investment in primates. *Journal of Zoology* 213:409–422.

Lee PC (1999) Comparative ecology of postnatal growth and weaning among haplorhine primates. In PC Lee (Ed) *Comparative Primate Socioecology* (Cambridge, Cambridge University Press), 111–139.

Lee PC, Bowman JE (1995) Influence of ecology and energetics on primate mothers and infants. In CR Pryce, RD Martin, D Skuse (Eds) *Motherhood in Human and Nonhuman Primates* (Basel, Karger), 47–58.

Lee PC, Majluf P, Gordon IJ (1991) Growth, weaning and maternal investment from a comparative perspective. *Journal of Zoology* 225:99–114.

Leigh SR (1995) Socioecology and the ontogeny of sexual size dimorphism in anthropoid primates. *American Journal of Physical Anthropology* 97:339–356.

Lindburg DG (1971) The rhesus monkey in North India: an ecological and behavioral study. In LA Rosenblum (Ed) *Primate Behavior* (New York, Academic Press), 1–106.

Livshits G, Kobyliansky E (1991) Fluctuating asymmetry as a possible measure of developmental homeostasis in humans: a review. *Human Biology* 63:441–466.

Low BS (1990) Fat and deception. *Ethology and Sociobiology* 11:67–74.

Maestripieri D (1994) Social structure, infant handling, and mothering styles in group-living Old World monkeys. *International Journal of Primatology* 15: 531–553.

Martin RD (1981) Relative brain size and metabolic rate in terrestrial vertebrates. *Nature* 293:57–60.

Martin RD (1990) *Primate Origins and Evolution* (Princeton, Princeton University Press).

Martin RD (1996) Scaling of the mammalian brain: the maternal energy hypothesis. *News in Physiological Sciences* 11:149–156.

Martin RD, MacLarnon AM (1985) Gestation period, neonatal size and maternal investment in placental mammals. *Nature* 313:220–223.

Martin RD, Willner LA, Dettling A (1994) The evolution of sexual size dimorphism in primates. In RV Short, E Balaban (Eds) *The Differences between the Sexes* (Cambridge, Cambridge University Press), 159–200.

Martorell R, Gonzalez-Cossio T (1987) Maternal nutrition and birth weight. *Yearbook of Physical Anthropology* 30:195–220.

Maynard Smith J (1980) A new theory of sexual investment. *Behavioral Ecology and Sociobiology* 7:247–251.

McMahon CA, Wigodsky HS, Moore GT (1976) Weight of the infant baboon *(Papio cynocephalus)* from birth to fifteen weeks. *Laboratory Animal Science* 26:928–931.

Meikle DB, Vessey SH (1988) Maternal dominance rank and lifetime survivorship of male and female rhesus monkeys. *Behavioral Ecology and Sociobiology* 22: 379–383.

Møller AP (1990) Fluctuating asymmetry in male sexual ornaments may reliably reveal male quality. *Animal Behavior* 40:1185–1187.

Moses RA, Boutin S, Teferi T (1998) Sex-biased mortality in woodrats occurs in the absence of parental intervention. *Animal Behavior* 55:563–571.

Muruthi P, Altmann J, Altmann S (1991) Resource base, parity, and reproductive condition affect females' feeding time and nutrient intake within and between groups of a baboon population. *Oecologia* 87:467–472.

Newall-Morris LL, Fahrenbruch CE, Sackett GP (1989) Prenatal psychological stress, dermatoglyphic asymmetry and pregnancy outcome in the pigtailed macaque *(Macaca nemestrina)*. *Biology of the Neonate* 56:61–75.

Norman AW, Litwack G (1997) *Hormones* (San Diego, Academic Press).

Novak JM, Rhodes OE, Smith MH, Chesser RK (1993) Morphological asymmetry in mammals: genetics and homeostasis reconsidered. *Acta Theriologica* 38(Suppl. 2):7–18.

Packer C (1979) Inter-troop transfer and inbreeding avoidance in *Papio anubis*. *Animal Behavior* 27:1–36.

Packer C, Collins DA, Sindinwo A, Goodall J (1995) Reproductive constraints on aggressive competition in female baboons. *Nature* 373:60–63.

Pagel M (1994) The evolution of conspicuous oestrous advertisement in Old World monkeys. *Animal Behavior* 47:1333–1341.

Palmer AR, Strobeck C (1986) Fluctuating asymmetry: measurement, analysis, patterns. *Annual Review of Ecology and Systematics* 17:391–421.

Parker GA (1983) Mate quality and mating decisions. In PPG Bateson (Ed) *Mate Choice* (Cambridge, Cambridge University Press), 141–166.

Parkes AS, Zuckerman S (1931) The menstrual cycle of the Primates, II: some effects of estrin on baboons and macaques. *Journal of Anatomy* 65:272–276.

Parsons PA (1992) Fluctuating asymmetry: a biological monitor of environmental and genomic stress. *Heredity* 68:361–364.

Paul A (1999) The socioecology of infant handling in primates: Is the current model convincing? *Primates* 40:33–46.

Paul A, Kuester J (1996) Differential reproduction in Barbary macaques. In JE Fa, DG Lindburg (Eds) *Evolution and Ecology of Macaque Societies* (Cambridge, Cambridge Unversity Press), 293–317.

Pond CM (1978) Morphological aspects and the ecological and mechanical consequences of fat deposition in wild vertebrates. *Annual Review of Ecology and Systematics* 9:519–570.

Resko JA, Ellinwood WE (1981) Testicular hormone production in fetal rhesus macaques. In MJ Novy, JA Resko (Eds) *Fetal Endocrinology* (New York, Academic Press), 253–267.

Reynolds V (1991) The biological basis of human patterns of mating and marriage. In V Reynolds, J Kellett (Eds) *Marriage and Mating* (Oxford, Oxford University Press, Oxford), 46–90.

Rhine RJ, Norton GW, Rogers J, Wasser SK (1992) Secondary sex ratio and maternal dominance rank among wild yellow baboons *(Papio cynocephalus)* of Mikumi National Park, Tanzania. *American Journal of Primatology* 27:261–273.

Richard AF (1985) *Primates in Nature* (New York, WH Freeman).

Ross C, MacLarnon A (1995) Ecological and social correlates of maternal expenditure on infant growth in haplorrhine primates. In CR Pryce, RD Martin, D Skuse (Eds) *Motherhood in Human and Nonhuman Primates* (Basel, Karger), 37–46.

Rowell TE (1967) Female reproductive cycles and the behavior of baboons and rhesus macaques. In SA Altmann (Ed) *Social Communication among Primates* (Chicago, University of Chicago Press), 15–32.

Rowell TE (1977) Variation in age at puberty in monkeys. *Folia Primatologica* 27:284–296.

Sade DS (1990) Intrapopulation variation in life-history parameters. In CJ DeRousseau (Ed) *Primate Life History and Evolution* (New York, Wiley-Liss), 181–194.

Saino N, Møller AP (1994) Secondary sexual characters, parasites and testosterone in the barn swallow *Hirundo rustica*. *Animal Behavior* 48:1325–1333.

Schmidt-Nielson K (1997) *Animal Physiology* (Cambridge, Cambridge University Press).

Schultz AH (1949) Sex differences in the pelves of primates. *American Journal of Physical Anthropology* 7:401–424.

Schultz AH (1969) *The Life of Primates* (New York, Universe Books).

Scott LM (1984) Reproductive behavior of adolescent female baboons *(Papio anubis)* in Kenya. In MF Small (Ed) *Female Primates* (New York, Alan R. Liss), 77–100.

Selander RK (1972) Sexual selection and dimorphism in birds. In B Campbell (Ed) *Sexual Selection and the Descent of Man, 1871–1971* (Chicago, Aldine), 180–230.

Shapiro S, Schlesinger ER, Nesbitt Jr, REL (1968) *Infant, Perinatal, Maternal, and Childhood Mortality in the United States* (Cambridge, Harvard University Press).

Short RV (1976) The evolution of human reproduction. *Proceedings of the Royal Society of London* B, 195:3–24.

Silk JB (1983) Local resource competition and facultative adjustment of sex ratios in relation to competitive abilities. *American Naturalist* 121:56–66.

Silk JB (1999) Why are infants so attractive to others? The form and function of infant handling in bonnet macaques. *Animal Behavior* 57:1021–1032.

Simpson MJA, Simpson AE (1982) Birth sex ratios and social rank in rhesus monkey mothers. *Nature* 300:440–441.

Sinclair D (1973) *Human Growth after Birth* (Oxford, Oxford University Press).

Sly DL, Harbaugh SW, London WT, Rice JM (1983) Reproductive performance of a laboratory breeding colony of patas monkeys *(Erythrocebus patas). American Journal of Primatology* 4:23–32.

Small MF (1993) *Female Choices* (Ithaca, New York, Cornell University Press).

Smith RJ, Jungers WL (1997) Body mass in comparative primatology. *Journal of Human Evolution* 32:523–559.

Smith RJ, Leigh SR (1998) Sexual dimorphism in primate neonatal body mass. *Journal of Human Evolution* 34:173–201.

Smuts BB (1985) *Sex and Friendship in Baboons* (Hawthorne, New York, Aldine).

Smuts B, Nicolson NA (1989) Reproduction in wild female olive baboons. *American Journal of Primatology* 19:229–246.

Stock MK, Metcalfe JM (1994) Maternal physiology during gestation. In E Knobil, JD Neill (Eds) *The Physiology of Reproduction*, Vol. 2, second ed. (New York, Raven Press), 947–983.

Strum SC (1994) Reconciling aggression and social manipulation as means of competition, I: life-history perspective. *International Journal of Primatology* 15: 739–765.

Strum SC, Western JD (1982) Variation in fecundity with age and environment in olive baboons *(Papio anubis). American Journal of Primatology* 3:61–76.

Tovée MJ, Maisey DS, Emery JL, Cornelissen PL (1999) Visual cues to female physical attractiveness. *Proceedings of the Royal Society of London*, B 266:211–218.

Trivers RL (1972) Parental investment and sexual selection. In B Campbell (Ed) *Sexual Selection and the Descent of Man, 1871–1971* (Chicago, Aldine), 136–179.

Trivers RL, Willard DE (1973) Natural selection of parental ability to vary the sex ratio of offspring. *Science* 179:90–92.

Ucko PJ, Rosenfield A (1967) *Paleolithic Cave Art* (New York, McGraw Hill).

van Hooff JARAM (1997) The socio-ecology of sex ratio variation in primates: evolutionary deduction and empirical evidence. *Applied Animal Behavior Science* 51:293–306.

van Noordwijk MA, van Schaik CP (1985) Male migration and rank acquisition in wild long-tailed macaques *(Macaca fascicularis). Animal Behavior* 33:849–861.

van Noordwikj MA, van Schaik CP (1999) The effects of dominance rank and group size on female lifetime reproductive success in wild long-tailed macaques, *Macaca fascicularis*. *Primates* 40:105–130.

van Schaik CP, Hrdy SB (1991) Intenstity of local resource competition shapes the relationship between maternal rank and sex ratios at birth in cercopithecine primates. *American Naturalist* 138:1555–1562.

van Schaik CP, Netto WJ, van Amerongen AJJ, Westland H (1989) Social rank and sex ratio of captive long-tailed macaque females *(Macaca fascicularis)*. *American Journal of Primatology* 19:147–161.

Van Valen L (1962) A study of fluctuating asymmetry. *Evolution* 16:125–142.

Wallen K (1990) Desire and ability: hormones and the regulation of female sexual behavior. *Neuroscience and Behavior Reviews* 14:233–241.

Wasser SK, Norton G (1993) Baboons adjust secondary sex ratio in response to predictors of sex- specific offspring survival. *Behavioral Ecology and Sociobiology* 32:273–281.

Wiley RH (1974) Evolution of social organization and life-history patterns among grouse. *Quarterly Review of Biology* 49:201–227.

Wiley RH, Poston J (1996) Indirect mate choice, competition for mates, and coevolution of the sexes. *Evolution* 50:1371–1381.

Wilson EO (1975) *Sociobiology* (Cambridge, Belknap Press of Harvard University).

Witelson SF (1976) Sex and the single hemisphere: specialization of the right hemisphere for spatial processing. *Science* 193:425–427.

Zahavi A, Zahavi A (1997) *The Handicap Principle: A Missing Piece of Darwin's Puzzle* (Oxford, Oxford University Press).

Zuk M (1994) Immunology and the evolution of behavior. In LA Real (Ed) *Behavioral Mechanisms in Evolutionary Ecology* (Chicago, University of Chicago Press), 354–368.

Zuk M, Johnsen TS, Maclarty T (1995) Endocrine-immune interactions, ornaments and mate choice in red jungle fowl. *Proceedings of the Royal Society of London*, B 260:205–210.

17

The Reproductive Ecology of Male Hominoids

MARTIN N. MULLER and RICHARD W. WRANGHAM

Ape mothers, like most mammalian females, invest more in parental effort than ape fathers do. This investment, in the form of internal gestation, lactation, and infant transport, reduces the mother's capacity to invest in subsequent reproduction. Theory therefore suggests that access to environmental resources such as food should be the primary constraint on female reproductive success, and an important determinant of female reproductive timing (Emlen and Oring 1977; Trivers 1972; Wrangham 1980). For example, females should conceive only when the resources necessary for successful pregnancy and parturition are available (Ellison 1990; Wasser and Barash 1983). In line with this expectation, in humans (reviewed in Ellison et al. 1993) and other great apes (Bentley 1999; Knott 1999, this volume) ovarian function is extremely sensitive to fluctuations in both energy balance and activity. This means that females have a lower probability of conception during periods when a successful reproductive outcome is less likely.

Adaptive mechanisms of this sort, sensitive to environmental energy availability, appear to be prominent in female apes, such as humans. By contrast, little is known about the factors affecting male gonadal function. One possibility is that, as in females, energy availability plays a major role. Preliminary evidence from western human populations, indeed, indicates that under some circumstances weight loss, dietary composition, and exercise can suppress testicular function (reviewed in Campbell and Leslie 1995). Consequently, Campbell and Leslie (1995) have argued that chronic environmental stress in nonwestern populations may adversely affect spermatogenesis and male fecundity. To date, however, there is little empirical support for the idea that testicular function is sensitive to local ecology in the way that ovarian function is (e.g., Ellison and Panter-Brick 1996). Nor is this surprising. Since the costs of gamete production for human males are small, energy balance is not expected to be the limiting factor on male reproductive success that it is for females.

Instead, male reproductive success is primarily constrained by access to mates. Thus, male gonadal function might be expected to be more responsive to social influences than to energetics. In accordance with this idea, a substantial body of research has shown that in vertebrates the steroid hormone testosterone (T) plays a critical role in facilitating male aggression, specifically in reproductive contexts (e.g., Higley et al. 1996; Lincoln et al. 1972; Moore 1986; Wingfield 1984). The evidence for this effect is particularly clear in birds, which show dramatic interspecific and individual differences in temporal patterns of T secretion, explicable by variation in the intensity of male mating competition (Beletsky et al. 1995; Wingfield et al. 1987, 1990). Basal T levels in free-ranging birds are slightly higher in the breeding season than in the nonbreeding season. This modest increase is sufficient to support basic reproductive functions, such as spermatogenesis and courtship behavior, but does not interfere with parental behavior. Following this initial rise in basal T, circulating levels of T increase further during periods of heightened male aggression, up to a maximum physiological level. According to the "Challenge Hypothesis" (Wingfield et al. 1990), T levels increase when males must respond to threats from conspecifics, particularly during territory formation and mate guarding. Experiments in the laboratory have shown that visual and auditory stimuli from male conspecifics are sufficient to induce changes in circulating T (Wingfield 1994). T levels decrease during periods when males need to provide parental care to offspring. Experimental manipulations of male birds have shown that high levels of T suppress parental behavior in favor of aggression (e.g., Hegner and Wingfield 1987).

Consistent with the predictions of the challenge hypothesis, polygynous birds maintain higher levels of circulating T during the breeding season than monogamous birds do (Wingfield et al. 1990). Furthermore, experiments in the wild have shown that T implants can induce polygyny in normally monogamous birds (Wingfield 1984). Bird species that exhibit high levels of paternal care, however, generally maintain low basal T levels. These species also show a greater T response to social challenges than do species with low paternal care, presumably because the latter are already maintaining T levels close to the physiological maximum (Wingfield et al. 1987, 1990).

The challenge hypothesis thus appears to have wide application for birds and some other vertebrates (e.g., spiny lizards: Moore 1986). It has rarely been applied to mammals, however. Preliminary data on ring-tailed lemurs (Cavigelli and Pereira 2000) are consistent with the predictions, while data on dwarf mongooses present a puzzling challenge (Creel et al. 1993). In this chapter we consider the reproductive ecology of male hominoids in the framework of the challenge hypothesis. Since none of the great apes is a seasonal breeder, and most male apes do not engage in parental care, the specific formulation of the hypothesis must be modified for these species. The emphasis will be on data collected from wild populations because captivity imposes dietary and demographic constraints that make it difficult to interpret variation in both behavior and hormone levels.

FIELD STUDIES OF ENDOCRINE FUNCTION IN THE GREAT APES

Although laboratory studies have examined the relationship between social factors and levels of circulating T in a variety of primates, few such data were available from the wild until recently. The most detailed information about endocrine function in a free-ranging primate comes from Sapolsky's studies of olive baboons in Kenya (Sapolsky 1983, 1991, 1992). Sapolsky took annual serum samples from darted baboons to examine individual variation in the stress response and its effects on the testicular axis. Stress analysis was possible because the anaesthetic used in the darting procedure was itself a stressor, assumed to be equivalently powerful across different individuals. Sapolsky's method was highly productive in showing, for example, how the stress response was related to social status and personality. It is not applicable, however, to species unsuitable for regular immobilization.

For example, although gorillas, chimpanzees, and orangutans have all been successfully darted in the wild, the risks associated with the procedure are considerably greater than for terrestrial baboons or smaller-bodied arboreal monkeys. Ethical considerations therefore preclude the darting of free-ranging apes for the collection of serum. Fortunately, methods for assaying steroid metabolites in urine and feces have recently been developed, allowing for noninvasive physiological monitoring in the field (Whitten et al. 1998).

Most of the field researchers studying endocrine function in great apes have chosen urine as an assay medium for both practical and theoretical reasons. First, apes urinate frequently and copiously. Second, they urinate predictably upon waking, so first morning samples are easy to collect. Third, since steroid metabolites accumulate in the bladder, urinary steroid levels represent an average of circulating levels between urinations. These averages are unaffected by the pulsatile release of hormones into the bloodstream that can confound basal measurements in serum. Finally, urinary assays are capable of detecting substantial acute increases in circulating steroid levels. In captive chimpanzees, for example, cortisol increases following anesthesia are apparent in both urinary and fecal assays (Whitten et al. 1998).

ENERGETICS AND VARIATION IN
REPRODUCTIVE FUNCTION

In women, acute increases in both workload and nutritional stress predictably reduce circulating levels of ovarian hormones (Ellison et al. 1993).
This reversible, short-term suppression can adversely affect fecundity.
Subfecund or anovulatory cycles and amenorrhea are common in western
women who are exercising heavily (e.g., Ellison and Lager 1985, 1986) or
losing weight (e.g., Schweiger et al. 1992). They are also prevalent in nonwestern populations, where workloads tend to be higher and seasonal
nutritional stress more severe (Ellison et al. 1989; Panter-Brick et al. 1993;
see also Jasienska, chapter 3, this volume).

In some clinical studies, human males show a similar pattern of suppressed gonadal function in response to extreme nutritional stress (e.g.,
Klibanski et al. 1981). Although it is conceivable that such suppression
could impact spermatogenesis, leading to decreased male fecundity
(Campbell and Leslie 1995), this effect is not likely to be of much consequence. First, the relationship between nutritional stress and decreased T
is ambiguous (Bentley et al. 1993) and consistently appears only under
pathological conditions (e.g., in anorexics). Second, rates of spermatogenesis are largely independent of circulating T concentrations, and testicular
T concentrations do not correlate with number of spermatozoa (Rommerts
1988; Weinbauer and Neischlag 1990). Finally, modest reductions in sperm
count do not appear to have a significant impact on male fecundity (Polanski and Lamb 1988). For further discussion of these issues in human males,
see Bribiescas (chapter 5) and Campbell et al. (chapter 7) in this volume.

In polygynous species, males can conceive in rapid succession compared with females. Conceptions that fail are therefore less costly for males
than for females (Wasser and Barash 1983). Accordingly, the benefits of
regulating fecundity in response to energetics are expected to be lower for
males than for females. Bribiescas (1996) has argued that under conditions
of chronic energy shortage, males might benefit by reducing levels of circulating T, because T promotes anabolism of metabolically expensive muscle tissue. He suggests that the suppression of testicular function in
response to nutritional stress may be an adaptive mechanism to optimize
somatic energy allocation and, therefore, increase survival.

However, the evidence that circulating levels of T are sensitive to either
acute or chronic changes in energy availability is weak. Relevant studies
have been conducted on a number of nonwestern human populations.
Ellison and Panter-Brick (1996) monitored salivary T levels in two populations of Nepalese men and found little response to seasonal nutritional
stress. Nepalese women in the same populations, by contrast, demonstrated pronounced variation in ovarian function between periods of high

and low energy availability (Panter-Brick et al. 1993). A similar pattern was observed among Lese horticulturalists in Zaire, with women showing pronounced seasonal variation in gonadal steroid production and men showing no such variation (Bailey et al. 1992; Bentley et al. 1993). Bribiescas (1997) monitored salivary T levels in two populations of Ache men in eastern Paraguay. He found no significant differences between a comparatively wealthy population, which enjoyed high net energy availability, and a poorer, more energetically stressed population.

The only comparable hormonal data from a nonhuman ape come from Knott's (1998, 1999) study of free-ranging orangutans in Gunung Palung National Park, Indonesia. Knott compared gonadal steroid levels in both males and females with data on seasonality in food availability and diet. She documented dramatic fluctuations in food availability between a mast-fruiting period, when both male and female orangutans consumed around 7,000 calories a day, and a non-mast period, when caloric intake fell by more than half (Knott 1998). During the food-poor season, orangutans were energetically stressed and lost weight. Preliminary hormonal data from this study appear consistent with results from human populations. Female orangutans showed significant seasonal differences in levels of urinary estrogen metabolites, suggesting reduced ovarian function during periods of food scarcity (Knott 1999). A comparison of urinary T levels between the same seasons in both adolescent and adult male orangutans, however, revealed no differences (Knott 1999). Further discussion can be found in chapter 18.

SEASONALLY BREEDING PRIMATES AND THE CHALLENGE HYPOTHESIS

Although the evidence for an acute effect of energetic status on gonadal function in male primates is equivocal, the influence of social interactions is relatively clear. In seasonally breeding primates, basal T levels tend to increase substantially during the breeding season (Dixson 1998). The timing of this increase appears to be coordinated by social cues rather than simply by changes in the physical environment (Herndon 1983). For example, troops of monkeys living in the same forest may show intergroup differences in the timing of the onset of mating, but intragroup synchrony is maintained (e.g., talapoin monkeys: Rowell and Dixson 1975). Furthermore, introducing estrogen-treated females to a free-ranging group before the breeding season begins can advance the onset of mating (e.g., rhesus monkeys: Vandenbergh and Drickamer 1974).

As with birds, some of the additional T produced by primate males during the breeding season may be necessary for spermatogenesis and the normal expression of sexual behavior (e.g., Zamboni et al. 1974). This requirement seems insufficient to explain the dramatic increases exhibited by some species, however, because relatively low concentrations of circulating testosterone are generally adequate to maintain male reproductive function (reviewed in Dixson 1998). A threshold effect of this kind is apparent in the rhesus macaque (*Macaca mulatta*). Non-breeding-season levels of T are sufficient to maintain sexual behavior in male rhesus monkeys. Researchers consistently report that intact males exposed to extraspecific females or receptive conspecifics outside of the breeding season immediately exhibit normal sexual behavior; sustained increases in circulating T occur subsequently (Bernstein et al. 1983; Michael and Zumpe 1993; Ruiz de Elvira et al. 1983). Castrated rhesus, on the other hand, show a gradual decline in sexual behavior over time (reviewed in Dixson 1998).

The challenge hypothesis posits that increases in male T during the breeding season facilitate male-male aggression in reproductive contexts. Although a number of primate studies have investigated the relationship between T and aggression, most of them have not tested the challenge hypothesis directly. Michael and Zumpe (1981), for example, compared T and aggression in a captive group of rhesus males over three years, but their subjects were housed in breeding pairs so the only possible recipients of aggression were female cagemates. Even under these unusual social conditions, high levels of circulating T were associated with increased aggression.

A more appropriate test of the challenge hypothesis requires data from free-ranging primate groups where male-male competition can occur during the breeding season. The best data of this kind come from a study by Higley and colleagues (1996), who measured cerebrospinal fluid (CSF) free T in free-ranging rhesus monkeys. They reported that individual levels of CSF free T were positively correlated with overall rates of aggression in their subjects. During the breeding season, both T levels and rates of aggression increased dramatically, as males competed for access to females (Mehlman et al. 1997). In captive studies where males have been allowed to interact in outdoor enclosures, both T levels and rates of aggression have also been found to increase during the breeding season (Gordon et al. 1976; Ruiz de Elvira et al. 1983). Thus, in the best-controlled studies, T tends to be positively correlated with aggression.

A more specific prediction of the challenge hypothesis suggested by work on birds is that species showing the most dramatic increases in aggression during the breeding season should also exhibit the largest increases in basal T during that time. The present paucity of hormonal data on free-ranging primates precludes a thorough test of this hypothesis. Data on fecal T in free-ranging muriquis (*Brachyteles arachnoides*), however, are suggestive. Like rhesus monkeys, muriquis are seasonal breeders that engage in intense sperm competition (Strier 1992). In contrast to rhesus, however, muriquis do not compete aggressively for access to females during the breeding season (Milton 1985; Strier 1992). Rather, males take turns copulating with receptive females in a relaxed atmosphere. Milton (1985) describes males lined up on a branch, peacefully awaiting an opportunity to copulate. As predicted by the challenge hypothesis, fecal T levels in wild male muriquis do not differ between breeding and nonbreeding seasons (Strier et al. 1999). This finding is consistent with the idea that acute changes in T have more to do with facilitating aggression in reproductive contexts than they do with sexual behavior, even in species that exhibit intense sperm competition (Strier et al. 1999). For further discussion of the reproductive ecology of muriquis, see Strier (chapter 15) in this volume.

Finally, a review of published serum T levels across species by Whitten (2000) suggests that, as with birds, interspecific patterns of T secretion in primates may be related to social systems. In cercopithecoids, species living in multimale groups show significantly higher T levels than those living in unimale groups. Male-male challenges are expected to be more persistent in mutimale groups. The comparison with birds suggests that in unimale groups, T responses to acute challenges should be more pronounced, but this has not been tested.

MALE-MALE COMPETITION IN THE GREAT APES

Among the extant great apes, operational sex ratios (Mitani et al. 1996), patterns of parental investment (Trivers 1972), and potential reproductive rates (Clutton-Brock and Vincent 1991) are all consistent with relatively high levels of male-male competition. This competition includes both sperm competition and aggressive competition, which takes two general forms. In the long-term, males can compete to maintain permanent access to females; in the short-term (i.e., a single reproductive cycle), males can compete to mate with estrous females. The relative intensity of these forms varies between species. For gorillas, male-male competition within any particular reproductive cycle is minimal, but competition to attract females to a group and retain them is pronounced (Watts 1996). For chimpanzees, who live in multimale communities, competition for access to estrous females is much more pronounced. The predictions of the challenge hypothesis should therefore vary between these species, according to the relative importance of short- and long-term mating competition. These predictions are reviewed below for each of the great apes, with relevant evidence from field studies of endocrine function. As very few field studies of endocrine function in male apes have been pursued, many of these predictions have yet to be tested.

Mountain Gorillas

Mountain gorillas (*Gorilla gorilla beringei*) live in relatively stable groups consisting of at least one silverback male, one or more unrelated females, and a variable number of offspring (Watts 1996). Both male and female mountain gorillas tend to emigrate from their natal groups (Harcourt 1978). Emigrating males either join an all-male band or range by themselves; females either join a new breeding group or take up with a solitary male (Watts 1996). Females do not range by themselves and normally leave a group only when a new group or a solitary male is nearby.

Silverbacks acquire females by attracting them from other males during intergroup encounters (Harcourt 1978; Watts 1996). Solitary males sometimes pursue established groups in order to challenge silverbacks (e.g., Yamagiwa 1986). Aggressive displays between solitary males and resident silverbacks may serve to advertise the fighting abilities of males for the benefit of females (Harcourt 1978; Sicotte 1993). During these encounters males also coerce females by committing infanticide; most mothers of infanticide victims transfer to the infanticidal male (Fossey 1984; Watts 1989).

To prevent their females from associating with other males, silverbacks employ two strategies. First, they sometimes herd females away from other males (Sicotte 1993). This is most likely to happen in newly formed, rather than well-established, groups. Second, they threaten or attack strange males.

More than 70% of encounters between strange male mountain gorillas in the wild involve aggression (Harcourt 1978; Sicotte 1993). Silverbacks perform threat displays against intruding males, which involve chest-beating, charging, and branch-breaking. Around 17% of these encounters escalate to full-contact aggression (Sicotte 1993). Fossey (1983) reported that 74% of silverback remains showed signs of healed head wounds, and 80% had broken or missing canines ($n = 64$), which she attributes primarily to fights between males. The intensity of male aggression in such encounters increases with the number of potential female emigrants (Sicotte 1993).

Short-term mating competition in mountain gorillas, on the other hand, is relatively subdued, partly because many groups have only one adult male (Harcourt et al. 1981). In groups with more than one male, a clear dominance hierarchy is evident; dominant males frequently interrupt copulations by subordinates and direct aggression towards them (Watts 1996).

The challenge hypothesis makes two predictions about levels of circulating T in male gorillas. First, dominant silverbacks should have higher T levels than subordinate males because they direct more aggression at subordinate males and are more involved in aggressive intergroup encounters. Preliminary data on urinary T values from three gorilla groups at Karisoke indicate that this is the case (Robbins and Czekala 1997). Second, silverbacks should show acute rises in circulating T levels during inter-group encounters, when their females are at risk. Tests of this hypothesis have not yet been attempted but should be possible because such encounters typically last between one and three days (Sicotte 1993). Since encounters between newly formed groups tend to be longer than those between well-established ones (Sicotte 1993), they are expected to lead to greater increases in circulating T.

Orangutans

Adult male orangutans *(Pongo pygmaeus)* occupy large and mutually overlapping home ranges that incorporate the overlapping ranges of multiple females. Resident males attempt to maintain exclusive access to sexually attractive females, reacting aggressively to rivals (Rodman and Mitani 1986). Not all adult males attempt to establish residency in a core area. Some range widely, seeking opportunistic matings with estrous females (Galdikas 1981; Rodman and Mitani 1986; te Boekhorst et al. 1990). Thus, van Schaik and van Hooff (1996) have characterized the orangutan social system as "roving male promiscuity."

Two relatively distinct morphs of adult male orangutan have been identified in captivity (Kingsley 1988) and the wild (te Boekhorst et al. 1990). "Developed" and "undeveloped" males are both sexually mature, but developed males exhibit a suite of secondary sexual characteristics that includes large body mass, fatty cheek pads, longer and thicker hair, and musty body odor. Developed males also emit a long-call vocalization which appears to mediate spacing between males. Low-ranking individuals avoid moving toward the calls of high-ranking individuals, and high-ranking individuals move toward the calls of low-ranking individuals (Mitani 1985a).

Relationships between developed male orangutans are consistently antagonistic (Galdikas 1981; Mitani 1985a). Developed males show a high rate of wounding and disfigurement from aggressive interactions with other males (Galdikas 1981; van Schaik and van Hooff 1996). Knott (1999) observed visible wounds from male-male competition in 6 of the 12 developed males in her study site at Gunung Palung National Park. Two of these individuals died during the study, both apparently from infected wounds inflicted by other males.

Relationships between developed males and undeveloped or subadult males are less consistently antagonistic. Galdikas (1979, 1981) reported that the presence or absence of females had a predictable effect on the level of aggression in these relationships. In the absence of females, developed males were more tolerant of undeveloped males and subadults. In the presence of females, especially consort partners, adult males were more aggressive, chasing other males, shaking branches at them, and making long-calls.

Most mating associations between a single male and female orangutan are short-term consortships (Galdikas 1981; van Schaik and van Hooff 1996). Dominant males often attempt to terminate associations between females and subordinate males. Undeveloped males will sometimes follow a consorting pair and attempt to mate when the male is distracted (van Schaik and van Hooff 1996). A large percentage of matings involving undeveloped males occurs as a result of male coercion (Galdikas 1981; Mitani 1985b).

The challenge hypothesis suggests that the occurrence of mate-guarding, high rates of long-calling, and high levels of aggression by developed male orangutans should correlate with high levels of circulating T. Unfortunately this hypothesis is difficult to test with data from the wild, because in the field it is often impossible to distinguish between subadult males, undeveloped adult males, and adult males who are in the process of developing secondary sexual characteristics (Cheryl Knott, personal communication 1999). Detailed endocrine studies of captive orangutans, however, provide preliminary support. Kingsley (1982, 1988) and Maggioncalda et al. (1999, 2000) examined T levels in juvenile orangutans, undeveloped adults, developing adults, and developed adults. In both studies, undeveloped adults exhibited significantly lower T levels than developed males. Males in the process of developing exhibited peaks of growth hormone (Maggioncalda et al. 2000), and in one study they were found to exhibit a peak in T slightly higher than that of the developed males (Maggioncalda et al. 1999). Kingsley (1982, 1988), however, reported T levels for developing males intermediate between developed and undeveloped males. Whether or not developing males exhibit a transitory increase in T, fully developed males appear to exhibit significantly higher levels than individuals in developmental arrest.

Maggioncalda et al. (1999) suggest that the risk of intense aggression from fully developed males makes it necessary for subadult males to carefully monitor their social environment before their final development. They suggest that the frequency of long-call vocalizations and rates of encounter with adult males give growing males a means of evaluating the density of their reproductive competitors, and adjusting their rates of development accordingly. For example, long-call vocalizations could modulate hormone production via neuronal connections from auditory receptors to the hypothalamus (Maggioncalda et al. 1999). Evidence for some mechanism of this sort in the wild comes from Ketambe, where four males were seen to exhibit developmental arrest for more than 10 years (te Boekhorst et al. 1990).

Anecdotal evidence from captivity (e.g., Maple 1980) suggests that subadults housed with developed males tend to experience delayed development. Caution is necessary in interpreting such reports, however, since in some cases subadults have been reported to develop in the presence of dominant males. Given that styles of dominance relationships between dyads can vary considerably, controlled experiments are needed to better understand the interaction between social context and male development.

Two more, specific hypotheses can be suggested for the acute effects of mating competition on T in developed male orangutans. First, dominant males should exhibit higher T levels when they are being challenged by subordinates. Such challenges can take place over a series of months and are accompanied by increased rates of aggression, including aggressive vocalizations and actual fighting (e.g., Utami and Setia 1995). Second, developed males consorting with females should show higher levels of T when they are mate-guarding.

Chimpanzees

Chimpanzees (*Pan troglodytes*) live in fission-fusion societies (Nishida 1979). Each individual belongs to a particular social community (or "unit group," Nishida 1968) containing from 20 to more than 140 individuals. Within communities individuals form temporary associations, traveling sometimes alone and sometimes in parties that may include all of the community's adult males, and many of the mothers. The range of a community is defined as the area used by its males, who are more gregarious and travel further than mothers (Nishida 1968; Goodall 1986; Wrangham 2000).

Males are philopatric—in other words, they live in the community where they were born—and they cooperate with each other to defend the community range as a territory, by expelling male intruders. In addition, males occasionally hunt and attack individuals on borders or in neighboring community ranges, apparently as part of a strategy to reduce the coalitionary power of neighbors and expand their own territory (Wrangham 1999a). Because the territory encompasses the ranges of numerous females, males appear to benefit in two ways from its expansion. Larger territories may lead to more females breeding with the resident males. For example, aggressors at Gombe and Mahale appropriated both territory and females from their defeated neighbors (Goodall et al. 1979; Nishida et al. 1985; Goodall 1986). In addition, there is evidence that in larger territories mothers have relatively high reproductive rates, through both shorter interbirth intervals and improved offspring survival (Williams 1999). Improved food density per mother is presumably partly responsible for this effect.

Within communities, reproductive competition among males occurs through sperm competition (Hasegawa and Hiraiwa-Hasegawa 1990) and aggression over mating opportunities (Watts 1998). Most copulations occur in multimale parties without male herding, aggression, or coercion. These opportunistic matings tend to be with nulliparous females, or early in the mid-follicular phase of parous females. Towards the end of the follicular phase—that is, in the peri-ovulatory period—parous females become more attractive to males, as shown by a marked increase in male coercion and male-male aggression (e.g., Watts 1998). Male-male aggressive competition is thus relatively intense around the time when parous females ovulate. Females can escape the aggressive attentions of males by accompanying a single adult male to a peripheral part of the range in an exclusive "consortship." The male then maintains exclusive access to her for several days, or occasionally more than a month (Goodall 1986). Although consortships vary in frequency among populations, they are never the predominant male strategy. For example, data from Gombe, Mahale, and Taï indicate that conceptions normally occur in multimale parties rather than in consortships (75–94% in parties: Boesch and Boesch 2000; Hasegawa and Hiraiwa-Hasegawa 1990; Wallis 1997).

Male-male contests over mating are therefore an important determinant of reproductive success. Victory in these contests is closely predicted by the dominance hierarchy, a set of dominance relationships which invariably includes a clear alpha-male, and often a linear set of relationships among all males (Bygott 1979; Goodall 1986; Hayaki et al. 1989; Nishida 1979). In larger groups, dominance relationships among some middle- or low-ranking dyads may be unresolved (Bygott 1979). Chimpanzee males employ frequent charging displays to maintain or to challenge the existing dominance hierarchy, including exaggerated locomotion, piloerection, slapping, stamping, branch swaying, and throwing (Bygott 1979). Dominance reversals are regularly preceded by a period of heightened aggression and increased rates of display by one or both members of the dyad. Reversals are normally the result of fights, which sometimes result in severe wounds (Goodall 1986). Although challenges are frequent, skilled use of coalitions, social grooming, and well-timed aggression normally allows an alpha male to maintain his top status for several years at a time. During this period, he is often able to dominate mating access to parous females in the peri-ovulatory period in multimale parties (below).

The nature of dominance relations among male chimpanzees therefore suggests two specific predictions from the challenge hypothesis. First, high-ranking males are expected to maintain higher levels of circulating T than low-ranking males. Second, males should show increased T during periods when parous females are in estrus in the late-follicular phase, which is a period of heightened aggression. Data collected between

November 1997 and December 1998 from the Kanyawara community in Kibale National Park, Uganda, support both of these hypotheses (Muller 2002).

In 1998 the Kanyawara community contained 11 adult male chimpanzees, all of whom could be ranked in a linear hierarchy. Rates of charging display by males were correlated with rank, and the alpha male displayed significantly more frequently than any other individual. Long-term data from Kibale indicate that during their tenures, two prior alpha males also exhibited the highest display rates in the group.

As has been reported for salivary T in humans, urinary T levels in chimpanzees were found to be higher and more variable in the morning than in the afternoon. Thus, morning and afternoon samples were analyzed separately. In both morning and afternoon samples, the alpha male exhibited higher T levels than any other individual. The beta male followed closely behind. For afternoon but not morning samples, T was correlated with rank across all 11 individuals (Figure 17.1). Additionally, permanent changes in rank were associated with changes in T in the appropriate direction. During their tenures, the two former alpha males had the highest T levels in the community. The first, Stocky, later plummeted to the bottom of the hierarchy. His T levels decreased dramatically, to the lowest in

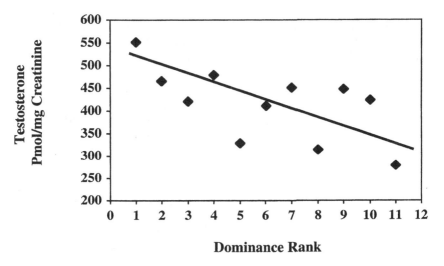

Dominance Rank

Figure 17.1.   The relationship between urinary testosterone levels and dominance rank in chimpanzees at Kanyawara, Kibale National Park. Data are from afternoon samples collected in 1998; mean male testosterone values are based on 5 to 39 samples, depending on the individual. (Percentage-bend correlation: $r = -.61$, $p < .05$, $n = 11$ males.)

the group. The second, Big Brown, fell to number four in the hierarchy and also showed dramatic reductions in urinary T. These changes in T with rank are consistent with those reported from experimental work with captive rhesus monkeys (reviewed in Bernstein et al. 1983), but unlike in those studies, the changes in chimpanzee T persisted over months. They were not transient changes that ended once the hierarchy stabilized.

It has been suggested that the failure to find a relationship between dominance rank and T levels in some species is an outcome of rank stability (Sapolsky 1983, 1991). In olive baboons, for example, Sapolsky reports a correlation between T and dominance during periods of rank instability that has never been seen during stable periods. Unstable periods in this species are associated with higher rates of aggression, particularly by high-ranking animals. Chimpanzees, on the other hand, appear to exhibit a relationship between rank and T, even during periods when the dominance hierarchy is relatively stable (e.g., in this study, for a period of at least 14 months).

There are two possible explanations for this discrepancy. First, chimpanzee dominance hierarchies might be less stable than those of baboons; individuals might always be subtly vying to rise in rank. The fission-fusion nature of chimpanzee society could exacerbate this phenomenon. Since dyads frequently break apart and come together after lengthy separations, it may be difficult for high-ranking individuals to know what kind of political maneuvering has been going on in their absence. Thus, it becomes important to reestablish one's rank when groups come together. This line of thinking is supported by Bygott's (1979) observation that a large percentage (39%) of contact aggression takes place during the context of reunions.

Alternatively, it is possible that the 14-month period of data collection at Kibale represented an unusually prolonged period of rank instability, and that the correlation between rank and T will not be found in other, more stable chimpanzee hierarchies. We are currently collecting hormonal data from two communities in Gombe National Park to test this hypothesis. We are also continuing data collection at Kibale to monitor long-term trends in that community.

A second prediction of the challenge hypothesis is that males should show acute increases in circulating T during periods when estrous females are maximally swollen. Chimpanzees do not have a breeding season, and the availability of estrous females varies temporally. Rates of male aggression increase when females are in estrus, and T is hypothesized to facilitate male-male aggression in the reproductive context. Few parous females were cycling during the 1998 study season, so few data are available from that time to examine short-term affects of mating competition on male T. However, one popular female, Lia, came into estrus after her infant son died. During one cycle she maintained a maximal swelling for 14 days, during which time she was followed by and mated with all but one of the community males. Both T levels and rates of escalated aggression (chases and attacks) in the males increased significantly during this period (Figure 17.2). Hormonal and behavioral data collected during 1999 are currently being analyzed. These data from additional cycles will allow a more complete test of this hypothesis.

Bonobos

The social lives of bonobos (*Pan paniscus*) are in many ways similar to those of chimpanzees. They also live in communities of 100 or more, within which individuals travel in parties of varying size and composition. Males are philopatric, and like chimpanzees they defend the community range as a territory. Within communities, males form dominance

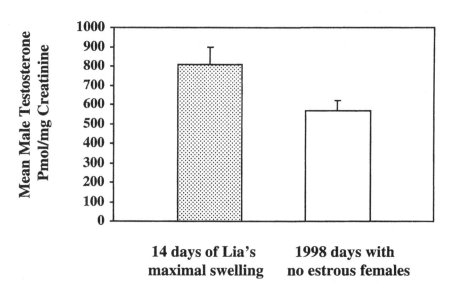

Figure 17.2. Effect of reproductive competition on urinary testosterone levels in male chimpanzees at Kanyawara, Kibale National Park. The stippled bar shows mean urinary testosterone for ten males during one 14-day period when a popular female (Lia) was in estrus. The white bar shows mean urinary testosterone for the same males on days when no estrous females were present. When each male is compared with himself, the differences between the two periods are statistically significant (Agresti-Pendergrast rank-based test: $p < .01$, $n = 10$ males). Error bars indicate the standard error of the mean. Both morning and afternoon samples are included.

hierarchies, and an alpha male is again recognizable. Most conceptions occur in multimale parties (Kano 1992).

Male bonobos are substantially less aggressive than male chimpanzees, however. As extreme examples, there is no evidence of infanticide, attempted infanticide, or coalitionary lethal aggression in bonobos, unlike in chimpanzees (Wrangham 1999a). Male bonobos rarely attempt to herd or coerce females, status competition is less frequent and dramatic among them than among chimpanzees, and there have been no reports of male bonobos competing aggressively over mating rights, even during the periovulatory period of parous females.

These differences suggest that sperm competition might be more important among bonobos than among chimpanzees. However, recent data indicate little if any difference in copulation rates between heterosexual pairs of chimpanzees and bonobos (Takahata et al. 1999). On the other hand, there is evidence that despite a lack of intense aggression, male copulation rate in small multimale parties is correlated with male rank (Kano 1996, see below). Possibly female choice plays a role in mediating this relationship.

Accordingly, the challenge hypothesis suggests that as in chimpanzees, high-ranking male bonobos will have higher levels of circulating T than low-ranking males. However, unlike chimpanzees, male bonobos are not expected to show increased T during periods when parous females are in estrus, given that there is no evidence for increased aggression. Finally, the reduced levels of aggression overall among male bonobos suggest either that circulating levels of T are lower or that peripheral sensitivity to T is reduced.

Humans

Humans are the only great ape in which males provide considerable paternal care. Thus, in contrast to the other apes, human males face a clear trade-off between parenting effort and mating effort (Trivers 1972). For men, then, the general predictions of the challenge hypothesis should closely parallel those for monogamous birds. First, men competing for an opportunity to mate should have higher levels of T than those who are not engaged in mating competition. Second, when men choose to invest in offspring rather than mating effort, they should exhibit decreases in circulating T.

The difficulty of obtaining long-term behavioral data on humans makes the testing of these predictions problematic. One approach to the first hypothesis is to compare married and unmarried men. In two studies of military personnel, married men were found to have slightly lower T levels than unmarried men, though the difference was modest (Booth and Dabbs 1993; Mazur and Michalek 1998). Although these results are suggestive, this approach is not ideal because it fails to take into account individual variation in mating effort. Some married men are presumably more committed to monogamous relationships than others, so significant variation in reproductive competition can be expected among married men.

The hypothesis that paternal care in men should correlate with decreased levels of T is somewhat easier to test. In birds periods of paternal care are predictably accompanied by decreases in male T (Beletsky et al. 1995). In mammals that exhibit paternal care, T levels also decrease from the period of gestation to lactation (e.g., prairie voles: Roberts et al. 1996; Mongolian gerbils: Brown et al. 1995; dwarf hamsters: Reburn and Wynne-Edwards 1999). In line with these findings, the challenge hypothesis predicts that T levels in men should decrease when they are caring for dependent offspring. Storey et al. (2000) tested this idea in 34 couples taking natal classes. Males in this sample, who presumably intended to invest in offspring, exhibited chronic declines in T production over the course of the pregnancy. They also exhibited acute decreases in circulating T in response to visual, tactile, olfactory, and auditory stimuli associated with paternal care (i.e., when listening to a tape of a crying baby, and holding a doll that had been wrapped in a blanket worn by a real baby).

Are high levels of T in men generally associated with higher rates of reproductive aggression, as they seem to be in the other great apes? The literature on T and aggression in humans is extensive, but on this point it is inconclusive. In general, studies that compare relatively aggressive groups with less aggressive groups have reported higher T levels in the aggressive groups (reviewed in Archer 1991). However, two widespread methodological difficulties make this test of the challenge hypothesis for human males problematic. First, most studies of human aggression utilize self-reports, peer reports, or psychological tests of aggressiveness, rather than behavioral data on rates of aggression (reviewed in Mazur and Booth 1998). Second, studies that do attempt to measure behavior directly rarely investigate aggression in the context of male-male reproductive competition. Instead, they commonly include aggression in nonreproductive contexts, such as stealing, or prison violence.

One of the few studies which avoids these pitfalls is Flinn's (1988) elegant work on mate-guarding in rural Dominica, an island in the Caribbean. Because houses in the village were quite open, Flinn was able to make direct behavioral observations of male-male competition, among other behaviors. Two related findings from this study are relevant here. First, males were found to exhibit higher rates of agonistic interactions with other males when their mates were fecund than when they were infecund. Flinn characterizes this as aggression in the context of mate-guarding. Second, males were involved in fewer agonistic interactions when their offspring were in early infancy. Unfortunately, no hormonal data were collected in this study. However, these represent the kind of rich behavioral data that are needed before a sophisticated account of T and aggression in men can be made.

Finally, one may expect the relationship among T, dominance, and aggression to be somewhat different in humans than in the other apes because male-male competition less routinely takes the form of contact aggression in humans. Among human foragers, for example, competitive aggressive displays are uncommon, and access to females and resources is not generally decided by threats or physical attacks (Boehm 1999). Mazur and Booth (1998) have suggested that T in humans should show stronger correlation with dominance behavior than it does with aggression, because humans strive for dominance in a variety of ways that do not involve aggression. The authors review a growing body of evidence that T in men responds in predictable ways to competition for status, that includes not only physical challenges, such as wrestling, but also contests such as chess or video games.

DOES DOMINANCE LEAD TO REPRODUCTIVE SUCCESS?

In theory, high male rank can be favored in at least three ways, by some combination of increasing the rate of reproduction, the probability of survival, or the fitness of relatives. The relative magnitude of these effects is unknown in the great apes, but as in other primates, reproductive benefits appear most important. However, the relevant data are largely behavioral rather than genetic.

The gorilla is the great ape in which the reproductive benefits of high male rank are clearest, to judge from mountain gorillas. Females mate principally in 2–3 day periods around ovulation, copulating only about 20 times per conception. Male aggression is more frequent and intense when more estrous or potentially emigrant females are available (Watts 1996). Between groups, males who win fights tend to attract females, and to defend them successfully against other males. Within groups, alpha males dominate mating access, for example by guarding estrous females and by interrupting subordinates' copulations. Subordinates do obtain some copulations, however. Tolerance towards rival males within groups is also shown in two circumstances. First, when their daughters reach reproductive age, silverbacks allow young males to mate them. Second, silverbacks sometimes develop tolerant relationships with "follower" males, subordinate adults who assist the alpha in intergroup encounters. "Follower" males are probably normally sons or brothers. Genetic data can therefore be expected to show that an alpha male's duration of tenure and the number of females in his group will predict male reproductive success rather closely. It is not yet known how often subordinate males sire offspring, but the benefits of rank appear mitigated to some extent by the value of sharing copulations with followers.

At the other extreme, the significance of high rank for male orangutans remains mysterious. Again, there are no paternity data. Evidence that developing males can undergo delayed maturation implies that survival falls when males become dominant, and since there is no hint that dominant males invest in kin, high rank should have reproductive benefits. Consistent with this idea is that developed and dominant males are totally intolerant of each other's presence, and developed males successfully supplant developing or subordinate males from consortships (van Schaik and van Hooff 1996). Nevertheless, females appear to mate several males per conception, and although theory and observational evidence both suggest that high-ranking males are attractive to females (Tanjung Putting: Galdikas 1985; Ketambe: Schürmann and van Hooff 1986), experimental data offer no support for this (Kutai: Mitani 1985a). Copulations by low-ranking males (probably including both developing and past-prime) are common and often involve coercion, but their reproductive significance is unknown. It is therefore uncertain whether subordinate status in male orangutans represents an inferior strategy or a balanced polymorphism.

Among chimpanzees and bonobos, mating patterns are also complex, but they are becoming better understood. Group mating is the predominant pattern, characterized by a female traveling with several males throughout her midcycle phase of maximal sexual swelling. Females tend to mate frequently with many or all community males, leading to several hundred copulations per conception. Much mating occurs without any attempts by males to mate-guard, with the result that there is often no relationship between male rank and total copulation rate (e.g., Gombe chimpanzees, Tutin 1979; Kanyawara chimpanzees, Wrangham in press; Mahale chimpanzees [data from 1980–1982, 1991], Hasegawa and Hiraiwa-Hasegawa 1990; Nishida 1997; Taï chimpanzees, Boesch and Boesch 2000). This led early observers to conclude that male rank would be unrelated to reproductive success. For example, Goodall (1986) suggested that the intense male dominance drive of chimpanzees is adapted to a different form of grouping than currently occurs in East Africa.

The apparent unimportance of male dominance rank turns out to be illusory, however. First, even in the absence of overt mate-guarding, the overall rate of copulation is sometimes related to dominance rank in the expected way, with higher-ranking males mating more often (e.g., Gombe chimpanzees in 1973–1974, Goodall 1986; Mahale chimpanzees in 1992, Nishida 1997; Wamba bonobos, Kano 1996). In chimpanzees this is more likely when there are few adult males in the community, and a stable hierarchy (Goodall 1986). There is a similar effect in bonobos within communities, in the sense that the relationship between male rank and copulation rate is most conspicuous within small parties (subgroups) containing only a few males (Kano 1996). Male rank is effective partly because dominant males sometimes interfere with subordinate's copulations (e.g., in 7% of bonobo copulations, Kano 1992).

Although male bonobos may compete over specific copulation opportunities, they show no possessiveness in the sense of consistently guarding access to a sexually receptive female. In contrast, mate-guarding occurs regularly in chimpanzees, associated with the peri-ovulatory period (within 2 days of a parous female's ovulation). Intensified aggression then means that dominance rank is more consistently related to mating success. Thus in Gombe, alpha males repeatedly had the highest mating success in peri-ovulatory periods (within 2 days of putative ovulation) (Tutin 1979; Goodall 1986). In Kanyawara, male rank was positively correlated with copulation rate with parous females (whereas nulliparous females were mated more often by low-ranking than high-ranking males) (Wrangham et al. in prep). In Mahale, copulation rate with parous females in the peri-ovulatory period was three times higher for the alpha-male than for any others (Hasegawa and Hiraiwa-Hasegawa 1990) and was correlated with dominance rank overall (Nishida 1997). In Ngogo, peri-ovulatory females were guarded by top-ranking males, either alone or in coalitions of two or three males (Watts 1998). In Taï, adolescent males were entirely prevented from copulating with conceptible ("fertile") females—in other words, females with an infant at least 40 months old. Furthermore, among the five adult males mating with conceptible females, the frequency of copulation was directly related to "coalition involvement" that is, males aiding each other to dominate rivals (Boesch and Boesch 2000).

Multimale groups are the only context of mating among bonobos, but in chimpanzees, female mating cycles can also take place wholly or partially in consortships, or isolated mating pairs (e.g., 8% of cycles; Boesch and Boesch 2000). Consortships have been estimated to be responsible for a small but significant proportion of conceptions (Gombe: 33%, Goodall 1986; 25%, Wallis 1997; Mahale: <20%, Hasegawa and Hiraiwa-Hasegawa 1990; Taï: 6%, Boesch and Boesch 2000). Consorting males in Taï were always high-ranking (Boesch and Boesch 2000). No clear effect of rank is known in Gombe. Whether consortships are associated with a high probability of conception is a matter of debate (Boesch and Boesch 2000). Consortships may, however, offer opportunities for males to escape the constraints of competing alliances of lower-ranking males (Boesch and Boesch 2000), or of domination by higher-ranking males (Goodall 1986). (The benefits to females are unclear but probably include reduced social stress and increased feeding time.) They illustrate the fact that low-ranking males have alternative strategies for achieving mating success.

For chimpanzees and bonobos, behavioral observations have now been corroborated by preliminary genetic data from three communities (Taï, Gombe, and Wamba). These data indicate that some low-ranking males do indeed achieve paternity but that, as expected, high-ranking males tend to do better. Reports from Gagneux et al. (1997, 1999) that 7 of 13 infants born into one community at Taï were sired by extracommunity males initially confused this picture. Although it was known that extracommunity copulations sometimes occur (i.e., when communities interact peaceably: Wamba bonobos; Kano 1992; when females make temporary visits to neighboring communities: Goodall 1986; or when consortships are formed with individuals from neighboring communities), it had generally been assumed that they were relatively rare. Gagneux and colleagues (1997, 1999), however, report that several mothers had disappeared for only a few days around the inferred time of conception, suggesting that they were purposefully seeking copulations with strange males during their most fertile periods. More recently, Constable et al. (in press) have reanalyzed the genetic data from Taï, identifying probable fathers within the community for six of the seven infants originally thought to have been sired outside the community. This casts doubt upon Gagneux et al.'s original conclusion that the Taï chimpanzees exhibit high rates of extragroup paternity.

Genetic data from Gombe are remarkably consistent with behavioral indications that high rank is reproductively advantageous (Constable et al. in press). Five of thirteen infants born there were likely to have been sired in the consortship context, while nine were sired in the group-mating context. Low- and middle-ranking males were responsible for all five paternities in the consortship context. Of the nine infants sired in a group setting, five were sired by the alpha male, two by males who subsequently became alpha, one by a high-ranking male, and one by a middle-ranking male. A similar result was reported from a genetic study of bonobos at Wamba (Gerloff et al. 1999). There between five and seven of ten infants were fathered by the two highest-ranking males in the community. The two lowest-ranking males fathered none of the offspring who were genotyped. In neither Gombe nor Wamba were any extracommunity conceptions detected.

In summary, all male great apes show more intense drives for intraspecific dominance than females do. Behavioral data suggest that male rank routinely confers reproductive benefits in gorillas, chimpanzees, and bonobos. Preliminary genetic data from chimpanzees and bonobos corroborate the behavioral data. In orangutans the benefits of male rank remain unclear.

COSTS OF MAINTAINING HIGH T

If high T facilitates aggression and dominance in male apes, and these are indeed associated with enhanced reproductive success, then why not maintain perpetually elevated T? In birds such elevation interferes with paternal care, but given that most male apes do not invest in offspring, this is not a constraint. The main problem with perpetually elevated T in apes appears to be the costly nature of frequent, escalated aggression. Combat between adult male apes is always risky, with high potential for severe or fatal wounds. Such a cost is seen in birds; for example, male brown-headed cow birds with T implants develop severe injuries from escalated fighting with other males (Beletsky et al. 1995). Thus, it is obvious why some individuals might, at times, accept low T and subordinate status to avoid the costs of male-male competition.

Do high-ranking males, though, suffer additional costs from maintaining increased levels of circulating T? Wingfield et al. (1997) have identified several costs associated with high T, three of which may apply to the great apes: direct energy costs, indirect energy costs, and immunosuppression. Direct energy costs refer to the fact that high T levels may increase metabolic rate and decrease fat reserves. Indirect energy costs of high T reflect the increased energetic expenditure associated with aggressive displays, territorial aggression, and fighting. Finally, there is some evidence that high levels of T may suppress the development of immune responses. This effect is not well-documented, however. One problem is that many studies compare T levels with some proxy of immune function, such as parasite load (e.g., Saino and Møller 1994). Experimental investigations using more sophisticated measures of immune function have failed to reveal a deleterious effect of high T on immune function in birds (Evans et al. 2000; Hasselquist et al. 1999). There is some evidence, however, that this effect may be more pronounced in the great apes. Women, for example, generally have stronger immune responses than men, and they exhibit a higher incidence of some autoimmune diseases (Grossman 1984; Talal and Ansar 1987); these patterns may be related to decreased levels of circulating androgens in women. For further discussion of androgens and immunity see Campbell et al. (chapter 7, this volume).

WHAT IS T DOING?

For both empirical and theoretical reasons, the proximate relationship between circulating testosterone and aggressive behavior is not well understood. The empirical problem is that although T is ultimately responsible for much male behavior, including aggression, the proximate relationship is not always predictable: high T may or may not be accompanied by frequent (or intense) aggression, and vice-versa. The theoretical difficulty is that specific neurochemical pathways linking testosterone with aggressive behavior have proven elusive.

Experimental studies on a range of species have shown that testosterone enhances directed attention (reviewed in Archer 1988); sustained attention to reproductive competitors presumably increases the likelihood of attack. Additional studies, mostly on rodents, have shown that testosterone activates vasopressin receptors in the hypothalamus (e.g., Delville et al. 1996). This is the clearest evidence to date that testosterone regulates a neurotransmitter known to be involved with offensive aggression. In general, however, the unpredictability of the correlation between T and aggression has frustrated efforts to identify a direct causal link from T to behavior.

With simple causal relationships rejected, researchers have increasingly focused on psychological, rather than physiological, effects of T on aggression. The suggestion that T is responsible for mood changes (e.g., Grinspoon et al. 2000; Rabkin et al. 2000) raises the possibility of psychological hypotheses for explaining the relationship between T and aggression. We propose one here, the positive-illusion hypothesis, in order to stimulate theoretical developments.

The positive-illusion hypothesis proposes that T modulates an individual's degree of illusion about its own competitive ability. Those with high T are predicted to have positive illusions, and therefore to fight more often, more intensely, and more successfully. Those with low T are predicted, by contrast, to have negative illusions, and therefore to avoid contests. The positive-illusion hypothesis does not imply that this action of T is the only pathway by which T influences aggression, or that positive illusions are influenced only by T. However, it does suggest that positive illusions may partly mediate the T-aggression correlation. The essential idea is that positive illusions are useful in contests, and that they are psychoendocrinologically supported by elevated T.

The importance of positive illusions is suggested by the contradiction between two observations. On the one hand, individuals in a contest are expected to be skillful at assessing the probable outcome, and to give up readily if they are outmatched; in other words, they are not expected to have illusions, whether negative or positive. On the other hand, individuals in fact routinely fight until they are badly damaged or dead. In the human context of contests between armies, the conflict between these two observations has led to the concept of "military incompetence." Thus, prolonged or escalated conflicts are seen as occurring because both opponents believe they will win. The losing opponent is proved wrong, however, and can therefore be said to have had a false illusion about its competitive ability, or to have been militarily incompetent. Military incompetence, or the failure to respond appropriately to an over-matched opponent, has traditionally been seen as resulting from a cognitive failure—in other words, a maladaptive positive illusion (Wrangham 1999b).

The positive-illusion hypothesis resolves the conflict by suggesting that positive illusions are adaptive because individuals who don't believe they will win are likely to lose (Wrangham 1999b). Accordingly, competitors with positive illusions are expected to stay in contests longer, and to fight harder, than those without such illusions. If this is correct, then selection should favor a mechanism that allows individuals to modulate their degree of positive illusion. Specifically, as individuals approach a contest, they should be able to increase their degree of positive illusion. During the contest, they should maintain their positive illusions. Following the contest, the winner can be expected to maintain his degree of positive illusion (because it has proved successful, and may do so again), whereas the loser should reduce his degree of positive illusion (because it has proved unsuccessful).

This account is of course similar to the time-course of T during contests between human males, as described in numerous "victory-effect" experiments (reviewed in Archer 1988; Mazur and Booth 1998). Men are able to regulate T over the short-term more precisely than women as a consequence of the more frequent pulsatile secretions of T by the testis than by the ovary or adrenal. It suggests that an increase in T might be responsible for an elevated degree of positive illusion. We know of no studies that have tested this directly in men, though several reports are suggestive (reviewed in Mazur and Booth 1998). Cashdan (1995) has reported that, in women, positive illusion was indeed correlated with T.

The positive-illusion hypothesis is thus based on the expected adaptive value of positive illusions for individuals in a fight, and it is supported by both the time-course of T during contests and the tentative correlation between T and positive illusions. It remains to be tested and refined. It is preliminary, but we propose it because we believe it illustrates the kind of hypothesis that will be most useful—in other words, one that considers the psychological rather than simply the physiological effects of T. Such hypotheses will have the advantage of accommodating variation relatively easily. Thus, they should be able to account for cases where correlations between T and behavior are absent because, for example, not all individuals with positive illusions are expected to be in fights (or to exhibit high T). If the positive-illusion hypothesis and similar kinds of explanation succeed in establishing psychological effects as mediating factors, the neurochemical effects of T and related hormones will then be easier to identify.

We thank the Uganda Wildlife Authority and Makerere University for sponsoring our research in Kibale. For assistance in the field we thank John Barwogeza, Christopher Katongole, Francis Mugurusi, Donor Muhangyi, Christopher Muruuli, and Peter Tuhairwe. For assistance in the laboratory, we are grateful to Cheryl Knott, Susan Lipson, Ross Wrangham, and Peter Ellison. Melissa Emery, Peter Gray, Cheryl Knott, and John Mitani provided valuable comments on the manuscript. Research was supported by NSF awards SBR-9729123 and SBR-9807448, and grants to MNM and RWW from the LSB Leakey Foundation.

REFERENCES

Archer J (1988) *The Behavioral Biology of Aggression* (Cambridge, Cambridge University Press).

Archer J (1991) The influence of testosterone on human aggression. *British Journal of Psychology* 82:1–28.

Bailey RC, Jenike MR, Bentley GR, Harrigan AM, Ellison PT (1992) The ecology of birth seasonality among agriculturalists in central Africa. *Journal of Biosocial Sciences* 24:393–412.

Beletsky LD, Gori DF, Freeman S, Wingfield JC (1995) Testosterone and polygyny in birds. In DM Power (Ed) *Current Ornithology* (New York, Plenum Press), 1–42.

Bentley GR, Harrigan AM, Campbell B, Ellison PT (1993) Seasonal effects on salivary testosterone levels among Lese males of the Ituri Forest, Zaire. *American Journal of Human Biology* 5:711–717.

Bentley GR (1999) Aping our ancestors: comparative aspects of reproductive ecology. *Evolutionary Anthropology* 7:175–185.

Bernstein IS, Gordon TP, Rose RM (1983) The interaction of hormones, behavior, and social context in nonhuman primates. In BB Svare (Ed) *Hormones and Aggressive Behavior* (New York, Plenum Press), 535–562.

Boehm C (1999) *Hierarchy in the Forest: The Evolution of Egalitarian Behavior* (Cambridge, Harvard University Press).

Boesch C, Boesch H (2000) *The Chimpanzees of the Tai Forest: Behavioral Ecology and Evolution* (Oxford, Oxford University Press).

Booth A, Dabbs J (1993) Testosterone and men's marriages. *Social Forces* 72:463–477.

Bribiescas RG (1996) Testosterone levels among Ache hunter-gatherer men: a functional interpretation of population variation among adult males. *Human Nature* 7:163–188.

Bribiescas RG (1997) *Testosterone as a Proximate Determinant of Somatic Energy Allocation in Human Males: Evidence from Ache Men of Eastern Paraguay.* PhD dissertation (Harvard University).

Brown RE, Murdoch T, Murphy PR, Moger WH (1995) Hormonal responses of male gerbils to stimuli from their mate and pups. *Hormones and Behavior* 29:474–491.

Bygott JD (1979) Agonistic behavior, dominance and social structure in wild chimpanzees of the Gombe National Park. In D Hamburg, ER McCown (Eds) *The Great Apes* (Menlo Park, California, Benjamin Cummings), 405–428.

Campbell BC, Leslie PW (1995) Reproductive ecology of human males. *Yearbook of Physical Anthropology* 38:1–26.

Cashdan E (1995) Hormones, sex and status in women. *Hormones and Behavior* 29:354–366.

Cavigelli SA, Pereira ME (2000) Mating season aggression and fecal testosterone levels in male ring-tailed lemurs (*Lemur catta*). *Hormones and Behavior* 37: 246–255.

Clutton-Brock TH, Vincent CJ (1991) Sexual selection and potential reproductive rates of males and females. *Nature* 351:58–60.

Constable JL, Ashley MV, Goodall J, Pusey AE (in press) Male and female reproductive strategies among Gombe chimpanzees evaluated by noninvasive paternity assignment. *Molecular Ecology*.

Creel SR, Wildt DE, Monfort SL (1993) Androgens, aggression and reproduction in wild dwarf mongooses: a test of the challenge hypothesis. *American Naturalist* 141:816–825.

Delville Y, Mansour KM, Ferris CF (1996) Testosterone facilitates aggression by modulating vasopressin receptors in the hypothalamus. *Physiology and Behavior* 60:25–29.

Dixson AF (1998) *Primate Sexuality: Comparative Studies of the Prosimians, Monkeys, Apes, and Human Beings* (New York, Oxford University Press).

Ellison PT, Lager C (1985) Exercise-induced menstrual disorders. *New England Journal of Medicine* 313:825–826.

Ellison PT, Lager C (1986) Moderate recreational running is associated with lowered salivary progesterone profiles in women. *American Journal of Obstetrics and Gynecology* 154:1000–1003.

Ellison PT, Peacock NR, Lager C (1989) Ecology and ovarian function among Lese women of the Ituri Forest, Zaire. *American Journal of Physical Anthropology* 78:519–526.

Ellison PT (1990) Human ovarian function and reproductive ecology: new hypotheses. *American Anthropologist* 92:933–952.

Ellison PT, Panter-Brick C, Lipson SF, O'Rourke MT (1993) The ecological context of human ovarian function. *Human Reproduction* 8:2248–2258.

Ellison PT, Panter-Brick C (1996) Salivary testosterone levels among Tamang and Kami males of central Nepal. *Human Biology* 68:955–965.

Emlen ST, Oring W (1977) Ecology, sexual selection, and the evolution of mating systems. *Science* 197:215–223.

Evans MR, Goldsmith AR, Norris RA (2000) The effects of testosterone on antibody production and plumage coloration in male house sparrows (*Passer domesticus*). *Behavioral Ecology and Sociobiology* 47:156–163.

Flinn MV (1988) Mate guarding in a Caribbean village. *Ethology and Sociobiology* 9:1–28.

Fossey D (1983) *Gorillas in the Mist* (Boston, Houghton Mifflin).

Fossey D (1984) Infanticide in mountain gorillas *(Gorilla gorilla beringei)* with comparative notes on chimpanzees. In G Hausfater, SB Hrdy (Eds) *Infanticide: Comparative and Evolutionary Perspectives* (Hawthorne, New York, Aldine), 217–235.

Gagneux P, Woodruff DS, Boesch C (1997) Furtive mating in female chimpanzees. *Nature* 387:358–359.

Gagneux P, Boesch C, Woodruff DS (1999) Female reproductive strategies, paternity and community structure in wild West African chimpanzees. *Animal Behavior* 57:19–32.

Galdikas BMF (1979) Orangutan adaptation at Tanjung Puting Reserve: mating and ecology. In DA Hamburg, ER McCown (Eds) *The Great Apes* (Menlo Park, Benjamin/Cummings), 195–234.

Galdikas BMF (1981) Orangutan reproduction in the wild. In CE Graham (Ed) *Reproductive Biology of the Great Apes* (New York, Academic Press), 281–300.

Galdikas BMF (1985) Adult male sociality and reproductive tactics among orangutans at Tanjung Puting. *Folia Primatologica* 45:9–24.

Gerloff U, Hartung B, Fruth B, Hohmann G, Tautz T (1999) Intracommunity relationships, dispersal pattern and paternity success in a wild living community of bonobos *(Pan paniscus)* determined from DNA analysis of faecal samples. *Proceedings of the Royal Society of London,* B 266:1189–1195.

Goodall J (1986) *The Chimpanzees of Gombe: Patterns of Behavior* (Cambridge, Harvard University Press).

Goodall J, Bandora A, Bergmann E, Busse C, Matama H, Mpongo E, Pierce A, Riss D (1979) Inter-community interactions in the chimpanzee population of the Gombe National Park. In DA Hamburg, ER McCown (Eds) *The Great Apes* (Menlo Park, Benjamin/Cummings), 13–54.

Gordon TP, Rose RM, Bernstein IS (1976) Seasonal rhythm in plasma testosterone levels in the rhesus monkey *(Macaca mulatta):* a three year study. *Hormones and Behavior* 7:229–243.

Grinspoon S, Corcoran C, Stanley T, Baaj A, Basgoz N, Klibanski A (2000) Effects of hypogonadism and testosterone administration on depression indices in HIV-infected men. *Journal of Clinical Endocrinology and Metabolism* 85:60–65.

Grossman CJ (1984) Regulation of the immune system by sex steroid. *Endocrine Reviews* 5:435–454.

Harcourt AH (1978) Strategies of emigration and transfer by primates, with particular reference to gorillas. *Zeitschrift für Tierpsychologie* 408:401–420.

Harcourt AH, Fossey D, Sabater-Pi J (1981) Demography of *Gorilla gorilla. Journal of Zoology* 195:215–233.

Hasegawa T, Hiraiwa-Hasegawa M (1990) Sperm competition and mating behavior. In T Nishida (Ed) *The Chimpanzees of the Mahale Mountains: Sexual and Life History Strategies* (Tokyo, University of Tokyo Press), 115–132.

Hasselquist D, Marsh JA, Sherman PW, Wingfield JC (1999) Is avian humoral immunocompetence suppressed by testosterone? *Behavioral Ecology and Sociobiology* 45:167–175.

Hayaki H, Huffman MA, Nishida T (1989) Dominance among male chimpanzees in the Mahale Mountains National Park, Tanzania: a preliminary study. *Primates* 30:187–197.

Hegner RE, Wingfield JC (1987) Effects of experimental manipulation of testosterone levels on parental investment and breeding success in male house sparrows. *Auk* 104:462–469.

Herndon JG (1983) Seasonal breeding in rhesus monkeys: influence of the behavioral environment. *American Journal of Primatology* 5:197–204.

Higley JD, Mehlman PT, Poland RE, Taub DM, Vickers J, Suomi SJ, Linnoila M (1996) CSF testosterone and 5-HIAA correlate with different types of aggressive behaviors. *Biological Psychiatry* 40:1067–1082.

Kano T (1992) *The Last Ape: Pygmy Chimpanzee Behavior and Ecology* (Stanford, Stanford University Press).

Kano T (1996) Male rank order and copulation rate in a unit-group of bonobos at Wamba, Zaire. In WC McGrew, LF Marchant, T Nishida (Eds) *Great Ape Societies* (Cambridge, Cambridge University Press), 135–145.

Kingsley S (1982) Causes of non-breeding and the development of secondary sexual characteristics in the male orangutan: a hormonal study. In L de Boer (Ed) *The Orangutan: Its Biology and Conservation* (The Hague, Junk Publishers), 215–229.

Kingsley S (1988) Physiological development of male orangutans and gorillas. In J Schwartz (Ed) *Orangutan Biology* (Oxford, Oxford University Press), 123–131.

Klibanski A, Beitins IZ, Badger T, Little R, McArthur JW (1981) Reproductive function during fasting in men. *Journal of Clinical Endocrinology and Metabolism* 53:258–263.

Knott CD (1998) Changes in orangutan caloric intake, energy balance, and ketones in response to fluctuating food availability. *International Journal of Primatology* 19:1061–1079.

Knott CD (1999) *Reproductive, Physiological and Behavioral Responses of Orangutans in Borneo to Fluctuations in Food Availability.* PhD dissertation (Harvard University).

Lincoln GA, Guinness F, Short RV (1972) The way in which testosterone controls the social and sexual behavior of the red deer stag *(Cervus elaphus). Hormones and Behavior* 3:375–396.

Maggioncalda AN, Sapolsky RM, Czekala NM (1999) Reproductive hormone profiles in captive male orangutans: implications for understanding developmental arrest. *American Journal of Physical Anthropology* 109:19–32.

Maggioncalda AN, Czekala NM, Sapolsky RM (2000) Growth hormone and thyroid stimulating hormone concentrations in captive male orangutans: implications for understanding developmental arrest. *American Journal of Primatology* 50:67–76.

Maple T (1980) *Orangutan Behavior* (New York, van Nostrand Reinhold).

Mazur A, Booth A (1998) Testosterone and dominance in men. *Behavioral and Brain Sciences* 21:353–397.

Mazur A, Michalek J (1998) Marriage, divorce, and male testosterone. *Social Forces* 77:315–330.

Mehlman PT, Higley JD, Fernald BJ, Sallee FR, Suomi SJ, Linnoila M (1997) CSF 5-HIAA, testosterone, and sociosexual behaviors in free-ranging male rhesus macaques in the mating season. *Psychiatry Research* 72:89–102.

Michael RP, Zumpe D (1981) Relation between the seasonal changes in aggression, plasma testosterone and the photoperiod in male rhesus monkeys. *Psychoneuroendocrinology* 6:145–158.

Michael RP, Zumpe D (1993) A review of hormonal factors influencing the sexual and aggressive behavior of macaques. *American Journal of Primatology* 30:213–241.

Milton K (1985) Mating patterns of woolly spider monkeys, *Bracyteles arachnoides:* implications for female choice. *Behavioral Ecology and Sociobiology* 17:53–59.

Mitani JC (1985a) Sexual selection and adult male orangutan long calls. *Animal Behavior* 33:272–283.

Mitani JC (1985b) Mating behavior of male orangutans in the Kutai Game Reserve, Indonesia. *Animal Behavior* 33:392–402.

Mitani JC, Gros-Louis J, Richards AF (1996) Sexual dimorphism, the operational sex ratio, and the intensity of male competition in polygynous primates. *American Naturalist* 147:966–980.

Moore MC (1986) Circulating steroid hormones during rapid aggressive responses of territorial male mountain spiny lizards, *Sceloporus jarrovi. Hormones and Behavior* 21:511–521.

Muller, MN (2002) Endocrine aspects of aggression and dominance in chimpanzees of the Kibale forest. PhD dissertation (University of Southern California).

Nishida T (1968) The social group of wild chimpanzees in the Mahali Mountains. *Primates* 9:167–224.

Nishida T (1979) The social structure of chimpanzees of the Mahale Mountains. In D Hamburg, ER McCown (Eds) *The Great Apes* (Menlo Park, Benjamin/Cummings), 73–122.

Nishida T (1997) Sexual behavior of adult male chimpanzees of the Mahale Mountains National Park, Tanzania. *Primates* 38:379–398.

Nishida T, Hiraiwa-Hasegawa M, Hasegawa T, Takahata Y (1985) Group extinction and female transfer in wild chimpanzees in the Mahale National Park, Tanzania. *Zeitschrift für Tierpsychologie* 67:284–301.

Panter-Brick C, Lotstein DS, Ellison PT (1993) Seasonality of reproductive function and weight loss in rural Nepali women. *Human Reproduction* 8:684–690.

Polanski FF, Lamb EJ (1988) Do the results of semen analysis predict future fertility? *Fertility and Sterility* 49:1059–1065.

Rabkin JG, Wagner GJ, Rabkin R (2000) A double-blind, placebo-controlled trial of testosterone therapy for HIV-positive men with hypogonadal symptoms. *Archives of General Psychiatry* 57:141–147.

Reburn CJ, Wynne-Edwards KE (1999) Hormonal changes in males of a naturally biparental and a uniparental mammal. *Hormones and Behavior* 35:163–176.

Robbins MM, Czekala NM (1997) A preliminary investigation of urinary testosterone and cortisol levels in wild male mountain gorillas. *American Journal of Primatology* 43:51–64.

Roberts RL, Zullo A, Gustafson EA, Carter CS (1996) Perinatal steroid treatments alter alloparental and affiliative behavior in prairie voles. *Hormones and Behavior* 30:576–582.

Rodman PS, Mitani JC (1986) Orangutans: sexual dimorphism in a solitary species. In BB Smuts, DL Cheney, RM Seyfarth, RW Wrangham, TT Struhsaker (Eds) *Primate Societies* (Chicago, University of Chicago Press), 146–154.

Rommerts FFG (1988) How much androgen is required for maintenance of spermatogenesis? *Journal of Endocrinology* 116:7–9.

Rowell TE, Dixson AF (1975) Changes in social organization during the breeding season of wild talapoin monkeys. *Journal of Reproduction and Fertility* 43:419–434.

Ruiz de Elvira M, Herndon J, Collins D (1983) Effect of estradiol-treated females on all female groups of rhesus monkeys during the transition between the nonbreeding and breeding season. *Folia Primatologica* 41:191–203.

Saino N, Møller AP (1994) Secondary sexual characters, parasites and testosterone in the barn swallow, *Hirundo rustica*. *Animal Behavior* 48:1325–1333.

Sapolsky RM (1983) Endocrine aspects of social instability in the olive baboon (*Papio anubis*). *American Journal of Primatology* 5:365–379.

Sapolsky RM (1991) Testicular function, social rank and personality among wild baboons. *Psychoneuroendocrinology* 16:281–293.

Sapolsky RM (1992) Cortisol concentrations and the social significance of rank instability among wild baboons. *Psychoneuroendocrinology* 17:701–709.

Schürmann CL, van Hooff JARAM (1986) Reproductive strategies of the orangutan: new data and a reconsideration of existing sociosexual models. *International Journal of Primatology* 7:265–287.

Schweiger U, Tuschl RJ, Platte P, Broocks A, Laessle RG, Pirke K-M (1992) Everyday eating behavior and menstrual function in young women. *Fertility and Sterility* 57:771–775.

Sicotte P (1993) Inter-group encounters and female transfer in mountain gorillas: influence of group composition on male behavior. *American Journal of Primatology* 30:21–36.

Storey AE, Walsh CJ, Quinton RL, Wynne-Edwards KE (2000) Hormonal correlates of paternal responsiveness in new and expectant fathers. *Evolution and Human Behavior* 21:79–95.

Strier KB (1992) *Faces in the Forest: The Endangered Muriqui Monkeys of Brazil* (Cambridge, Harvard University Press).

Strier KB, Ziegler TE, Wittwer DJ (1999) Seasonal and social correlates of fecal testosterone and cortisol levels in wild male muriquis *(Brachyteles arachnoides)*. *Hormones and Behavior* 35:125–134.

Takahata Y, Ihobe H, Idani GI (1999) Do bonobos copulate more frequently and promiscuously than chimpanzees? *Human Evolution* 14:159–167.

Talal N, Ansar AS (1987) Sex hormones and autoimmune diseases: a short review. *International Journal of Immunotherapy* 3:65–70.

te Boekhorst IJA, Schurmann CL, Sugardjito J (1990) Residential status and seasonal movements of wild orang-utans in the Gunung Leuser Reserve (Sumatra, Indonesia). *Animal Behavior* 39:1098–1109.

Trivers RL (1972) Parental investment and sexual selection. In B Campbell (Ed) *Sexual Selection and the Descent of Man, 1871–1971* (Chicago, Aldine), 136–179.

Tutin CEG (1979) Mating patterns and reproductive strategies in a community of wild chimpanzees. *Behavioral Ecology and Sociobiology* 6:39–48.

Utami S, Setia TM (1995) Behavioral changes in wild male and female Sumatran orangutans *(Pongo pygmaeus abelii)* during and following a resident male takeover. In RD Nadler, BFM Galdikas, LK Sheeran, N Rosen (Eds) *The Neglected Ape* (New York, Plenum Press), 183–190.

van Schaik CP, van Hooff JARAM (1996) Toward an understanding of the orang-utan's social system. In WC McGrew, LF Marchant, T Nishida (Eds) *Great Ape Societies* (Cambridge, Cambridge University Press), 3–15.

Vandenbergh JG, Drickamer L (1974) Reproductive coordination among free-ranging rhesus monkeys. *Physiology and Behavior* 13:373–376.

Wallis J (1997) A survey of reproductive parameters in the free-ranging chimpanzees of Gombe National Park. *Journal of Reproduction and Fertility* 109: 297–307.

Wasser SK, Barash DP (1983) Reproductive suppression among female mammals: implications for biomedicine and sexual selection theory. *Quarterly Review of Biology* 58:513–538.

Watts DP (1989) Infanticide in mountain gorillas: new cases and a reconsideration of the evidence. *Ethology* 81:1–18.

Watts DP (1996) Comparative socio-ecology of gorillas. In WC McGrew, LF Marchant, T Nishida (Eds) *Great Ape Societies* (Cambridge, Cambridge University Press), 16–28.

Watts DP (1998) Coalitionary mate guarding by male chimpanzees at Ngogo, Kibale National Park, Uganda. *Behavioral Ecology and Sociobiology* 44:43–55.

Weinbauer GF, Nieschlag E (1990) The role of testosterone in spermatogenesis. In E Nieschlag, HM Behre (Eds) *Testosterone: Action, Deficiency, Substitution* (Berlin, Springer-Verlag), 23–50.

Whitten PL (2000) Evolutionary endocrinology of the cercopithecoids. In P Whitehead, C Jolly (Eds) *Old World Monkeys* (Cambridge, Cambridge University Press), 269–297.

Whitten PL, Brockman DK, Stavisky RC (1998) Recent advances in noninvasive techniques to monitor hormone-behavior interactions. *Yearbook of Physical Anthropology* 41:1–23.

Whitten PL, Stavisky R, Aureli F, Russell E (1998) Response of fecal cortisol to stress in captive chimpanzees *(Pan troglodytes)*. *American Journal of Primatology* 44:57–69.

Williams J (1999) *Female Strategies and the Reason for Territoriality in Chimpanzees: Lessons from Three Decades of Research at Gombe*. PhD dissertation (University of Minnesota).

Wingfield JC (1984) Androgens and mating systems: testosterone-induced polygyny in normally monogamous birds. *Auk* 101:665–671.

Wingfield JC (1994) Control of territorial aggression in a changing environment. *Psychoneuroendocrinology* 19:709–721.

Wingfield JC, Ball GF, Dufty AM, Hegner RE, Ramenofsky M (1987) Testosterone and aggression in birds. *American Scientist* 75:602–608.

Wingfield JC, Hegner RE, Dufty AM, Ball GF (1990) The "challenge hypothesis": theoretical implications for patterns of testosterone secretion, mating systems, and breeding strategies. *American Naturalist* 136:829–846.

Wingfield JC, Whaling CS, Marler P (1994) Communication in vertebrate aggression and reproduction: the role of hormones. In E Knobil, JD Neill (Eds) *The Physiology of Reproduction* (New York, Raven Press), 303–342.

Wingfield JC, Jacobs J, Hillgarth N (1997) Ecological constraints and the evolution of hormone-behavior interrelationships. *Annals of the New York Academy of Sciences* 807:22–41.

Wrangham RW (1980) An ecological model of female-bonded primate groups. *Behavior* 75:262–300.

Wrangham RW (1999a) The evolution of coalitionary killing: the imbalance-of-power hypothesis. *Yearbook of Physical Anthropology* 42:1–30.

Wrangham RW (1999b) Is military incompetence adaptive? *Evolution and Human Behavior* 20:3–17.

Wrangham RW (2000) Why are male chimpanzees more gregarious than mothers? A scramble competition hypothesis. In PM Kappeler (Ed) *Primate Males* (Cambridge, Cambridge University Press), 248–258.

Wrangham RW (in press) The cost of sexual attraction; is there a trade-off in female *Pan* between sex appeal and received coercion? In C. Boesch, G. Hohmann, L. Marchant (Eds) *Behavioural Diversity in Chimpanzees and Bonobos* (Cambridge, Cambridge University Press).

Yamagiwa J (1986) Activity rhythm and the ranging of a solitary male mountain gorilla *(Gorilla gorilla beringei)*. *Primates* 27:273–282.

Zamboni L, Conaway CH, van Pelt L (1974) Seasonal changes in production of semen in free-ranging rhesus monkeys. *Biology of Reproduction* 11:251–267.

18

Female Reproductive Ecology of the Apes
Implications for Human Evolution

CHERYL KNOTT

Long-term research on great apes is now revealing that a wide range of variation exists both within and between species in reproductive parameters such as age at menarche, age at first birth, and interbirth interval. However, a clear understanding of what ecological factors may influence these female reproductive parameters and the relative importance of each factor has been lacking from great ape studies. We know much more about the ecology of reproduction in female humans than we do for any of the great ape species.

Owing to the close kinship between humans and great apes, research on the ecological context of human ovarian function is extremely relevant to understanding the variability in great ape reproductive parameters. I argue that recent evidence suggests that the same ecological variables that are regulating reproduction in humans also influence the great apes. Outside of lactation, the key ecological mediators of fecundity in human females are nutritional intake, energetic expenditure, and net energy balance (Ellison et al. 1993). A thorough understanding of the ecology of reproductive functioning in the great apes can help us make sense of interindividual variation, interpopulation variation, and to some extent, interspecies variability. Furthermore, if great ape and human reproductive physiology share similar adaptive responses to the environment, then we can develop more accurate models for human, as well as great ape, evolution.

I begin by reviewing the variability in reproductive parameters within each species of the great apes. Specifically, I examine age at menarche, length of adolescent subfecundity, age at first birth, and the components of the interbirth interval in wild as well as captive ape populations. Then, I outline evidence from my study of wild orangutans to demonstrate how female energy intake and expenditure influence hormonal functioning in the wild. I present evidence that orangutans experience dramatic changes in energetic status owing to fluctuations in fruit availability and that these changes result in significant differences in hormonal levels. I review evidence in the literature that supports the conclusion that chimpanzees are influenced by these same ecological factors. Finally, I discuss how parallels between ape and human reproductive functioning help us to understand human evolution. In particular, I explore changes in the interbirth interval and the period of juvenile dependency during hominid evolution.

VARIABILITY IN REPRODUCTIVE PARAMETERS

Apes of the same species living under different ecological conditions display wide variability in their reproductive timetables. This is true in the extreme in the altered ecological conditions of captivity. Most captive apes, living under conditions of nutritional abundance and low energy expenditure, have dramatically earlier ages at menarche and shorter interbirth intervals than are seen in any wild population. This variability in reproductive patterns demonstrates that the timing of reproduction occurs within a range for each species and is not a fixed parameter. We can no longer, for example, talk about the interbirth interval of "the" chimpanzee. Instead, it is much more informative to explore what causes this reproductive parameter to vary both within chimpanzees and among the great ape species.

Most studies of variability in reproductive patterns within great ape populations focus on males and the effectiveness of male mating strategies in achieving paternity (e.g. Tutin 1979; Tutin and McGinnis 1981). Until recently, there has been little focus on how ecological factors might influence a female ape's ability to conceive—largely because of the difficulty of measuring nutritional status and reproductive functioning in the field. Additionally, wild apes cannot be sampled as reliably as those in captivity. Tutin (1994) points out that female transfer in gorillas and chimpanzees makes it difficult to track these individuals longitudinally during development and to know the ages at which they go through menarche and reproduce. In orangutans, the size and fluidity of their residence patterns also makes tracking individuals over their reproductive lifespan extremely difficult.

Below I review what we know about female reproductive parameters in captivity and in the wild. New data are provided from my study of wild orangutans in Gunung Palung National Park, West Kalimantan, Indonesia. For gorillas, captive data come from members of the western lowland gorilla subspecies (*Gorilla gorilla gorilla*) whereas wild data are from mountain gorillas (*Gorilla gorilla beringei*). Where more than one study has taken place at a single field site, I only report the most recent figures. Medians are presented where available and data are converted into comparable units (e.g. years, months) to facilitate these comparisons when possible. Data are summarized in Table 18.1.

Age at Menarche

Unlike human studies, where first menstrual bleeding provides the obvious marker of menarche, great ape studies, particularly in the wild, normally rely on other indicators of reproductive maturity, such as first sexual swelling, sexual behavior, or first successful copulation with an adult male.

Orangutans. In captive orangutans menarche can be assessed through the presence of menstrual bleeding. Markham (1990, 1995) found that menarche occurred between 5.8 and 11.1 years. Within the seven individuals in her sample, menarche was earliest in a large, overweight female and latest in two females with eating disorders. Asano (1967) provides data for one female who reached menarche at 4.5 years and first began mating at 5.5 years. Lippert (1977) states that first sexual activity occurs at 7–9 years in captivity. The age of menarche is particularly difficult to determine in wild orangutans owing to the absence of a sexual swelling. Galdikas (1981) defines menarche as the advent of proceptivity and describes a wild female from Tanjung Putting, Borneo, who began approaching adult males at an estimated age of 10–11 years. In the future, with field application of chemstrips (Knott 1996), menarche may be able to be determined by the presence of blood in urine.

Gorillas. In captivity, the first menstrual flow reportedly occurs between 6 and 7 years of age (Dixson 1981). Menstrual bleeding has not been observed in wild mountain gorillas at Karisoke; thus menarche has been determined from the first evidence of labial tumescence (Harcourt et al. 1980) or first sexual activity (Watts 1991). After their first swellings, according to Harcourt et al. (1981) it took 5 months for two females to mate with a fully adult male. Watts (1991) reports that the first sexual activity among mountain gorillas occurs between 5.7 and 7.1 years (median = 6.3 years).

Bonobos. The median age at menarche for three captive-born females (known birth date) and six wild-born females (estimated birth date) was 7.7 years (Thompson-Handler 1990). Kuroda (1989) states that bonobo females at Wamba, Zaire, experience their first swellings at the age of 8 or 9 years. Females transferred into the intensively studied E-group at an estimated age of 13–15 years.

Table 18.1. Reproductive Parameters of Wild and Captive Female Apes. Means are given, followed by medians in parentheses. Ranges and sample sizes, when available, are provided in parentheses below (n is the number of samples or intervals and f is the number of females).

Species	Site	Age at menarche (yrs.)	First Sexual Behavior (yrs.)	Adolescent Subfecundity (yrs.)	Age at First Birth (yrs.)	Interbirth Interval (yrs.)	Postpartum Amennorhea (yrs.)	Waiting Time to Conception (mths.)
Orangutan	Captive	7.7 (7.6)[1,19,20,a] (4.5–11.1, n=8)	5.5–9[1,18]	0.8 (0.6)[1,19,a,f] (0.6–1.2, n=3)	9–9.9[20] (mode) (5.2–32.7, n=372)	6.3[19] (n=1)	4.7[19] (n=1)	1[17]–10[19] (n=1)[19]
Orangutan	Tanjung Putting	—	10–11[10] (estimated age, n=1)	12–4[10,g] (n=2)	15.7 (16.0)[28] (15–16, n=3)	7.7 (7.7)[11,i] (5.2–10.4, n=23, f=11)	6+[8]	10.3 (2)[8,9,a] (1–28, n=3, f=3)
Orangutan	Ketambe	—	—	5[22,g] (n=1)	14.7 (16.0)[28] (12–16, n=3)	8.6(8.4)[29,k] (5.7–12.8, n=9, f=5)	—	—
Orangutan	Gunung Palung	—	—	—	—	7.0 (7.0)[2] (6–8, n=4, f=3)	5.7[2] (4.5–7, n=2, f=2)	2.5[2] (n=1)
Gorilla	Captive	6–7[6] (n=3)	—	2.1[6,f] (see text)	9.3[6]	4.2 (4.0)[23] (2.3–6.4, n=16, f=13)	2.7 (2.4)[23] (1.5–5.2, n=13, f=8)	2.0 (2.0)[23] (0.07–8, n=9, f=8)
Gorilla	Karisoke	—	(6.3)[31] (5.7–7.1)	0.9–1.5[13,h] (n=3)	(10.0)[13,31] (8.7–12.7, n=13)	(3.9)[31] (3–7.2, n=26)	(3.2)[31] (2.2–4.2, n=12)	3–4 (5)[31] (1–10+)
Bonobo	Captive	8.2 (7.7)[27] (6.0–11.2, n=9)	—	4.4 (4.2)[27] (1.9–8.4, n=7)	10.8 (10.0)[16,27,a] (7.7–20.0, n=20)	3.6[27] or 5.1 (5.2)[14] (1.9–7.6, n=21, f=14)[14]	1.3–2.7[14] (n=3)	2.4–37.2[14,27] (calculated, see text)
Bonobo	Wamba	8–9[16]	—	5.0[16,h] (calculated)	14.2 (14.0)[16] (13–15, n=6)	4.5[26] (n=10)	1 or 3–4[15] (see text)	0–33.6[15] (calculated, see text)

Species	Site							
Bonobo	Eyengo, Lomako	—	—	—	—	8.0 (9.0)[7,1] (4–9, n=19)	—	—
Chimpanzee	Captive	8.0[24,33,a,e,f] (6.3–10.2, n=25)	—	0.93[3,f] (0.3–1.4, n=7)	10.8[24] (n=17)	3.8[5] (1.5–6.3, n=15, f=8)	2.3[5] (1.2–3.2, n=11, f=7)	10.5[5] (calculated)
Chimpanzee	Gombe	10.8[30,c] (8.5–13.5, n=8)	—	2.4[30,i] (0.6–4.9, n=4)	13.3[30] (11.1–17.2, n=4)	5.5[12] (4.0–6.5, n=21, f=13)	3.9[30] (2.4–5.7, n=12)	4.7[30] (0.5–13.4, n=17)
Chimpanzee	Mahale	10.6 (10.0)[21,c] (9–13, n=33)	10.9 (10.7)[21] (9.1–13.4, n=20)	2.3 (2.1)[21,i] (0.3–6.9, n=13)	14.6 (15.0)[21] (12–20, n=22)	6.0 (6.0)[21] (4.4–7.3, n=19, f=16)	4.4 (4.6)[21] (2.5–5.6, n=18, f=15)	10.6 (8.9)[21,m] (1.4–32.4, n=18, f=15)
Chimpanzee	Tai	—	—	2.6 (2.2)[3,i] (1.4–5.7, n=7)	14.3 (14.0)[3] (12.5–18.5, n=8)	5.8 (5.4)[3] (4.0–10.0, n=33, f=19)	2.0 (1.9)[3,4] (0.2–5.1, n=26, f=19)	26.9[3,m] (n=33, f=19)
Chimpanzee	Kanywara, Kibale	11.1[32,c] (n=1)	11.1[32] (n=1)	1.6 (1.6)[32,i] (0.3–2.5, n=5)	15.4 (15.0)[32] (14–18, n=5)	6.2 (6.0)[32,1] (2.3–10.0, n=31)	4.4 (4.0)[32] (1.7–6.5, n=11)	15.3 (18.9)[32] (calculated)
Chimpanzee	Bossou	—	—	—	12–14[25]	5.1 (5.0)[25] (3.0–11.0, n=15)	—	—

Sources: [1]Asano, 1967.; [2]author's data; [3]Boesch and Boesch-Achermann, 2000; [4]Boesch, pers. comm., 2000; [5]Courtney, 1987; [6]Dixson, 1981; [7]Truth, pers. comm; [8]Galdikas, 1981; [9]Galdikas, 1980; [10]Galdikas 1995; [11]Galdikas and Wood, 1990; [12]Goodall, 1986; [13]Harcourt et al., 1981; [14]Harvey, 1997; [15]Kano, 1992; [16]Kuroda, 1989; [17]Lippert, 1974; [18]Lippert, 1977; [19]Markham, 1990; [20]Markham, 1995; [21]Nishida et al., 1990; [22]Schurrmann and van Hoof, 1986; [23]Sievert et al., 1991; [24]Smith et al., 1975; [25]Sugiyama, 1994; [26]Takahata et al., 1996; [27]Thompson-Handler, 1990; [28]Tilson et al., 1993; [29]Utami, pers. comm..; [30]Wallis, 1997; [31]Watts, 1991; [32]Wrangham, pers. comm.; [33]Young and Yerkes, 1943. [a]Age at first full swelling. [b]Age at first full swelling. [c]Age at first menstruation. [d]The mean and median were calculated by pooling all the original raw data from the multiple studies, thus I weighted the sample means by the sample sizes to calculate the overall mean. [e]The raw data were not available from the multiple studies cited, thus I weighted the sample means by the sample sizes to calculate the overall mean. [f]Period between first menstruation and conception. [g]Period between first copulation and conception. [h]Period between first swelling and conception. [i]Period between first full swelling and conception. [j]Period between first copulation and conception. [k]Excluding data from one interval with a known miscarriage. [l]Median computed using a Kaplan-Meier analysis with censored and uncensored intervals. [m]Subtracting gestation length from published figures.

Chimpanzees. In captivity, mean ages of menarche (defined as first menstruation) in female chimpanzees have been reported as 7.6 (Smith et al. 1975) and 8.9 (Young and Yerkes 1943) years, although some individuals may show swellings as early as 5 years (Wallis, personal observation). Wallis (1997) reports that the first *full-sized* swellings in Gombe (Tanzania) chimpanzees occur at a mean age of 10.8 years. Menarche (first menstruation) occurs 1–3 years after the first sexual swelling (at age 11–14; Tutin and McGinnis 1981) and 1–6 months after the first *full- sized* swelling (Goodall 1986). At Mahale, Tanzania, the median age of first maximal swelling is 10.0 years (6 of 33 individuals are of known birth year; calculated from Nishida et al. 1990). Age at first mating occurred at a median age of 10.7 years. The apparent first menstrual blood was seen in one Mahale chimpanzee at 11 years of age (Nishida et al. 1990). At Kanyawara, in the Kibale Forest of Uganda, one female of known birth date had her first swelling at 10.2 years, and her first *full* swelling and first copulation at 11.1 years (Wrangham, personal communication 2000).

Adolescent Subfecundity

The terms *adolescent subfecundity* and *adolescent sterility* have both been used to describe the period between menarche or the beginning of sexual activity and conception. In most species there is normally only a brief period in which cycles are truly sterile. Succeeding cycles are variably fecundable, with ovulation sometimes occurring but often without an adequate luteal or follicular phase. As in humans, ovulation may occur but progesterone secretion may not be adequate to support pregnancy (Young and Yerkes 1943).

Orangutans. Markham (1990) reports on two captive females of known ages at menarche and first parturition. Asano (1967) provides similar figures for one female. From these I calculate a median period of adolescent subfecundity of 0.6 years (subtracting 8.1 months of gestation [Markham 1995]). Menstrual cycle lengths were longer in females during the first two years after menarche than in older females (Markham 1990). However, after analyzing urinary estrone, Masters and Markham (1991) found a pattern similar to adults in an adolescent female only eight months past menarche. In the wild at Tanjung Putting, Galdikas (1995) describes one female with an estimated age at first sexual activity of 10–11 years and first birth at 14–15 years, giving a four-year period of adolescent subfecundity. A second female had at least a one-year cycling period before conceiving. Schürmann and van Hooff (1986), working at Ketambe, Sumatra, have data on one female. She did not conceive for five years after the onset of sexual activity, despite an estimated 130–210 copulations.

Gorillas. Dixson (1981) reports a mean age at first conception of 8.6 years for captive gorillas. With an average age at menarche of approximately 6.5 years (Dixson 1981), this indicates a period of adolescent subfecundity of about 2.1 years. At Karisoke, wild mountain gorillas experienced adolescent subfecundity for 10.5–18.5 months (Harcourt et al. 1980). Watts (1991) states that more recent data from Karisoke also support a period of adolescent subfecundity of about two years.

Bonobos. Thompson-Handler's (1990) survey of the captive literature gives a median period of adolescent subfecundity of 4.25 years. In the wild population at Wamba, I calculate a mean length of adolescent subfecundity of 5.0 years from Kuroda's (1989) estimates of mean age at first birth (14.2 years) minus mean age at first swelling (8.5 years) minus gestation length (255 days).

Chimpanzees. In captivity, female chimpanzees reportedly have a mean period of adolescent subfecundity of 0.9 years (Young and Yerkes 1943). In four females at Gombe where menarche (first full swelling) and first birth were observed, conception occurred on average 2.4 years later (Wallis 1997). At other study sites, where menarche and first birth have not been observed in the same individuals (owing to female transfer), the time between immigration and first conception has been called the period of adolescent subfecundity. However, values calculated in this manner should be viewed as minimums since females reach menarche and start copulating before they transfer between communities. Using this method gives a median of 2.1 years at Mahale for 13 females (subtracting a 228 day gestation period [Martin et al. 1978] from Nishida et al.'s [1990] figures). At Taï, the median was 2.2 years for seven females (Boesch and Boesch-Achermann 2000) and at Kanyawara, 1.6 years for five females (Wrangham, personal communication 2000).

Age at First Birth

Orangutans. International Orangutan Studbook data show mean age at first birth in captivity over the past 50 years as 11.2 years (Markham 1995). However, it is not known how many of these animals were housed with fertile males. Thus, Markham (1995) provides a modal range of 9–9.9 years (when 20% of first parturitions occurred) as a more indicative figure. In Tilson et al. (1993), age at first birth is reported at a median of 16 years at both Tanjung Putting and Ketambe. Details about the age determination of these females is not provided, although most or all were probably not followed from birth and therefore are estimates.

Gorillas. First birth in captive lowland gorillas (some of estimated age) occurs at a mean age of 9.3 years (extrapolated from age at first conception provided by Dixson 1981). In the wild, Harcourt et al. (1981) report a median age at first parturition of 10.0 years for five females. Watts (1991) found the same 10.0 median for eight additional females in the same population.

Bonobos. In captivity, three intervals from Kuroda (1989) and 17 intervals from Thompson-Handler (1990) indicate a median age at first birth of 10.0 years. The median age at first birth for six females at Wamba (estimated ages) was 14.0 years (Kuroda 1989). However, Kuroda notes that two females over 15 years old had not yet given birth; thus, he feels that this figure will increase.

Chimpanzees. Reports from captivity place age at first birth for chimpanzees as 10.8 years (Smith et al. 1975). Kuroda (1989) reports that the earliest age at first birth in Japanese zoos was 7 years. Age at first birth is higher at all wild chimpanzee sites, although female emigration means that most ages are only estimates. Wallis (1997) reports a mean age at first birth of 13.3 years for four females at Gombe. Sugiyama (1994) reports an age at first birth of 12–14 years at Bossou, Guinea (some estimated ages). Nishida et al. (1990) place this figure at a median of 15.0 years (all estimated ages) for chimpanzees of Mahale. At Taï, Ivory Coast, the median was 14 years (all estimated ages), which includes one unusual female who did not emigrate and who gave birth at 18.5 years (Boesch and Boesch-Achermann 2000). The median for Kanyawara chimpanzees was 15.0 years (estimated ages; Wrangham, personal communication 2000).

Interbirth Intervals

Interbirth intervals can be prematurely shortened by death or removal of the first infant before it has been weaned. Unless otherwise noted, I only report intervals where the infant was known to have remained with the mother until weaning. Some authors use a Kaplan-Meier analysis, which has the advantage of taking into account long intervals that have not been completed.

Orangutans. International Studbook records give the mean interbirth interval of captive orangutans as 3.0 years. Thirty-six percent of the interbirth intervals occurred within a modal range of 1–1.9 years (Markham 1995). Lippert (1977) also reports captive orangutan interbirth intervals as less than 3 years. However, these figures do not distinguish between mothers who were allowed to rear their infants and those that had infants taken away after birth. Markham (1990) presents data for one "natural" interbirth interval for a female who remained continuously with her infant and had access to a male. Her interbirth interval was 6.3 years. In contrast, wild orangutans gave birth after a median of 7.7 years at Tanjung Putting (computed using a Kaplan-Meier analysis on 11 censored and 12 uncensored intervals; Galdikas and Wood 1990). This figure is 8.4 years for 9 intervals at Ketambe when data from one female who had a miscarriage is excluded (Utami, personal communication 2001). At Gunung Palung, Borneo, I can estimate the length of four intervals, giving a median of 7.0 years.

Gorillas. Sievert et al. (1991) surveyed gorillas in 24 captive institutions and found the median interbirth interval for mother-reared infants was 4.0 years. The median interval between surviving births for 26 intervals in wild mountain gorillas at Karisoke was 3.9 years (Watts 1991). Sievert and colleagues (1991) attribute the similarity of captive and wild interbirth intervals primarily to problems with infertility in captive gorillas. For example, Beck and Power (1988) found that only 61% of captive female gorillas in North America had given birth to a live infant. Factors accounting for this high degree of infertility in captivity have included lack of prior social experience, environmental constraints, social stress, diet, and incompatibility with the paired male (Maple and Hoff 1982; Nadler 1977). Testicular atrophy (Dixson 1981) and early sterility of males (Beck 1982) are also common.

Bonobos. Thompson-Handler (1990) surveyed the captive bonobo population and reports a mean interbirth interval of 3.6 years. These were all females who kept their infants until the birth of their next infant and were continuously housed with a male. Harvey (1997) calculates the interbirth interval for captive bonobos as 5.1 years for females who remained with their infants, but it is not clear if all of these individuals were constantly housed with a male. In the wild, Takahata et al. (1996) report a mean interbirth interval of 4.5 years at Wamba. However, Kano (1992) argues that the mean interbirth interval will end up being over 5 years. In contrast, using a Kaplan-Meier survival analysis, Barbara Fruth (personal communication, 2000) found that the median interbirth interval between 1990 and 1998 in the Eyengo community of bonobos in Lomako, Democratic Republic of the Congo, was 9.0 years.

Chimpanzees. In captivity, chimpanzees who were allowed to rear their offspring had a mean interbirth interval of 3.8 years in the Taronga Zoo in Sydney (Courtenay 1987). Similarly, a range of 3.5–4.0 years is reported from the University of Texas Chimpanzee colony (Bloomsmith, personal communication [to Wallis] 1997). Goodall's (1986) analysis of the Gombe data shows a mean interbirth interval of 5.5 years. At Mahale, Nishida et al. (1990) report a median interbirth interval of 6.0 years. Chimpanzees at Bossou had a median interbirth interval (in mothers whose first offspring survived at least 3 years) of 5.0 years (Sugiyama 1994). In Taï, the interval was a median of 5.4 years (Boesch and Boesch-Achermann 2000). The latest calculation by Wrangham (personal communication, 2000) gives a median of 6.0 years for Kanyawara using a Kaplan-Meier analysis on 11 censored and 20 uncensored intervals. A mean of 6.2 years was obtained for just uncensored intervals.

Postpartum Amenorrhea

Postpartum amenorrhea is defined here as the time between birth and the first subsequent onset of menstrual cycling. This period has also been called lactational amenorrhea. However, because lactation may extend after cycling has resumed, the former term is preferred here. Data below are for mothers with living infants.

Orangutans. In captivity, Masters and Markham (1991) monitored a female who had been suckling an infant for 4 years and showed no signs of menstruation. Another adult female did not menstruate for 4.7 years after her infant's birth (Markham 1990). In the wild, with the lack of an estrous swelling and the difficulty of detecting menstruation, this reproductive parameter is particularly hard to assess. Thus, I report here on age at first completed mating after parturition. This period has been estimated as over 6 years in the wild (Galdikas 1980). At Gunung Palung, I found that the time from birth to the first known completed mating was 4.5 years for one female (KR). This interval followed the birth of her third known infant. Another female (MR) was first seen mating after an estimated 7 years since the birth of her last offspring. Both undeveloped and developed males had attempted to mate with this female 18 months before, and thus it is possible that an earlier mating was not observed.

Gorillas. Sievert et al. (1991) found that in captive female gorillas the median length of time until first postpartum sexual behavior was 2.4 years. They attribute this to the recognized problems with breeding gorillas in captivity. Watts (1991) reports that in 23 such intervals in wild mountain gorillas the median was 3.2 years.

Bonobos. Resumption of menses following parturition for females who kept their infants was 1.3–2.7 years in captivity (Harvey 1997). However, Harvey cautions that this does not necessarily indicate regular cycling since Vervaecke and colleagues (unpublished data cited in Harvey

1997) describe the menstruation of captive bonobos as irregular for 0.3–3.1 years after parturition. Vervaecke and colleagues (unpublished data) record that the resumption of swelling was 1 month to 0.8 years after parturition. *Full* swelling occurred 0.3–1.4 years post-parturition. Kano (1989, 1992) was not able to detect menstruation but found that females at Wamba resume genital swelling and begin to copulate within one year of parturition. He speculates, however, that these cycles are nonovulatory for 3–4 years because lactation lasts until the infant is about 4 years old (Kano 1989, 1992). Thus, sexual swellings may not indicate regular cycling and ovulation in bonobos, and more precise hormonal measurements are necessary to establish this parameter.

Chimpanzees. Courtenay's (1987) study of 11 captive chimps indicated a mean postpartum amenorrhea of 2.3 years. Wallis (1997) found that at Gombe the mean length of postpartum amenorrhea in mothers with living infants was 3.9 years. Most females were still nursing when they resumed postpartum cycling (Tutin and McGinnis 1981). This period has been reported as a median of 4.6 years at Mahale (Nishida et al. 1990), 1.9 years at Taï (Boesch and Boesch-Achermann 2000), and 4.0 years at Kanyawara (Wrangham, personal communication 2000). At Mahale, wild chimpanzees normally do not show sexual swellings while lactating (Nishida et al. 1990). However, one exceptional female resumed swellings within 7 months of parturition while continuing to lactate (Takasaki et al. 1986).

Waiting Time to Conception

Following parturition and postpartum amenorrhea, the period from the resumption of regular cycles/sexual activity to the next conception is called the waiting time to conception. Data below are for mothers with living infants.

Orangutans. Lippert (1974) reports that orangutans in captivity cycle for one or two months before conception. Markham (1990) presents data for one 36-year-old female who conceived again 10 months after weaning her ninth infant. Her cycles were on average 58 days long, and she may not be representative. Galdikas (1981) describes one wild female who consorted for two months before a possible conception. A second female was seen to mate while in the process of weaning her offspring and did not get pregnant. Then, six months later during the first cycle of another consortship she apparently conceived. A third female resumed postpartum sexual activity in 1976 and did not give birth again until 1979 (Galdikas 1980). Given an 8.1-month gestation length (Markham 1995), this individual would have had a waiting time to conception of approximately 2.3

years. At Gunung Palung, I found that one female (MR) conceived after 2.5 months of sexual activity.

Gorillas. In captive gorilla mothers who raised their infants, the median length of time between sexual behavior and conception was 2.0 months (Sievert et al. 1991). In the wild, Watts (1991) reports a median of five cycles until conception for 23 females who had a surviving infant.

Bonobos. The waiting time to conception has not been reported specifically for bonobos in either captivity or the wild. However, we can determine a maximum and minimum range by subtracting the lengths of postpartum amenorrhea from the interbirth intervals (minus a gestation length of 225 days [Kuroda 1989]) reported above to obtain a mean range of 2.4–37.2 months in captivity and 0–33.6 months for the wild at Wamba. As discussed above, because of the difficulty of determining when ovulatory cycles actually resume, the waiting time to conception in bonobos cannot be reliably determined until hormonal measurements are made.

Chimpanzees. I calculated chimpanzee waiting time to conception from Courtenay's (1987) postpartum amenorrhea and interbirth interval figures, subtracting a gestation length of 228 days (Martin et al. 1978). This gives a mean waiting time to conception in captivity of 10.5 months. In the wild, the mean time between resumption of postpartum cycles and conception was 4.7 months at Gombe (Wallis 1997). Nishida et al. (1990) found that the median period between the resumption of swelling and the next birth was 16.5 months. Subtracting 228 days of gestation gives an 8.9-month waiting time. Data from Taï (Boesch and Boesch-Achermann 2000) indicate a mean of 34.5 months from resumption of cycling to birth. Subtracting gestation length gives a waiting time of 26.9 months. At Kanyawara, the waiting time can be calculated from the median interbirth interval minus the median period of postpartum amenorrhea and the length of gestation to arrive at a figure of 18.9 months.

WHAT ACCOUNTS FOR CAPTIVE VS. WILD DIFFERENCES?

The Ecological Energetics Hypothesis

The above data show a striking contrast in reproductive parameters between captive and wild populations of chimpanzees and orangutans. The captive apes of these two species have accelerated reproductive timetables for age at menarche, adolescent subfecundity, age at first birth, interbirth interval, length of postpartum amenorrhea, and waiting time to conception relative to their wild counterparts. Where sufficient data exist at more than one study site for each species, intersite variability also exists. This difference also appears to be the case in bonobos for age at first birth, but interbirth interval differences are unresolved. Reproductive parameters do not appear to differ between captive and wild gorillas, a peculiarity that will be discussed later.

What may account for this variation in reproductive parameters? What I propose here is that the recent, extensive anthropological research into human reproduction which attempts to understand ovarian function within an adaptive, ecological context (e.g., Ellison 1990, Ellison et al. 1993) provides a guiding framework with which to approach the study of reproductive variance within the great apes. As in the apes, human populations show tremendous population variability in reproductive parameters. Some of this variance is due to cultural practices, such as differences in the duration and patterning of lactation. However, a growing body of evidence suggests that outside of lactation and age, energetic differences, caused by varying local ecologies, are the major modifiers of female reproductive function (Ellison et al. 1993). Energetics plays a role both in development and in short-term modulation of reproductive function. Humans growing up under conditions of energy deficit have slower reproductive maturation, accompanied by slower overall maturation (Ellison 1990). In the short term, female ovarian function is finely modulated to respond to environmental perturbations on a continuum ranging from luteal and follicular suppression to complete amenorrhea (Ellison 1990). For example, in normal weight women with adequate fat reserves, small degrees of weight loss cause a reduction in reproductive hormones (Schweiger et al. 1987; Lager and Ellison 1990). This ovarian responsiveness is also seen in seasonal reductions in ovarian function of nonwestern women in response to short-term nutritional stress (Ellison et al. 1986; Panter-Brick et al. 1993). These studies suggest that rather than simply nutritional status or fatness per se, it is positive or negative energy balance that affects ovarian function (Ellison 1990). Furthermore, moderate levels of exercise (Ellison and Lager 1986) and heavy workload independent of weight loss (Jasienska and Ellison 1998) can reduce ovarian function in women. This ability of ovarian function to respond to energetic conditions is interpreted as an adaptive response to time reproductive effort to occur when it has the highest probability of success (Ellison et al. 1993).

In contrast, other models of primate reproduction come from studies of seasonally breeding animals in the temperate zone. In many of these mammals it appears that conception is timed so that births occur during the period of highest food production (Bronson 1989). This may be a good strategy for a temperate zone animal that lives in a highly seasonal but *predictable* environment, where the timing of high food availability can be anticipated and conception timed accordingly. But for many long-lived, tropical animals like great apes, food availability is sufficiently unpredictable that conception cannot be timed so that birth will occur during such periods (van Schaik and van Noordwijk 1985). Instead, I would predict that, just as in humans, conception is more likely to occur during periods of positive maternal energy balance in order to begin the period of intensive reproductive investment when energy availability is sufficient.

Evidence from Orangutans

To test this hypothesis, which I refer to as the "Ecological Energetics Hypothesis," I began a study of the reproductive ecology of wild orangutans in Gunung Palung National Park. In this study I tested the hypothesis that nutritional intake, energy expenditure, and energy balance have a significant effect on orangutan ovarian function.

Based on approximately 6,000 hours of observation over 14 months I found that significant changes in fruit availability were correlated with changes in nutritional intake (Knott 1997a, 1997b, 1998, 1999). These changes in availability were assessed through monthly monitoring of 558 orangutan fruit trees. From December of 1994 through February of 1995 the forest at Gunung Palung experienced a "mast fruiting" period of high flower and fruit availability. During the three months of peak fruit abundance, orangutans spent 98–100% of their feeding time eating energy-rich seeds and pulp. In contrast, when fruit availability reached a low several months later, seeds and pulp composed only 24% of the diet. The remainder was made up of 37% bark, 23% leaves, 9% pith, and 6% insects. All foods eaten by orangutans were analyzed for metabolizable energy, revealing that caloric intake was significantly higher during the mast period than in the other periods.

Activity patterns and energy expenditure varied in accordance with fluctuations in diet and fruit availability. During periods of high fruit availability, orangutans spent significantly more time foraging, but did so within a small day range. As fruit availability decreased, average day range increased as they searched for fruit over a larger area. During severe fruit shortage, however, day range shrank as orangutans fed on low quality, but abundant, bark and leaves.

The effects of these energetic changes on orangutan physiology were assessed through a number of noninvasive techniques. More than 400 urine samples were obtained from >40 orangutans by placing plastic sheets beneath individuals during urination. Ketones, a measure of fat metabolism, were present in significantly more urine samples during the non-mast period of low fruit availability. Estrone conjugates (E1C) were measured using radioimmunoassay to assess changes in ovarian function as a result of changing energetic status. Two nonpregnant females were followed extensively during periods of high and low fruit availability, and both showed a significant decrease in E1C levels during the low fruit availability period. Comparisons of weekly mean E1C values in 12 nonpregnant females showed a significant decrease in E1C when fruit availability decreased. Several conceptions also occurred during the period of high fruit availability. The importance of E1C levels for conception was shown by Masters and Markham (1991), who found that higher peak, as well as mean, levels of estrone conjugates were associated with increased fecundity of orangutan ovarian cycles in captivity. These data from the wild suggest that changes in nutritional intake and energy balance have a significant effect on orangutan ovarian function, much as they do in humans.

Does the Model Apply to Other Apes?

Intrapopulation variability. The relationship between caloric intake and hormonal functioning has not yet been studied in other wild great apes. However, other researchers have speculated about the importance of nutrition in explanations of reproductive variance in these species (Bentley 1999; Courtenay 1987; Galdikas 1995; Markham 1995; Nishida et al. 1990; Sugiyama 1994; Tutin 1994; Wallis 1995, 1997). Here I present several lines of evidence indicating that nutrition is an important modulator of reproduction in the most studied of the great apes—chimpanzees.

First, just as in orangutans, chimpanzees have an earlier age at menarche and first birth and shorter interbirth intervals in captivity than in the wild. It seems abundantly clear that this is due to energetic differences between the two conditions. Given the ready availability of food and the lower levels of energy expenditure inherent in captivity, one can logically conclude that captive apes have a more consistent and positive energetic status than their wild counterparts.

Second, Wallis (1997) points out in her review of reproductive parameters in chimpanzees at Gombe National Park that the individuals with the shortest interbirth intervals were all descendants of one female, named Flo. These family members were the most frequent visitors to the banana feeding station, and thus Wallis speculates that they may have received better nourishment. No data were available on the relative food availability in the forest when the chimpanzees came to the feeding station, but such visitation may have been important for making up any caloric deficits.

Alternatively, it may have been that Flo and her descendants had access to better foraging areas (Pusey et al. 1997). Using 35 years of field data from Gombe, Pusey et al. (1997) found that high-ranking chimpanzee females were more reproductively successful in a number of dimensions.

They reached sexual maturity sooner (which was significantly correlated with age at first birth), they had significantly higher offspring survival, their annual production of offspring surviving to weaning age was significantly greater—indicating shorter interbirth intervals, and they tended to live longer. The daughters of high-ranking females reached sexual maturity earlier owing to their higher rates of weight gain. The authors attribute these differences primarily to the ability of high-ranking females to maintain access to the best foraging areas, which gave them higher nutritional status than subordinates.

Third, Uehara and Nishida (1987) provide evidence that periods of low fruit availability are associated with negative energy balance in chimpanzees. They weighed wild chimpanzees at Mahale and found that body weights decreased when fruit was scarce. In humans, small changes in body weight are sufficient to have measurable effects on progesterone levels (Bullen et al. 1985). Lipson and Ellison (1996) found that a relatively small increase in body weight in women was associated with higher midfollicular estradiol levels, which were correlated, in turn, with conception cycles. Thus, a decline in chimpanzee energetic status during periods of low fruit availability may likewise lower their ovarian function.

Fourth, seasonality linking food availability with a variety of reproductive parameters has been found at several wild chimpanzee field sites. Conceptions are reportedly seasonal at Gombe and Mahale, with the majority occurring during the dry season (Goodall 1983, 1986; Nishida et al. 1990; Wallis 1992, 1995). Wallis (1997) found that *all* postpartum cycles that led to conception occurred during the dry season. She also reports that "paradoxically" more births in Gombe chimpanzees occurred during the wet season, which she states is the riskier time of year owing to higher rates of deaths and other health problems (Wallis 1995). Thus, chimpanzees do not time conceptions so that births occur during the optimum period.

A number of other reproductive states also peak in the late dry season at Gombe: the first full anogenital swelling in adolescents, the appearance of anogenital swellings in lactating and pregnant females, maximal swelling in cycling females (Wallis 1995), resumption of cycling after weaning (Goodall 1986), and peak number of swellings (Tutin 1975). Cycling females were more likely to show just partial swellings during the early wet season (Wallis 1995). These partial swellings probably reflect low or insufficient levels of the ovarian hormones necessary for reproduction. This assertion is based on Emery and Whitten's (in review) work, which has shown strong correlations between the size of sexual swellings and levels of estrogen and progesterone.

A similar seasonal pattern is reported by Nishida et al. (1990) from Mahale, where first sexual swellings after postpartum amenorrhea occurred significantly more often during the late dry season (September–October). These authors point out that this is also when the food supply increases, and they suggest that the first postpartum swelling is triggered by increased food availability. Uehara and Nishida (1987) show that body weights increased between the early and late dry seasons. Births showed a significant bimodal distribution, with peaks in May and January. While the January peak is unexplained, the May birth peak suggests a late dry season conception peak in September coincident with the increased food supply (Nishida et al. 1990).

What is happening during the dry season to influence reproductive physiology? These data strongly suggest an ecological effect because of the influence of season on the timing of female swellings in all reproductive stages: cycling, lactation, pregnancy, menarche, and postpartum resumption of cycles. Reproductive events are spread throughout the year but concentrate during this time. Is there evidence that the dry season in Gombe and Mahale is associated with greater food availability? First, the dry season has larger party sizes than the wet season (Nishida 1974; Sakura 1994; Wrangham 1977). In turn, at all major chimpanzee field sites there is an observed relationship between party size and food abundance, (Boesch 1996; Chapman et al. 1995; Goodall 1986; Nishida 1974; Sakura 1994; Wrangham 1986, 2000). These larger group sizes during the dry season are also associated with the presence of females with sexual swellings (Riss and Busse 1977; Wallis and Matama 1993; Wrangham 2000). Thus, the dry season is associated with increased food abundance, larger party sizes, and a greater number of maximally swollen females.

To test this relationship in chimpanzees further, data are needed on hormonal functioning, fluctuations in preferred foods, the caloric content of those foods, and ideally, actual differences in caloric intake and energy balance. Thus, we must look to future fine-grained studies of individuals within populations that incorporate both nutritional and hormonal information to investigate this hypothesis in chimpanzees. In addition, as suggested by Nishida et al. (1990), because nutrition is important in regulating chimpanzee reproductive events, quantification of seasonal changes in food supply is needed. I have focused here primarily on nutritional intake and energy balance. Investigation of differences in energetic expenditure between and within the great apes also warrants further inquiry, although we may not find the kinds of extreme energetic expenditure found in some human populations with heavy workloads.

Interpopulation variability. Between-site comparisons are also intriguing, particularly in chimpanzees for which a good deal of data exist. Bossou, for example, has the shortest interbirth intervals and Kanyawara has the longest. Sugiyama (1994) attributes this to differences in food availability between Bossou and the other sites. Boesch and Boesch-Achermann (2000) found that Taï chimpanzee females have increased infant survivorship with longer interbirth intervals and thus speculate that different chimpanzee populations may be adapted to different infant mortality rates. Wrangham et al. (1996) speculate that the low reproductive rate of Kanyawara chimpanzees may be due to greater fruit scarcity and heavier reliance on fallback foods such as figs and terrestrial herbaceous vegetation. However, the Kanyawara chimpanzees are relatively large and do not appear to suffer from seasonal weight loss.

As more data are collected these apparent study site differences are narrowing. An initial estimate of the interbirth interval at Bossou was 4.2 years (Sugiyama 1989) whereas the most recent analysis puts it at 5.1 years (Sugiyama 1994). At the other extreme, in Kanyawara, the early estimate of interbirth intervals was 7.2 years (Wrangham et al. 1996), but with the addition of more intervals the figure has fallen to 6.0 years (Wrangham, personal communication 2000). Additionally, the length of postpartum amenorrhea and the waiting time to conception are also quite markedly variable between sites, with Taï being particularly relevant (Table 18.1). It remains to be seen whether these differences are real or just differences in definition. Clearly, detailed studies that examine hormonal levels and energetics in the wild are needed to investigate these interpopulation differences.

In bonobos, the difference in interbirth intervals between the two wild study sites is striking. As with chimpanzees, these differences may narrow with additional sampling; alternatively, they may reflect real differences between the sites. Two possibilities come to mind. First, the bonobos at Wamba are provisioned for 2 to 3 months each year (Kano 1992), which would be expected to result in improved nutritional status. Alternatively, Kano (1992) attributes the good nutritional status of Wamba bonobos to a decrease in human pressure since the initiation of the study. He argues that without the threat from humans, bonobos are now able to forage at will in preferred locations from which they were previously restricted by human presence.

Gorillas. Finally, what can we make of the interesting finding that gorillas do not appear to have faster reproductive timetables in captivity? Tutin (1994) suggests that the similarity in reproductive parameters between wild and captive gorillas indicates that they are reproducing up to their species potential in the wild. Wild mountain gorillas subsist primarily on readily available herbs and vegetation and no seasonality in births or conceptions has been discovered (Watts 1998), suggesting that wild mountain gorillas may not suffer the same intensity of food shortage found in orangutans and chimpanzees (Tutin 1994). Alternatively, the problems with captive breeding in gorillas (Beck 1982; Beck and Power 1988; Maple and Hoff 1982; Nadler 1982; Sievert et al. 1991; Watts 1990) may have resulted in a lengthening of these reproductive variables in captivity. Because captive researchers see these difficulties as a constraint on gorilla reproduction, it is difficult to know if they are really breeding at their full "captive potential." Comparable data on wild western lowland gorillas are not yet available.

Alternative Explanations

Immigration Stress Hypothesis.   Several alternative hypotheses have been put forward to explain variation in great ape reproductive parameters. Nishida et al. (1990) note that the period of adolescent subfecundity is longer at Mahale than at Gombe. They tie this to the finding that female chimpanzees at Mahale are much more likely to emigrate than are Gombe females and suggest that Mahale females have longer periods of adolescent subfecundity owing to increased stress from immigration. However, even *resident* Mahale females who are no longer experiencing the stress of immigration have longer periods of postpartum amenorrhea, waiting time to conception, and interbirth intervals than do Gombe chimpanzees. The fact that these other reproductive parameters are extended in Mahale females does not support the immigration stress hypothesis. An alternative explanation is that Gombe chimpanzees that remain in their natal group have better access to and better knowledge of local food resources.

Critical Fatness Hypothesis.   Tutin (1994) suggests that the critical fatness hypothesis postulated by Frisch and Revelle (1970) for humans may apply to menarche in chimpanzees. However, as Ellison (1981, 1982) has shown, menarche in humans is better predicted by increase in skeletal maturation than by attaining a certain fatness level. Both, of course, may be directly influenced by nutrition, but in humans there does not appear to be a critical level of body fat at which females either start or stop menstruating (Ellison 1990). It appears more likely that positive or negative changes in weight (energy balance), rather than a critical level of fatness, influence reproductive function.

Reproductive Synchrony Hypothesis.   Wallis (1997) proposes that there may be an *indirect* influence of food availability on chimpanzee ovarian function—the effect of social contact on menstrual synchronization in females. She suggests that owing to larger feeding parties in the dry season, more females would be associating with each other and stimulating each other to cycle. However, even if females are likely to synchronize with each other (Wallis 1985, 1992), this would not necessarily influence their *levels* of ovarian hormones or the probability of conception. As suggested earlier, a more likely explanation is that larger feeding parties and the presence of females with sexual swellings are both correlated with greater food availability, the latter as a result of improved energy availability.

Phytoestrogen Hypothesis. Wallis (1997) has also suggested ingestion of plant estrogens as a possible explanation for seasonal variation in reproduction. However, no phytochemical studies have been conducted on chimpanzee (or other ape) foods. Additionally, given the strong association between food availability and reproduction in humans, orangutans, and chimpanzees, it is difficult to accept this association as a spurious correlation and argue that the ingestion of phytoestrogens is the causal agent. Radically different diets and plant species are eaten by humans and the other apes, and it is unlikely that a phytochemical in each of these diets is responsible for this relationship.

Competition Hypothesis. Watts (1990, 1991) suggests that social factors might affect reproduction since birth rates in gorillas decline with increasing group size, apparently because of competition between females for access to adult males. However, it may not be competitive stress per se that affects ovarian function but the energetic consequences of competition. For example, increased competition for mates or food may negatively impact female nutritional intake and result in lower ovarian function. Thus, it may not be competition itself, but the interaction between competition and energetics, that affects reproductive functioning.

Photoperiod Hypothesis. Photoperiod is thought to be the primary reproductive cue for many temperate zone mammals (Tamarkin et al. 1985). However, photoperiod is not a likely regulator of reproductive events in tropical apes because day length only varies slightly throughout the year in the equatorial regions where apes are found. For example, at Gombe, Tanzania, there is just a 36 minute annual variation in photoperiod (Wallis 1995). Photoperiod varies even less in sites closer to the equator. Temperate zone animals may use photoperiod as a proxy measure of upcoming changes in food availability, but this is not a predictor of food availability in tropical forests. It is thus unlikely to be a factor regulating ape reproduction.

Interspecies Comparisons

Ecological Energetics Hypothesis. I have focused primarily on what may cause variation in reproductive patterns *within* a given species. However, the Ecological Energetics Hypothesis may ultimately be important in explaining differences *among* ape species as well. The degree of predictability in the food supply may be one of the factors that led to the evolution of differences in the apes' reproductive parameters (Tutin 1994). This can be seen by comparing gorillas, on one end of the food predictability spectrum, with orangutans, on the other. Although there is variability in the fruit supply eaten by gorillas (Goldsmith 1999), their more regular consumption of leaves and other herbaceous vegetation means that their diet does not fluctuate as much in quality as does the more fruit-rich diet of chimpanzees and orangutans. Owing to mast fruiting in Southeast Asia, orangutans are subject to the greatest fluctuations in fruit availability among the apes (Knott 1999). Thus, the species with the greatest variability in food resources (orangutans) has the longest interbirth interval whereas the species with the most predictable food supply (gorillas) has the shortest. Western lowland gorillas incorporate significantly more fruit in their diet than do mountain gorillas (Goldsmith 1999); it will be interesting to see how this difference affects the reproductive parameters of these western populations when such data become known.

Tutin (1994) makes the argument that the greater demands of chimpanzee infants, particularly infant carrying, help explain why they have longer interbirth intervals than gorillas. I would argue that this is consistent with the Ecological Energetics Hypothesis—that the constraints imposed by infant carrying and investment have an energetic cost that affects the interbirth interval. This may be especially true for orangutans. Orangutans, with their almost exclusive use of the canopy (particularly by females), may bear heavier energetic costs than gorillas or chimpanzees because of arboreal infant carrying. This may constrain their ranging patterns and their ability to sample more widely dispersed foods. Mountain gorilla mothers with their readily abundant, terrestrial food supply may not be as constrained by infant travel and may be able to range more easily without this encumberment. Fossey (1979) reports that once gorillas reach age two they are carried very little by their mothers. Orangutans at least occasionally carry their infants up to age 7 or older (Knott, personal observation). Similarly, Wrangham (2000) has proposed that the travel costs imposed on females by traveling with and carrying infants may be a critical factor in explaining grouping differences between bonobos and chimpanzees. Thus, since the degree of infant carrying varies among the ape species we can expect it to be a factor in maternal energetics.

While I argue that energetic factors are particularly important in determining great ape reproductive parameters, other hypothesis are discussed below.

Paternal Investment Hypothesis. Galdikas and Wood (1990) point out that the average interbirth interval in the great apes is negatively associated with paternal investment. They argue that male gorillas invest by protecting their offspring from infanticide, and chimpanzee males may occasionally share food with females and thus indirectly invest in offspring. Chimpanzee males also engage in border patrols that can help protect young from infanticidal neighbors. Orangutan juveniles, on the other hand, receive no direct or indirect paternal care. Galdikas and Wood (1990:190) thus suggest that "differences in paternal investment may have an important effect on the pace of reproduction."

Cost of Vigilance Hypothesis. Tutin (1994) argues that chimpanzee mothers, compared with gorilla mothers, must bear greater costs of vigilance against infanticide which contributes to longer interbirth intervals in chimpanzees. However, consideration of orangutans indicates that the cost of vigilance is probably not a very good explanation for differences in interbirth intervals. Orangutans have the longest interbirth intervals and yet engage in almost no vigilant behavior (Setiawan et al. 1996).

Immigration Stress Hypothesis—between ape species. Tutin (1994) argues that a version of the "Immigration Stress Hypothesis" may account for shorter interbirth intervals and earlier age at menarche and first birth in gorillas compared with chimpanzees. She argues that female immigration into a new group is more stressful for chimpanzees than it is for gorillas, thus delaying the onset of fertile cycles and causing a high rate of first pregnancy loss. When orangutans are brought into this comparison, however, this explanation falters since orangutans have longer interbirth intervals than either of these other apes and yet they do not have to face any stresses related to immigration into a new social group.

Suckling Hypothesis. Galdikas and Wood (1990) propose that the suckling period may be longer in orangutans than in the other great apes, which may account for the variance in interbirth interval between them. In humans, maternal nutritional status may modulate the length of the suckling period (Perez-Escamilla et al. 1995). Thus, if differences in suckling do exist among the apes, these differences may again relate to basic ecological differences between species. The long lactation period in orangutans may be due to negative female energetic status caused by extended periods of low fruit availability. An additional factor here is the availability of fallback foods for young apes. Fallback foods, in particular bark eaten by orangutans, may be more difficult to access and process by juveniles than the terrestrial herbaceous vegetation relied upon by chimpanzees during fruit scarcity. Thus, orangutan juveniles may need to suckle for a longer period given the inadequacy of their diet during fruit-poor periods. Mountain gorillas show very little variation in their standard herbaceous diet (Watts 1998).

Finally, there is no reason to assume that all apes should have the same reproductive timetables. Different environmental and social conditions in each species have undoubtedly selected for different reproductive potentials. Investigation of these factors is an important step in our understanding of ape evolution and will be a fruitful area for future comparative inquiry. What we now know is that apes and humans appear to have many similarities in the way reproduction responds to ecological conditions. We have just begun to investigate reproductive ecology in the apes (Bentley 1999), and future studies will reveal the extent to which these responses are shared across species and with humans. Below I discuss how knowledge of the mechanisms that regulate ape reproduction can help us understand human evolution.

IMPLICATIONS FOR HUMAN EVOLUTION

Compared with the other great apes, humans have the shortest interbirth intervals. Studies of natural fertility populations have reported median interbirth intervals of 3.4 years for the !Kung of South Africa (Howell 1979), 3.0 years for the Gainj of Papua New Guinea (Wood 1994), 2.8 years for the Matlab of Bangladesh (Wood 1994), 1.6 years for the Hutterites (a North American Anabaptist sect; Wood 1994), and approximately 3.0 years for the Hadza of Tanzania (Frank Marlowe, personal communication 2000). Depending on local ecological constraints, the optimal interbirth interval may vary among these different populations (Blurton Jones 1993), but all natural fertility human societies appear to have interbirth intervals that are shorter than those found among wild great apes.

In apes, the interbirth interval represents the period during which the offspring is nutritionally dependent on its mother. This is accomplished through lactation, which eventually tapers off as juvenile apes gradually incorporate other foods in their diet. Once nursing is over juvenile apes are, for the most part, nutritionally independent. Although there may be occasional food sharing and juveniles may continue to stay close to their mothers and learn from them, ape mothers do not directly provide nourishment to more than one offspring at a time. This is not the case with humans. Humans are characterized by having overlapping, nutritionally dependent offspring (Lancaster and Lancaster 1983). We do this by providing nutrition outside of lactation to our offspring. We can nurse an infant, have a four-year-old to whom we are providing weaning foods, and have an eight-year-old who helps to collect and prepare food but is still reliant on adults to meet some of his or her nutritional needs. We have thus broken from the anthropoid pattern of only being able to provide nutritionally for one offspring at a time.

Human children have the longest period of juvenile dependency of any of the apes, but the shortest period of lactation. Draper and Cashdan (1988) report that !Kung childhood lasts from about 5 to 15 years during which time they rarely forage and derive almost all of their food from adults. Among the Hadza of northern Tanzania, children over 8 sometimes help their mothers gather and children left in camp can sometimes forage on their own when the food supply is rich (Blurton Jones 1993), but children still rely heavily on adult assistance. Thus, if humans were to follow the great ape pattern, supplementing offspring nutrition with lactation and not conceiving again until juveniles were totally nutritionally independent, we would expect 10- to 15-year interbirth intervals—a severe constraint on human reproductive potential.

How have humans managed to have the shortest interbirth interval of any of the apes and yet the longest period of juvenile dependency? Insight derived from human and ape reproductive ecology can help us understand how early hominids may have moved from an apelike pattern to the human pattern we see today. Studies of human and ape reproductive ecology suggest that ovarian hormonal levels can be increased and interbirth interval shortened by improving female energetic status: in other words, by increasing nutritional intake, decreasing energy expenditure, or both. Any changes that ameliorated the energetic burden on human females would have had important reproductive consequences.

In addition to maternal condition, the length of the interbirth interval is also governed by the needs of dependent offspring. Suckling is very energetically costly to mothers and has a suppressive effect, at least in the initial stages, on female ovarian function. It is the primary factor influencing the length of interbirth interval (Valeggia and Ellison, chapter 4, this volume). Thus, any changes that would have shortened the period of suckling would also have had a direct effect on interbirth intervals.

Thus, I propose here that a critical suite of hominid adaptations involved finding ways to extract more energy from the environment in order to reduce female energetic burdens and shorten the period of lactational dependence of juveniles on their mothers. A number of authors have recently explored ways in which early hominids were able to overcome the nutritional constraints operating on other apes (Aiello and Wheeler 1995; Conklin-Brittain et al. in press; Leonard and Robertson 1997; Milton 1987; Wrangham et al. 1999). These arguments, however, have not focused on the consequences of increased energy efficiency on female reproductive physiology and the spacing of births.

When might this transition have occurred? Australopithecines were probably similar to great apes in many of their life history characteristics (Smith 1992); thus it is unlikely that the human pattern had emerged at that time, although it is possible that incipient changes could already have appeared. Conklin-Brittain et al. (in press) argue that the first stage in a transition to improved dietary quality occurred with the exploitation of roots, and reduced dietary fiber in australopithecines. If australopithecines exploited roots that were difficult for juveniles to access (O'Connell et al. 1999) there may have been increased food sharing between mothers and offspring. Conklin-Brittain et al. (in press) suggest that australopithecines had an improved dietary quality relative to chimpanzees that set the stage for further improvements in dietary quality with the advent of *Homo*. The emergence of *Homo*, or more specifically *Homo erectus* at 1.9 mya, has been postulated as representing a major shift in evolutionary strategy and increased dietary quality (Aiello and Wheeler 1995; Wrangham et al. 1999). The genus *Homo* is associated with increased body size, reduced sexual dimorphism, reduction in dentition (Walker and Leakey 1993), increased brain size (Holloway 1979), and the presence of flaked stone tools and cut-marked bones (Klein 1984) among other features. I would propose that a shift towards shorter interbirth intervals was part of this complex of new behaviors emerging at that time.

A suite of behaviors that can be inferred to have emerged with early *Homo* would have had a significant impact on interbirth interval: (1) exploitation of new foods; (2) development of new methods of food acquisition and processing—in particular, cooking; (3) provisioning and introduction of appropriate weaning foods; and (4) changes in social structure with an increase in non-maternal child care. These changes would have allowed hominid females to successfully shorten their interbirth intervals and would have permitted, for the first time, the occurrence of overlapping, nutritionally dependent offspring. Furthermore, I argue that rather than being just a *consequence* of changing hominid behavior, decreasing interbirth interval, increasing fertility, and increasing juvenile survivorship could themselves have been selective forces driving the changes seen in the *Homo* clade.

Exploitation of New Foods

The transition between an apelike ancestor and modern *Homo sapiens* has been punctuated by periods of environmental change in which the climate became cooler, drier, and perhaps more seasonal—thereby either forcing or enabling early hominids to shift into new habitats and exploit new dietary resources (O'Connell et al. 1999). Humans have much higher-quality diets (defined as lower in fiber) than do other apes (Conklin-Brittain et al. in press). This is associated with an overall reduction in gut size (Aiello and Wheeler 1995), an enlarged small intestine, and a shortened colon relative to apes (Milton 1999). Aiello and Wheeler (1995) propose that this shift in dietary quality allowed for more energy to be diverted to brain development. Increased energy availability may also have been important in the increase in overall body size, particularly in females, which is seen in the transition between australopithecines and *Homo erectus* (Wrangham et al. 1999). However, an as-yet-overlooked aspect of this increased energetic efficiency would have been its positive effect on maternal energy reserves and hence female ovarian function.

What dietary changes would have provided increased energy availability for females? Two food sources have been proposed as critical in this transition: meat (e.g., Dart 1953; Milton 1999; Washburn and Lancaster 1968) and tubers (O'Connell et al. 1999; Wrangham et al. 1999). Supporters of the meat-eating hypothesis draw attention to evidence of increased reliance on hunting within the *Homo* genus. The tuber argument looks to the prevalence of underground storage organs, which were a relatively unexploited and reliable food source, on the African plains (O'Connell et al. 1999; Wrangham et al. 1999). The critical feature of both foods is that they are easily digestible and could have lowered the fiber content of the diet, thus improving female energetic status.

Changes in Tool Use: Food Acquisition and Food Preparation

The ability of hominids to exploit these new foods would have been contingent upon the development of technologies to extract and process them. Indeed, the advent of *Homo* is accompanied by a huge increase in the variety and sophistication of tools found in the archaeological record (Klein 1984). In the meat-eating scenario, the development of weapons for hunting and tools for processing of animals, including those for extracting bone marrow, would have greatly opened up this food resource to hominid exploitation.

Tools would also have been extremely important in the acquisition and processing of plant foods such as tubers. O'Connell et al. (1999) argue that stone tools found after 2.5 mya would have been suitable for making digging sticks. Perhaps most important is the possible advent of cooking at this time, fully elaborated upon by Wrangham et al. (1999) and supported by O'Connell et al. (1999) as well. Cooking greatly increases the digestibility of foods and would have been a significant way that hominids were able to increase energy availability. Wrangham et al. (1999) argue that cooking increases energy intake to a greater extent than does the replacement of plants in the diet with meat.

Changes in food and feeding technologies are also evidenced in the dentition of early hominids. Several of the earliest *Homo* species have quite enlarged dentition, similar to that of the australopithecines (Walker and Leakey 1993). This gradually evolved to the reduced dentition seen in *Homo erectus*. Food processing techniques, in particular cooking, could have reduced the emphasis on oral preparation of the food and selected for this reduced dentition (Wrangham et al. 1999). Other techniques such as grinding and pounding could also have been important.

Such new methods of food acquisition and preparation would have been essential in enabling these hominids to shift to a more energy-rich diet. The effect of tools on increasing the efficiency of food processing and enhancing female energetic status is also suggested by studies of chimpanzees. For example, Bossou, one of the nutcracking sites, has the shortest interbirth intervals.

Provisioning and Introduction of Weaning Foods

All human societies provide food to dependent offspring and prepare some sort of special weaning foods. In contrast, apes rarely share food with dependent offspring and provide no special "transition" foods. The human ability to provide foods to juveniles would have allowed mothers to stop nursing sooner and thus shorten their interbirth intervals. Galdikas and Wood (1990) also suggest that supplementation may have resulted in shorter interbirth intervals in humans. O'Connell et al. (1999) propose that it was primarily the labor of grandmothers that enabled this pattern of provisioning. However, although the labor of grandmothers could have helped, I argue that it is primarily the labor reduction for mothers themselves from the use of new tools and the exploitation of new, superior foods that would have been central to shortening the interbirth interval.

Milton (1987, 1999) and others (Dart 1953; Washburn and Lancaster 1968) have argued that meat was the important new food addition with *Homo*. Meat may have been an important weaning food. Moir (1994) points out that all mammals are initially carnivorous—subsisting at first solely on mother's milk. Single plant foods are inadequate for juvenile growth because they are deficient in certain amino acids and vitamins (Moir 1994). This can be remedied through eating a diverse plant diet, but meat consumption is an even more efficient solution. Meat provides the full complement of amino acids needed by growing children. It would not be necessary for children to consume great quantities of this food, but small portions (as seen for Hadza children; Frank Marlowe, personal communication 2000) could have been an important dietary supplement. Marrow could also have served this purpose. The increased digestibility of cooked meat would have made it even more accessible to young children.

The incorporation of new foods and new food processing techniques could have been important for preparing plant foods for weanlings as well. Cooking food and thus making it more digestible would have allowed juveniles to be weaned onto adult plant foods much more quickly than if these same foods were consumed in their natural, whole state.

Study of a more recent human subsistence transition, between hunting and gathering and agriculture, provides an analogy for what might have changed in human evolution. Buikstra et al. (1986) argue that the development of large, thin-walled cooking vessels facilitated the cooking of starchy weaning foods, enabling native populations in the American Southwest to wean their children onto maize at an earlier age. This transition between hunting-gathering and agriculture has been associated with a decrease in interbirth interval (Bentley et al. 1993), thus providing a historic model for how technological change could have reduced interbirth interval during earlier hominid evolution.

O'Connell et al. (1999) propose that the trend towards a cooler/drier climate around 1.8 mya led to seasonal reductions in the plant foods easily available to juveniles, which then led to the provisioning of juveniles, particularly by grandmothers. Again, grandmothers may have assisted, but I argue that the primary focus should be on what mothers themselves did to improve their energetic status and reduce their own interbirth intervals.

One of the commonalties of the meat and tuber/plant food arguments for weaning foods is that juveniles would not have been able to obtain these foods solely by themselves. Manufacture of stone tools, hunting, and animal carcass preparation would be beyond the scope of young children. Similarly, most tubers would have required the manufacture and use of a digging stick. Cooking also requires adult involvement. O'Connell et al. (1999) point to their experiences among the Hadza, where young children require adult assistance to start a fire.

Thus the use of new foods, application of new technologies, and preparation of weaning foods were dramatic breakthroughs that enabled early hominids to (1) increase the energetic quality of the diet and thus female energetic status and (2) allow a woman to wean her offspring sooner than an ape mother normally would. These two biological consequences of changing feeding technology would have enabled a female to resume full fecundity more quickly than she would if she were more energetically stressed or had a longer period of obligate lactation. Thus, interbirth interval could have shortened at the same time as juvenile dependency increased.

Changes in Social Structure

In all the great apes, care of offspring rests primarily with females. Except for a few examples of paternal care, such as gorillas protecting offspring from infanticide, other adults do not actively assist a mother in raising her young. Ape females are unable to invest nutritionally in multiple dependent offspring. Shorter interbirth intervals and longer periods of juvenile dependency in humans would have had to be coupled with changes in group structure that would allow females to care for these closely spaced dependent offspring. The precise social structure of early hominids is unknown, but sexual dimorphism is clearly reduced between the australopithecines and later *Homo*. This implies multimale/multifemale groups rather than the single male breeding systems associated with pronounced sexual dimorphism. Wrangham et al. (1999) suggest that this is the period when the human mating system of pair bonds enmeshed within multimale, multifemale communities (Rodseth et al. 1990) first came into being. Hrdy (1999) argues that humans are "cooperative breeders" in order to meet the needs of offspring care. Regardless of the exact nature of the social structure, maternal support from a male partner, female relatives, or other group members would clearly have been essential to this adaptation.

CONCLUSION

From comparative studies of great apes we can see that energetics plays a central role in regulating reproductive parameters. Now we can project how they might have affected early hominid reproductive ecology. Ape females are more heavily constrained by the needs of dependent offspring than are humans. Our technological and social adaptations have allowed us to have phenomenal reproductive success. We have moved into almost all imaginable environments and increased our numbers at exponential rates. This could not have been accomplished if humans had retained an apelike interbirth interval and the need for one offspring to be nutritionally independent before producing the next. Once some individuals exploited new foods or processed existing foods in new ways, the resultant increase in dietary quality would have had dramatic effects on interbirth intervals. The cooking of plant foods, possibly tubers, is one likely candidate for this new resource. The consumption of some quantity of meat or marrow may have been an important weaning supplement as well.

Thus, changes in foods consumed, the development of technology for processing them, and the introduction of weaning foods would have had dramatic effects on female energetics, juvenile nutritional dependency, and the interbirth interval. First, it would have increased the energetic quality of the human diet, having a net positive effect on female energetic status. This would have improved female reproductive condition and allowed females to recoup energetic investment in offspring more quickly. Second, for the first time it would have allowed a hominoid to provision offspring outside of lactation. Third, the associated reduction in sexual dimorphism and a postulated change in social structure would have made the care of these closely spaced, dependent offspring feasible. Ultimately,

I see this complex of hominid adaptations as an important driving force in human evolution through their effects on female energetics and reductions in interbirth interval.

I would like to thank Peter Ellison for asking me to contribute to this volume and for his encouragement to extend the field of reproductive ecology to the study of apes. I am grateful to Richard Wrangham, Barbara Fruth, Christophe Boesch, and Suci Utami for providing their unpublished data to me. Lori Perkins at Zoo Atlanta and Lisa Ellis at the Milwaukee Zoo helped provide data on captive apes. Catherine Smith, Melissa Emery, and Tim Laman provided valuable comments on the manuscript. I also thank the Directorate of Nature Conservation (PHPA) for permission to conduct research in Gunung Palung National Park and the Indonesian Institute of Sciences (LIPI), the Center for Research and Development in Biology, and PHPA for their sponsorship. Grants from the National Geographic Society, the L.S.B. Leakey Foundation, the National Science Foundation, the Wenner-Gren Foundation, the Conservation, Food and Health Foundation and Harvard University made my field research in Gunung Palung possible.

REFERENCES

Aiello LC, Wheeler P (1995) The expensive tissue hypothesis: the brains and the digestive system in human and primate evolution. *Current Anthropology* 36:199–221.

Asano M (1967) A note on the birth and rearing of an orang-utan *Pongo pygmaeus* at Tama Zoo, Tokyo. *International Zoo Yearbook* 7:95–96.

Beck BB (1982) Fertility in North American lowland gorillas. *American Journal of Primatology* (Suppl. 1):7–11.

Beck BB, Power ML (1988) Correlates of sexual and maternal competence in captive gorillas. *Zoo Biology* 7:339–350.

Bentley GR (1999) Aping our ancestors: comparative aspects of reproductive ecology. *Evolutionary Anthropology* 7:175–185.

Bentley GR, Goldberg T, Jasienska G (1993) The fertility of agricultural and non-agricultural traditional societies. *Population Studies* 47:269–281.

Blurton Jones N (1993) The lives of hunter-gatherer children: effects of parental behavior and parental reproductive strategy. In ME Pereira, LA Fairbanks (Eds) *Juvenile Primates: Life History, Development, and Behavior* (New York, Oxford University Press), 309–326.

Boesch C (1996) Social grouping in Taï chimpanzees. In WC McGrew, LF Marchant, T Nishida (Eds) *Great Ape Societies* (Cambridge, Cambridge University Press), 101–113.

Boesch C, Boesch-Achermann H (2000) *The Chimpanzees of the Taï Forest: Behavioural Ecology and Evolution* (New York, Oxford University Press).

Bronson FH (1989) *Mammals and Reproductive Biology* (Chicago, University of Chicago Press).

Buikstra JE, Konigsberg LW, Bullington J (1986) Fertility and the development of agriculture in the prehistoric Midwest. *American Antiquity* 51:528–546.

Bullen BA, Skrinar GS, Beitins IZ, vonMering G, Turnball BA, McArthur JW (1985) Induction of menstrual disorders by strenuous exercise in untrained women. *New England Journal of Medicine* 312:1349–1353.

Chapman CA, Wrangham RW, Chapman LJ (1995) Ecological constraints on group size: an analysis of spider monkey and chimpanzee subgroups. *Behavioral Ecology and Sociobiology* 36:59–70.

Conklin-Brittain NL, Wrangham R, Smith CC (in press) A two-stage model of increased dietary quality in early hominid evolution: the role of fiber. In *Human Diet: Perspectives on Its Origin and Evolution* (Greenwood Publications).

Courtenay J (1987) Post-partum amenorrhoea, birth intervals and reproductive potential in captive chimpanzees. *Primates* 28:543–546.

Dart RA (1953) The predatory transition from ape to man. *International Anthropological and Linguistic Review* 1:201–218.

Dixson AF (1981) *The Natural History of the Gorilla* (New York, Columbia University Press).

Draper P, Cashdan E (1988) Technological change and child behavior among the !Kung. *Ethnology* 27:339–365.

Ellison PT (1981) Threshold hypotheses, developmental age, and menstrual function. *American Journal of Physical Anthropology* 54:337–340.

Ellison PT (1982) Skeletal growth, fatness and menarcheal age: a comparison of two hypotheses. *Human Biology* 54:269–281.

Ellison PT (1990) Human ovarian function and reproductive ecology: new hypotheses. *American Anthropologist* 92:952–993.

Ellison PT, Lager C (1986) Moderate recreational running is associated with lowered salivary progesterone profiles in women. *American Journal of Obstetrics and Gynecology* 154:1000–1003.

Ellison PT, Panter-Brick C, Lipson SF, O'Rourke MT (1993) The ecological context of human ovarian function. *Human Reproduction* 8:2248–2258.

Ellison PT, Peacock NR, Lager C (1986) Salivary progesterone and luteal function in two low-fertility populations of northeast Zaire. *Human Biology* 58:204–207.

Emery MA, Whitten PL (in review) Size of sexual swellings reflects ovarian function in chimpanzees (*Pan troglodytes*).

Fossey D (1979) Development of the mountain gorilla (*Gorilla gorilla beringei*): the first thirty-six months. In DL Hamburg, ER McCown (Eds) *The Great Apes* (London, WA Benjamin), 139–186.

Frisch RE, Revelle R (1970) Height and weight at menarche and a hypothesis of critical body weights and adolescent events. *Science* 169:397–399.

Galdikas BMF (1980) Living with the great orange apes. *National Geographic Magazine* 157:860–852.

Galdikas BMF (1981) Orangutan reproduction in the wild. In CE Graham (Ed) *Reproductive Biology of the Great Apes* (New York, Academic Press), 281–300.

Galdikas BMF (1995) Social and reproductive behavior of wild adolescent female orangutans. In RD Nadler, BFM Galdikas, LK Sheeran, N Rosen (Eds) *The Neglected Ape* (New York, Plenum Press), 163–182.

Galdikas BMF, Wood JW (1990) Birth spacing patterns in humans and apes. *American Journal of Physical Anthropology* 83:185–191.

Goldsmith ML (1999) Ecological constraints on the foraging effort of western gorillas (*Gorilla gorilla gorilla*) at Bai Hokou, Central African Republic. *International Journal of Primatology* 20:1–23.

Goodall J (1983) Population dynamics during a 15-year period in one community of free-living chimpanzees in the Gombe National Park, Tanzania. *Zeischrift für Tierpsychologie* 1–60.

Goodall J (1986) *The Chimpanzees of Gombe: Patterns of Behavior* (Cambridge, Harvard University Press).

Harcourt AH, Fossey D, Stewart KJ, Watts DP (1980) Reproduction in wild gorillas and some comparisons with chimpanzees. In RV Short, BJ Weir (Eds) *The Great Apes of Africa. Journal of Reproduction and Fertility* (Suppl 28):59–70.

Harcourt AH, Stewart KJ, Fossey D (1981) Gorilla reproduction in the wild. In CE Graham (Ed) *Reproductive Biology of the Great Apes* (New York, Academic Press), 265–279.

Harvey NC (1997) Gestation, parturition, interbirth intervals, and lactational recovery in bonobos. In J Mills, G Reinartz, H De Bois, L Van Elsacker, B Van Puijenbroeck (Eds) *The Care and Management of Bonobos in Captive Environments* (Milwaukee, Zoological Society of Milwaukee County), 6.1–6.11.

Holloway RL (1979) Brain size, allometry, and reorganization: toward a synthesis. In ME Hahn, C Jenson, BC Dudek (Eds) *Development and Evolution of Brain Size* (New York, Academic Press), 61–88.

Howell N (1979) *Demography of the Dobe !Kung* (New York, Academic Press).

Hrdy SB (1999) *Mother Nature* (New York, Pantheon Books).

Jasienska G, Ellison P (1998) Physical work causes suppression of ovarian function in women. *Proceedings of the Royal Society of London*, B 265:1847–1851.

Kano T (1989) The sexual behavior of pygmy chimpanzees. In PG Heltne, LA Marquardst (Eds) *Understanding Chimpanzees* (Cambridge, Harvard University Press), 176–183.

Kano T (1992) *The Last Ape: Pygmy Chimpanzee Behavior and Ecology* (Stanford, Stanford University Press).

Klein RG (1984) *The Human Career: Human Biological and Cultural Origins* (Chicago, University of Chicago Press).

Knott CD (1996) Field collection and preservation of urine in orangutans and chimpanzees. *Tropical Biodiversity* 4:95–102.

Knott CD (1997a) The effects of changes in food availability on diet, activity, and hormonal patterns in wild Bornean orangutans *(Pongo pgymaeus). American Journal of Physical Anthropology* 24 (Suppl):145.

Knott CD (1997b) Interactions between energy balance, hormonal patterns and mating behavior in wild Bornean orangutans *(Pongo pygmaeus). American Journal of Primatology* 42:124.

Knott CD (1998) Changes in orangutan diet, caloric intake and ketones in response to fluctuating fruit availability. *International Journal of Primatology* 19:1061–1079.

Knott CD (1999) *Reproductive, Physiological and Behavioral Responses of Orangutans in Borneo to Fluctuations in Food Availability.* PhD dissertation (Harvard University).

Kuroda S (1989) Developmental retardation and behavioral characteristics of pygmy chimpanzees. In PG Heltne, LA Marquardst (Eds) *Understanding Chimpanzees* (Cambridge, Harvard University Press), 184–193.

Lager C, Ellison PT (1990) Effect of moderate weight loss on ovarian function assessed by salivary progesterone measurements. *American Journal of Human Biology* 2:303–312.

Lancaster JB, Lancaster CS (1983) Parental investment: the hominid adaptation. In D Ortner (Ed) *How Humans Adapt* (Washington DC, Smithsonian), 33–58.

Leonard WR, Robertson ML (1997) Comparative primate energetics and human evolution. *American Journal of Physical Anthropology* 102:265–281.

Lippert W (1974) Beobachtungen zum Schwangerschafts- und Geburtsverhalten beim Orang-Utan *(Pongo pygmaeus)* im Tierpark Berlin. *Folia Primatalogia* 21:108–134.

Lippert W (1977) Erfahrungen bei der Aufzucht von Orang-Utans *(Pongo pygmaeus)* im Tierpark Berlin. *Zoologische Garten* 47:209–225.

Lipson SF, Ellison PT (1996) Comparison of salivary steroid profiles in naturally occurring conception and non-conception cycles. *Human Reproduction* 11:2090–2096.

Maple TL, Hoff MP (1982) *Gorilla Behavior* (New York, Van Nostrand Reinhold).

Markham R (1990) Breeding orangutans at Perth Zoo: twenty years of appropriate husbandry. *Zoo Biology* 9:171–182.

Markham R (1995) Doing it naturally: reproduction in captive orangutans (*Pongo pygmaeus*). In RD Nadler, BFM Galdikas, LK Sheeran, N Rosen (Eds) *The Neglected Ape* (New York, Plenum Press), 273–278.

Martin DE, Graham CE, Gould KG (1978) Successful artificial insemination in the chimpanzee. *Symposium of the Zoological Society of London* 43:249–260.

Masters A, Markham R (1991) Assessing reproductive status in orangutans by using urinary estrone. *Zoo Biology* 10:197–208.

Milton K (1987) Primate diets and gut morphology: implications for hominid evolution. In M Harris, EB Ross (Eds) *Food and Evolution: Toward a Theory of Human Food Habits* (Philadelphia, Temple University Press), 93–116.

Milton K (1999) A hypothesis to explain the role of meat-eating in human evolution. *Evolutionary Anthropology* 8:11–21.

Moir RJ (1994) The "carnivorous" herbivores. In DJ Chivers, P Langer (Eds) *The Digestive System in Mammals* (Cambridge, Cambridge University Press), 87–102.

Nadler RD (1977) Sexual behavior of the chimpanzee in relation to the gorilla and orangutan. In GH Bourne (Ed) *Progress in Ape Research* (New York, Academic Press), 191–206.

Nadler RD (1982) Laboratory research on sexual behavior and reproduction of gorillas and orangutans. *American Journal of Primatology* (Suppl 1):57–66.

Nadler RD, Graham CE, Gollins DC, Gould KG (1979) Plasma gonadotropins, prolactin, gonadal steroids and genital swelling during the menstrual cycle of lowland gorillas. *Endocrinology* 105:290– 296.

Nishida T (1974) Ecology of wild chimpanzees. In R Ohtsuka, J Tanaka, T Nishida (Eds) *Human Ecology* (Tokyo, Kyoritsu-suppan), 15–60.

Nishida T, Takasaki H, Takahata Y (1990) Demography and reproductive profiles. In T Nishida (Ed) *The Chimpanzees of the Mahale Mountains: Sexual and Life History Strategies* (Tokyo, University of Tokyo Press), 63–97.

O'Connell JF, Hawkes K, Blurton Jones NG (1999) Grandmothering and the evolution of *Homo erectus*. *Journal of Human Evolution* 36:461–485.

Panter-Brick C, Lotstein DS, Ellison PT (1993) Seasonality of reproductive function and weight loss in rural Nepali women. *Human Reproduction* 8:684–690.

Perez-Escamilla R, Cohen RJ, Brown KH, Rivera LL, Canahuati J, Dewey KG (1995) Maternal anthropometric status and lactation performance in a low-income Honduran population: evidence for the role of infants. *American Journal of Clinical Nutrition* 61:528–534.

Pusey A, Williams J, Goodall J (1997) The influence of dominance rank on the reproductive success of female chimpanzees. *Science* 277:828–831.

Riss D, Busse C (1977) Fifty day observation of a free-ranging adult male chimpanzees. *Folia Primatologica* 28:283–297.

Rodseth L, Wrangham RW, Harrigan AM, Smuts BB (1990) The human community as a primate society. *Current Anthropology* 31:1–38.

Sakura O (1994) Factors affecting party size and composition of chimpanzees (*Pan troglodytes*) at Bossou, Guinea. *International Journal of Primatology* 15: 167–183.

Schurmann CL, van Hooff JARAM (1986) Reproductive strategies of the orangutan: new data and a reconsideration of existing sociosexual models. *International Journal of Primatology* 7:265–287.

Schweiger U, Laessle R, Pfister H, Hoehl C, Schwingenschloegel M, Schweiger M, Pirke KM (1987) Diet-induced menstrual irregularities: effects of age and weight loss. *Fertility and Sterility* 48:746–751.

Setiawan E, Knott CD, Budhi S (1996) Preliminary assessment of vigilance and predator avoidance behavior of orangutans in Gunung Palung National Park, Indonesia. *Tropical Biodiversity* 3:269– 279.

Sievert J, Karesh WB, Sunde V (1991) Reproductive intervals in captive female western lowland gorillas with a comparison to wild mountain gorillas. *American Journal of Primatology* 24:227–234.

Smith B (1992) Life history and the evolution of human maturation. *Evolutionary Anthropology* 1:163–164.

Smith AH, Butler TM, Pace N (1975) Weight growth of colony-reared chimpanzees. *Folia Primatologica* 24:29–59.

Sugiyama Y (1989) Population dynamics of chimpanzees at Bossou, Guinea. In PG Heltne, LA Marquardst (Eds) *Understanding Chimpanzees* (Cambridge, Harvard University Press), 134–145.

Sugiyama Y (1994) Age-specific birth rate and lifetime reproductive success of chimpanzees at Bossou, Guinea. *American Journal of Primatology* 32:311–318.

Takahata Y, Ihobe H, Idani G (1996) Comparing copulations of chimpanzees and bonobos: do females exhibit proceptivity or receptivity? In W McGrew, T Nishida, L Marchandt (Eds) *Great Ape Societies* (Cambridge, Cambridge University Press), 146–155.

Takasaki H, Hiraiwa-Hasegawa M, Takahata Y, Byrne RW, Kano T (1986) A case of unusually early postpartum resumption of estrous cycling in a young female chimpanzee in the wild. *Primates* 27:517–519.

Tamarkin L, Baird CJ, Almeida OFX (1985) Melatonin: a coordinating signal for mammalian reproduction? *Science* 277:714–720.

Thompson-Handler (1990) *The Pygmy Chimpanzee: Sociosexual Behavior, Reproductive Biology and Life History.* PhD dissertation (Yale University).

Tilson R, Seal US, Soemarna K, Ramono W, Sumardja E, Poniran S, van Schaik C, Leighton M, Rijksen H, Eudey A (1993) *Orangutan Population and Habitat Viability Analysis Report* (Medan, North Sumatra, Indonesia, Orangutan Population and Habitat Viability Analysis Workshop).

Tutin CEG (1975) *Sexual Behaviour and Mating Patterns in a Community of Wild Chimpanzees.* PhD thesis (University of Edinburgh).

Tutin CEG (1979) Mating patterns and reproductive strategies in a community of wild chimpanzees *(Pan troglodytes schweinfurthii). Behavioral Ecology and Sociobiology* 6:29–38.

Tutin CEG (1994) Reproductive success story: variability among chimpanzees and comparisons with gorillas. In RW Wrangham, WC McGrew, FBM de Waal, PG Heltne (Eds) *Chimpanzee Cultures* (Cambridge, Harvard University Press), 181–193.

Tutin CEG, McGinnis PR (1981) Chimpanzee reproduction in the wild. In CE Graham (Ed) *Reproductive Biology of the Great Apes* (New York, Academic Press), 239–264.

Uehara S, Nishida T (1987) Body weights of wild chimpanzees *(Pan troglodytes schweinfurthii)* of the Mahale Mountains National Park, Tanzania. *American Journal of Physical Anthropology* 72:315–321.

Van Schaik CP, van Noordwijk MA (1985) Interannual variability in fruit abundance and the reproductive seasonality in Sumatran long-tailed macaques *(Macaca fascicularis). Journal of Zoology, London* A 206:533–549.

Walker A, Leakey R (1993) *The Nariokotome* Homo erectus *Skeleton* (Cambridge, Harvard University Press).

Wallis J (1985) Synchrony of estrous swelling in captive group-living chimpanzees *(Pan troglodytes). International Journal of Primatology* 6:335–350.

Wallis J (1992) Chimpanzee genital swelling and its role in the pattern of sociosexual behavior. *American Journal of Primatology* 28:101–113.

Wallis J (1995) Seasonal influence on reproduction in chimpanzees of Gombe National Park. *International Journal of Primatology* 16:435–451.

Wallis J (1997) A survey of reproductive parameters in the free-ranging chimpanzees of Gombe National Park. *Journal of Reproduction and Fertility* 109: 121–154.

Wallis J, Matama H (1993) Social and environmental factors influencing sleep/ wake patterns in wild chimpanzees. *American Journal of Primatology* 30:354.

Washburn SL, Lancaster CS (1968) The evolution of hunting. In RB Lee, I DeVore (Eds) *Man the Hunter* (Chicago, Aldine), 293–303.

Watts DP (1990) Mountain gorilla life histories, reproductive competition, and sociosexual behavior and some implications for captive husbandry. *Zoo Biology* 9:185–200.

Watts DP (1991) Mountain gorilla reproduction and sexual behavior. *American Journal of Primatology* 24:211–225.

Watts DP (1998) Seasonality in the ecology and life histories of mountain gorillas *(Gorilla gorilla beringei). International Journal of Primatology* 19:929–948.

Wood JW (1994) *Dynamics of Human Reproduction: Biology, Biometry, Demography* (New York, Aldine de Gruyter).

Wrangham RW (1977) Feeding behaviour of chimpanzees in Gombe National Park, Tanzania. In TH Clutton-Brock (Ed) *Primate Ecology* (London, Academic Press), 503–538.

Wrangham RW (1986) Ecology and social relationships in two species of chimpanzee. In DI Rubenstein, RW Wrangham (Eds) *Ecology and Social Evolution: Birds and Mammals* (Princeton, Princeton University Press), 352–370.

Wrangham RW (2000) Why are male chimpanzees more gregarious than mothers? A scramble competition hypothesis. In P Kappeler (Ed) *Primate Males: Causes and Consequences of Variation in Group Composition* (Cambridge, Cambridge University Press), 248–258.

Wrangham RW, Chapman C, Clark-Arcadi AP, Isabirye-Basuta G (1996) Social ecology of Kanywara chimpanzees: implications for understanding the costs of great ape groups. In WC McGrew, LF Marchant, T Nishida (Eds) *Great Ape Societies* (Cambridge, Cambridge University Press), 45–57.

Wrangham RW, Jones JH, Laden G, Pilbeam D, Conklin-Brittain N (1999) The raw and the stolen: cooking and the ecology of human origins. *Current Anthropology* 40:567–594.

Young WC, Yerkes RM (1943) Factors influencing the reproductive cycle in the chimpanzee: the period of adolescent sterility and related problems. *Endocrinology* 33:121–154.

Index

Printed in the United States
by Baker & Taylor Publisher Services